SPORTS
SUPPLEMENTS

Jose Antonio, PhD
Rexall Sundown - Active Nutrition
6111 Broken Sound Pkwy NW
Boca Raton, Florida

Jeffrey R. Stout, PhD
Director of Sport Science
Scientific Affairs Department
Nutricia USA
Boca Raton, Florida

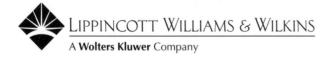
LIPPINCOTT WILLIAMS & WILKINS
A **Wolters Kluwer** Company

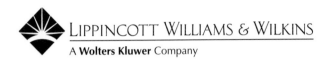

Editor: Pete Darcy
Managing Editor: Eric Branger
Marketing Manager: Christen DeMarco
Project Editor: Jennifer Pirozzoli
Indexer: Mary Kidd
Designer: Armen Kojoyian
Typesetter: TechBooks
Printer: Courier-Kendallville

530 Walnut Street
Philadelphia, Pennsylvania 19106

351 West Camden Street
Baltimore, Maryland 21201-2436 USA

The publisher is not responsible (as a matter of product liability, negligence or otherwise) for any
injury resulting from any material contained herein. This publication contains information relating to
general principles of medical care which should not be construed as specific instructions for individual patients. Manufacturers' product information and package inserts should be reviewed for current
information, including contraindications, dosages and precautions.

Printed in the United States of America

Library of Congress Cataloging-in-Publication Data

Sports supplements / [edited by] Jose Antonio, Jeffrey R. Stout.
    p. ; cm.
  Includes index.
  ISBN 0-7817-2241-1
  1. Dietary supplements. 2. Athletes–Nutrition. 3. Sports. I. Antonio, Jose, PhD.
II. Stout, Jeffrey R.
[DNLM: 1. Dietary Supplements. 2. Sports. QU 145.5 S764 2001]
RM258.5 .S67 2001
613.2′088′796—dc21
                                               2001029213

*The publishers have made every effort to trace the copyright holders for borrowed material. If they have inad-
vertently overlooked any, they will be pleased to make the necessary arrangements at the first opportunity.*

To purchase additional copies of this book, call our customer service department at **(800) 638-3030**
or fax orders to **(301) 824-7390**. For other book services, including chapter reprints and large quantity sales, ask for the Special Sales department.

For all other calls originating outside of the United States, please call **(301)714-2324**.

Visit *Lippincott Williams & Wilkins* on the Internet: http://www.lww.com. Lippincott Williams &
Wilkins customer service representatives are available from 8:30 am to 6:00 pm, EST, Monday
through Friday, for telephone access.

01 02 03 04
1 2 3 4 5 6 7 8 9 10

Dedication

To the most important people,

Our wives Karla and Martha and children Brooke, Brandi, Jeffrey and Nicole

Foreword

The sports supplement industry, primarily in the past few years, has experienced an unprecedented expansion involving the introduction and availability of ergogenic aids (substances that may enhance athletic performance or improve body composition). What was once considered an industry inundated with useless and even fraudulent products, now offers an abundance of effective compounds that are supported by research and "real-world" success. The heightened national interest in the area of sports supplementation has also been controversial, because the circulation of accurate, reputable information is lacking. Much of the information disseminated in popular fitness magazines is often a result of user trial and error. Only recently have the standards of science been used to assess the efficacy of various supplements; however, many popular fitness magazines still tend to hyperbolize the usefulness of various supplements. The proper selection and administration of supplements for desired benefits is an area of ambiguity for both the layperson and qualified personnel in the field of exercise and nutritional counseling. Accordingly, increased awareness in the fitness industry, as well as public and media interest, has led to the need of a book that addresses key issues of natural ergogenic compounds. To date, no publication exists that effectively summarizes the research behind these supplements, as well as offers expert opinion and experience from scientists in the field of ergogenic aids. The text, *Sports Supplements,* offers the clinician, professor, or educated layperson applicable information regarding ergogenic aids. The book covers the entire spectrum of supplements and their effectiveness (or lack thereof), including proper dosages and applications to specific goals, as well as recommendations from the author(s). As a clinician who works daily with athletes, this text could not have come at a better time. I know my fellow colleagues in sports medicine will find this an invaluable resource.

Eric Serrano, MD
Associate Clinical Professor
Ohio State University

Preface

"Sure, not every piece of research is in . . .
[But] men buy companies, run political campaigns,
wage wars . . . all based on the best available—but incomplete—data."
–Bob Arnot, M.D., Medical Correspondent, in his book
"The Prostate Cancer Protection Plan."

The above quote is in response to Dr. Arnot's dietary advice concerning prostate cancer. As with any book related to diet or supplementation, a healthy dose of criticism always follows. Certainly, we have attempted to provide similar advice to athletes regarding the use of dietary supplements. Yes, we *know* that the data are incomplete. Yes, we *know* that they are often inconclusive. And yes, we *know* that more data are needed. In fact, as scientists, we make a living in part by convincing others (i.e., those with research dollars) that more data are always needed. And we've become so good at it that we *still* have studies that are funded showing that exercise is needed for permanent weight loss. (Is that still a mystery?) Of course, the same cannot be held true for the field of nutrition, particularly sports nutrition.

So, we admittedly have incomplete and inconclusive data regarding sports nutrition and supplements. Does that mean we should hide behind the ivory tower and refrain from giving practical advice to athletes? We think not. Yet, from our experience, that seems to be the case with many scientists. As scientists, we are often caught between those seeking practical advice (athletes) and our colleagues (fellow scientists) who are very disinclined to give an opinion regarding supplementation other than "eat a balanced diet and drink plenty of water." In fact, several of our colleagues subscribe to the notion that taking dietary supplements is largely ineffectual, costly, and a waste of time. On the other hand, it is clear that many common foods we eat are in fact "supplemented." We have orange juice fortified with vitamin C and calcium. We have refined bread fortified with B vitamins, milk fortified with vitamin D, and so on.

So why does the use of dietary supplements by athletes provoke such a negative response? As scientists, is it wrong to provide opinions based on incomplete data? And if scientists are the "experts" who the public seeks advice from, then should we not provide such information? Or should we leave that to the teenage boy working behind the counter at your local health food store? From whom would *you* seek advice?

We realize this book might contain controversial statements, but we also realize that an attempt to please everyone is a formula for failure. However, as academicians ourselves, we realize how insular our field can be. The lay public is often more confused concerning dietary supplements when the "experts" themselves cannot agree. Should you take supplemental vitamin C or not? Does creatine harm you or not? With such confusion, is it any wonder that athletes might be averse to listening to scientists who refuse to give practical "how-to" advice?

There is a tremendous need for scientists to bridge the gap (and it can be a wide one) between laboratory findings and real-world athletics. As we've stated previously, the data are far from complete. But we believe it would be irresponsible not to provide information to athletes regarding supplement use. Leaving such advice to the untrained salesman behind the health food store counter is sheer folly. We certainly will not lay claim to a monopoly on sports supplement knowledge, far from it. Indeed, it is far better to try to give well-intentioned advice, rather than hiding behind the clichéd "more research is needed" answer.

As you know, more research is *always* needed. That isn't new.

Nonetheless, we hope that you will find this book a valuable resource. We have attempted to provide an extensive literature review on a wide variety of dietary supplements. However, we know that new information on dietary supplements is published at an astonishing rate. Thus, some of you may view this text as being slightly behind the times.

We also hope that this text will be a great resource for the undergraduate and graduate student in the exercise sciences and nutrition as well as academicians and clinicians (i.e., physicians, dietitians).

For many of the chapters, we have attempted to cover *in vitro* and animal data (where appropriate) related to various dietary supplements (as well as human work). Though many in the exercise science community might cringe at the use of non-human data to "support" the claims made concerning certain supplements, it is clear that the best way to understand the purported mechanism of action regarding these supplements is via animal/in vitro studies. Regardless of how many human studies are performed, it is highly unlikely that one will get to a mechanistic understanding of the interplay between dietary supplementation (and nutrition in general) and exercise performance/body composition alterations.

Of interest to the athlete and coach is the section of each chapter entitled "Author(s) Recommendations." This section will set this book apart from other similar texts. In spite of the limited data, we have attempted to provide something useful . . . a take-home message. We believe that, without such a section, those in the "real world" (i.e., those who actually incur the benefits or costs of choosing to use [or *not use*] dietary supplements) might find the text just another pointless academic exercise.

We hope that you find this text useful. Because of the rapidity of change in this field, you may find recent, cutting-edge research missing. Such is the nature of print publishing.

Jose Antonio, PhD
Jeffrey R. Stout, PhD

Acknowledgments

We gratefully acknowledge the contributors to this book. Without their input, this book would not have been possible. In addition, we thank all of the experts who provided numerous sidebars in our book.

We would like to thank the staff of Lippincott Williams & Wilkins for their perseverance and dedication to our project. We know that this project will be successful considering the tremendous effort put forth by the contributors, editors, and the LWW staff.

We would also like to thank our mentors (Peter Lemon, William J. Gonyea, Terry Housh) who helped in our development as scientists. They laid the foundation for our future success. For that we are especially grateful.

Contributors

Jose Antonio, PhD, CSCS, FACSM
Rexall Sundown - Active Nutrition
6111 Broken Sound Pkwy NW
Boca Raton, Florida 33487-2799

Ash Batheja, MPT, CSCS
Licensed Physical Therapist
Allegiance Health
Omaha, Nebraska

John M. Berardi, BS, CSCS
Doctoral Student
University of Western Ontario
Ontario, Canada

Nancy Betts, PhD, RD
Professor
Department of Nutritional Science and Dietetics
University of Nebraska-Lincoln
Lincoln, Nebraska

Greg E. Bradley-Popovich, DPT, MSEP, MS, CSCS
Director of Clinical Research
Northwest Spine Management, Rehabilitation &
    Sports Conditioning
Portland, Oregon

Joseph Chromiak, PhD, FACSM, MS, CSCS
Assistant Professor
University of Mississippi
Exercise Science and Leisure Management
Oxford, Mississippi

Conrad Earnest, PhD, CSCS
Research Scientist
Cooper Institute for Aerobics Research
Dallas, Texas

Thomas Incledon, MS, RD, LD/N, CSCS, NSCA-CPT
Human Performance Specialist, Inc.
Plantation, Florida

Douglas Kalman, MS, RD
Research Scientist
Miami Research Associates
Miami, Florida

Marian Kohut, PhD
Assistant Professor
Department of Health and Human Performance
University of Iowa
Iowa City, Iowa

Richard B. Kreider, PhD, FACSM
Professor & Director of Exercise & Sport Nutrition Lab
Department of HMSE
University of Memphis
Memphis, Tennessee

Peter W.R. Lemon, PhD, FACSM
Professor
Exercise Nutrition Research Laboratory
University of Western Ontario
Ontario, Canada

Brian Leutholtz, PhD, FACSM
Professor
Department of Exercise Science, Physical Education,
    and Recreation
Old Dominion University
Norfolk, Virginia

Lonnie Lowery, PhD
Assistant Professor
Kent State University
Kent, Ohio

Jun Ma, MS
Doctoral student
University of Nebraska-Lincoln
Lincoln, Nebraska

Chuck Rudolph, MS, RD
Research and Development
Metabolic Response Modifiers
Newport Beach, California

Jeffrey R. Stout, PhD, CSCS, FACSM
Director of Sports Science
NUTRICIA USA
Boca Raton, Florida

Chris Street, MS, CSCS
Writer and Sports Nutrition Consultant

Darin Van Gammeren, MA, CSCS
Doctoral student
University of Florida
Gainesville, Florida

Matthew Vukovich, PhD, FACSM
Assistant Professor
Director of Applied Physiology Lab
South Dakota State University
Brookings, South Dakota

Tim N. Ziegenfuss, PhD, CSCS, EPC
Chief Scientific Officer
Phoenix Labs - Division of Nutrition, Metabolism & Exercise
Adjunct Research Scientist
Human Nutrition Laboratory
Kent State University
Kent, Ohio

Table of Contents

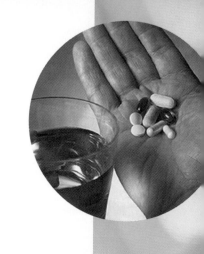

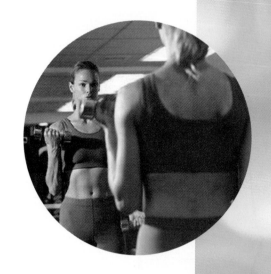
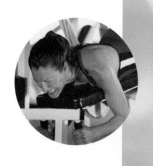

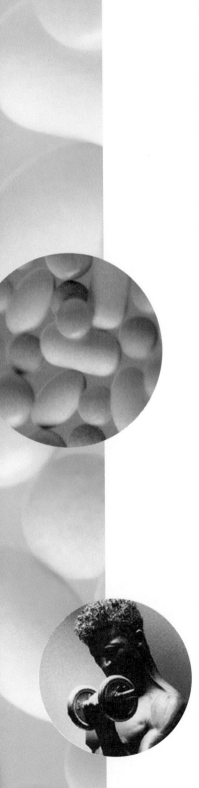

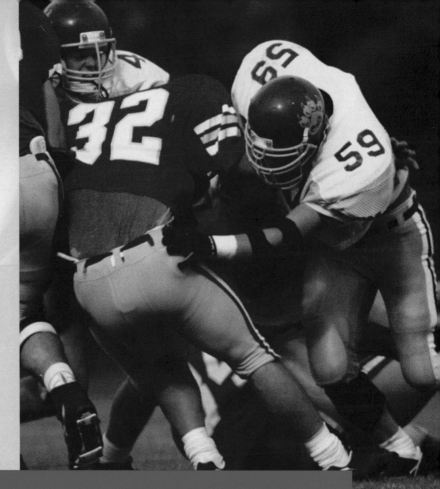

CHAPTER

1

Sports Supplements: Evolution and Revolution

Greg Bradley-Popovich, Jeffrey R. Stout, and Jose Antonio

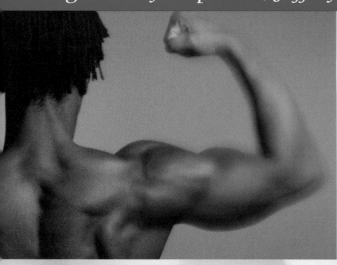

Introduction

B y nature, athletics demand a competitive attitude. The athlete may desire to outperform the opponent, or the athlete may compete with oneself while striving to maximize personal potential. This drive to succeed has fueled the development of several performance-enhancing resources. Tools intended to enhance athletic performance are referred to as "ergogenic aids," a term derived from the Greek words "ergon," meaning "work," and "gennan" meaning "to produce." Ergogenic aids may take several forms, including nutritional, pharmacological, physiological, biomechanical, and psychological.[1] The purpose of this book is to provide an in-depth treatment of the dynamic field of nutritional ergogenic aids, which is rapidly accumulating new scientific evidence.

Origin and Successful Evolution of Sports Supplementation

The quest for reaching the pinnacle of physical performance and aesthetics can be traced to ancient times. Long before the pervasive use of illicit drugs in modern sports, or the popularity of surgical augmentation techniques such as implants or liposuction, our ancestors also sought ancillary means to achieving a body that was ideal in form and function.

The Primitive Beginnings: Mythology, Mysticism, and Mushrooms

The earliest use of natural preparations can be traced to the Chinese, who have used various concoctions for over 5,000 years. The Babylonians and Egyptians documented drug use approximately 4,000 years ago. In these cultures, using such substances was usually accompanied by rituals, chanting, and superstition.[2]

The ancient Greeks may have first pondered how to gain a competitive athletic "edge" through proper diet and supplementation. Indeed, a keen interest in the physique and athletic prowess may have best been exemplified by the ancient Greeks, who embraced and celebrated athletic competition, and who speculated about the ideal diet for optimum athletic performance.[3]

Greek trainers and athletes sought nutritional aids and may have believed that certain animal organs held special properties. For example, gladiators may have thought a lion's heart conferred courage upon those who consumed it.[1,4] Use of such substances, however, was scrutinized by athletic officials. Similar to the controversy surrounding some modern dietary supplements, in 300 BC three

Olympic athletes were banned from competing for ingesting mushrooms and animal protein.[5]

A well-known Greek athlete of mythological proportions was Milo of Croton. Milo, a champion wrestler, was said to have built tremendous strength by lifting a calf daily until it was fully mature. What may not be as well known was Milo's voracious appetite. One version of the story tells of Milo parading around the stadium at Olympia while holding the bull above him. Milo's relationship with the bull is said to have ended when he butchered the animal and devoured it in a single day! This feat may not be so surprising because the legend is that Milo's typical daily diet included 20 pounds of meat, 20 pounds of bread, and 8 quarts of wine.[3]

Although we may laugh at such superstition and exaggeration, some of the advice from this period still applies today. For instance, writings of antiquity (circa 400 AD) reveal a suspected incompatibility of overeating and excessive alcohol consumption with athletic performance. Also, athletes of this period were advised to shy away from desserts.[3]

The Turning Point

Despite its early beginnings, the science of sports nutrition evolved little over the next millennium because the primary interest of those knowledgeable in medicine and nutrition was the prevention of debilitating or life-threatening nutrient deficiencies. By the mid-1800s, surprisingly little was known about the most fundamental aspects of sports nutrition. For example, the German researcher von Liebig wrote in 1842 that protein was the primary energy source for muscular work, when in fact, it is not.[4]

The isolation of vitamins in the early 1900s marked an exciting, dramatic turning point in nutrition science. Several studies would demonstrate in the next few decades an ergogenic, or work-enhancing benefit to dietary supplementation. Around the same time that vitamins were discovered, caffeine was recognized as possessing fatigue-masking qualities, and protein provided a minimal contribution to the body as a fuel for physical activity.[4]

In the 1920s, scientists began testing the effects of dietary carbohydrate manipulation on performance. One such experiment was conducted by Harvard Medical School on participants in the Boston Marathon. The researchers found that a supplemental carbohydrate— partly in the form of sugary candy—helped to decrease fatigue among the participants when consumed before and during the event.[4]

By the 1940s, it was well established that protein was not a significant source of energy during exercise and did not enhance endurance performance. However, supplemental protein was found to enhance muscle mass gains in strength athletes.[4] It was outside the scientific community, however, where supplemental protein would gain an enthusiastic endorsement. This resounding endorsement from the forefathers of a fledgling sport would have far-reaching implications for the future of the supplement industry.

Industry experts recognize that it was the niche of strength training and body building that espoused the special dietary needs of athletes. York Barbell Company founder Bob Hoffman (1899–1985) ushered in the sports supplement movement. Hoffman began publishing *Strength & Health* in 1932, followed by the successful *Muscular Development* in 1964, which still thrives today. Another icon of the physical culture movement was Joe Weider. In the late 1930s, Joe Weider (1923–) began publishing his newsletter, *Your Physique,* which evolved into the well-known *Muscle & Fitness* magazine. Both Hoffman and Weider began using their publications to market sports nutrition supplements, particularly protein supplements.[6] Although scientific evidence supporting the use of these early nutrition supplements, like wheat germ oil and bee pollen, was minimal to nonexistent, such propaganda helped plant the seeds from which a prosperous sports supplement industry would grow.

The next big boost for the use of nutritional ergogenic aid occurred not as the result of a single person, but rather, a concept. Based on Scandinavian research that showed the fatigue-delaying qualities of carbohydrates, Gatorade created a new market in sports beverages in the 1960s.[4,7] In addition to supplying carbohydrates to combat fatigue, the beverage was designed to be absorbed quickly to prevent dehydration. Gatorade was developed by researchers at the University of Florida at Gainesville to improve the performance of the "Gators" football team. Because of the research behind its development and the specificity of its objective, Gatorade may be regarded as the first sports nutrition product.[4]

The marketing of sports supplements continued through the 1970s and 1980s, but was still limited to the narrow weight training niche. New products abounded with endorsements from popular body builders, yet most were without scientific merit. In addition to the ever-present wheat germ products and bee pollen, protein supplements were still heavily marketed. Eventually, protein supplements were first chemically digested and then sold as their building blocks under the alias of *amino acid* or *peptide* capsules and pills. During this era, high-calorie, weight-gain powders flourished as did *steroid replacement kits* and a questionable assortment of miscellaneous products such as smilax, dibencozide, gamma-oryzanol, and inosine.

The late 1980s was also characterized by the misrepresentation of scientific studies to market products. Before this point, consumers bought supplements on good faith. Now, supplement companies sought to develop an advantage by creating the illusion that their products were backed with science. Perhaps the best example of such a product is the fraudulent marketing of the mineral boron, which was shown in a study to increase testosterone production in undernourished menopausal women, but which was marketed to weight training enthusiasts.[2,8]

The 1990s, a breakthrough de[...] ergogenic aids, was the period duri[...] plement companies retained their h[...] expanded the consumer base to in[...] letes, casual athletes, and people livi[...] This broadening of audience was sl[...] ment of a sports nutrition bar duri[...] the popular television series Seinfeld. In addition to the expanding consumer base, some companies attempted to expand the research base by voluntarily offering grants to fund university research.

The advent of "engineered foods," spearheaded by Met-Rx in the early 1990s, provided fitness enthusiasts and athletes with a useful meal-replacement supplement that was quick, relatively palatable, and nutrient dense without many calories. Though initial expectations and claims were somewhat unrealistic, the practicality and convenience of meal-replacement products were undeniable for a bustling health and appearance-conscious society. The engineered-food movement began as powders but has spawned several different products, most notably meal-replacement bars. Also during this time, creatine emerged from obscurity to become the most popular and most studied ergogenic aid of all time. In 1997, better products and aggressive marketing led the way to a record $1.27 billion in sales of sports nutrition supplements in the United States alone.[7]

If there was ever a golden age of nutritional ergogenic aids, it is now. Increasingly well-researched products and a better-educated public have led to nothing less than a supplement explosion. However, this revolution has not yet stamped out bogus supplements completely. For example, one of the most exotic nutritional supplements ever consumed by athletes was ground bull testes, which claimed to enhance testosterone production. What is remarkable about this unfounded supplement is that it was marketed to athletes as recently as the 1990s![2]

The Future Illuminated

Realizing how much the field has progressed in recent years, what are the exciting possibilities for sports supplementation in the future? Unfortunately, it is likely that less scrupulous companies will continue to manufacture an endless array of ill-conceived, ineffective supplements that will come and go, eventually ending up in the supplement graveyard like countless others before them. However, there is much to look forward to as more university research focuses on sports nutrition, proving the worth of many new and exciting supplements while ironing out the details of many effective supplements already in use.

Industry experts anticipate a continued broadening of the market, including using vending machines to dispense certain products. The number of middle-age users will likely increase as a result of men becoming concerned with cardiac health and women, with preventing porosis. In addition, supplement regimens will likely designed to fit the needs of particular activities.[7] Specifically, endurance athletes will see many new supplement options appear because endurance athletes outnumber strength athletes by at least 3 to 1.

In the future, look for a decrease in endorsements from big-name athletes; progressively more enlightened consumers are interested in science rather than hype. Any future endorsements may instead recruit medical professionals and researchers.[7]

Expect the medical community to become more accepting of sports supplements and to implement use of these supplements within certain patient populations, such as cardiac patients, given that current creatine research has already veered in that direction. Following the trend in Europe, American pharmaceutical companies, with their great financial resources, may become a powerful force in the development and marketing of new ergogenic aids. These progressive pharmaceutical companies may develop their own ergogenic aid division, or may acquire well-established sports nutrition companies. This widespread growth of the industry will lead to a greater public awareness, which will in turn result in more growth within the industry.

Legal Aspects of Nutrition Supplementation

What would a supplement revolution be without a change in government policy? The Nutrition Labeling and Education Act (NLEA), followed by the Dietary Supplement Health and Education Act (DSHEA) had a significant impact on the sports supplement industry.

The Nutrition Labeling and Education Act (NLEA)

President Bush signed the NLEA on November 8, 1990; it took effect 2 years later. The NLEA brought many changes for not only packaged foods, but also nutritional supplements; nutrition labels have appeared on nearly all packaged foods. United States recommended dietary allowances (USRDAs) have been replaced by reference daily intakes (RDIs) and daily reference values (DRVs); RDIs and DRVs have been combined on labels as daily values (DVs); the nutrition label format has been standardized and simplified; previously vague terms such as *low, light, have been reduced,* and *good source of* defined; and disease-specific claims have been authorized.[9] Disease-specific claims will be addressed later in this chapter.

The NLEA also modified the definition of "dietary supplement." Traditionally, the Food and Drug Administration (FDA) regarded nutritional supplements to contain only essential nutrients such as vitamins, minerals, and protein. The NLEA amended this definition of dietary supplement to include "herbs, or similar nutritional substances."

The Dietary Supplement Health and Education Act (DSHEA)

Even more influential with regard to dietary supplements, the DSHEA, legally known as Public Law 103-417, was signed by President Clinton on October 25, 1994 in response to concerned nutritional supplement consumers and manufacturers who needed reassurance that safe dietary supplements would remain available to those who want to use them.[10,11] In fact, for the 2 years preceding the DSHEA, many congressmen reported that they received more correspondence and phone calls regarding dietary supplements than on any other subject, including the national deficit, healthcare reform, and abortion. Consequently, members of Congress approved the measure unanimously.[9]

The DSHEA basically allows supplement manufacturers the freedom to market more products as dietary supplements and to provide information about product benefits so that consumers can make informed choices.[12] Although the DSHEA was welcomed by manufacturers and consumers alike, in the eyes of some consumer advocates, it "weakened" the enforcement ability of the FDA, but not as much as its original sponsors had intended.[9,13]

Ingredient and Nutrition Information Labeling

The most visible DSHEA-mediated change is written on the packaging of nutritional supplements. Through requirements of the DSHEA, dietary supplement labels have been redesigned to be more consumer friendly. A dietary supplement is easy to recognize because the product label reads "dietary supplement." Among other requirements, supplement labels will provide a "Supplement Facts" panel, a clear identity statement, and a complete list of ingredients. Supplement labels will be further described in this chapter under "Consumer Savvy."

Distinguishing Among Foods, Food Additives, and Nutritional Supplements

Historically, the FDA regulated dietary supplements as foods for several decades. This was done to ensure that their labeling was accurate and that the supplements were safe and "wholesome." Under the 1958 Food Additive Amendments to the Federal Food, Drug, and Cosmetic Act (FD&C Act), any new dietary ingredients for use in food or supplements were evaluated for safety. Frequently, the FDA previously viewed ingredients contained within dietary supplements as being analogous to substances that are added to foods. This perspective was problematic for supplement manufacturers because if a substance was not recognized as safe (GRAS) based on ample scientific literature, then the substance was categorized as a food additive; categorizing it in this way had several consequences for a dietary supplement.

According to the FD&C Act, to market a food additive required petitioning the FDA for permission. To successfully petition often required much new research, money, and patience; it sometimes took the FDA more than 5 years to approve a new food additive. Because this previous system seemed unnecessarily complex, Congress amended the FD&C Act with the DSHEA to incorporate many provisions for dietary supplements. One major provision of the DSHEA is the precise clarification that the term "food additive" does not apply to dietary supplements. Hence, the DSHEA excludes the ingredients in dietary supplements (and therefore sports supplements) from the premarket safety assessment that is mandated for food additives or for new uses of previously established food ingredients. Binders, fillers, diluents (substances used to dilute), preservatives, and colors that may be used in nutritional supplements are still subject to food additive regulations.[9] (*New* and *old* ingredients are defined by the FDA with respect to whether they were marketed for nutritional supplement use in the U.S. before or after October 15, 1994.)

The Supplement Police

With the new legislation, the regulatory role of the FDA was changed from that of evaluating premarket safety to policing the industry.[9] Essentially, the FDA went from playing the role of the teacher granting a hall pass to assuming the role of the principal patrolling the hallways for violators. Thus, the burden of proof now rests on the FDA. However, dietary supplements are not exempt from all safety provisions.[10]

What is a "Safe" Supplement?

The DSHEA categorizes a nutritional supplement as *adulterated* (impure, or of questionable safety) if it or one of its ingredients poses "a significant or unreasonable risk of illness or injury" when used as indicated on its label. If there are no directions on the label, then the supplement must not present a risk when used under normal conditions. Also, any new ingredient may be considered unsafe if there is inadequate information from which to draw conclusions about its safety.[10]

The government did receive some new authorization as a result of the DSHEA. For example, the Secretary of Health and Human Services may proclaim a dietary supplement "to pose an imminent hazard to public health or safety," which would effect an immediate ban on sales of the product.[9]

Using Literature to Inform Consumers

Before the DSHEA, any publications used to promote dietary supplements could be regulated by the FDA as labels when used at the time of a prospective sale. Literature that claimed any role in the cure, mitigation, treatment, or prevention of any disease was particularly targeted. These claims, though not made on the product itself, would have made the supplement subject to regulation as a drug. So according to the old statutes, supplement salesclerks should not have promoted products by showing customers any publications that claimed disease-prevention benefits.[9] This restriction was even true of scientific publications. Despite these restrictions, however, these marketing strategies were widely practiced.

The new legislature offers significant freedom to those who wish to use literature to market nutritional supplements. The DSHEA says that a "third-party" publication, such as "an article, a chapter in a book, or an official abstract of a peer-reviewed publication," "shall not be defined as labeling" and may be "used in connection with the sale of a dietary supplement to consumers" if the literature is "reprinted in its entirety." Furthermore, the publication must meet several criteria: it must not be false or misleading; it must not promote a particular brand or manufacturer; it must be presented with similar material in a balanced fashion that illustrates the sum of the available scientific literature; when displayed, it must be physically separate from the supplements; it must not have any additional information, such as product promotional literature, affixed to it.[9,10] Given these amendments, a supplement salesclerk may now legally promote supplements by showing consumers scientific literature detailing the health benefits of particular supplements.[9]

What is the Difference Between a Supplement and a Drug?

What exactly is a dietary supplement, and how does it differ from a drug? Generally, a nutritional supplement provides a substance that is a component of a normal physiological or biochemical process. In contrast, a drug alters a physiological or biochemical process. Of course, more complex legal definitions have been established to distinguish between these two entities.

As previously mentioned, the NLEA expanded the traditional definition of "dietary supplement" to include not just essential nutrients, but also to encompass "herbs, or similar nutritional substances." The DSHEA further expanded the definition of dietary supplements to include nonessential nutrients to encompass substances such as garlic, ginseng, fish oils, enzymes, psyllium (a fiber laxative), glandulars (extracts from animal glands or tissues), and combinations of these.[10]

The following is an abbreviated, nontechnical definition of "dietary supplement" provided by the Office of Dietary Supplements at the National Institutes of Health (NIH), an office itself established as stipulated by the DSHEA: "The Dietary Supplement Health and Education Act defines dietary supplements as a product (other than tobacco) intended to supplement the diet that bears or contains one or more of the following dietary ingredients: a vitamin, mineral, amino acid, herb or other botanical; or a dietary substance to supplement the diet by increasing the total dietary intake; or a concentrate, metabolite, constituent, extract, or combination of any ingredient described above; and intended for the ingestion in the form of a [liquid,] capsule, powder, softgel, or gelcap, and not represented as a conventional food or as a sole item of a meal or the diet."[10]

According to the FD&C Act, a "drug" is legally defined as any article (excluding a device) "intended for use in the diagnosis, cure, mitigation, treatment or prevention of disease" and "articles (other than food) intended to affect the structure or function of the body."

An additional distinction between a dietary supplement and a drug is the FDA premarket evaluation process. Before it is marketed, a drug must undergo clinical studies to determine its effectiveness, possible interactions with other substances, safety, and appropriate dosage. Then the FDA must analyze the generated data and authorize the drug's use before marketing it. In contrast, the FDA does not test or authorize nutritional supplements.[12]

Legalizing Health Claims

At first, the distinction between *dietary supplement* and *drug* may appear straightforward. According to the definition of *drug,* a dietary supplement cannot claim to diagnose, cure, mitigate (alleviate), treat, or prevent a specific disease. For example, a dietary supplement could not carry the claim *reverses heart disease* or *cures cancer* or treats *high blood pressure.* However, to the public, the line between a nutritional supplement and a medicine is sometimes a thin one, depending on the claims made. Under the DSHEA and prior labeling legislature, there are three types of claims that can possibly be made by supplement manufacturers when justified: nutrient-content claims, disease claims, and nutrition support claims. No longer is a manufacturer required to obtain FDA approval to make these three types of health claims, as long as the manufacturers follow some simple guidelines, as described in the following paragraphs.

Nutrient-content claims tout the amount of nutrient contained in a supplement. For example, a supplement's label could claim the product to be *high in calcium* if it contained a minimum of 200 milligrams of calcium. Similarly, a supplement label could read "Excellent source of vitamin C" in a supplement having at least 12 milligrams of vitamin C.[12]

Disease-specific claims make an association between a substance and a disease or health-related condition. These claims are pre-authorized by the FDA based on its thorough review of the scientific evidence. Alternatively, disease claims can be based on a consensus statement from certain scientific bodies, such as the National Academy of Sciences, describing a proven link between a nutrient or food and health. Only certain nutrients are pre-approved

for such claims. For example, a disease claim could make a link between calcium intake and decreased risk of osteoporosis if the supplement contains sufficient levels of calcium.[12] To date, just a few disease-specific claims have been authorized, and only two of these associations allow for nutritional supplements in addition to food: calcium and osteoporosis, and folic acid and neural tube defects. Currently, wordy, model-label statements are required for a product marketed with a disease-specific claim. Thus, many manufacturers may be deterred from making such claims given the limited space on supplement labels.[9]

Nutrition support claims describe a link between a nutrient and its deficiency disease. For example, a vitamin C supplement's label could legally state that vitamin C prevents scurvy if the product contains sufficient levels. When nutrition support claims are made, the prevalence of the deficiency disease in the U.S. must appear on the label. Certain nutrition support claims, called structure-function claims, can refer to the supplement's effect on the structure or function of the human body. An example of a structure-function claim would be "adequate protein is necessary to build muscle." To use structure-function claims, manufacturers do not need FDA approval. Supplement manufacturers base these claims on their interpretation of the scientific literature. But, as with all label claims, structure-function claims must be truthful and not misleading. To detect a structure-function, simply look for the label disclaimer that reads "This statement has not been evaluated by the Food and Drug Administration. This product is not intended to diagnose, treat, cure, or prevent any disease." Interestingly, even though the manufacturer must be able to substantiate its claim, it need not furnish it to either the FDA or the public.[12] This scenario beckons the phrase "There is no truth, just data to be manipulated."

Playing by the Rules

Note, however, that just because the U.S. federal government recognizes a supplement as legal does not guarantee that other regions or organizations will recognize it as such. Each state in the U.S. reserves the right to ban the sale of a particular substance, such as the weight-loss aid ephedrine. Of course, the sale, possession, and use of dietary supplements varies among different countries, and other countries such as Canada do not enjoy the same degree of dietary supplement freedom as does the U.S. An example is the formation of the Canadian Coalition for Health Freedom (CCHF), composed of manufacturers and consumers, whose purpose is to battle "the oppressive and discriminating regulation being enforced against natural health care products in Canada. . . ."[14] Indeed, Canadians do not have access to many nutritional ergogenic aids that Americans use frequently. Furthermore, importing a banned or restricted dietary supplement into a country may violate that country's laws, even if the supplement was legally

Dietary Supplement Science: How Much Research is Enough?

Shawn M. Talbott, PhD

Achieving the right balance between business/marketing objectives and scientific considerations is always a difficult goal. On the one hand, government regulations are flexible in their allowance of claims that can be made for dietary supplements, so many companies are reluctant to commit large financial investments for research that can be "poached" by competitors. On the other hand, consumers of dietary supplements, particularly athletes, are beginning to ask for (demand) high-quality, well-controlled scientific evidence of a product's safety and effectiveness before they will make a purchase. The idea of science as a compelling marketing tool has become popular within the past few years—and it is likely to become a much more important consideration as consumers become further educated about supplements and as supplements become more sophisticated in their mechanism and mode of action.

The existing regulations governing dietary supplements permit manufacturers and marketers to make claims for particular ingredients based on the structure or function that they may have in the body (e.g., glucosamine for joints or amino acids for protein synthesis). For these types of structure/function claims, little to no research is required, and a good biochemistry text is the only requirement for generating many claims. Only a handful of supplement companies take the initiative (and spend the money) to go beyond the basic structure/function claims and support their product or ingredient claims with *good* research, including both safety/toxicity studies (in animals) and clinical trials (randomized, double-blind, placebo-controlled studies conducted in an appropriate population of human subjects). Anything less is considered of questionable value from a scientific perspective and (hopefully) will soon be of little value from a marketing/business perspective also.

So how much research is enough for dietary supplements? The answer may ultimately come from consumers and marketers, rather than from scientists. As reliably as the sun rises each morning, scientists and health professionals will insist on *more* research for a particular supplement—a position of critical importance that will undoubtedly help to refine our understanding of the mechanisms by which many supplements work or don't work. Unfortunately, *more* research is not necessarily the most prudent approach when viewed in light of the market pressures under which most supplement companies operate. From one viewpoint, *enough* research could be defined as the amount needed to convince a skeptical consumer to become a regular user.

At this point in the evolution of dietary supplements, for better or worse, a simple structure/function claim is often enough "evidence" for enthusiastic "early adopters" to take the plunge and start using a new supplement (even though many aspects of safety and effectiveness may not be fully addressed). As consumers become more educated, however, and learn to ask the *right* questions about ingredients, dosages, and mechanisms they will also become more skeptical (of product claims) and more demanding (for the actual evidence), which will force supplement companies to conduct more research to "prove" their products to potential customers.

obtained in another country. At the other extreme is China, where numerous unfounded concoctions abound.[15]

Athletic governing bodies also vary in their list of banned substances, which includes many legal over-the-counter drugs and dietary supplements. Perhaps the most obvious discrepancy between what is considered legal according to the law but illegal according to doping guidelines is the use of caffeine. Caffeine, a chemical naturally found in food, has had upper limits imposed on its use in athletics, but acceptable doses have still been shown to be ergogenic.[16] Similarly, the ephedrine-containing herb ma huang is a legal dietary supplement, but is completely banned by the International Olympic Committee (IOC). The guidelines for prohibited methods and substances formulated by the IOC serves as the basis for the doping policies of most other sport governing bodies, including the National Collegiate Athletic Association (NCAA). However, inconsistencies remain between athletic organizations. For example, at the time of this writing, the prohormone androstenedione is banned by most sports federations, with the notable exception of professional baseball.

Olympic athletes who have questions regarding the imposed restrictions on medicines or ergogenic supplements they may be taking are encouraged to contact the United States Olympic Committee's Drug Education Hotline at 1-800-233-0393. The hotline provides information regarding only the IOC status of a substance, not its legality. Again, some perfectly legal substances are banned by the IOC and other organizations. Keep in mind that this number may change. All athletes who use or may use over-the-counter (OTC) drugs or dietary supplements are encouraged to contact their specific athletic associations, whose doping policies may vary subtly from those of the IOC.

Ethical Aspects of Nutrition Supplementation

Allegations in popular literature that illicit performance-enhancing drug use remains rampant among elite and professional athletes and may still be rising; the media has given organized athletics a black eye.[17] Evidence of epidemic ergogenic drug abuse is supported in the scientific literature as well. Illicit drug use transcends all levels of athletics, reaching even junior high and high school students.[18,19]

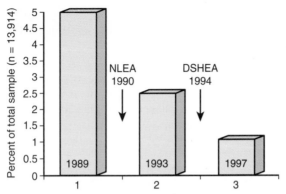

Figure 1-1. Trends of anabolic steroid usage among NCAA college athletes. Note how legislation (NLEA and DSHEA) providing greater dietary supplement availability and promotion coincides with a decrease in steroid use. This decrease in doping also overlaps with the development and marketing of increasingly more effective nutritional ergogenic aids. Data from the 1997 NCAA Study of Substance Use and Abuse Habits of Athletes.

Fortunately, there is at least a partial solution to this pervasive drug problem. As more effective, scientifically based dietary supplements have become available in recent years, individuals may be less likely to resort to illicit drug use, opting instead for legal supplements. FIGURE 1-1 shows the findings of a study conducted by the National Collegiate Athletic Association, which reports that anabolic-androgenic steroid use across all sports decreased 78% between 1989 and 1997. Interestingly, the decline in drug use closely followed the NLEA and DSHEA. Furthermore, the NCAA study indicates that nutritional supplements are most appealing to individuals who experiment with ergogenic drugs. Thus, those athletes who seek an "edge" have an opportunity to discontinue drug use in favor of implementing a regimen of nutritional ergogenic aids. Another promising fact is that most coaches and personal trainers encourage athletes to experiment with nutritional supplements,[20] which sets the stage for the abandonment of illicit drugs for safer, legal alternatives.

Although nutritional ergogenic aids present the obvious advantages of legality and safety over illicit or banned performance-enhancing drugs, for some athletes, an ethical dilemma may still exist. The collective morals of the athletic governing bodies are expressed in their doping guidelines; any methods or substances thought to confer an unfair advantage are banned. Therefore, the use of any nutritional ergogenic aid that is not banned could be considered ethical because using it would not violate the law. However, the ethical qualities of such aids is ultimately determined by an individual's code of ethics. Frankly, given that many athletes, by nature, are willing to take risks and do almost anything to improve their chances of winning, it is unlikely that many athletes will wrestle with

the issue of using dietary supplements. But those who have issues with the use of supplements may ultimately find themselves at a competitive disadvantage as more effective supplements are discovered.

One complicated factor in the discussion of ethics is the seemingly inherent contradiction between the IOC definition of doping and its list of banned substances. Doping is generally defined by the IOC as any substance taken in abnormal quantity with the intended purpose of artificially and unfairly enhancing performance. Yet, a long list of nutritional ergogenic aids are taken in quantities greater than what can be obtained through diet alone. Thus, such quantities would logically be considered *abnormal*. Similarly, it could be argued that eating ten chicken breasts a day to enhance muscle growth in a weightlifter is *abnormal*. Yet, where does one draw the line? At this point, it is difficult to predict how sport-governing bodies will continue to react to new ergogenic aids. Will they ban any aid that is found to be effective, or will they permit the use of otherwise legal ergogenic aids that have been proven to be safe and effective? Certainly, the next few years will play a pivotal role in how nutritional ergogenic aids will be used by athletes and perceived by them, their peers, and the public.

Supplement Manufacturers: The Major Players

Sales of general nutritional supplements have more than doubled in the past decade.[12] In the U.S. sales of nutritional supplements increased 50% between 1994 and 1998, bringing the total annual sales of nutritional supplements to well over $6 billion.[21] Of that $6 billion, over $1 billion can be attributed to sports supplements.[12] Manufacturers of sports supplements, when able to firmly establish themselves, have enjoyed similar growth.

A 1998 analysis of the sports nutrition market revealed that six manufacturing companies had annual sales of over $80 million, typically closer to $100 million. Ten companies had sales of $10–80 million and 94 other companies comprised the rest of the market.[7]

The top six companies, in no particular order, were Met-Rx, Weider, Twin Labs, Experimental and Applied Sciences (EAS), Power Foods, and General Nutrition Center (GNC). These six companies represented 56% of the market.[7]

The above-mentioned market study omitted sales of sports beverage companies. Of sports beverage companies, Gatorade dominated the market, controlling 85% of the share, while Pepsi's All Sport and Coca-Cola's Powerade each had 12% of sales.[7]

The future looks bright for the sports supplement industry as the market expands in response to legislative change, scientific endeavor, and consumer education.

Consumer Savvy

Because the DSHEA requires less premarket review for dietary supplements than for other substances it regulates, such as drugs and food additives, a greater burden is placed on the shoulders of both manufacturers and consumers in determining the safety of a product and the truth of its label claims.[12] Ultimately, though, it is the consumer who decides whether to introduce a particular product into his/her body. Thus, consumers need to educate themselves with unbiased information, rather than marketing propaganda, to exercise consumer savvy, or discretion.

Interpreting Scientific Studies

At one time, published scientific studies on dietary supplements were available to researchers and health care practitioners to interpret. Now, however, the consumer is constantly confronted with a barrage of scientific studies. The evening news, radio and television commercials, and magazines are full of references to scientific studies. Some supplement manufacturers have even cited studies right on the jars of their products! Today's savvy consumer must be equipped to gain at least a cursory meaning of scientific studies and the jargon that accompanies them.

The scientific method consists of asking a question, developing a hypothesis (tentative explanation), designing a study to test the hypothesis, controlling as many extraneous (interfering) variables as possible, manipulating only one variable at a time, statistically analyzing the results, and submitting the study to a peer-reviewed science journal for publication. The term *peer-reviewed*, sometimes called *refereed*, indicates that a manuscript submitted for publication in a journal will first be scrutinized by other experts in the field before it is accepted. Abstracts, which are brief study results that have been presented at a conference, are also published in peer-reviewed journals, but are not as rigorously reviewed as full journal articles. Abstracts are usually readily identified in a citation by the appearance of the word *abstract* in brackets. The term *abstract* also applies to a one-paragraph summary that appears at the beginning of a full journal article.

Commonly, when the media reports studies, their results are reported as *significant* or *nonsignificant*. These terms, used extensively throughout scientific literature, refer to whether chance may have played a large role in the results of a study. The generally accepted level of significance is P < 0.05, where "P" stands for "probability," and means that the probability of the outcome occurring by chance is less than 5%. Expressed another way, at least 95% of the time, the findings are truly the result of the variable that was manipulated.

An important reminder for the athlete, coach, or nutritionist is that statistical significance does not guarantee functional significance. For example, a particular endurance supplement may be shown to significantly increase maximum exercise duration by 10% at a given level of intensity. But, one must ask if this 10% increase will have

---

Table 1-1 Sorting Out the Truth From the Hype: Asking the Right Questions of Scientific Studies

1. Is there a legitimate rationale for the dietary supplement? Theoretically, the dietary supplement should be able to influence physiological processes involved in physical performance or physique development.

2. Were appropriate subjects studied? Subjects should be similar to the consumers to whom the product will be marketed. Thus, mode, type, intensity, and duration of physical activity should be similar, as should other variables such as subject age.

3. How were the changes in performance or body composition evaluated? The tests used should be valid and reliable. A valid test measures what it is supposed to measure, and a reliable test gives consistent results when the test is repeated. For example, was an increase in muscle size evaluated by a tape measure or more accurate stacked MRI scans?

4. Was a placebo used? The dietary supplement should be provided in the appropriate amount and for an appropriate time period to the experimental group of subjects, but a placebo (inactive substance) should be used with a control group of subjects. A dietary supplement may work for some individuals, not because of any bona fide physiological effect, but a psychological placebo effect may modify personal behaviors conducive to performance or physique enhancement.

5. Were the subjects randomly assigned to the treatments? Subjects should be randomly assigned to the dietary supplement or placebo groups. If the study is a crossover design in which all subjects take both the dietary supplement and placebo during different phases, the order of giving the supplement should be balanced; that is, half of the subjects should take the dietary supplement first, and half, the placebo. In the second phase of the study, the subjects switch treatments.

6. Was the study double-blind? Neither the subjects nor the investigators should know which group receives the dietary supplement or placebo. This is known as a double-blind protocol.

7. Were extraneous factors controlled? Investigators should attempt to control other factors besides the treatment that may influence what is being measured. Diet, exercise, and daily physical activities need to be controlled.

8. Were the data analyzed properly? Appropriate statistical techniques should be used to minimize the chance of statistical error.

Data from Williams, MH. ACSM's Health & Fitness Journal [Online]. October 19, 1998

any meaningful effect on performance. For example, if an endurance athlete never has to compete to the point of total exhaustion, will a slight delay in fatigue offer any advantage? Does the increase in performance justify the cost of the supplement or any potentially negative side effects? A similar example could be made for a bodybuilding supplement that claims to have been shown to significantly increase testosterone production. Such an increase does not guarantee that a significant change in strength, muscle mass, or body fat will occur.

Another important aspect of the scientific method is reproducibility. Too often, a new nutritional ergogenic aid is aggressively marketed with only one scientific study to support its use. A single study does not constitute conclusive evidence that a supplement is or is not effective for its intended purpose. Again, there is always a slight probability that the results were due to nothing more than chance. The possibility that the original researcher was biased and could have unconsciously or consciously influenced the outcome of the study also exists. Therefore, most reputable scientists prefer to evaluate the sum results of several well-controlled research studies. It is best if the studies are conducted by different researchers. For example, skepticism would ensue if a particular researcher demonstrated twice that a miraculous form of a mineral he invented could build muscle and decrease body fat, yet many other competent researchers subsequently failed time and time again to reproduce the findings.

When evaluating nutritional ergogenic aid research, or any other research, there are many additional considerations. TABLE 1-1 demonstrates several questions that should be raised when evaluating research. It can be difficult to sort out the hype from the truth, and the ability to properly analyze a study's methods, results, and conclusions will depend somewhat on the evaluator's educational background.

Flex, Lies, and Measuring Tape: Evaluating Supplement Claims

Unfortunately, some marketing strategies still prey on a person's vulnerability. Athletes are faced with a constant supply of supplement advertisements that often include complex terminology, skewed graphs, diagrams of foreign biochemical reactions, and impressive claims. Is this legal? The answer is "yes," because this kind of material is protected under the First Amendment, which guarantees the freedom of speech. As long as this type of material—however unreasonable the claims—does not make drug-like claims and is physically separate from any supplements, then the law is not violated. Consumers need to be reminded that although something is written down does not mean that it is true. Magazines, books, and editorials in magazines often contain nothing more than fictional advertisements disguised as information. TABLE 1-2 gives

---

Table 1-2 Tips for Developing Sports Supplement Savvy

Critically evaluate ads that tell only part of the story. For example, an ad may emphatically proclaim that high-quality protein is required for muscle growth, but make no mention of the importance of the interactions of resistance exercise or total caloric intake.

Be suspicious of a single substance that claims to enhance performance or physique in multiple ways. For instance, a suspicious endorsement may claim that a single substance can build muscle, increase strength, burn fat, increase stamina, increase concentration, strengthen the immune system, enhance sex drive, and speed recovery. However, some elaborate products may contain a combination of different ergogenic aids and therefore may exert multiple effects.

Be wary of any company that implies that it is okay to eat poorly as long as a person takes his or her supplement. Everyone should recognize that the best sports supplement regimen cannot compensate for the worst dietary habits. For example, using an effective fat-loss supplement will not do a person any good if that person is consuming twice as many calories as he or she should.

Be skeptical of ads that claim it is easy to reduce body fat while making no mention of the importance of proper diet and exercise. If it were simple to alter body composition, a book of this magnitude would not need to be written. Only when used in the context of a proper diet, exercise, and patience can fat loss be optimal, and even in such an ideal situation, fat loss will be challenging for most.

Recognize that in most instances, a *natural* supplement is neither more effective nor safer than a *synthetic* supplement. Regardless of its source, for example, vitamin C is still vitamin C, whether it is was synthesized in a scientist's laboratory or in a flower's laboratory. An additional consideration is that many herbal or natural products may contain additional, unidentified substances that may have undesirable effects.

Carefully scrutinize claims of products that promise miraculous results in a brief period of time. A select few products such as those that affect fluid balance or the nervous system show results in relatively short order. However, when using most effective ergogenic aids, success is not achieved overnight, and it is the meticulous application of a long-term strategy that yields the best results.

Look for products that support their claims with only anecdotes and testimonials, as opposed to scientific studies. Testimonials are unreliable and frequently fraudulent. A consumer should ask oneself or a qualified individual if there could be an alternative explanation for a particular result.

Dismiss a product that claims to be equal or superior to anabolic steroids in its ergogenic properties. Such a claim is not only unreasonable, but also unverifiable. Because of the negative side effects and controlled status of anabolic steroids, it is extremely unlikely that these drugs will ever be directly compared against the effectiveness of a legal ergogenic aid in a university study.

Challenge ads that support a product with a single study. Good scientists (and consumers) rely on the data generated by several studies to ensure that the results are reproducible and not a fluke.

Mistrust ads that may cite a scientific study but give inadequate referencing information to locate the study. For example, a

Table 1-2 (continued)

publication may state that "A study by Smith et al. revealed that yams increase testosterone production." A similar tactic could appear as "Researchers at West Virginia University found that our product is absorbed 600% better than that of other brands." At minimum, citation information should include the last name of the first author, the year of publication, the journal title, and the volume, issue, and page numbers. Also helpful is the inclusion of other authors' names, and the title of the study.

Whether or not a manufacturer cites any studies, ask the manufacturer for full journal references or actual copies of the journal articles supporting their claims.

Evaluate if a supplement claim is measurable. It is difficult to analyze the purported benefits of a substance if it is claimed to make you *feel better* or *feel more energetic*. Drug-using athletes may be attracted to a product that claims to *detoxify the liver*, yet have no means of assessing the supposed effectiveness. Purposefully vague claims do not allow a consumer to determine if the supplement was worthy of the hype.

In sports supplement ads, look for dubious credentials that are not recognized by mainstream science and education. If a supplement company cannot find anyone with a reputable background to stand behind their product, steer clear of it.

Ignore products that make you self-conscious or vulnerable. Some advertisers may manipulate consumers by alienating them, convincing them that everyone else is using a particular product.

Don't allow obsession or desperation to cloud one's judgment. Some athletes, desperate to beat the competition, will use every supplement available to reassure themselves that they've explored every option. Stick with scientifically based products.

Use common sense. If the claim appears to be too good to be true, it probably is.

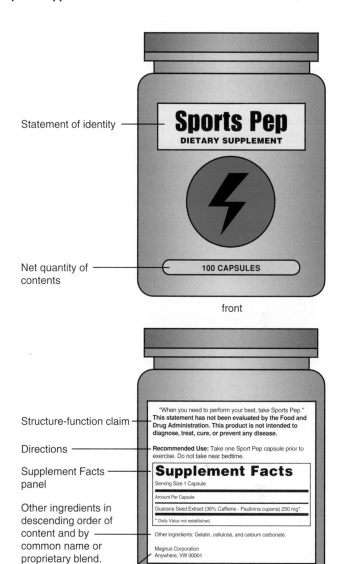

Figure 1-2. Anatomy of the new requirements for a dietary supplement label. This new format is more consumer friendly, and the "Supplement Facts" panel closely resembles the "Nutrition Facts" panel found on food items. (Data from Kurtzwei P. An FDA guide to dietary supplements. FDA Consumer 1998;32(5):30.)

suggestions for how consumers can avoid being taken advantage of by a supplement marketer.

Understanding Dietary Supplement Labels

As of March 1999, dietary supplement labels were required to meet certain expectations developed as a result of the DSHEA. The new standards make supplement label information more complete with the inclusion of an information panel entitled "Supplement Facts," a clear identity statement listing the name of the product and its ingredients. The supplement facts panel should show the manufacturer's suggested serving size, the specific nutrients contained in the product, percent daily value for nutrients with an established reference amount, and the part of the plant used in herbal preparations.[22] FIGURE 1-2 illustrates the basic anatomy of the new supplement labels. FIGURE 1-3 shows variations of the

supplement facts panel and explains some of the new labeling rules.

Finding a Reputable Source of Sports Supplement Information

Charlatans thrive in the field of nutrition perhaps more so than in any other area of medical science. A quick glance through the business pages of the phone book will likely reveal many nutritionists who claim to be qualified nutrition-related consultants. Some sports supplement consumers will undoubtedly wish to consult with a nutrition

Dietary supplement containing dietary ingredients with and without RDIs and DRVs:

Supplement Facts

Serving Size 1 Packet

Amount Per Packet		% Daily Value
Vitamin A (from cod liver oil)	5,000 IU	100%
Vitamin C (as ascorbic acid)	250 mg	417%
Vitamin E (as d-alpha tocopherol)	150 IU	500%
Thiamin (as thiamin mononitrate)	75 mg	5000%
Riboflavin	75 mg	4412%
Niacin (as niacinamide)	75 mg	375%
Selenium	20 mcg	28%
Vanadium	10 mcg	*

* Daily Value not established.

Other ingredients: Cellulose, stearic acid, and silica.

Dietary supplement containing an herb:

Supplement Facts

Serving Size 1 Capsule

Amount Per Capsule

Guarana Seed Extract (36% Caffeine - Paulinina cupana) 250 mg*

* Daily Value not established.

Other ingredients: Gelatin, cellulose, and calcium carbonate.

A proprietary bland of dietary ingrediants:

Supplement Facts

Serving Size 1 Tbsp (9 g) (makes 8 fl oz prepared)
Servings Per Container 24

	Amount/Serving	% Daily Value
Calories	10	
Total Carbohydrates	2 g	1%*
Sugars	2 g	†
Proprietary blend	6 g	
Creatine Monohydrate		†
HMB (calcium β hydroxy β methylbutyrate monohydrate)		†
Glutamine		†

* Percent Daily Values are based on a 2,000 calorie diet.
† Daily Value not established.

Other ingredients: Fructose, stearic acid, and red 40.

With a little room for stylistic preferences, the following labeling rules apply as of March 1999:

1. Title, "Supplement Facts," will allow for easy identification.

2. Information must be listed "per serving." Serving sizes are determined by the manufacturer's recommendations for consumption at one occasion.

3. Nutrients required in nutrition labeling of conventional foods must be listed when present and omitted when not present.

4. "Other dietary ingredients" (such as botanicals, phytochemicals) that do not have recommendations for daily consumption are listed beneath a bar. They are required to state the quantity present and to be identified as having no recommendation for consumption.

5. The list of dietary ingredients in the nutrition label (nutrients and non-nutrients) may include the source ingredient; if it does, the source ingredient need not be listed again on the ingredient list.

6. Botanicals (herbs) must state the part of the plant present and be identified by their common or usual name. In addition, their Latin binomial name is needed if the common or usual name is not published in Herbs of Commerce, published by the American Herbal Products Association.

7. Proprietary (secret) blends may be listed with the weight given for the total blend only, as opposed to the weight of each individual ingredient. When this is done, components of the blend must be listed in descending order of predominance by weight.

Figure 1-3. Summary of nutrition labeling rules for dietary supplements and examples of labels for three different supplements.

professional to individualize and optimize their supplement program. But to whom should one turn to for accurate, unbiased sports supplement advice?

TABLE 1-3 provides a list of individuals (along with credentials) who may advise athletes about nutritional ergogenic aids. A listing in the table does not imply endorsement for an included credential, as many questionable credentials have been included. Rather, the table features an array of possible sports supplement advisors, despite whether or not they are truly qualified.

As used in Table 1-3, *accreditation* refers to a distinction granted by various government-approved organizations that are specific to a particular field. In most instances, accreditation means that an educational institution's course credits will transfer to another school. Accreditation does not guarantee scientific accuracy, but does demonstrate that the program is well organized. All respected educational institutions are accredited.[23]

Some institutions grant degrees, such as BS, MS, and even PhD degrees, but are not accredited. And unfortunately, some dishonest individuals use titles that they have not earned.

Because certain titles are not legally defined in all states, the person bearing a given title may or may not have obtained a degree through an accredited institution. For example, some states have reserved the title of *nutritionist* for practitioners who have completed an appropriate college degree, whereas in other states anyone can call himself or herself a nutritionist regardless of educational background. Fake degrees that have been accredited by phony accrediting agencies add to the confusion. A legitimate accreditation agency must be recognized by the US Department of Education. To find out if a degree is from a properly accredited institution, a person may refer to the Accredited Institutions of Post-secondary Education Programs Candidates, which is published by the American Council on Education. This directory is available at many libraries, and lists accredited institutions, professionally accredited programs, and candidates for accreditation. Additional information can be obtained by writing to the Council for Higher Education Accreditation, One Dupont Circle NW, Suite 501, Washington, DC 20036-1135 or visiting their web site at www.chea.org. To specifically discover if a correspondence school is accredited and to receive a free listing of accredited correspondence programs, write to the Distance Education and Training Council, 1601 Eighteenth Street NW, Washington, DC 20009 or call (202) 234-5100.

Licensure refers to a particular state's recognition of an individual's competence. Competence is commonly determined by passing a state licensure examination. Licensing provides a way to ensure that practitioners have met minimal standards of education and experience. A revocation of licensure does not negate a person's academic credentials. For example, an unlicensed medical doctor, although unable to practice medicine, can still use the

Table 1-3 Some Credentials of Those Who Offer Sports Supplementation Advice

Title	Abbreviation	Accredited	Licensed
Registered Dietitian	RD	yes	variable
Licensed Dietitian	LD	yes	yes
Doctor of Osteopathy	DO	yes	yes
Doctor of Medicine	MD	yes	yes
Doctor of Chiropractic	DC	yes	yes
Doctor of Pharmacy	PharmD	yes	yes
Registered Pharmacist	RPh	yes	yes
Doctor of Philosophy	PhD	yes	no
Doctor of Science	DSc	yes	no
Doctor of Education	EdD	yes	no
Master of Science	MS	yes	no
Master of Arts	MA	yes	no
Bachelor of Science	BS	yes	no
Bachelor of Arts	BA	yes	no
Certified Athletic Trainer	ATC	yes	variable
Licensed Athletic Trainer	LAT	yes	yes
Exercise Physiologist	EP	variable	variable
ASEP[1] Master Level Nutrition & Weight Control Certified	—	yes	no
IART[2] Certified Nutrition Advisor	CNA	yes*	no
ACE[3] Certified Lifestyle & Weight Management Consultant	—	no	no
Nutritionist	—	variable	variable
Dietitian	—	variable	variable
Sport(s) Nutritionist	—	no	no
Certified Nutritionist	CN	no	no
Certified Clinical Nutritionist	CCN	no	no
Certified Nutrition Consultant	CNC	no	no
Homeopathic Medical Doctor	HMD	variable	variable
Nutrition Counselor	NC	variable	variable
Doctor of Naturopathy	ND	variable	variable
Doctor of Nutrimedicine	NMD	no	no

[1]American Sport Education Program
[2]International Association of Resistance Trainers
[3]American Council on Exercise
*IART, a Canadian-based nonprofit organization, is recognized by the Canadian government as an educational institution

designation of MD and, in some states, may still be able to provide services as a *nutritionist*. To find out if a nutrition practitioner is licensed in the state in which he or she practices, the consumer should contact that particular state's health-licensing agency. A standard name for such an agency does not exist, so a consumer may have to search the state government pages of the phone book for the appropriate agency.

Traditionally, the primary health professional who dispenses nutritional information is the registered dietitian (RD), which requires the completion of a bachelor's or master's degree approved by the American Dietetic Association (ADA). However, the distinction of RD alone may not be sufficient enough to prepare a dietitian to become familiar with all of the sports supplements because of its rapid progression. Therefore, an RD should ideally be a member of the Dietary Practice Group (DRG) for Sports, Cardiovascular, and Wellness Nutritionists (SCAN), a section of the ADA having over 5000 professionals devoted to the application of sports nutrition. Becoming a SCAN member requires nothing more of the RD (or other ADA member) than paying a fee, but it does ensure that the RD has access to the latest scientific information in the field. The public can verify whether a provider using the RD credential is a registered dietitian by calling the ADA at 1-800-877-1600, ext. 5500.

Other scholastically qualified individuals who may be good resources for scientific information on ergogenic aids include exercise physiologists, pharmacists, nutrition researchers, and physicians. These degrees alone are insufficient if the individuals have not specialized in nutrition as it relates to sport or if they have not actively and intensively self-studied such information. For example, the most desirable MDs and DOs for sports supplement consultation are those who have completed residencies in bariatrics (obesity), sports medicine, and endocrinology, or who have specialized in clinical nutrition. The academic/research degrees of BS, BA, MS, MA, PhD, and EdD offer expertise in any number of fields, from history to psychology and so on. Therefore, qualified individuals who hold these degrees should have specific backgrounds in biochemistry, nutritional biochemistry, nutritional physiology, nutrition, nutrition science, muscle physiology, exercise physiology, exercise science, or sports pharmacology.

The most common credentials of nonrecognized nutritionists are attained through certification rather than formal education. The difficulty of becoming certified varies greatly among the certifying bodies, but most certification organizations are not as rigorous as those that offer programs for becoming licensed. In fact, many certification organizations are correspondence courses that allow open-book examinations, which are graded liberally. In the past, some certifying bodies charged a fee in exchange for a fancy certificate, which led to household pets becoming recognized certificate holders.

Fortunately for the consumer, the days of unreliable nutritional consultation are numbered. The ADA has been leading a successful movement to restrict or prohibit unlicensed individuals from disseminating nutritional information. Essentially, the ADA is making dispensing nutritional information by an unqualified person analogous to practicing medicine without a license.

To summarize, the consumer can check the qualifications of an individual providing sports supplement information by first looking for the credential or degree abbreviations listed after the person's name. Next, the reputation of the degree-granting institution can be checked through directories of accredited institutions. The consumer can also contact the health-licensing agency of the state in which the consultant practices to find out if the consultant meets the state requirements to advise clients in nutrition. To find out if a person is qualified as an RD, the consumer may contact the ADA.

Recourse for the Dissatisfied Customer

Fortunately, several organizations are available in which a dissatisfied supplement consumer can appeal. The consumer should first start with the store in which the product was purchased. Many nutritional supplement companies now guarantee customer satisfaction, with their guarantee appearing on the product packaging or label along with a company address or phone number. With such a guaranteed product, the retailer where the product was purchased may be able to provide some satisfaction. Individuals should keep their receipts to facilitate an exchange or

---

Table 1-4 Where to Report Sports Supplement Dissatisfaction

Chief Postal Inspector
US Postal Service
Washington, DC 20260

FDA
5600 Fishers Lane
Rockville, MD 20857

FTC Bureau of Consumer Protection
Washington, DC 20580

National Advertising Division, Council of Better Business Bureau
845 Third Ave.
New York, NY 10022

National Council Against Health Fraud, Inc.
PO Box 1276
Loma Linda, CA 92354

National Council Against Health Fraud Task Force
on Victim Redress
PO Box 1747
Allentown, PA 18105
(610) 437-1795

National Fraud Information Center Hotline
(800) 876-7060

In addition to these offices, the consumer should contact local and regional offices of federal agencies. To do so, they should be directed to the US Government section of the phone book.

Table 1-5 **Sports Supplement Buzzwords and Essential Terminology**

anabolic—Referring to something that causes a building-up of tissue, or anabolism. Anabolism generally refers to an increase in lean tissue, particularly muscle.

anticatabolic—Referring to something that causes a building-up of tissue through the inhibition of catabolic mechanisms, thus allowing anabolic processes to prevail.

bioavailability—The ease with which something is absorbed from the digestive tract. The higher the bioavailability, the greater the total absorption and rate of absorption.

catabolic—Referring to something that causes a tearing-down of tissue, or catabolism. Catabolism generally refers to a decrease in lean tissue, particularly muscle.

chelating agent—An organic (hydrogen and carbon-containing) compound that binds to charged metallic atoms (ions) to increase absorption.

coenzyme—An organic (hydrogen and carbon-containing) compound that binds to a specific type of enzyme to activate it. A coenzyme is a type of cofactor. B vitamins commonly act as coenzymes.

cofactor—An inorganic or organic substance that binds to a specific type of enzyme to activate it. Vitamins and minerals frequently serve as cofactors.

effervescent—Possessing the quality of giving off gas bubbles. Effervescence provides a means of some drug or dietary supplement delivery systems and is intended to enhance absorption of the active ingredient(s).

efficacy—A term borrowed from pharmacology describing the maximum response of an administered supplement, regardless of the dose. At a certain point, consuming more of a particular substance fails to elicit any greater effect. For example, the chemically dissimilar supplements A and B have each been shown to increase lean body mass by different mechanisms. However, product A always results in greater total increases in lean body mass than does supplement B. So, no matter how much supplement B a person consumes, he/she cannot expect greater increases in lean body mass with B when compared with an optimal dose of A. Similarly, for a person in excruciating pain, no quantity of aspirin will be as efficacious as an optimal dose of morphine. Efficacy is much more important than either bioavailability or potency.

endogenous—Originating from within the body. In the most simple terms, anything produced inside the body, such as the hormone testosterone, is endogenous. However, exogenous substances can have endogenous influences. For example, a supplement that could increase the testicular production of testosterone would be said to increase "endogenous" testosterone secretion.

engineered food—A kind of nutrition supplement that is designed to augment the diet or to replace a meal. Typically contains carbohydrate, fat, protein, vitamins, and minerals. May be sold as a powder, meal-replacement bar, or even specially designed foods such as pizza.

ergogenic—Possessing the ability to enhance work output, particularly as it relates to athletic performance.

ergolytic—Possessing the ability to decrease work output. Sometimes what is intended to enhance physical performance inadvertently hinders performance. For example, alcoholic beverages consumed immediately before an event were once thought to be ergogenic for endurance athletes, but may have actually been ergolytic.

ergostatic—Having no effect on physical performance. This is not a part of the current sports nutrition vocabulary, but should be because it is the category in which most failed ergogenic aids fit; failed ergogenics are not necessarily ergolytic. Whereas *ergogenic* and *ergolytic* represent opposites like black and white, *ergostatic* represents gray. *Ergostatic* could replace clumsy phrases such as "not ergogenic," "has no effect," and "makes no difference."

exogenous—Referring to substances originating outside the body. For example, taking a hormone supplement would be consuming an *exogenous* form of the hormone.

free radicals—A highly reactive atom or compound having an unpaired electron. Free radicals are produced during metabolism and are believed to cause cellular damage. Free radicals may play a role in aging and disease. Antioxidants are consumed to help neutralize free radicals by sacrificing themselves to react with the free radicals so that the free radicals do not react with the body's cells.

functional foods—Foods that may provide medical or health benefits beyond basic nutrition because of the presence of physiologically active compounds such as phytochemicals.

GRAS (Generally Recognized as Safe)—Food ingredients not evaluated by the FDA-prescribed testing procedure fall under the regulatory status of GRAS. GRAS also includes common food ingredients that were used before the 1959 Food Additives Amendment to the Food, Drug and Cosmetic Act was enacted.

isolates—Substances that have been separated, or isolated, from their original source.

metabolism—The sum total of all anabolic and catabolic reactions in the body. Metabolism also refers to the ridding of the body of foreign substances, during which lipid-soluble compounds are converted into more water-soluble metabolites for facilitated excretion.

metabolite—Any product of metabolism, such as an intermediate or waste product. For example, the popular supplement beta-hydroxy beta-methylbutyrate (HMB) is a metabolite, or breakdown product, of the amino acid leucine.

natural—Referring to foods or supplements that have not been greatly refined (processed) and which do not contain *artificial* chemicals such as fertilizers, colors, etc. The term *natural* presently has no legal definition.

(continued)

Table 1-5 (continued)

nutraceuticals—Substances in a food that may provide medical or health benefits beyond basic nutrition, including disease prevention. Research indicates this term does not appeal to most consumers possibly because it reminds them of medicine.

organic—Pertaining to agricultural products that are grown using biological, mechanical, and cultural methods as opposed to synthetic methods to control pests, enhance soil quality, and/or improve processing. The United States Department of Agriculture (USDA) is presently drafting a legal definition for what may be considered organic. The currently accepted definition permits farmers to use natural pesticides, but no synthetic products.

oxidation—Process by which oxygen is added to a compound and/or electrons are lost. Oxidation is involved in the derivation of energy from compounds and causes the release of free radicals.

patent—A numeric distinction granted to an invention, process, etc. by the US Patent Office. A patent gives exclusive rights, or a monopoly, to the inventor for production, use, sale, and profit. In regard to dietary supplements, a patent signifies only that a product is unique, not that it is effective. The US Patent Office does not test effectiveness.

pharmaceutical grade—Implying purity. This term has no legal or trade definition but is frequently used on sports supplement labels.

phytochemical—Substances found in fruits and vegetables that may be consumed by humans daily in gram quantities. Phytochemicals exhibit a potential for reducing the risk of cancer.

potency—A term borrowed from pharmacology describing the absolute amount (dose) of a substance to produce a specified ergogenic effect. This term is commonly confused with the terms *efficacy* and *bioavailability*. Potency is often overemphasized during marketing hype. For example, if supplement X requires a dose that is twice that of supplement Y, it does not necessarily follow that Y is any more effective. Cost of the supplement per unit weight may be an additional consideration.

prohormone—A compound that can be converted into a hormone within the body. Prohormones are produced by glands in the body in which they await further processing to become functional hormones. Some prohormones are now sold as sports supplements.

pure—Referring to a supplement that contains nothing but the ingredients stated on the label. This term has no legal definition.

reduction—The counterpart to oxidation, in which electrons are gained by a compound.

stacking—Consumption of two or more supplements during the same time frame in an attempt to maximize results. This term originated with anabolic steroid regimens.

supraphysiological—Consumption or accretion of a substance in amounts greater than what is required for normal physiological processes. For example, eating supraphysiological amounts of protein has been shown to positively influence muscle growth.

synergistic—Having the property of enhancing or multiplying the effectiveness of another substance. For example, carbohydrates consumed with creatine monohydrate have a synergistic relationship.

refund, and should attempt any returns before the "best if used by" date on the product, if one is provided. If the retailer can't help, then contacting the manufacturer is the next possible avenue. If the consumer is still dissatisfied, having not received an exchange or refund, then that person may wish to contact the Better Business Bureau.

Although the previous tactics apply to simple consumer dissatisfaction, numerous other agencies and organizations exist for the pursuit of more serious complaints regarding fraud. For products sold by mail-order, the U.S. Postal Service can block the exchange of orders and goods in circumstances when the products have been falsely advertised, but there are ways for unscrupulous companies to get around the laws. If a manufacturer has made any drug claims on its dietary supplement product that were disapproved, the FDA may seize the product and impose criminal charges on its manufacturer, provided that the claim is somehow traceable to the manufacturer. The Federal Trade Commission (FTC) has jurisdiction over false advertising and has the authority—but not necessarily the manpower—to file complaints and negotiate settlements. Another organization, the National Council Against Health Fraud (NCAHF) can help victimized

dietary supplement consumers file lawsuits. Contacting one's state attorney general is also an option.[13] TABLE 1-4 provides contacts for any disgruntled consumers of sports supplements. Perhaps the best advice for the consumer can be found in the Latin phrase, "Caveat emptor," or "Let the buyer beware."

Staying Informed: The DSHEA at Work (Again) and Current Buzzwords

In 1999, the Office of Dietary Supplements, created by the DSHEA, successfully carried out a mandate in the DSHEA to launch a database for dietary supplement research. This exciting development, called the International Bibliographic Information on Dietary Supplements (IBIDS) database, is a database of published scientific literature from around the world. The IBIDS database is free of charge through the Office of Dietary Supplements home page at http://dietary-supplements.info.nih.gov and is intended to assist both scientists and the lay public in finding credible scientific publications on dietary supplements.[24]

Finally, to exemplify the meaning of consumer savvy, a person must understand the meaning of the most current nutritional and sports supplement jargon, or *buzzwords*, as well as some basic terminology. TABLE 1-5 provides definitions of some current buzzwords in the sports supplement industry.

SUMMARY

Nutritional ergogenic aids have evolved over several thousand years, but did not approach being a subject of scientific endeavor until the early twentieth century. Many sports supplements originated with weight trainers, but the market has grown significantly, partly as a result of legislative change. Among other provisions, the Dietary Supplement Health and Education Act of 1994 defines dietary supplements, establishes guidelines for the display of literature, creates a new framework for ensuring safety, and requires certain criteria of supplement labels. The DSHEA also changes the emphasis of FDA regulation from premarket safety to policing. Effective sports supplements have offered alternatives to illicit performance-enhancing drug use, but ethical considerations remain unsettled. Today's consumer must be well informed, but is equipped with several avenues of recourse should there be dissatisfaction with a sports supplement product.

REFERENCES

1. Williams MH. The Ergogenics Edge: Pushing the Limits of Sports Performance. Champaign, IL:Human Kinetics, 1998.
2. Barron RL, Vanscoy GJ. Natural products and the athlete: Facts and folklore. Ann Pharmacother 1993;27:607–615.
3. Grivetti LE, Applegate EA. From Olympia to Atlanta: a cultural-historical perspective on diet and athletic training. J Nutr 1997;127:860S–868S.
4. Applegate EA, Grivetti LE. Search for the competitive edge: a history of dietary fads and supplements. J Nutr 1997;127:869S–873S.
5. Wagner JC. Abuse of drugs used to enhance athletic performance. Am J Hosp Pharm 1989;46:2059–2067.
6. Barret S, Herbert V. The Vitamin Pushers: How the "Health Food" Industry is Selling America a Bill of Goods. Amherst, MA: Prometheus Books, 1994.
7. Anonymous. Sports nutrition on track for growth. Nutr Bus J 1998;3(7):1–24.
8. Williams MH. Nutrition for Fitness and Sport. 4th ed. Baltimore: Williams and Wilkins, 1995.
9. Forbes AL, McNamara SH. Food labeling, health claims, and dietary supplement legislation. In: Shils ME, Olson JA, Shike M, Ross AC, eds. Modern Nutrition in Health and Disease. 9th ed. Baltimore: Williams & Wilkins, 1999.
10. Anonymous. Dietary Supplement Health and Education Act of 1994. [Online] US Food and Drug Administration, 1999. http://vm.cfsan.fda.gov/~dms/dietsupp.html.
11. Anonymous. What are dietary supplements? [Online] Office of Dietary Supplements, 1999. http://odp.od.nih.gov/ods/whatare/whatare.html.
12. Kurtzwell, P. An FDA guide to dietary supplements. FDA Consumer 1998;32(5):28–35.
13. Barret S, Herbert V. Fads, fraud, and quackery. In: Shils ME, Olson JA, Shike M, Ross AC, eds. Modern Nutrition in Health and Disease. 9th ed. Baltimore: Williams & Wilkins, 1999.
14. Anonymous. About the Canadian Coalition for Health Freedom. [Online] Canadian Coalition for Health Freedom, 1999. http://www.cchf.com.
15. Bidlack WR, Wang W. Designing functional foods. In: Shils ME, Olson JA, Shike M, Ross AC, eds. Modern Nutrition in Health and Disease. 9th ed. Baltimore: Williams & Wilkins, 1999.
16. Eichner ER. Ergogenic aids: what athletes are using—and why. Phys Sportsmed 1997;25(4):70–79,83.
17. Begley S, Brant M. The real scandal. Newsweek 1999;133(7):48–54.
18. Catlin D, Wright J, Pope H Jr, et al. Assessing the threat of anabolic steroids. Phys Sportsmed 1993;21(8):37–44.
19. NCAA study of substance use and abuse habits of college student-athletes. September, 1997.
20. Survey: The Use of Dietary Supplements in Sports Training. NSCA Bulletin 19:4, 1998.
21. World vitamin, diet supplement sales soar: A report of Reuters Health, 1999.
22. Anonymous. Dietary supplements now labeled with more information. [Online] US Department of Health and Human Services, 1999. http://www.fda.gov/bbs/topics/NEWS/NEW00678.html.
23. Anonymous. About CHEA. [Online] Council for Higher Education Accreditation, 1999. http://www.chea.org/About/index.html.
24. Anonymous. NIH office of dietary supplements announces [sic] new database of scientific literature on dietary supplements. [Online] National Institutes of Health. http://odp.od.nih.gov/ods/news/releases/dsrdb.html[1999, Jan 19].

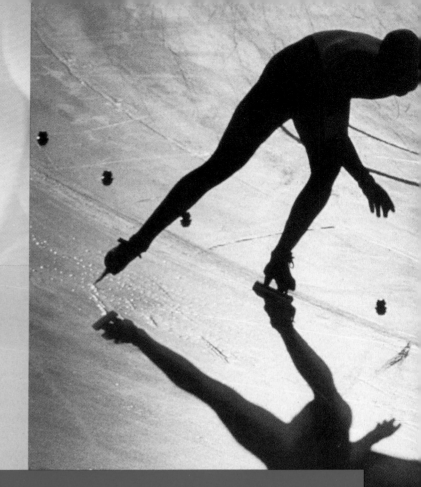

Food: The Ultimate Drug

Ash Batheja and Jeffrey R. Stout

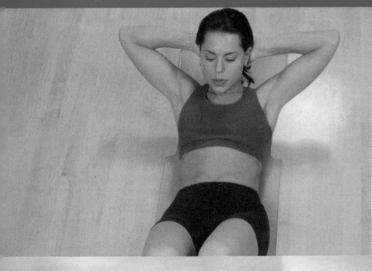

Research Review

Increased Protein Retains Nitrogen during Energy Restriction

A study by Walberg and colleagues examined the effects of varied dietary strategies on body composition, nitrogen retention, and muscular endurance in weight lifters during periods of reduced energy intake. After a 1-week maintenance period to normalize diet and exercise programs, 19 experienced male weight lifters were assigned to one of three groups: a control diet; a moderate protein (0.8 g/kg/day), high carbohydrate hypoenergy diet; or a high protein (1.6 g/kg/day), moderate carbohydrate hypoenergy diet. Both hypoenergy diets provided 18 kcal/kg/day. Following the 1-week experimental period, the researchers discovered that, although body composition did not change, nitrogen balance significantly differed between the two hypoenergy groups. Specifically, the moderate protein group had a balance of −3.19 g/day, whereas the nitrogen balance in the high protein group was a positive 4.13 g/day. In both groups, isometric muscular endurance was unaffected in the biceps, but quadriceps endurance declined in the high protein group. In conclusion, a hypoenergy diet providing twice the recommended daily allowance (RDA) of protein was more effective in preserving body protein than was a higher carbohydrate diet providing the RDA for protein.

Commonly, athletes and exercise enthusiasts limit caloric intake in hopes of losing body weight, either for athletic pursuits or aesthetic intentions. Of course, the goal is to reduce body fat while maintaining or even increasing lean body mass. Because nitrogen balance measures the body's anabolic (or catabolic) condition, it is reasonable to conclude that a positive nitrogen balance is conducive to maximizing muscular mass.

The study by Walberg indicates that retaining body protein is possible even under conditions of intense energy restriction (a 70-kg male would receive only a meager 1260 kcal daily). Because weight lifters and those involved in anaerobic sports (gymnastics, wrestling) do not have the luxury of a high-energy expenditure, they must rely primarily on dietary restriction to decrease body fat levels. Therefore, it appears that elevating protein intake is an efficient method for avoiding the potentially detrimental effects of incurring lean tissue losses while dieting. Furthermore, it is likely that including resistance activity may lead to net muscle protein synthesis.

In contrast, the lack of sufficient carbohydrate (50% of calories) in the high-protein diet may diminish muscular endurance. This can be attributed to the corresponding glycogen depletion that presumably occurred in this group. Obviously a factor that cannot be overlooked, athletes must carefully consider this drawback when initiating a restrictive dietary regimen. Perhaps a gradual reduction in energy intake or a less drastic caloric decline can offset the potential performance decrements associated with this diet.

Finally, the authors also surmise that the combination of a higher protein intake combined with weight training may provide enough amino acids to allow net protein synthesis, while the moderate protein/high carbohydrate diet led to the catabolization of more protein for energy. They concluded that this is consistent with the theory that the high-protein content of a low calorie diet maintains protein synthesis while energy needs are met primarily through the oxidation of fat. Additionally, it underscores the importance of increasing protein intake during energy restriction to conceivably promote losses in body fat.

Walberg JL, Leidy MK, Sturgill DJ, et al. Macronutrient content of a hypoenergy diet affects nitrogen retention and muscle function in weight lifters. Int J Sports Med 1988;9:261–266.

Introduction

Before any endeavor into sports supplementation, a sound nutritional program is an indispensable prerequisite to athletic success and physique enhancement. Whereas dietary supplements have for years seen their value fulfilled as replacements for dietary deficiencies (i.e., vitamins and minerals), in the realm of athletics and fitness pursuits their potential is truly achieved as powerful additions to already ideal nutritional regimens. Thus, without knowledge and adherence to appropriate nutritional principles, the myriad of compounds on today's market cannot legitimately be termed *supplements*.

In recent years, both athletes and fitness enthusiasts have benefited from the significant advancements made in sports nutrition. In fact, sports nutrition has become one of the most heavily researched areas of nutrition, and as a result, many concepts are currently being re-examined. Now, it is common for nutritionists to endorse increasing protein intake beyond the recommended daily allowance (RDA) for those involved in many fitness endeavors, and it is also readily accepted that poor nutrition is a primary contributor to overtraining. At the same time, preliminary research, and frequently misinterpreted research, has provided the impetus for recommendations that are often incorrect, unsubstantiated, and even detrimental to health or sports performance.

To make educated recommendations regarding nutritional choices, the basics of energy intake and expenditure must be examined. Instrumental to these calculations is the importance of the proper consumption of carbohydrates, proteins, and fats as they relate to athletic enhancement. Subsequently, this chapter will explore special topics in the field of sports nutrition, such as the dietary relationship between nutrients and hormones. Finally, energy intake as it pertains to body composition goals, such as fat loss or increasing lean body mass, will also be outlined.

Energy Requirements

Determining adequate caloric intake to maintain body weight depends primarily on resting metabolic rate and activity level. Furthermore, energy cost also depends on the amount of lean body mass, intensity of exercise, and cardiorespiratory efficiency. Specifically, in two individuals with the same body weight, the individual with the greater proportion of lean body mass would possess a higher resting energy expenditure. Moreover, as intensity of exercise increases, energy cost does also. These factors must be considered before determining an appropriate caloric intake, training program, and macronutrient (carbohydrate, protein, and fat) ratio.

Ensuring proper nutrient intake should be reflected through optimal health and athletic performance, and maintenance of body mass and composition. An undesired gain or loss of body weight, adverse changes in body composition, or poor exercise or sports performance all indicate potentially inappropriate caloric intake.

Only rough estimates of daily caloric cost can be made because it is impractical for all athletes and fitness enthusiasts to use sophisticated methods of determining energy expenditure (i.e., activity monitors, calorimetry). Furthermore, daily energy requirements may vary depending on exercise intensity and other less understood factors, such as fluctuations in hormonal levels, especially in females. Regardless of the procedure used to determine daily energy expenditure, a consistent and reliable method for monitoring body weight and composition (accurately calibrated weigh scales, underwater weighing, skinfold calipers, etc.) should be used on a regular basis to assess the effects of a combined nutrition and training program. Thus, involuntary changes in weight and/or composition would signal the need for dietary alterations.

Determining resting energy expenditure (REE) can be ascertained from the equations listed in TABLE 2-1. However, these estimates are the sum of energy expended at rest only, and do not account for activity level. Furthermore,

Table 2-1 Estimates of Resting Energy Expenditure (kcal/day)

Age	Males	Females
10–18	$(17.5 \times BW) + 651$	$(12.2 \times BW) + 746$
18–30	$(15.3 \times BW) + 679$	$(14.7 \times BW) + 496$
30–60	$(11.6 \times BW) + 879$	$(8.7 \times BW) + 829$

BW = body weight in kg.
Data from McArdle WD, Katch FI, Katch VL. Exercise Physiology: Energy, Nutrition, and Human Performance. 3rd ed. Philadelphia: Lea & Febiger, 1991.

because fat is considerably less metabolically active than muscle, individuals with greater lean body mass (all bodily constituents except fat) would possess relatively higher resting energy expenditures. Table 2-1 reveals that resting metabolism is approximately 10–15% lower in females than in males. This lower metabolism occurs primarily because women, in general, possess more body fat than do men of similar size. Consequently, as activity level and lean body mass (LBM) vary among individuals, total daily energy expenditure does as well.

Table 2-1 represents the resting metabolic rate, a total of an individual's sleeping, basal, and arousal metabolism.[1] For an average person, this sum comprises approximately 60–75% of the daily energy expenditure.[1] The remaining energy consumption includes the thermic effect of food intake, which comprises approximately 5–10% of energy intake,[1,2] and the thermic effect of physical activity, which constitutes roughly 15–30%.[1] Accordingly, the energy allowance for athletes may range between approximately 1.6 to 2.4 × REE.[2]

As stated previously, energy requirements vary extensively depending on the volume of daily activity, particularly among athletes. Economos et al.[3] recommend, as a general guideline, that male athletes consume at least 50 kcal/kg/day and females consume approximately 45 to 50 kcal/kg/day when training for more than 90 minutes daily. Based on these estimates, a 110-kg (242-lb.) football player training for 1.5 hours daily would require over 5500 kcal daily, whereas a 50-kg (110-lb.) female tennis player training for the same duration would require approximately 2350 kcal/day.

Accounting for intensity of exercise also greatly influences daily energy intake. Obviously, an individual who walks for 60 minutes will expend considerably less energy than if he/she were to undergo a more intense activity, such as jogging, for the same duration. But even among athletes who train consistently for a given sport, energy consumption can vary drastically on a daily basis. For example, a triathlete undergoing a particularly difficult training session may expend as much as 2000 kcal in a workout, whereas in a session of lesser intensity expends only 1000 kcal.

As an approximate guide, TABLE 2-2 can be used to estimate energy expenditure for various activities. In turn, daily energy expenditure can then be calculated by using

Table 2-2 Energy Cost of Various Activities (kcal/min/kg BW)

Activity	kcal/min/kg BW	Activity	kcal/min/kg BW
Aerobics (medium)	.103	Running (cross-country)	.163
Aerobics (intense)	.135	Running (9 min/mile)	.193
Badminton	.097	Running (8 min/mile)	.208
Basketball	.138	Running (7 min/mile)	.228
Boxing	.222	Running (6 min/mile)	.252
Cycling (9.4 mph)	.100	Swimming (back stroke)	.169
Cycling (racing)	.169	Swimming (breast stroke)	.162
Field Hockey	.134	Tennis	.109
Football	.132	Volleyball	.050
Gymnastics	.066	Walking (normal pace)	.080
Jumping Rope (125/min)	.177	Weight Training (circuit)	.091
Racquetball	.178		

Data from McArdle WD, Katch FI, Katch VL. Exercise Physiology: Energy, Nutrition, and Human Performance. 3rd ed. Philadelphia: Lea & Febiger, 1991:804–811.

determinations of resting metabolic rate (see Table 2-1). As an example, a 25-year-old, 70-kg (154-lb.) male would possess a resting energy expenditure of 1750 kcal/day [(15.3 × 70 kg) + 679]. Adding 20% to the REE to account for the thermic effect of physical activity brings the total to 2100 kcal. Accounting for the thermic effect of food consumption adds an additional 90 kcal (~5% of REE). Finally, if he engages in running at a pace of 8 min/mile for 30 minutes, he would expend approximately 437 kcal (70 kg × .208 × 30 min). Therefore, the sum total for daily energy expenditure for this individual is approximately 2627 kcal/day.

Of course, vigorous daily activities (i.e., strenuous labor) could potentially increase the daily energy expenditure. Also, lean body mass was not counted in the preceding calculation, which can radically alter expenditure calculations. Perhaps a more accurate method of estimating energy expenditure would involve determining macronutrient requirements and ratios that are based on resting metabolism, activity level, and lean body mass. Such methods will be addressed in subsequent sections, and will use protein, carbohydrate, and fat requirements of various athletic pursuits. Regardless of the calculations made, however, an appropriate dietary strategy is one that balances energy intake and expenditure, which will ultimately maintain body weight and composition.

Weight Loss

For many athletes, and also those who seek physique enhancement, weight loss is often the primary goal of a combined training and nutrition regimen, especially in sports such as wrestling, boxing, and weightlifting, in which stringent body weight requirements necessitate weight loss in many cases. Likewise, in sports such as gymnastics and distance running, in which there are no weight limitations, low body fat levels are considered optimal for performance.

Indeed, weight and body fat loss is frequently the primary objective for anyone pursuing physique improvement. In pursuit of weight loss, many individuals, including athletes, adopt nutritional principles that are ineffective and potentially harmful. For instance, drastically reducing caloric intake is not only associated with a reduction in performance, but it can also cause adverse changes in vitamin and mineral status.[4] Accordingly, improper rates of weight loss can encourage a loss of lean body mass and glycogen stores, and increase the likelihood of dehydration.[4–6]

Simultaneously losing body fat and gaining lean body mass is possible through appropriate training and caloric restriction.[6] However, in the case of the individual who has a relatively low body fat content before losing weight it is possible that reductions in lean body mass will accompany fat losses. Additionally, large and/or rapid weight reductions following caloric restriction likewise result in losses of lean body mass.[7,8] Therefore, to counteract the potential for muscular losses and a subsequent decrease in metabolic rate during caloric restriction, resistance training and an increase in dietary protein should accompany attempts at weight loss.[7,8] Note that initial weight loss incurred from undergoing caloric restriction is mostly water loss, especially within the first 3 days. In fact, as much as 70% of weight loss achieved through reducing calories by 1000 kcal/day can be attributed to water loss.[9]

As a general guideline, an acceptable rate of weight loss appears to be approximately 1% per week, which can be achieved through a caloric deficit of 500 to 1000 kcal/day. Because 3500 kcal comprise 0.45 kg (1.0 lb.) of fat, weight reductions should proceed at, but not surpass, 0.5–1.0 kg/wk.[5,6]

The most effective approach to weight loss involves a regimen that both reduces dietary caloric intake and also burns calories through exercise. Numerous studies have shown that adding exercise to a weight loss program results in a greater loss of body fat, while maintaining or increasing lean body mass.[7,10,11] For example, a program of weight control that expended 250 kcal daily through exercise and an additional 250 kcal through dietary restriction would be more effective than a program that simply limited caloric intake by 500 kcal. Furthermore, when weight is reduced by diet alone, there is a greater likelihood that there will be a loss of lean tissue,[12] subsequently promoting a drop in resting metabolic rate.

AUTHORS' RECOMMENDATIONS REGARDING WEIGHT LOSS

The profound reduction in resting metabolic rate that often accompanies caloric restriction is a primary cause of failed attempts at weight loss.[13] Specifically, as a dieter undergoes successive bouts of reduced energy intake, the body counteracts these attempts by slowing the body's metabolic processes.[13] In essence, the body strives to maintain a *set point,* using an internal control mechanism to maintain body weight and fat. Thus, even though caloric intake may be reduced to starvation-like proportions, body weight is held constant, making weight loss nearly impossible.

Compounding matters is the rapid weight gain that often occurs when an appropriate caloric intake is resumed following periods of depressed metabolism. In essence, the body has created a reservoir of enzymes that favor the deposition of calories, particularly those that promote fat synthesis and storage.[14] Not only does this add to the difficulty of losing weight, it facilitates undesired weight gain.

A plausible explanation for this unwanted phenomenon is illustrated in an evolutionary sense. Essentially, the present human form is a product of millions of years of adapting to environmental stresses, including periods of famine. To survive these food shortages, those who had a larger amount of fat stores prevailed. As a result, humans have evolved into beings that preferentially hoard fat to offset potential periods of famine. From a more scientific standpoint, the human body has *learned* to survive intervals of decreased energy intake by slowing metabolic processes and increasing the number of enzymes that promote fat storage.

This is basically what occurs during prolonged attempts at weight loss through drastically reduced caloric intakes. Although losses of weight may occur rapidly during initial stages of dieting, they also become stagnant quite abruptly. As an attempt to continue the celebrated weight loss, the innocent dieter simply reduces caloric intakes further, often with limited success. By this stage, the body has compensated for the inadequate energy intake by kicking in the aforementioned *starvation* mode.

As stated previously, exercise (a combination of endurance and resistance training in particular) is a successful formula for offsetting the drastic reductions in resting metabolic rate that occur during caloric restriction. From a dietary standpoint, an additional counteractive measure might be a cyclical or periodic caloric intake, in which energy ingestion is not reduced linearly; rather, it is decreased, as outlined in TABLE 2-3. Through diet and caloric deficit that

varies weekly, and by readjusting energy intake after 3 weeks, an average weekly deficit of 4900 kcal is attained. In this manner, ideally, the body does not adapt to a constant or sequentially decreasing caloric intake.

The estimates used in TABLE 2-3 are neither perfect nor absolute. Further adjustments may be required, specifically in the category of dietary intake, to ensure weight loss. Maintenance of body weight, or even weight gain, is possible, and minor reductions in energy intake may be required if the expected weight loss is not achieved. Conversely, rapid reductions in weight ($>1.5-2.0$ kg/wk) should signal the need for increasing caloric consumption. Of course, once a desirable weight and body composition has been achieved, the individual may return to an energy intake that is commensurate with maintenance of weight and body fat.

These recommendations signify the importance of periodic assessments of weight and body composition to ensure that weight loss occurs primarily in the

---

Table 2-3 Example of a Periodized Dietary Regimen

Subject: Female, Age 23
Body Weight: 61.36 kg (135 lbs.)
Total Daily Energy Expenditure:

    2480 kcal/day (REE)
 + 495 kcal/day (thermic effect of physical activity and food
                  intake)
    2975 kcal/day

	Caloric Intake	Energy Cost of Exercise	Sum Caloric Deficit (daily)
Week 1	2875	300	400 kcal
Week 2	2675	400	700 kcal
Week 3	2375	400	1000 kcal

Total Caloric Deficit for First Three Weeks = 14,700 kcal
Estimated Weight Loss = 14,700 kcal/3500 kcal/lb. = 4.2 lbs.
New Body Weight = 59.45 kg (130.8 lbs.)
New Total Daily Energy Expenditure = 2902 kcal/day

	Caloric Intake	Energy Cost of Exercise	Sum Caloric Deficit (daily)
Week 4	2802	300	400 kcal
Week 5	2602	400	700 kcal
Week 6	2302	400	1000 kcal

Week 7 Reassess Weight and Daily Energy Expenditure and Modify Dietary Regimen

form of fat. Correspondingly, regular dietary adjustments are necessary as body weight and composition change. An example is provided in TABLE 2-3, in which an updated total daily energy expenditure is calculated and caloric intake is modified accordingly. Also, forthcoming sections of this chapter will address the effects of differing body compositions (percentage body fat) on energy requirements in those who want to lose weight. They will also emphasize the importance of proper macronutrient ratios and other dietary attributes that promote weight and fat reductions.

Weight Gain

Just as athletes want to lose weight for competitive purposes, many attempt to gain weight to obtain athletic superiority. For most, this means improved strength and power, which can also lead to increased speed and greater resistance to opponents' movements. This would be especially advantageous in sports such as football, heavier classes in weightlifting and wrestling, and track and field events (specifically the javelin and other *throwing* events).

However, athletes are not the only ones who desire body mass gains. Many recreational weight trainers also strive to gain weight, and the protocol used to achieve this goal should be no different from that used by athletes. Also, from a health standpoint, weight gain is often necessary for proper physical and metabolic maturation.[15] Such is the concern in the extremely lean individual or amenorrheic female who risks bone loss.[16] Regardless, the goals of weight gain should maximize increases in lean body mass while minimizing gains in fat mass. But, just as a loss of lean tissue often accompanies weight loss, the accrual of fat is usually an undesired addition to muscular gains. In either instance, optimal physique enhancement is always accomplished by appropriate dietary and training practices.

In the case of weight gain, this is best accomplished through resistance training. Such exercise promotes an anabolic environment by enhancing protein synthesis, stimulating the release of muscle-building hormones, and encouraging muscle growth through adaptation to strenuous training. As this is achieved, the body is primed for the acceptance of additional calories (beyond that required to maintain body weight) that presumably favor lean body mass gains.

The appropriate caloric intake required to stimulate lean body mass gains is approximately 500 to 1000 kcal in excess of the total daily energy expenditure. The approach is similar to weight loss in terms of manipulating energy intakes. However, whereas exercise can be used to increase the daily caloric deficit during attempts to lose weight, it must receive compensation in the dietary regimen of those who seek to gain weight. For example, if an individual expends 2500 kcal daily as a result of REE and regular activities, and an additional 300 kcal from weight training (a total of 2800 kcal daily), this individual's program of weight gain should contain 3300 to 3800 kcal daily.

As with weight loss, weight gains should proceed slowly, at the rate of approximately 0.5–1.0 kg/wk. Rapid weight gain is typically associated with gains in water weight initially, followed by fat gains. This is especially the case when one desires to gain a significant amount of weight. To prevent this, weight gain should be prolonged further, such that individuals proceed at approximately 0.25–0.5 kg/wk. This approach would likely ensure primarily lean body mass gains. Finally, as with attempts at weight loss, body weight and composition should be monitored regularly (every 1–2 wks) to signal necessary dietary changes.

Choosing macronutrient ratios that favor muscular gains is also an important but often overlooked strategy for physique and athletic improvement. Proper manipulation of these dietary variables is a substantial tool in establishing an anabolic environment, thus promoting muscular growth. Also, pre and post-exercise feedings are also crucial to attaining a desired goal, be it to gain/lose weight or enhance athletic achievement. Accordingly, these topics will be addressed in forthcoming sections of this chapter.

Conclusions

Regardless of the method used to determine caloric intake, factors such as weight and body composition management/improvement, achievement of desired performance, and realization of subjective goals ultimately establish an appropriate diet. However, if one is unable to fulfill the preceding factors, he/she will need to modify his/her diet or use appropriate supplementation. Knowledge of sports supplements is imperative, as is a detailed understanding of nutritional concepts in the pursuit of achieving dietary success.

Carbohydrate Requirements

Carbohydrate, which carries 4 kilocalories per gram, is the macronutrient needed in greatest amounts during training and competition. The primary function of carbohydrates is to fuel the body's energy to power muscular contractions and numerous physiological functions. This is accomplished via the breakdown of ingested carbohydrate and stored glycogen to its active energy form, glucose.

However, relative to fat, the stored glycogen present in liver and muscle is relatively small. This becomes apparent during endurance exercise in particular, where a lack of available energy can be detrimental to performance.

However, endurance exercise is not the only form of training and competition in which carbohydrate depletion can compromise performance; it can also occur during high-intensity exercise as well,[17] especially during activities that involve high quantities of repeated anaerobic bouts. This depletion can then trigger a phenomenon known as gluconeogenesis, a process by which additional energy is formed by the synthesis of glucose from protein and fats. Unfortunately, a prevailing disadvantage of this compensatory energy-producing mechanism is the potential loss of muscle tissue. This, of course, flags the significance of adequate carbohydrate intake and its role in the maintenance of the body's protein stores.[18]

Furthermore, a dangerous side effect of inadequate carbohydrate intake is impaired central nervous system (CNS) function, considering that the brain uses glucose almost exclusively as its primary fuel. This is apparent during starvation and prolonged endurance exercise, when depleted glycogen stores can induce feelings of dizziness and general malaise. In the case of low-carbohydrate diets, prevalent side effects are symptoms of fatigue, weakness, and hunger.[19] Conversely, excess carbohydrate intake can lead to undesired weight gain. Because ingested carbohydrates are converted to muscle and liver glycogen, once their carrying capacity is achieved, the rest is converted to fat. Obviously, this is an unwanted result for those who want to lose weight and improve body composition. It is also critically disadvantageous for those athletes engaged in events in which weight gain can diminish performance (i.e., distance running). Therefore, this signifies the extreme importance of a dietary regimen that strikes a balance between adequate energy production and physique maintenance or improvement.

The Glycemic Index

The nutritional goals of athletes must include the use of carbohydrates to provide prolonged energy for exercise sessions, improve performance, and restore glycogen for optimal recovery. The attention paid to the type of carbohydrate, however, has only recently become an area of focus in sports nutrition, and has given rise to an effective classification system. Apparently, not all carbohydrates are created equal because the use of carbohydrates spans further than its function as an energy fuel (such as in its potentially large and varied influence on fat usage). Thus, both the relevance and guidelines of categorizing carbohydrates can be revealed via the body's ensuing glucose and insulin (a hormone released from the pancreas) responses following food ingestion.

All carbohydrates are eventually broken down into glucose and released to the bloodstream. The amount and speed of glucose entering the blood determines the corresponding insulin response. Naturally, a large and rapid glucose response will spark a considerable surge of insulin, which stimulates the transport of glucose, proteins, and fats out of the blood and into cells. Consequently, this creates a reduction of readily available energy as a result of the banishment of glucose; the condition has been termed *rebound hypoglycemia*.[20] Particularly before exercise, this outcome diminishes the energy potential that can be gleaned from glucose and fats. Furthermore, the resulting increased fat storage presents a profound disadvantage for those seeking weight loss. Ideally, to provide sufficient energy for training (and possibly the optimal environment for physique enhancement), the glucose response should be gradual and maintained. Not only does this ensure adequate energy for sustained exercise bouts, but it also attenuates the corresponding insulin response.

Traditionally, classifying carbohydrates into *simple* and *complex* was the norm in educating athletes and lay people about the alleged benefits and pitfalls of this macronutrient. According to accepted sports nutrition dogma, simple carbohydrates, such as those found in fruits and high-sugar foods, reportedly triggered a rapid and large rise in blood glucose levels, which was followed by a rapid and often greater fall.[21] In contrast, complex carbohydrates, such as pasta and starchy vegetables, were labeled as nutrient rich and seemingly induced a more sustained blood glucose response.[21]

Unfortunately, this system does not accurately account for the delicate diversity of carbohydrate-rich foods, nor does it provide meaningful information to direct food selection. In fact, the preceding characterizations are largely inaccurate and oversimplified. For example, although fruits contain primarily simple carbohydrates, there exists considerable disparity in the corresponding glucose responses following their ingestion. Interestingly, many kinds of fruit provide an ideal glucose response, whereas many forms of pasta (a complex carbohydrate) spawn an unfavorably rapid one. Confusing matters further is the fact that many foods contain both simple and complex carbohydrates. Moreover, numerous foods that contain simple sugars are often incorrectly labeled as unhealthy, and many complex carbohydrates are in fact nutrient poor.

As a successful alternative, the glycemic index (GI) has emerged as an accepted tool to guide nutritional selections. The GI is a ranking of foods based on their actual blood glucose response following consumption.[21] The ranking of a particular food is determined by its blood glucose response relative to a reference food, either glucose or white bread. Therefore, the GI reflects the rate of digestion and absorption of carbohydrate-rich food,[21] and by using the GI, one can reliably form appropriate meals to potentially promote enhanced fitness.

TABLE 2-4 summarizes the GI of common foods and partitions them into high, moderate, and low categories. The

Table 2-4 The Glycemic Index of Common Foods

High	Moderate	Low
Glucose (137)	Muffins (88)	Grain bread (69)
Instant rice (128)	Ice cream (87)	Grapefruit juice (69)
Crispix cereal (124)	Cheese pizza (86)	Green peas (68)
Baked potato (121)	White rice (83)	Grapes (66)
Cornflakes cereal (119)	Popcorn (79)	Linguine (65)
Rice Krispies cereal (117)	Oatmeal cookies (79)	Macaroni (64)
Pretzels (116)	Brown rice (79)	Orange (63)
Total cereal (109)	Spaghetti, durum (78)	Peach (60)
Donut (108)	Sweet corn (78)	All-Bran cereal (60)
Watermelon (103)	Oat bran (78)	Spaghetti, white (59)
Bagel (103)	Sweet potato (77)	Apple juice (58)
Cream of Wheat (100)	Banana (77)	Apple (54)
Grapenuts cereal (96)	Special K cereal (77)	Vermicelli (50)
Nutri-grain bar (94)	Orange juice (74)	Barley (49)
Macaroni and cheese (92)	Cheese tortellini (71)	Fettucine (46)
Sucrose (92)	Pumpernickel (71)	Lentils (41)
Raisins (91)	Chocolate (70)	Fructose (32)

Index based on reference to white bread (GI = 100)

Data from Van Erp-Baart AMJ, Saris WHM, Binkhorst RA, et al. Nationwide survey on nutritional habits in elite athletes. Part 1: Energy, carbohydrate, protein, and fat intake. Int J Sports Med 1989;10:S3–S10.

number assigned to each food represents the speed at which the food is digested and subsequently absorbed, with higher numbers reflecting faster introduction of glucose into the bloodstream. Generally, these values represent the average indices as ascertained from a number of studies and laboratories.[22] The table also illustrates the obvious unpredictability of making nutritional choices based on traditional belief and/or subjective appeal. For instance, fructose possesses a surprisingly low index, while apparent *powerhouse* energy sources such as potatoes and bagels rank rather high. Because the GI also, albeit indirectly, indicates the ensuing insulin response of food consumption, high-GI foods eaten in isolation are not recommended before training. They are also considered disadvantageous for those who seek to lose weight and body fat, though these individuals do see the value of high-GI foods fulfilled in post-exercise meals. These and other practical applications regarding the GI will be covered in upcoming sections of this chapter.

Foods are usually eaten in combinations; therefore, it is important to note that the glycemic index of a meal is usually lower than the glycemic index (stituent. For instance, if equal calories apple are combined, the glycemic in becomes a more acceptable 79. Protein it efficiently decreases the total glycem the absorption rate of carbohydrates, ing the insulin response. Because those seeking weight loss should strive for a reduced insulin response, this emphasizes the importance of combining protein and carbohydrates in each meal.

Finally, the GI provides clinical practicality in that a low-GI diet improves glucose control in diabetics[23] and reduces hyperlipidemia.[24] Low-GI foods are also indicated as increasing satiety,[25] furthering their benefit for those involved in weight control regimens. Overall, therefore, the GI has become an accepted nutritional tool not only for athletes, but also for anyone aspiring to improve his or her health.

Carbohydrate Needs of Endurance Athletes

Endurance competitors (i.e., distance runners, soccer players, rowers, etc.), perhaps more than other athletes, must not overlook the distinct advantage provided by adequate carbohydrate intake. As defined by the authors, endurance activities are those activities that include prolonged, continuous, low- to moderate-intensity exercise that is principally aerobic in nature. Endurance athletes expend an inordinate amount of energy in training and competing, and, because carbohydrates are the preferred fuel source in most sports, they therefore must be the first macronutrient accounted for in any dietary regimen. Many studies have demonstrated the undeniable relationship between high-carbohydrate diets and ample pre-exercise glycogen stores, improved endurance, and optimal performance.[26–28]

A review of the scientific literature at the International Consensus Conference in 1991 examined the connection between food, nutrition, and sports performance, and consequently devised carbohydrate recommendations for athletes.[29] The most significant contributor to endurance capacity was pre-exercise glycogen concentration. Therefore, a recommendation was made that athletes should allow carbohydrates to comprise approximately 60–70% of their daily energy intake. However, it was also advised that this high level of carbohydrate intake should not be part of the athlete's normal diet—but simply preparation for heavy exercise. For example, only athletes who train exhaustively on successive days or compete in prolonged endurance events should follow a dietary program that consists of 70% carbohydrates.[30]

Regarding an endurance athlete's routine diet, a common recommendation is to ingest approximately 60% of daily calories from carbohydrates. Although this guideline may be accurate, it neglects the recommended mandate the total amount of carbohydrates required for ideal performance, replenishing glycogen stores, and assisting in recovery. Specifically, carbohydrate needs of all athletes should be expressed relative to body weight. The importance of this is illustrated by a study by Walberg-Rankin.[31] In their research, the authors computed the daily carbohydrate intake and dietary macronutrient ratios of a number of athletes from both aerobic and anaerobic sports. Surprisingly, they found that even in those athletes who consumed 60% of their total calories from carbohydrates, most still fell short of their projected total when carbohydrate requirements were formed on the basis of body weight.

Furthermore, as gleaned from dietary surveys, it is apparent that endurance athletes are not meeting their daily carbohydrate requirements.[32-34] In many cases, daily energy and carbohydrate requirements to support strenuous training may even surpass those required for competition.[34] Consequently, most studies support the notion that endurance athletes should consume carbohydrates (CHO) on the order of −10 g/kg body weight/day to restore and maintain glycogen levels.[35,36] This total also represents an ideal quota for optimal sports performance, as depicted in a study by Sherman et al.[37] The authors examined runners and cyclists who completed 70 minutes of intense interval training over 7 days. They found that the subjects who consumed 10 g CHO/kg/day maintained significantly higher glycogen levels than those who ingested 5 g/kg/day. The goal of carbohydrate intake is to maximize available energy throughout exercise; therefore, inadequate glycogen stores will likely reduce training intensity and eventually lead to premature fatigue.

For athletes involved in strenuous training, it appears that maximum benefits are derived from a carbohydrate intake of 500 g daily (TABLE 2-5).[38] According to Costill et al,[39] an intake of 524 to 648 g CHO/day is ideal for maximal muscle glycogen replenishment following strenuous exercise. In fact, intake beyond this range does not appear to provide additional benefit.[39] Additionally, even if this ideal amount makes up less than the recommended 60% of the athlete's total daily calories, it still appears sufficient for glycogen restoration and optimal performance. Hawley et al.[40] demonstrated that athletes who consume 550 g CHO/day or more can adequately replenish glycogen stores, although this amount may only make up 45% of total daily calories. They also point out that there is little research to support the use of chronically high carbohydrate diets to enhance training in athletes with high-energy intake. Furthermore, because elevating carbohydrate ingestion to 70% of total energy may result in insufficient protein and fat ingestion, this type of diet is strongly discouraged for those athletes who are restricting caloric intake (figure skaters, distance runners, gymnasts).[41] The practices of athletes who habitually reduce fat or protein intake could potentially jeopardize their health and

Table 2-5 Carbohydrate and Total Kcal Needs of Endurance Athletes

Body Weight	Daily Carbohydrate Requirement	Total Kcal
50 kg (110 lbs.)	400 g/1600 kcal	2667 kcal
60 kg (132 lbs.)	480 g/1920 kcal	3200 kcal
70 kg (154 lbs.)	560 g/2240 kcal	3733 kcal
80 kg (176 lbs.)	640 g/2560 kcal	4267 kcal
90 kg (198 lbs.)	720 g/2880 kcal	4800 kcal
100 kg (220 lbs.)	800 g/3200 kcal	5333 kcal

Note: Table uses a carbohydrate requirement of 8.0 g/kg body weight/day, and this quantity makes up 60% of total daily kcal.

performance (i.e., significant low-fat intakes may promote deficiencies in fat-soluble vitamins).[41]

Carbohydrate Loading

Carbohydrate loading is a technique used to increase muscle glycogen stores beyond the maximum attained through the conventional dietary methods as previously outlined. Traditionally, carbohydrate loading is performed in two stages: a glycogen depletion stage and a carbohydrate loading phase. During glycogen depletion (which begins about 6 days before endurance competition), the athlete performs intense, exhaustive exercise over a period of 2 to 3 days while eating a low-carbohydrate diet. Specifically, exercise should target the muscles to be used during competition, and should consist of approximately 90 minutes of intense submaximal exercise. The athlete will also maintain a daily carbohydrate intake of only 60 to 100 g during this period.

Essentially, the depletion phase is used to create a *glycogen debt* in the chosen muscles. Then, at least 3 days before competition, the carbohydrate loading phase begins, and creates what is termed *glycogen supercompensation*. This is a phenomenon in which glycogen storage is enhanced significantly, and is likely a result of the increased concentration of glycogen-storing enzymes created by the previous glycogen debt. In addition to abundant water, vitamins, minerals, and protein, carbohydrate intake during the loading phase increases to 50–600 g/day.

Carbohydrate loading has resulted in significant increases in endurance capacity (the time taken from the start of exercise to exhaustion), although large improvements in endurance performance (the time taken to complete a predetermined workload) have not been reported.[42] In other words, carbohydrate loading may allow athletes to maintain a chosen pace for longer periods than if they had not carbohydrate loaded. These results have increased recommendations that carbohydrate loading is only beneficial for endurance activities lasting 1 hour or more.

Possible disadvantages of carbohydrate loading typically occur during the glycogen depletion stage, and occasionally produce such undesirable side effects as weight gain, irritability, and mental and physical fatigue.[43] Of course, all of these adverse reactions may be detrimental to performance. Because of these side effects, the authors recommend that athletes follow a modified procedure if undergoing carbohydrate loading for the first time. This may consist of a truncated depletion phase (1 day instead of 2 or 3), or may involve a more agreeable carbohydrate intake of 150 to 250 g/day during depletion.

Nevertheless, many athletes derive success from consuming a normal mixed diet and simply tapering their training in the days leading to competition. In fact, this procedure can generate higher than normal pre-exercise muscle glycogen levels, even without carbohydrate loading.[42] Another modified approach involves a 50% carbohydrate diet and no exhaustive exercise during the depletion phase, and a loading phase in which carbohydrate intake is increased to 70% of total calories and training is tapered.[44] Perhaps surprisingly, this procedure results in an accumulation of glycogen reserves to approximately the same level as attained with the classic protocol. Regardless of the method used, however, athletes should become well informed about carbohydrate loading before manipulating their dietary and exercise habits to achieve glycogen supercompensation.

Pre-Exercise Carbohydrate Intake

Adequate carbohydrate intake is especially important before endurance training or competition. Given that many endurance events last 2 hours or longer, and that glycogen stores are sufficient for approximately 2 hours of intensive exercise, pre-exercise carbohydrate feedings carry utmost significance. When properly ingested before exercise, carbohydrates have been shown to improve performance,[45] especially when combined with during-exercise feedings.[46] Additionally, ingesting carbohydrates during these two critical time periods also induces a glycogen-sparing effect,[47,48] which prolongs intensive exercise.[49,50]

The goals of pre-training nutrition are to maximize glycogen stores, avoid a significant increase in plasma insulin concentrations (resulting in a hypoglycemic state), and avoid gastrointestinal upset during exercise.[51] The pre-exercise period can be defined as the 4-hour period before an activity and can be further delineated into two distinct phases: 2 to 4 hours before and 30 to 60 minutes prior to exercise.[51]

The 2- to 4-hour period preceding exercise takes on special significance in cases in which glycogen concentrations may be depleted as a result of intense exercise or insufficient carbohydrate ingestion in the days before an event. In these instances, the intake of a sizable amount of carbohydrates, approximately 300 g, 4 hours before exercise

has been shown to increase work output and performance.[52] Similar findings, along the same lines of enhanced endurance and work output, have also been reported when greater than 200 g CHO were consumed 3 to 4 hours before endurance-type exercise.[53,54] Therefore, research indicates that athletes should ingest 200 to 300 g CHO in the 2 to 4 hours preceding exercise. The case can even be made for a greater intake in special circumstances (before significantly long endurance events, following a fasted state, and following successive days of intense endurance exercise).

To promote sustained carbohydrate availability throughout an exercise session, the 30 to 60 minutes before an event is significant not only in that a sufficient intake must be achieved, but the proper type of carbohydrate must also be consumed. In light of this importance, properly manipulating the glycemic index of this meal may optimize carbohydrate availability for ensuing exercise. Because a potential disadvantage of pre-exercise carbohydrate intake is an exaggerated insulin response, which suppresses fat metabolism and curtails available glucose for subsequent exercise, the glycemic index becomes an indispensable tool. For example, Foster et al.[55] reported that feeding 75 g of glucose (a high-glycemic carbohydrate) 30 minutes before exercise impaired the resulting cycle time to exhaustion.

In contrast, Thomas and colleagues[56] noted that consuming 1 g CHO/kg body weight of a low-GI food (lentils) 1 hour before endurance exercise prolonged work capacity when compared with the ingestion of an equal amount of a high-glycemic food (potatoes). The authors suggested that this performance increase was attributable to glycogen sparing following the consumption of low-glycemic carbohydrates. Thus, according to this study, low-GI meals appear to elicit a sustained source of energy throughout exercise and recovery.[21] However, other studies[57,58] have expressed no differences in performance following ingestion of low- or high-glycemic foods, although the investigators did find that high-GI meals caused a decline in blood glucose concentration before exercise. Perhaps these differences in glucose concentration during the early phases of exercise are short-lived and do not negatively affect the performance of most athletes. Further research is needed in this area, but it is clear that low-GI foods definitely promote a more favorable metabolic environment for exercise.

Regardless of glycemic index, it is evident that adequate glycogen stores before exercise is the predominant nutritional factor in subsequent performance. In the 30- to 60-minute window preceding exercise, most studies suggest that 60 to 75 g of carbohydrates consumed in this period are sufficient to *top off* glycogen stores and improve performance.[56,59,60] One should make sure that these feedings do not cause excessive fullness or gastrointestinal upset, however, which can actually impair exercise performance.

Carbohydrate Intake During Exercise

The primary goals of carbohydrate feedings during exercise are to maintain glucose levels to sustain energy and work output, and spare liver glycogen. When ingested in sufficient quantity, elevated carbohydrate availability during endurance exercise can improve work capacity in events lasting more than 1 hour.[61] Also, the manner in which carbohydrates are ingested during exercise, specifically in terms of feeding schedule and composition (solid or liquid), is an important performance-related variable.

With regard to quantity, research indicates that the maximal oxidation rate for exogenous carbohydrate is approximately 60 g/hr.[62] It is this finding that gives rise to the common belief that carbohydrates ingested at a rate of 45 to 75 g/hr are sufficient to improve exercise performance. Accordingly, various types of carbohydrates, including glucose, sucrose, and maltodextrins, are all effective choices to make to enhance training and competition. In fact, the glycemic index does not appear to elicit any physiologically important differences.[21] Ingesting fructose, however, because it is slowly absorbed,[63] is not advised during exercise because of the increased risk of gastrointestinal distress.

Although the effect of feeding frequency does not seem to influence subsequent carbohydrate oxidation during endurance exercise, withholding carbohydrates until late in an exercise bout will impair performance.[51] Similarly, this points to the necessity of ingesting carbohydrates throughout exercise not only to sustain energy, but to avoid possible gastrointestinal disturbance. Correspondingly, consuming carbohydrates in liquid or solid form elicits similar effects, although liquid solutions provide the added benefit of maintaining hydration. To coincide with the 45 to 75 g/hr recommendation, this would typically involve ingesting approximately 1 liter of sports drink (carbohydrate-electrolyte solution) per hour. Fortunately, these solutions play a dual role of providing both adequate energy and hydration without causing excessive fullness.

Post-Exercise Carbohydrate Intake

The primary objective of ingesting carbohydrates following exercise is to replenish glycogen stores for subsequent exercise bouts. In doing so, overtraining is prevented and adequate energy is again available for forthcoming exercise. It was previously thought that full restoration of muscle glycogen stores takes approximately 48 hours. If performed properly, however, research now indicates that this process can be accomplished in approximately 20 hours.[64]

Research also confirms that glycogen restoration occurs most rapidly when carbohydrates are consumed immediately post-exercise.[64] In fact, when carbohydrate feedings ensue immediately following exercise, the rate of muscle glycogen storage is almost twice that of when they are consumed after a 2-hour delay.[64] However, because full glycogen restoration can still be achieved via adequate intake (regardless of timing), these results indicate the importance of immediate feedings only when further exercise is imminent. Therefore, this strategy is most important when only 4 to 8 hours of recovery pass between exercise sessions.[51] As the time for recovery increases (longer than 24 hours), the importance of carbohydrate quantity takes precedence over feeding frequency or timing. Interestingly, the frequency of feedings does not significantly alter muscle glycogen restoration rates as long as the daily carbohydrate needs of endurance athletes (7–10 g/kg body weight) are met.[51]

The optimal rate of glycogen storage appears to be achieved when at least 0.7–1.0 g CHO/kg body weight is consumed every 2 hours in the early stages of recovery, leading to a daily total of 7 to 10 g/kg body weight.[36,65] Although this can be achieved with solid or liquid forms of carbohydrate, particular glycemic types seem to have differing effects on subsequent glycogen restoration. Glucose and sucrose feedings have been shown to induce similar rates of glycogen recovery, whereas fructose produces a lower rate of storage.[66] These findings have sparked suggestions that post-exercise carbohydrate intake should consist mainly of moderate- to high-glycemic foods. Given their more rapid introduction to the bloodstream, it appears that these types of carbohydrates are more beneficial in achieving swift glycogen restoration. Indeed, studies have indicated that high-glycemic carbohydrate foods consumed post-exercise promote greater glycogen storage than do an equal amount of low-GI foods.[67,68] Specifically, it has been suggested that foods with a low glycemic index should not make up more than one-third of recovery meals.[69]

Carbohydrate Needs of Strength/Power Athletes

Compared with prolonged endurance activity, much less has been researched and written regarding the influence of carbohydrate intake on high-intensity sporting events. The authors define high-intensity events, also termed *strength/power sports,* as exercise requiring high power or force output. This includes events in which power output leads to muscular fatigue in a few minutes of activity or less, and exercise that requires repetitive, high-force production from specific muscles. High-intensity exercise, therefore, cannot be sustained for extended periods of time, and frequent or prolonged rest periods are required. Fortunately for strength/power athletes, rest periods are usually included in such sports, owing to the depletion of energy substrates (i.e., phosphocreatine, glycogen) and accumulation of metabolic products (i.e., lactate, ammonia).

Although the performance benefits of carbohydrate ingestion are well documented in endurance athletes, strength and power athletes must also be aware of this macronutrient's potential ergogenic effects. Whereas glycogen use is insignificant during brief anaerobic events (i.e., Olympic weightlifting), in situations that call on

AUTHORS' RECOMMENDATIONS REGARDING CARBOHYDRATE INTAKE

Although exact recommendations are not available for carbohydrate intake, a safe approach would be to consume approximately 5 to 7 g CHO/kg body weight/day. This total could make up roughly 60% of a strength/power athlete's diet. For example, an 80-kg (176-lb.) football player consuming 6 g CHO/kg would ingest a daily total of 480 g CHO, which could make up 60% of a 3200 kcal daily total. As for pre-exercise carbohydrate intake, even less has been researched, but recommendations can nevertheless be based on the strategy outlined above. Specifically, one fourth to one third of the daily carbohydrate total should be ingested approximately 2 hours before an event or particularly intense training session. Therefore, for the 80-kg athlete consuming 480 g CHO/day, the pre-event meal would consist of roughly 120 to 160 g of carbohydrates.

Interestingly, the rate of glycogen resynthesis following high-intensity exercise is faster than that following prolonged endurance exercise. This surprising phenomenon is likely caused by higher plasma insulin and glucose concentrations, lactate levels (which can be converted to glycogen), and increased glycogen synthase (an enzyme that promotes glycogen resynthesis) activity following high-intensity training. In fact, the rate of resynthesis induced by carbohydrate feeding can actually be two to four times greater following high-intensity exercise than after prolonged exercise.[73] This finding may point to the presumably minor contribution of high carbohydrate feedings towards glycogen resynthesis following intense exercise.

Although this may be true, strength/power athletes can still benefit from proper carbohydrate intake post-exercise. High-glycemic carbohydrates should remain the norm for these athletes and endurance competitors, because they promote an enhanced post-exercise insulin response. This would be beneficial to an athlete performing resistance exercise, because it may attenuate muscle protein degradation[74] and enhance muscle protein synthesis.[75] Therefore, in the first 1 to 2 hours following intense exercise, an intake of 0.5 to 1.0 g CHO/kg body weight should be sufficient. Beyond that, as long as daily carbohydrate needs are met, augmented intake post-exercise is likely not advantageous. Only in the case of multiple training sessions/competitions in 1 day would an increased intake be warranted. In these special cases, an athlete can follow the same recommendations made for endurance athletes following training (0.7–1.0 g CHO/kg body weight every 2 hours post-exercise).

---

athletes to perform repeated anaerobic exercise bouts (i.e., repetitive sprints, basketball, football), proper carbohydrate ingestion becomes increasingly significant. Too often, adequate carbohydrate intake is overlooked and the resulting glycogen debt becomes the culprit when premature fatigue surfaces in strength/power sports. In contrast, the energy attained via glycogen use in many prolonged low-intensity endurance sports (i.e., marathon running) is aided by the oxidation of fats. However, in the case of such anaerobic sports as basketball and ice hockey, the repetitive nature (and correspondingly high-glycogen use) does not physiologically allow for surplus energy production from fats. Thus, the ample glycogen availability demanded by these sports necessitates an augmented carbohydrate intake. Certainly, the carbohydrate requirements for high-intensity sports are not as great as those for endurance events, although some studies have noted the ability to maintain higher training intensities when greater than normal intakes were consumed.[70,71] However, as the intensity of the event increases (and thus the duration decreases), higher than normal glycogen concentrations do not appear to offer any additional benefits. Therefore, a supplemental carbohydrate intake is most advantageous for those athletes involved in repetitive high-intensity events or training regimens of a similar nature. As an example, ice-hockey players who consumed a carbohydrate supplement (360 g/day for 3 days) in addition to their normal diet before a competition possessed muscle glycogen levels that were twice as high as those in players who were not given the supplement.[72] It may also be important for similar athletes to ingest a high-carbohydrate diet during periods of intense training.

Protein Requirements

There still exists considerable confusion and controversy regarding the protein requirements for athletes—particularly for those who are involved in high-intensity training. Even scientists have disagreed on exact protein requirements, and thus many strength and conditioning professionals who desire muscular enhancement in their athletes have increased their protein intake well beyond the recommended daily allowance (RDA). Much of the confusion arises from poorly designed research studies and a lack of understanding of protein metabolism, resulting in recommendations that are unnecessary and occasionally harmful.

Proteins are complex molecules that have many enzymatic and structural functions related to the promotion of body growth, maintenance, and repair. The function of dietary protein in the athlete, fitness enthusiast, or sedentary individual is to contribute the amino acids necessary for the body to assimilate proteins that comprise skeletal structures (including muscle) and hormones, function as cell membrane receptors, and maintain fluid balance. Protein, which carries 4 kilocalories per gram, also makes a minor contribution (~5–10%) to energy production, but this offering may increase in episodes of decreased energy intake.

The basic building blocks of protein are amino acids, which contain nitrogen. The body's nitrogen status can be determined by measuring dietary nitrogen intake (via protein intake) and subtracting nitrogen loss (sweat, urine, and feces). Measuring the body's nitrogen balance provides a valuable estimate of a person's overall protein balance because muscle protein is in a constant state of turnover. For example, impaired protein synthesis allows catabolic (breakdown) effects to predominate, resulting in an increased excretion of nitrogen. If protein is ingested in excessive amounts, it can be oxidized for energy or converted to fat. Therefore, the amount of protein in muscle is determined in large part by the balance between a positive nitrogen balance, which promotes protein anabolism (growth or build-up), and a negative nitrogen balance, which promotes catabolism.

Protein quality is an important factor in establishing its daily requirement. Of the 22 distinct amino acids required for protein synthesis, 9 are essential and 13 are nonessential. Essential amino acids are those that the body cannot synthesize and thus they must be obtained from the diet. Nonessential amino acids are synthesized as long as there is an adequate source of nitrogen in the body, but can also be acquired from the diet. Individuals must obtain a sufficient amount of essential amino acids for the proper synthesis of human tissue protein. Dietary proteins that contain all the necessary amino acids are known as complete proteins, and are generally derived from meat, fish, and dairy products. Incomplete proteins lack one or more of the essential amino acids and are the constituents of such plant foods as nuts, grains, and legumes. Consequently, this signifies the need to eat a balanced diet containing a variety of protein-rich foods. Also, it is apparent that vegetarians may become deficient in one or more essential amino acids and thus may benefit from protein supplementation.

Protein Needs of Athletes

The RDA for protein in adults is 0.8 g/kg body weight per day.[76] A margin of safety is also included in this recommendation to account for individual differences in protein metabolism, variations in the biological value of protein, and nitrogen loss via urine and feces. Intake beyond this amount is therefore unnecessary. However, as the demands of training increase, so do caloric needs and protein requirements. Furthermore, athletes and those who seek weight and muscular gains also demand increased energy and corresponding protein intake.

During exercise, protein synthesis is depressed and protein degradation may be increased.[77] Because this may result in catabolism, training may increase the need for dietary protein.[78] In fact, research has discovered that both intensive aerobic[79] and anaerobic[80] training may lead to a negative nitrogen balance, which could produce losses in lean body mass. This could also increase the chances of injury.

An additional factor influencing protein and nitrogen balance is pre-exercise muscle glycogen concentrations.[81] If initial concentrations are low, the use of protein for energy takes on added importance. Specifically, during aerobic activity, 10% or more of total energy demands may be derived from protein in the face of inadequate muscle glycogen stores.[81] Therefore, the potential for lean tissue loss is increased in the case of overexercise and/or inadequate diet.[82] Consequently, because carbohydrates typically represent 60% of an athlete's total caloric intake, protein (PRO) should make up approximately 15% of the daily total.

Using these ratios for a 70-kg endurance athlete ingesting 490 g CHO daily, an amount that represents 60% of total calories (3267 total daily kcal), a 15% protein total would be 122 g, or 1.74 g PRO/kg body weight. In fact, this estimate falls in line with most research-based recommendations for protein intake of endurance athletes. For such competitors, it is advised that they ingest between 1.2 and 2.2 g PRO/kg body weight.[79,83,84] Much of the impetus behind this recommendation appears to be based on the increased oxidation of branched-chain amino acids during endurance training.[79]

As for strength/power athletes, although there exist numerous research studies that have examined the topic of protein needs, there remains considerable ambiguity as to what exact requirements should be. It is clear, however, that athletes involved in high-intensity sports or heavy resistance training can benefit from an increased protein intake. Research by Tarnopolsky et al.[85] presents evidence suggesting that the protein requirement for such athletes is approximately 1.76 g PRO/kg body weight per day. The total represents an amount that is necessary to maintain or enhance a positive nitrogen balance, thus potentially promoting gains in strength and muscle mass. Further research by Tarnopolsky also indicates that weight lifters were able to maintain nitrogen balance on 1.0 g/kg, but those consuming 2.77 g/kg attained a positive balance that was greater than twice that of the lower protein group.[86] However, a discrepancy does exist between this finding

and the investigators' previous research,[83] which suggested that bodybuilders may require only 0.82 g/kg to maintain nitrogen balance. Possibly, in the case of these conflicting results, and in other contradictory research in this area, the culprit may be the considerable variation in test subjects and training programs used in the studies.

Research by Lemon et al.[84,87] provides evidence in agreement with previous studies on protein needs of strength/power athletes. Their research supports a requirement of 1.5 to 2.0 g PRO/kg body weight to maintain a positive nitrogen balance in athletes involved in high-intensity training. Also, the authors recommend an intake of at least 1.7 g/kg for subjects who are just initiating a strength-training regimen. An elevated intake may also be a necessity for athletes who make large adjustments or add volume to their exercise programs, given that the potential for slipping into a negative nitrogen balance is increased during these periods.

Studies have examined the protein needs of athletes undergoing periods of increased volume or intensity of training. Perhaps surprisingly in one study, protein intakes as high as 2 g PRO/kg body weight were not sufficient enough to maintain a positive nitrogen balance.[88] Therefore, inadequate protein intake during heavy training could exacerbate the overtrained state. As a result, in the case of especially intense training, the percentage of protein making up total calories can be increased to 20% or more. This increase would also be suitable for athletes in a hypocaloric state or those involved in sports where weight loss is necessary (i.e., making weight in wrestling), thus offsetting the negative nitrogen balance and loss of lean tissue.[89] This was confirmed in a study by Walberg et al.,[90] who concluded that, during energy restriction, experienced weightlifters consuming a moderate-protein intake (0.8 g/kg) possessed a negative nitrogen balance, whereas those who consumed 1.6 g/kg maintained a positive balance.

Current Controversy: Protein Intake

Commonly, many athletes and strength coaches believe that protein is the sole determinant influencing strength and muscle mass gains. Given its relation to nitrogen balance and presence in muscle tissue, protein has thus taken on a *more is better* attribute among those attempting to increase body weight and strength. Although total ingested calories and carbohydrate intake (for its protein-sparing effect) also carry extreme significance for these athletes, it is protein intake that often increases to unnecessary proportions. The popular belief that high intakes lead to health risks, however, has not been established in healthy individuals.

The media often state that a chronically high protein intake may result in metabolic strain on kidney and liver function; however, this has not been reported in healthy individuals. In general, amino acids are renal vasodilators that can elevate the pressure in the glomerular capillary, which has been purported to lead to glomerulosclerosis (Brenner et al., 1982). Protein metabolism also leads to an increased output of urea by the kidneys, therefore increasing their physiological exertion. Nevertheless, the kidneys do adapt morphologically to sustain increased urea output. Only in the unhealthy individual does this pose a risk. For example, high-protein diets have been linked to renal degeneration in patients with pre-existing kidney pathology.[91] As of yet, there exist no definitive data to confirm that excessive protein intakes are harmful to healthy athletes.

Determining an exact amount of protein that might be considered excessive, given individual genetic differences, variation in protein quality, and training status is difficult. However, it is likely that protein intakes that exceed 4 g/kg is grossly unnecessary. Although this amount still may not be harmful to some individuals, the fact that most of it will be excreted or converted to fat makes this practice pointless. Similarly, high-protein diets can induce water loss (via increased urea production and excretion, which draws additional fluid into the urine) and thus contribute to dehydration in athletes.

Although it appears safe to ingest approximately 2 g PRO/kg body weight per day or slightly more, many high-protein sources also contain high amounts of fat. High-fat diets, prevalent in the United States, are associated with an increased incidence of heart disease and certain types of cancer. Identification of foods containing high-quality protein while limiting fat content will permit athletes to achieve adequate protein intake without endangering their health.

Brenner BM, Meyer TW, Hostetter TH. Protein intake and the progressive nature of kidney disease: the role of hemodynamically mediated glomerular sclerosis in aging, renal ablation, and intrinsic renal disease. N Eng J Med 1982;307:652.

Fat Requirements

Relative to carbohydrates and protein, fat has received considerably less attention as a credible macronutrient for athletic improvement. In fact, the recommendation to avoid fats is a prevailing suggestion. Often fueled by public misconception, fats have taken on an unfavorable reputation as strictly harmful. Much of the trepidation arises from the fact that high intakes of fat are associated with heart disease and cancer, and that fat contains more than twice as many calories (9 calories per gram) as do carbohydrates and protein. What is neglected, however, are the many essential physiological functions that are accomplished through the ingestion of fats. Furthermore, although some types of fats can be delineated into harmful categories, others, when used correctly, can be deemed beneficial.

Fats are important for many metabolic processes, including energy production and as transporters of lipid-soluble vitamins. They are also instrumental in the synthesis of vitamin D, cholesterol, and related steroid hormones, such as estradiol and testosterone. Finally, fats find additional value in providing the structural components of cell membranes and nervous tissue.

Fatty acids and triglycerides (the storage form of lipids) compose the fats that are known as simple lipids. Fatty acids may be saturated (contain single bonds between carbon atoms) or unsaturated (contain double bonds between carbons). Unsaturated fatty acids can be further classified as monounsaturated, having one double bond, or polyunsaturated, containing multiple double bonds between carbon atoms. The significance is that saturated fatty acids have been linked to cardiovascular disease and increased blood pressure, and thus are recommended to make up no more than 10% of total daily calories. Conversely, unsaturated fatty acids are more instrumental in the described positive attributes of lipids, and therefore most ingested fat should be of this variety. This also includes essential fatty acids, which are synthesized in tiny amounts by the body. Linoleic, linolenic, and arachidonic acids are all essential fatty acids and must be eaten in the diet.

Fat Needs of Athletes

Given the recommendation that total daily caloric intake should consist of no more than 30% fat, and that the average diet contains a significantly greater percentage, much of the perils attributed to fat can be charged to excessive fat consumption. In fact, most recommendations made by nutritionists suggest that a safer fat intake would be approximately 20–25% of total calories. Of this amount, roughly two-thirds should be comprised of unsaturated fatty acids, with saturated fats making up the final one-third.

In most cases, athletes and lay people alike consume more fat than is required. From an athletic standpoint, it may be that fat intake is not of dire concern if carbohydrate needs are met and adequate glycogen stores are maintained. Furthermore, the energy that can be derived from triglycerides in stored adipose tissue is sufficient for nearly interminable periods of moderately intense exercise. For the most part, therefore, as long as carbohydrate and protein ratios are met, athletes should allow fats to make up the remaining percentage. For example, because carbohydrates will typically make up roughly 60% of total calories and protein, 15–20%, fats would comprise the aforementioned 20–25% of total energy.

Although ample amounts of energy are stored as fat, the relative contribution of fat to energy production is limited by the delay in which it can be mobilized and ultimately oxidized. In the case of high-intensity exercise, this delay is increased and fat oxidation can eventually become unattainable. That is, as exercise intensity increases, the contribution of fat towards energy production decreases. Because low-intensity training uses a greater percentage of fat than does high-intensity exercise, it would appear that fat intake is a significant concern for endurance athletes. However, many endurance competitors can maintain an exercise intensity level that still derives a majority of energy from glycogen, thus reducing the importance of fats. Even in the occurrence of ultra-endurance events (i.e., triathlons, ultramarathons), in which fat metabolism increases in significance, the near-endless supply of stored fats makes the need for further supplementation unnecessary.

The significance of proper fat intake for the high-intensity sporting athlete is found in the fact that fatty acids are continually oxidized to provide energy for muscular function, although the contribution of fat is minimal during exercise itself. For this athlete, it is between repeated high-intensity exercise bouts when benefits are derived from fat oxidation and adequate intake. For example, the enormous caloric expenditure that results from repeated sprints means that increased fat will be oxidized at rest and during low-intensity phases of training. Although performance benefits are doubtful following fat supplementation, inadequate fat intake (less than 15–20% of total calories) has the potential to hinder performance. Such is the case for both endurance and high-intensity athletes.

Those individuals who are severely limiting fat intake (less than 10% of calories) run the risk of becoming deficient in essential fatty acids, particularly linoleic acid. This may jeopardize health in the long-term, especially because this practice may also cause deficiencies in fat-soluble vitamins. Many athletes and exercise enthusiasts restrict fat intake for physique-related reasons, and this practice is also discouraged, given that total calories are much more significant in reaching body composition goals. Severely restricting fat intake, as stated in previous sections, has the potential to limit subsequent fat mobilization and oxidation. Of course, this is highly undesirable for those individuals who want to lose fat.

Fat Loading

Considering that the body possesses an enormous reservoir of energy from fat stores, attracting interest is the concept of increasing fat intake to potentially allow mobilization of these reserves for performance enhancement. For example, some studies have suggested that an adaptation to a high-fat diet (greater than 50% of calories) can increase muscle triglyceride stores and decrease glycogen stores, promoting the use of fat as an energy source during rest and moderate-intensity training.[91–94] Whether these changes positively affect performance, however, is still undetermined.

The only study to report an improvement in work capacity while on a high-fat diet was an investigation by Lambert et al. involving trained cyclists.[95] The researchers concluded that a diet consisting of 70% fat for 2 weeks led to enhanced endurance during prolonged exercise and no impairment in performance, despite significantly reduced initial glycogen levels. Another study, however, has refuted these findings. In particular, research by Johannessen et al. reported that participants on a high-fat diet (76% of energy) reached exhaustion quicker when running on a treadmill compared with their high-carbohydrate (76% of energy) counterparts.[96]

Although supporting fat loading for athletes is speculative, perhaps benefits can be derived from this practice when initial glycogen stores are significantly reduced. This may have been the case in the study by Lambert et al. Regardless of these findings, there still exist insufficient data to support fat loading for athletes. Although further studies are warranted, the relationship of high fat intakes and cardiovascular disease makes this practice questionable. For instance, studies have indicated that even in athletes who are involved in vigorous training, cholesterol levels may be negatively affected by a high-fat diet.[97,98]

In two recent literature reviews, both groups of investigators discouraged the practice of fat loading, citing ineffectiveness in enhancing athletic performance.[99,100] One review[100] even concluded that short-term (3–5 days) ingestion of a high-fat diet actually deteriorates endurance performance. Taken together, it appears that fat loading is inadvisable and that carbohydrates should remain the primary energy fuel for all athletic pursuits.

Influence of Differing Macronutrient Ratios

Disseminated throughout the public and athletic communities, fairly conclusive evidence has extolled the virtues of carbohydrates, protein, and fat intake on ath-

letic enhancement. Recently, research has focused on alternative methods of improving performance. One of these methods is the manipulation of macronutrient ratios and its subsequent effects on, among other factors, mood, performance, and hormone release. Specifically, modifying macronutrient ratios involves varying the percentage of carbohydrate, protein, and fat content in the diet and examining its effects on the aforementioned factors. Additionally, macronutrient ratio studies have explored such topics as weight loss, weight gain, and recovery from exercise with encouraging results. Although most positive evidence can only be viewed as preliminary, it is nevertheless promising and warrants future study.

Recent studies examining the effects of different macronutrient ratios have worked under the assumption that providing necessary energy for physiological function is not the only purpose of a meal or dietary regimen. Instead, investigators have speculated that content, size, and timing of the meals themselves play a complex role in subsequent mood, alertness, and performance. If indeed food does have an effect on these factors, it still remains unknown as to why, although speculation also suggests that food may elicit hormone- and neurotransmitter-related changes that affect performance.

Effects on Alertness and Mood

Experimental studies have indicated that in the few hours following lunch, people feel drowsier than they do before eating.[101,102] Although several factors may be involved, this response can be related to the macronutrient content of the meal, or other circumstances such as time of day and size of the meal. More specifically, other studies have found that alertness and performance are significantly lower following a high-fat, low-carbohydrate meal than after a meal containing equal calories from both fat and carbohydrates (protein was held constant).[103,104] A follow-up study by Wells et al.[105] demonstrated that, in the morning, fat exerts a greater depression on alertness and mood than does carbohydrate, regardless of total energy content. The authors also stated that the depressive effects of fat were more pronounced in the morning than later in the day.

Finally, some evidence suggests that when protein and carbohydrates dominate the caloric content of a meal, they also induce lethargy and mental slowness.[101] In one study, a carbohydrate-to-protein ratio of 3 to 1 (55% CHO, 18% PRO) was the optimal balance for promoting positive changes in mood and performance of night-shift work, in comparison to diets rich in either carbohydrate (70%) or protein (52%).[106] The authors did indicate, however, that the high-protein diet produced the best subjective ratings of mood and nevertheless correlated with increased alertness. This finding also coincides with reports that subjects feel happier following a meal containing protein than they do after a meal without protein.[107] These conclusions may be a result of the possible relationship between protein and the augmented uptake of the amino acid tyrosine (and thus the resultant catecholamine neurotransmitter formation), which enhances feelings of alertness.[106]

Preliminary data, therefore, would indicate that overconsumption of any macronutrient, especially fat and carbohydrates, in a particular meal can have detrimental effects on alertness and mood. The exact role of protein, however, is less understood. Although further research is needed, perhaps a slightly elevated amount of protein per meal (in the range of 18–25%) is the optimal balance for sustaining alertness without incurring the performance decrements associated with overconsumption.

Effects on Exercise

Only a small number of studies have investigated the effects of manipulating the macronutrient content of a diet on physical performance. Given that an accepted axiom of sports nutrition is that carbohydrates are the preferred and prevailing fuel source for exercise (and thus the macronutrient percentages outlined previously should be the norm for such dietary regimens), altering macronutrient ratios for this purpose has only recently sparked interest in the literature. Not surprisingly, therefore, the results of these studies are far from unanimous.

An investigation by Scott et al.[108] studied the effects of two different energy-restricted diets, one that was 40% CHO, 40% fat, and 20% PRO, versus a diet that contained 60% CHO, 20% fat, and 20% PRO. The authors concluded that the subjects showed no differences in aerobic power, body weight/composition, or other physical performance measures after 8 weeks. The authors also stated that to induce any negative changes in performance, a more extreme variation in carbohydrate and fat content may be necessary. A comparable study that also gives credence to the traditional macronutrient percentages for optimal athletic performance (approximately 60–65% CHO, 20–30% fat, 15% PRO) was done by Greenhaff et al.,[109] who suggested that acute variations in macronutrient content can adversely affect physical performance. In fact, they concluded that diets high in fat and protein produced alterations in muscle biochemistry that resulted in metabolic acidosis during exercise, which can negatively affect exercise performance. It appears at this time, therefore, that athletes should still allow carbohydrates to remain their primary macronutrient constituent.

Effects on Hormone Release and Selected Compounds

Likewise in its infancy stages, research on the effects of macronutrient manipulation on hormone release and other compounds (i.e., enzyme activity) has commenced in recent years. The surging interest in this area of investigation has primary implications on potential athletic performance enhancement and recovery, body composition improvement, and effects on substrate use during exercise and rest. For example, some studies have explored the effects of dietary manipulation on the hormones testosterone, growth hormone, and insulin, which promote strength and muscular increases. Thus, such research triggers particular interest for those involved in strength/power sports or who wish to increase strength and muscularity through resistance training. Other studies have examined the effect of macronutrient manipulation on such factors as fat loss and metabolic rate (which may be related to hormones and other compounds), with considerable implications for those intending to improve body composition. Again, although no definite conclusions can be made, initial research has certainly sparked additional interest in this realm of physique and athletic enhancement.

The goal of many athletes and exercise enthusiasts is to increase muscular strength and size; therefore, optimal conditions for recovery following training sessions are necessary. Optimal recovery is mandatory because heavy-resistance exercise damages certain muscle fibers that must subsequently undergo remodeling. Recovery, in fact, involves the function of many physiological processes that are influenced by the availability of specific hormones and nutrients.[110] Together, hormones, nutrients, and other growth factors regulate this remodeling of skeletal muscle proteins.[111]

Independent of exercise, nutrients also have the power to influence hormonal concentrations that may positively affect athletes and those who wish to improve body composition. A simple increase in caloric intake above energy requirements enhances growth hormone, testosterone, and insulin-like growth factor-I (IGF-I) concentrations.[112] In contrast, energy and protein restriction has produced negative effects on serum IGF-I concentrations,[113] and diets with low percentages of dietary fat are associated with lower testosterone concentrations.[114]

Research regarding nutritional supplementation's effects on the hormonal response to resistance exercise has been performed by Chandler et al.,[115] who demonstrated that insulin and growth hormone (GH) release can be influenced by the diet. The researchers concluded that, following a resistance training session, insulin and growth hormone concentrations were significantly higher and testosterone concentrations were lower when subjects consumed a protein-carbohydrate supplement immediately before and 2 hours after the workout. In agreement with these findings was a study by Fahey et al.,[116] who reported a significant increase in insulin concentrations following exercise when subjects consumed a protein-carbohydrate supplement 30 minutes before and intermittently during a weight-training session.

A similar study by Kraemer et al.[110] also coincided with previous findings, and in this case involved 3 consecutive days of resistance training. The investigators found that ingesting a protein-carbohydrate supplement (33% protein or ~30 g; 67% carbohydrate or ~60 g) 2 hours before and immediately after workouts significantly increased serum concentrations of insulin, growth hormone, and IGF-I while testosterone decreased below resting levels. The authors predicted that these responses could enhance glycogen and protein synthesis during recovery. They also proposed diet-related factors that could explain the drop in testosterone concentrations that occurred in this and aforementioned studies. A primary factor, according to the authors, was that percent dietary fat ranged from nonexistent to 14% in the supplements administered in the studies, which correlates with decreased testosterone levels.[114] Secondly, the protein-to-carbohydrate ratio during supplementation was significantly higher than during the placebo conditions. This is also a potential factor because a high protein-to-carbohydrate ratio is also associated with lower testosterone concentrations in healthy active men.[117]

Further research examining the influence of diet on testosterone has been performed by Volek et al.,[117] who simultaneously studied the effects of nutrients on cortisol, a catabolic hormone. According to their research, results indicate that specific nutrients may have the potential to alter the regulation and metabolism of testosterone, whereas effects on cortisol remain unclear.[117] Their evidence verifies that testosterone levels positively correlate with percentages of dietary fat and negatively correlate with percentages of energy that is protein. Likewise, it appears that the protein-to-carbohydrate ratio is negatively correlated with testosterone levels.[117] Regarding fat, a previous investigation has also observed a significant positive correlation between percent energy fat and testosterone in young athletic men,[118] and preliminary evidence also suggests a positive relationship between monounsaturated and saturated fatty acids on resting testosterone concentrations.[117] In contrast, a negative correlation between the polyunsaturated-to-saturated fatty acid ratio and testosterone was reported.[117]

A study by Raben et al.[119] also found similar results when studying the hormonal responses to a meat-rich diet versus a vegetarian diet. In a study of male endurance athletes, the investigators reported a significant decrease in testosterone concentrations and an attenuation of the exercise-induced increase in testosterone when the subjects switched to vegetarian diets. These results may be explained by the likelihood that vegetarians consume less fat, saturated fatty acids, and a higher polyunsaturated-to-saturated fatty acid ratio than meat-eaters, and therefore exhibit lower concentrations of testosterone.[117,119] Interestingly, both diets in this study derived equal amounts of energy from protein, carbohydrates, and fat, indicating that the supply of energy from the macronutrients was not responsible for the effect on testosterone.[117] Thus, the composition (in this case, vegetarian versus animal sources) of the energy-providing macronutrients may also modify testosterone concentrations.[117]

The findings of these studies are particularly important for athletes and exercise enthusiasts who are attempting to increase or maintain strength and muscle mass, especially during periods of intense training, which can elevate levels of cortisol. Overtraining may also be responsible for a decline in resting testosterone concentrations, further signifying the need for appropriate dietary habits. Accordingly, such debilitating effects of overtraining may be exacerbated by a diet low in fat, which many athletes (i.e., wrestlers, gymnasts) consume.[117]

Further studies have examined the ratio of carbohydrate to fat in the diet and its effect on nitrogen retention. Such an investigation was performed by McCargar et al.,[118] who also studied this ratio's effects on substrate use and hormone response in healthy males. The researchers found that the high-fat diet (45% of total calories) increased nitrogen retention, especially when maintenance energy intakes were consumed. The authors also stated that their findings indicated a potentially increased fat oxidation in those subjects consuming a high-fat diet, and that the nitrogen-sparing effect of such a diet was likely substrate mediated (as opposed to being hormonally mediated). The results also indicated that the high-carbohydrate diet (60% of energy) induced elevated triglyceride levels, which may be a reflection of additional fat synthesis in the liver owing to the presence of excess glucose.[118] The significance here is that once energy and glycogen needs are met, surplus carbohydrates may lead to hypertriglyceridemia.[118]

Studies examining the impact of caloric intake on resting testosterone levels have discovered a depressive effect on such concentrations. For instance, one study showed that fasting for 5 days can lower testosterone levels by as much as 30–50%.[120] It also appears that severe caloric restriction, even if induced by excessive exercise, lowers testosterone levels.[121] Combine these revelations with the possibility that increased fat intake may enhance testosterone levels, and the importance of adequate fat, as in the overtrained state, becomes paramount.

Yost and colleagues[122] investigated the effects of macronutrient composition on the activities of adipose tissue lipoprotein lipase (an enzyme that breaks down fat) and insulin sensitivity. The researchers studied the reaction of these compounds to both a high-carbohydrate (55% of total kcal) and high-fat (50%) diet. They concluded that after 16 days of the high-carbohydrate diet only the responsiveness of adipose tissue lipoprotein lipase was increased. There was no effect on insulin sensitivity, although other researchers have found that diets containing a higher percentage of energy from fat produce insulin resistance.[123,124] Of course, if such findings are conclusive, the development of type 2 diabetes, hypertension, and cardiovascular disease are possible adverse consequences.

Considerations for Weight Loss

As stated previously, attempts at weight loss must satisfy the condition that energy expenditure must exceed energy intake. In addition, exercise increases caloric output and may also raise metabolic rate. Although neither of these facts are recent discoveries, the newly investigated role of nutrient timing and macronutrient balance may also be significant in attempts at weight loss. For example, a study by Keim et al.[125] concluded that consumption of large morning meals (70% of daily energy intake consumed in the AM) resulted in greater weight loss than consumption of large evening meals. This could be the result of a higher metabolic rate in the morning, and potentially a more effective metabolic use of ingested calories at this time period. However, fat-free mass loss was also greater in this instance, and was better preserved with the consumption of large evening meals. Speculation, therefore, may lead to the recommendation that an enhanced protein intake in the evening may work to counterbalance the high-percentage morning caloric consumption required in this weight loss regimen.

Macronutrient specificity may also be an additional weight loss factor. For example, although protein contributes only a small portion to energy intake and expenditure, its ingestion could be influential in subsequent energy turnover. Forslund et al.[126] concluded that 6 days of a high-protein (2.5 g/kg/day) regimen resulted in a positive protein and carbohydrate balance, and a negative fat balance, in relation to a *normal protein* intake (1.0 g/kg/day). This also corresponds to a higher relative contribution to energy turnover from fat with the high-protein diet.

In contrast, with respect to carbohydrates, it appears that the ratio of this macronutrient in the diet has little influence on subsequent weight loss. Numerous studies have concluded that total energy intake more effectively determines weight loss than does the carbohydrate makeup (which ranged from 15–75% of total kcal in these studies) of a diet.[127–129] The reason for this may be the numerous mechanisms by which the body can adapt to and maintain glycogen stores in the face of fluctuating carbohydrate intakes, such as mobilization of liver glycogen stores and gluconeogenesis.[129] Even with regard to fat, it is likely that total energy restriction is a more significant predictor of weight loss than is simply limiting fat intake. A 24-week study by Harvey-Berino found that subjects who restricted total energy lost twice as much weight (11.5 kg vs. 5.2 kg) as those that only restricted fat.[130]

The Effect of Macronutrient Manipulation on Hormones

Jeff S. Volek, PhD

To enhance the development of muscular strength and size with heavy resistance training, optimal conditions for recovery from the individual exercise training sessions are necessary. Recovery involves the coordinated functioning of several physiological processes that are heavily influenced by the availability and actions of specific hormones and nutrients. Qualitative and quantitative changes in skeletal muscle contractile proteins are all supported and signaled by a host of systematic trophic influences from hormones to nutrient availability. Clearly, heavy resistance exercise disrupts or damages certain muscle fibers that later must undergo a repair and remodeling process. Dietary nutrients, hormones, and growth factors act upon each other and regulate this remodeling of skeletal muscle proteins. Manipulation of these variables to favor anabolism over catabolism during recovery may enhance training adaptations.

Resistance exercise is a potent stimulus for altering certain hormones; however, there is much less information on the effects of manipulating macronutrients on hormonal responses, especially in athletes training intensely. Hormonal responses to changes in diet are time dependent. For example, the hormonal responses to consumption of a fat-rich meal could differ substantially from the hormonal responses to a prolonged fat-rich diet. A distinction should also be made between diets that alter the exercise-induced response, the postprandial response (i.e., after a meal), and the postabsorptive (i.e., fasting) concentrations of a hormone. In theory, any elevation in an anabolic hormone (e.g., insulin, growth hormone, testosterone), whether for minutes, hours, days, or weeks, could be viewed as positive because the exposure time of the target cell to an increased concentration of a particular hormone is extended.

The majority of research that examines the effects of macronutrients on hormones has altered the amount of carbohydrate and fat consumed. Hormonal and metabolic adaptations to a eucaloric carbohydrate-reduced diet mirror many of the responses usually seen with fasting. Hormonal adaptations induced by consuming a low-carbohydrate diet favor an environment that enhances mobilization of energy stores via increased sympathoadrenal activity, which may be related to blood concentrations of glucose, fatty acids, ketone bodies, or tissue glycogen content.

Insulin

Insulin is a peptide hormone secreted by the pancreas, which plays a critical role in the regulation of blood glucose levels and stimulation of amino acid uptake for incorporation into skeletal muscle proteins. Carbohydrate ingestion leads to an increase in blood glucose and a relatively similar increase in insulin concentrations. A meal rich in fat results in lower insulin responses compared with meals rich in either carbohydrate or protein. Also, there is a decrease in resting glucose and insulin concentrations in response to 3 to 4 days of a eucaloric low-carbohydrate diet high in fat and low in carbohydrate. Three weeks of a low-carbohydrate diet may significantly lower resting insulin but not glucose concentrations in healthy men. Although insulin stimulates protein synthesis, maximizing insulin concentrations may not be advantageous because of the potent antilipolytic (i.e., blocks mobilization of fat from storage) and lipogenic (i.e., promotes storage of fat) effects of insulin.

Growth Hormone

Growth hormone is a major anabolic peptide hormone secreted from the anterior pituitary that is involved in many anabolic functions (e.g., increases muscle and skeletal growth) and metabolic regulation (e.g., increases protein synthesis, lipolysis, and glucose conservation). Dietary nutrients may indirectly modulate the resting and exercise-induced responses of growth hormone by altering the plasma concentrations of different energy substrates (i.e., glucose, free fatty acids, and ketone bodies). Acute ingestion of a liquid supplement rich in fat did not affect resting values of growth hormone, but attenuated the exercise-induced increase compared with a high-carbohydrate supplement. Prolonged intake of a diet higher in fat results in a much different response. Merimee et al. examined the 24-hour growth hormone response to diets rich in either fat (75%), carbohydrate (80%), or protein (70%) consumed for 10 to12 days. Although the fat and protein-rich diets had no apparent effect, the carbohydrate-rich diet clearly suppressed growth hormone concentrations in men. A similar reduction in growth hormone was detected in men who consumed diets that contained 65% of energy from carbohydrate compared with diets that were lower in carbohydrate but similar in total calories. Thus, the absolute fat content may not be as important as the absolute amount of carbohydrate. Others have also reported that resting and exercise-induced growth hormone concentrations are elevated when preceded by a high-fat diet. Exercise-induced increases in growth hormone are also higher after fasting but decreased when energy intake is moderately restricted. Exercise-induced elevations in growth hormone caused by a high-fat diet or fasting are accompanied by a more rapid decline in plasma insulin and glucose concentrations during exercise, suggesting that glucose-sensitive receptors may modulate the growth hormone response to exercise. Glucose infusion at the end of exercise does not attenuate the greater growth hormone response observed after a fat-rich diet, suggesting that other substrates (i.e., glycogen, ketones, fatty acids) or hormones (insulin, catecholamines) may also be involved in the regulation of growth hormone secretion. Elevated levels of free fatty acids have also been shown to inhibit growth hormone secretion; however, this effect appears to be minimal when blood glucose concentrations are simultaneously decreased.

Testosterone

Testosterone is a steroid hormone secreted from the Leydig cells of the testes that has both anabolic and anticatabolic effects upon muscle tissue. Dietary nutrients, in particular fat, have been shown to affect testosterone. Individuals consuming a diet containing about 20% fat compared with a diet containing 40% fat have significantly lower concentrations of testosterone. Also, replacing dietary carbohydrate with protein has been shown to decrease testosterone concentrations. Men consuming a vegetarian or meatless diet have lower circulating concentrations of testosterone compared with men consuming a mixed Western or a high-meat diet. These studies indicate that the distribution of macronutrients has a significant influence on testosterone concentrations. The specific type or quality of macronutrient may also impact testosterone independent of a change in diet composition. Volek et al. reported significant positive correlations between dietary fat, specifically saturated and monounsaturated fatty acids, and resting testosterone concentrations in a group of young resistance-trained men. Raben et al. reported a significant decrease in resting testosterone concentrations and an attenuation in the exercise-induced increase in testosterone in male endurance athletes who switched from a meat-rich diet to a lacto-ovo vegetarian diet. The diets contained equal percentages of calories derived from protein, carbohydrate, and fat; however, the source of protein in the vegetarian diet was derived mainly from vegetable sources (83%), whereas the mixed diet contained significantly less vegetable protein (35%). The exact mechanism linking nutrition to testosterone is unknown. Increasing anabolic hormone concentrations at rest, after a meal, or after exercise may enhance adaptations to resistance training. Manipulation of the distribution of carbohydrate and fat in the diet may alter the hormonal environment (e.g., habitual consumption of a fat-rich diet has been shown to elevate fasting testosterone and growth hormone concentrations). Thus, macronutrient manipulation should be considered a potential strategy to enhance the adaptations to exercise training programs. However, until further research is performed that documents specific training outcome markers in athletes under a variety of dietary regimens, generalizations should be made with caution. Practically no information exists regarding the practical application of increasing circulating anabolic hormones on muscle size and strength; the potential differential effects in different populations (e.g., men vs. women, young vs. old, trained vs. sedentary); the interaction of different hormone responses; the effects at the target tissue (e.g., potential down-regulation of receptors); and the impact of "nutrient cycling" (e.g., consuming a carbohydrate-rich diet followed by a fat-rich diet). Considering the enormous complexity in which the endocrine system operates in the regulation of cellular function and the diverse mechanisms that control homeostasis, the optimal dietary strategy to maximize an athlete's natural production of anabolic hormones will require extensive research.

Volek JS, Kraemer WJ, Bush JA, et al. Testosterone and cortisol in relationship to dietary nutrients and resistance exercise. J Appl Physiol 1997;82(1):49–54.

Raben A, Kiens B, Richter EA, et al. Serum sex hormones and endurance performance after a lacto-ovo vegetarian and a mixed diet. Med Sci Sports Exerc 1992;24:1290–1297.

Lovejoy J, DiGirolamo M. Habitual dietary intake and insulin sensitivity in lean and obese adults. Am J Clin Nutr 1992;55:1174–1179.

Merimee TJ, Pulkkinen AJ, Burton CE. Diet-induced alterations of hGH secretion in man. J Clin Endocrinol Metab 1976;42:931–937.

Forslund AH, El-Khoury AE, Olsson RM, et al. Effect of protein intake and physical activity on 24-h pattern and rate of macronutrient utilization. Am J Physiol 1999;276:E964–E976.

AUTHORS' RECOMMENDATIONS

Before an appropriate, individualized diet can be incorporated, an accurate reading of body fat percentage must first be performed. Daily calorie requirements depend both on the amount of lean body mass and activity level of an individual; therefore, this is a necessary estimation. This is because of the radically different metabolic processes required to maintain muscle as opposed to fat. Specifically, muscle requires a great deal of energy to sustain it, whereas fat does not. As a result, the daily calorie intake should be sufficient to maintain muscle, not fat. Bear in mind, however, that this method of determining energy requirements remains unexplored in the literature. As a result, the forthcoming recommendations are based on extrapolation of research, but are nevertheless subject to judgment.

Currently, numerous methods exist to estimate body fat percentage. Although underwater weighing is considered the gold standard, its accessibility to the population at large hinders its effectiveness. A more accessible and efficient method, as well as being both valid and reliable, is the use of skinfold measurements. This technique involves the use of special pincer-type calipers to measure subcutaneous fat folds at selected sites on the body. The measurements are then placed into an equation to determine body density and ultimately body fat percentage. The authors recommend that all measurements be taken by an experienced fitness professional, and the resulting totals be placed in the equations provided in TABLE 2-6.

Once body fat percentage is known, lean body mass should then be calculated. This can be determined by multiplying body weight in kilograms by the lean body percentage of the individual. For example, an individual with 15% body fat would have a lean body percentage of 85% (100 − 15 = 85). Therefore, if this person weighs 70 kg (154 lbs.), his lean body mass would be 59.5 kg (70 kg × 0.85 = 59.5 kg). Next, this calculation will be used in TABLE 2-7 to determine a suitable daily protein intake based on activity level.

If, for example, this particular individual falls into the *highly active* category, he would therefore require a protein intake of 2.2 g PRO/kg lean body weight daily.

Table 2-6 Estimating Body Fat Percentage by Measurement of Subcutaneous Fatfolds

A. Jackson and Pollock[128,129] equations for estimating body density (D_b):

1. Men: $D_b = 1.10938 - 0.0008267x + 0.0000016x^2 - 0.0002574A$

    x = sum of chest, abdomen, and thigh skinfolds
    A = age in years

2. Women: $D_b = 1.0994921 - 0.0009929x + 0.0000023x^2 - 0.0001392A$

    x = sum of tricep, suprailiac, and thigh skinfolds
    A = age in years

B. Siri[130] formula for estimating percent body fat:

1. Percent body fat = $495/D_b - 450$

This equates to a daily protein total of approximately 131 g protein (59.5 kg × 2.2 g/kg = 130.9 g protein). Because protein carries four calories per gram, this individual would receive 524 daily calories from protein (131 g × 4 = 524). Finally, this amount can be used in TABLE 2-8, where an appropriate daily energy intake and macronutrient profile can be determined based on physique modification goals.

As listed in TABLE 2-8, a daily caloric intake can be developed for an individual seeking weight gain, weight loss, or maintenance of body weight. However, even in the maintenance category, the macronutrient ratios provided are geared toward achieving loss of body fat and enhancement of lean tissue. To determine total caloric intake, one can simply use the daily caloric total derived from protein and divide its appropriate percentage into this amount. For example, if the 70-kg male depicted previously desired weight gain, his protein total would make up 16% of daily calories. He should consume 524 calories from protein; therefore, his total daily caloric intake would be 3275 kcal (524/0.16). Carbohydrates would then comprise 56% of this total (1834 kcal, 459 g), and fat, 28% (917 kcal, 102 g).

If this same individual desired weight loss, the protein total would then make up 26% of daily calories.

Table 2-7 Determination of Daily Protein Intake Based on Activity Level and Lean Body Mass

Activity Level	Daily Protein Intake (g PRO/kg lean body mass)
Sedentary (no additional exercise beyond normal daily activities)	1.1 g
Light Activity (approximately 3 hours/week of light endurance and/or resistance activity)	1.4 g
Moderately Active (approximately 6 hours/week of light activity or 3 hours of intense training)	1.8 g
Highly Active (approximately 6 to 8 hours of intense training weekly)	2.2 g
Extremely Active (10 or more hours of intense training weekly)	2.6 g

Note: Light activity refers to endurance training at approximately 60–70% of maximum heart rate or resistance training at less than 75% of one-repetition maximum. Intense activity would be considered endurance or resistance training beyond these ranges. Please also note that the preceding protein recommendations are not only arbitrary, but certain individuals may feel that they fall into intermediary categories. For example, it is possible to fall between the highly active and extremely active categories, and as such a protein intake of 2.4 g/kg daily would be appropriate.

The total daily energy intake in this scenario then becomes 2015 kcal (524/0.26). In this instance, carbohydrates will comprise 50% of the total (1008 kcal, 252 g), and fat, 24% (484 kcal, 54 g). In TABLE 2-9, a sample diet, with a goal of physique enhancement and weight maintenance, is provided for this individual.

Note that the dietary regimen outlined in Table 2-9 contains five meals per day. This was included as a possible means to stimulate metabolic rate increases via an increased thermic effect of food consumption. It is recommended that consuming multiple daily meals should be a method used regardless of physique modification goals. In this way, potential enhancements in the efficiency of the body's metabolic processes may ensue.

As an added note, it cannot be stressed enough that the information provided in Tables 2-7 and 2-8 are rec-

Table 2-8 Recommended Macronutrient Ratios for Weight Gain, Loss, and Maintenance

	Weight Gain	Weight Loss	Maintenance
Protein	16%	26%	20%
Carbohydrate	56%	50%	54%
Fat	28%	24%	26%

Table 2-9 A Sample Maintenance Diet

Body Weight: 70 kg   Percent Body Fat: 15%
Lean Body Mass: 59.5 kg   Macronutrient Ratio: 20% PRO, 54% CHO, 26% FAT

	Protein (g)	Carbs (g)	Fat (g)	Total kcal
Meal 1				
2 whole eggs plus 4 egg whites	22	2	12	204
Oatmeal, 1 cup	10	52	6	302
Banana	1	27	0	112
Meal 2				
Tuna, 1 can	33	0	1	141
Mayonnaise, 1 tbsp	0	2	7	71
Apple	0	25	0	100
Wheat Bread, 2 slices	4	30	2	154
Meal 3				
Peanut Butter, 2 tbsp	8	8	16	208
Jelly, 1/2 tbsp	0	7	0	28
Wheat Bread, 2 slices	4	30	2	154
Orange	0	25	0	100
Meal 4				
Yogurt w/fruit, 1 cup	8	38	3	211
Mixed vegetables, 1 cup	4	24	0	112
Rice, 1 cup	4	27	0	124
Butter, 1/2 tbsp	0	0	4	36
Meal 5				
Extra Lean Ground Beef, 4 oz.	28	0	18	274
Spaghetti, 1 cup	7	42	1	205
Spaghetti Sauce, 1/2 cup	2	15	2	86
Totals	135	354	74	2622

ommendations based on limited research and the authors' discretion. Individual tinkering of the daily caloric total is likely for the achievement of desired goals. For example, rapid weight loss is a sign that caloric intake is deficient, and subsequent losses in weight are more likely the result of water and lean tissue losses than fat. In this case, a slight increase in daily calories is necessary, as weight loss (and gain) should be a consistent, gradual process. Similarly, frequent (roughly every 2 weeks) reassessments of body weight and composition should be performed, and appropriate dietary modifications should be implemented based on these findings.

SUMMARY

Not unlike the majority of the research on sports supplementation, there still exist many nebulous facets of sports nutrition that require constant investigation and re-examination. Nevertheless, the wealth of knowledge contained within the field of sports nutrition, although constantly evolving, far surpasses the relatively recent surge of evidence supporting nutritional supplements. With this fact in mind, any individual seeking the physique and sport-related advantages offered by nutritional supplementation must first take stock of his or her personal nutritional profile. Once the basic tenets of sound nutritional planning are satisfied, only then can appropriate supplements be introduced and used effectively, and ultimate physique or athletic enhancement achieved.

Chapter Highlights:

1. To achieve desired body composition goals, individuals can determine an appropriate caloric intake by using estimates of resting energy expenditure and activity level. Weight gain, weight loss, and maintenance are influenced primarily by these two factors.

2. Macronutrient (carbohydrate, protein, and fat) intake can also be determined based on desired objectives, whether for physique or athletic enhancement. Each macronutrient possesses unique characteristics, and may be manipulated slightly to potentially improve performance.

3. Carbohydrate intake should be increased to enhance endurance activities, and an increased protein intake can benefit strength/power athletes and those who seek muscular gains. Recommendations are made regarding carbohydrate intake before, during, and after exercise. Carbohydrate loading, a technique used to increase glycogen stores beyond normal capacity, is effective in events lasting more than 1 hour.

4. The glycemic index, which measures digestion and absorption rates of various carbohydrates, can be used to promote increased energy for athletic events, spare protein breakdown, and replenish glycogen after exercise.

5. Although research is limited, manipulating macronutrient ratios can also elicit alterations in alertness and mood, hormone release, and physical performance.

6. The authors made final recommendations concerning weight gain and loss, and a sample system is outlined for achieving such goals. This system uses body fat percentage and activity level to arrive at appropriate macronutrient percentages to achieve the desired physique-related goal.

REFERENCES

1. McArdle WD, Katch FI, Katch VL. Exercise Physiology: Energy, Nutrition, and Human Performance. 3rd ed. Philadelphia: Lea & Febiger, 1991.
2. Food and Nutrition Board, Recommended Dietary Allowances, 10th ed., National Academy of Sciences, Washington DC, 1989;30.
3. Economos CD, Bortz SS, Nelson ME. Nutritional practices of elite athletes. Sports Med 1993;16:383.
4. Fogleholm GM, Koskinen R, Laasko J, et al. Gradual and rapid weight loss: Effects on nutrition and performance in male athletes. Med Sci Sports Exerc 1993;25(3):371–377.
5. American College of Sports Medicine. Weight loss in wrestlers. Med Sci Sports Exerc 1976;8:xi–xiii.
6. American College of Sports Medicine. Proper and improper weight loss programs. Med Sci Sports Exerc 1983;15:534–539.
7. Ballor DL, Katch VL, Beque MD, Marks CR. Resistance weight training during caloric restriction enhances lean body weight maintenance. Am J Clin Nutr 1988;47:19–25.
8. Walberg JL, Leidy MK, Sturgill DJ, et al. Macronutrient needs in weightlifters during caloric restriction. Med Sci Sports Exerc 1987;19(Suppl):70.
9. Grande F. Nutrition and energy balance in body composition studies. In Techniques for Measuring Body Composition. Washington, DC: National Academy of Sciences, National Research Council, 1961.
10. Bouchard C, Tremblay A, Moorjani S, et al. Long-term exercise training with constant energy intake: Effect on body composition and selected metabolic variables. Int J Obesity 1990;14:57.
11. Zuti WB, Golding LA. Comparing diet and exercise as weight reduction tools. Phys Sportsmed 1976;4:49.
12. Moyer CL, et al. Body composition changes in obese women on a very low calorie diet with and without exercise. Med Sci Sports Exerc 1985;17:292.
13. Elliot DL, Goldberg L, Kuchl KS, Bennett WM. Sustained depression of the resting metabolic rate after massive weight loss. Am J Clin Nutr 1989;49:93.
14. Kern PA, Ong JM, Saffari B, Carty J. The effects of weight loss on the activity and the expression of adipose-tissue lipoprotein lipase in very obese humans. N Engl J Med 1990;322:1053.
15. Roemmich JN, Sinning WE. Weight loss and wrestling training: Effects of nutrition, growth, maturation, body composition, and strength. J Appl Physiol 1997;82:1751.
16. Drinkwater BL, et al. Menstrual history as a determinant of current bone density in young athletes. JAMA 1990;263:545.
17. Boobis L, Williams C, Wootton S. Human muscle metabolism during brief maximal exercise. J Physiol 1982;338:21.
18. Lemon PWR. Protein and exercise: Update 1987. Med Sci Sports Exerc 1987;19(Suppl):179–190.
19. Stone MH, Keith R, Kearney JT, et al. Overtraining: A review of the signs and symptoms of overtraining. J Appl Sports Sci Res 1991;5(1):35–50.
20. Yannick C, et al. Oxidation of corn starch, glucose, and fructose ingested before exercise. Med Sci Sports Exerc 1989;21:45.
21. Burke LM, Collier GR, Hargreaves M. Glycemic Index – A new tool in sports nutrition? Int J Sports Nutr 1998;8:401–415.
22. Foster-Powell K, Brand Miller J. International tables of glycemic index. Am J Clin Nutr 1995;62(Suppl):871–893.
23. Brand JC, Colagiuri S, Crossman S, et al. Low glycemic index foods improve long-term glycemic control in NIDDM. Diabetes Care 1991;14:95–101.

24. Jenkins DJA, Wolever TMS, Kalmusky J, et al. Low glycemic index carbohydrate foods in the management of hyperlipidemia. Am J Clin Nutr 1985;42:604–617.

25. Holt S, Brand J, Soveny C, Hansky J. Relationship of satiety to postprandial glycemic, insulin, and cholecystokinin responses. Appetite 1992;18:129–141.

26. Karlsson J, Saltin B. Diet, muscle glycogen, and endurance performance. J Appl Physiol 1971;31:203–206.

27. O'Keeffe K, Keith RE, Blessing DL, et al. Dietary carbohydrate and endurance performance. Med Sci Sports Exerc 1987;19:S538.

28. Snyder AC, Lamb DR, Baur T, et al. Maltodextrin feeding immediately before prolonged cycling at 62% VO2 max increases time to exhaustion. Med Sci Sports Exerc 1983;15:126.

29. Devlin JT, Williams C. Foods, nutrition, and sports performance; a final consensus statement. J Sports Sci 1991;9:S9:iii.

30. Costill DL. Carbohydrate nutrition before, during, and after exercise. Fed Proc 1985;44:364–368.

31. Walberg-Rankin J. Dietary carbohydrate as an ergogenic aid for prolonged and brief competitions in sport. Int J Sports Nutr 1995;5:S13.

32. Short SH, Short WR. Four year study of university athletes' dietary intake. J Am Diet Assoc 1983;82:632–645.

33. Van Erp-Baart AMJ, Saris WHM, Binkhorst RA, et al. Nationwide survey on nutritional habits in elite athletes. Part 1: Energy, carbohydrate, protein, and fat intake. Int J Sports Med 1989;10:S3–S10.

34. Burke LM, Collier GR, Hargreaves M. Muscle glycogen storage following prolonged exercise: Effect of the glycemic index on carbohydrate feedings. J Appl Physiol 1993;75:1019–1023.

35. American Dietetic Association. Position stand of the American Dietetic Association and the Canadian Dietetic Association: Nutrition for physical fitness and athletic performance for adults. J Am Diet Assoc 1993;93:691–696.

36. Costill DL. Carbohydrates for exercise: Dietary demands for optimal performance. Int J Sports Med 1988;9:1.

37. Sherman WM, Doyle JA, Lamb DR, Strauss RH. Dietary carbohydrate, muscle glycogen, and exercise performance during 7 days of training. Am J Clin Nutr 1993;57:27.

38. Ivy JL. Muscle glycogen synthesis before and after exercise. Sports Med 1991;11:6.

39. Costill DL, Sherman WM, Fink WJ, et al. The role of dietary carbohydrates in muscle glycogen resynthsesis after strenuous running. Am J Clin Nutr 1981;34:1831–1836.

40. Hawley JA, Dennis SC, Lindsay FH, et al. Nutritional practices of athletes: Are they sub-optimal? J Sports Sci 1995;13:75S–87S.

41. Clarkson PM. Nutrition for improved sports performance: Current issues on ergogenic aids. Sports Med 1996;6:393–401.

42. Williams C. Dietary macro- and micronutrient requirements of endurance athletes. Proc Nutr Soc 1998;57:1–8.

43. Keith RE, O'Keefe KA, Blessing DL, Wilson GD. Alterations in dietary carbohydrate, protein, and fat intake and mood state in trained female cyclists. Med Sci Sports Exerc 1991;23:212.

44. Sherman WM, Costil DL, Fink WJ, Miller JM. Effect of exercise-diet manipulation on muscle glycogen and its subsequent utilization during performance. Int J Sports Med 1981;2:114.

45. Sherman WM. Metabolism of sugars and physical performance. Am J Clin Nutr 1995;62:228S.

46. Wright D, Sherman WM, Dernbach AR. Carbohydrate feedings before, during, or in combination improve cycling endurance performance. J Appl Physiol 1991;71:1082.

47. Leatt PB, Jacobs I. Effect of glucose polymer ingestion on glycogen depletion during a soccer match. Can J Sports Sci 1989;14:112.

48. Simard J. Effects of carbohydrate intake before and during an ice hockey game on blood and muscle energy substrates. Res Quart Exer Sport 1988;59:144.

49. Kirkendall D, Foster C, Dean J, et al. Effect of a glucose polymer supplementation on performance of soccer players. In Science and Football. Reilly T, Lees A, David K, Murphy W, eds. London: E&FN SPON, 1988;33.

50. Rehunen S, Littsola S. Modification of the muscle-glycogen level of ice-hockey players through a drink with high carbohydrate content. Z Sportsmed 1978;2:15.

51. Hawley JA, Burke LM. Effect of meal frequency and timing on physical performance. Br J Nutr 1997;77(Suppl):91–103.

52. Sherman WM, Brodowicz G, Wright DA, et al. Effects of 4h pre-exercise carbohydrate feedings on cycling performance. Med Sci Sports Exerc 1989;21:598–604.

53. Wright D, Sherman WM, Dernbach AR. Carbohydrate feedings before, during, or in combination improve cycling endurance performance. J Appl Physiol 1991;71:1082.

54. Neufer PD, Costill DL, Flynn MG, et al. Improvements in exercise performance: Effects of carbohydrate feedings and diet. J Appl Physiol 1987;62:983–988.

55. Foster C, Costill DL, Fink WJ. Effects of pre-exercise feedings on endurance performance. Med Sci Sports Exerc 1979;11:1–5.

56. Thomas DE, Brotherhood JR, Brand JC. Carbohydrate feeding before exercise: Effect of glycemic index. Int J Sports Med 1991;12:180–186.

57. Sparks MJ, Selig SS, Febbraio MA. Pre-exercise carbohydrate ingestion: Effect of the glycemic index on endurance exercise performance. Med Sci Sports Exerc 1998;30:844–849.

58. Febbraio MA, Stewart KL. Carbohydrate feeding before prolonged exercise: Effect of glycemic index on muscle glycogenolysis and exercise performance. J Appl Physiol 1996;81:1115–1120.

59. Gleeson M, Maughan RJ, Greenhaff PL. Comparison of the effects of pre-exercise feeding of glucose, glycerol and placebo on endurance performance and fuel homeostasis in man. Eur J Appl Physiol 1986;55:645–653.

60. Okano G, Takeda H, Morita I, et al. Effect of pre-exercise fructose ingestion on endurance performance in fed men. Med Sci Sports Exerc 1988;20:105–109.

61. Coyle EF, Coggan AC. Effectiveness of carbohydrate feeding in delaying fatigue during prolonged exercise. Sports Med 1984;1:446.

62. Hawley J, Dennis S, Noakes T. Oxidation of carbohydrate ingested during prolonged endurance exercise. Sports Med 1992;14:27.

63. Craig BW. The influence of fructose feeding on physical performance. Am J Clin Nutr 1993;58(S):815S.

64. Ivy JL, Katz AL, Cutler CL, et al. Muscle glycogen synthesis after exercise: Effect of time carbohydrate ingestion. J Appl Physiol 1988;4:1481–1485.

65. Coyle EF. Timing and method of increased carbohydrate intake to cope with heavy training, competition and recovery. J Appl Physiol 1991;9:29–52.

66. Blom PC, Hostmark AT, Vaage O, et al. Effect of different post-exercise sugar diets on the rate of muscle glycogen synthesis. Med Sci Sports Exerc 1987;19:491–496.

67. Burke LM, Collier GR, Hargreaves M. Muscle glycogen storage after prolonged exercise: Effect of the glycemic index of carbohydrate feedings. J Appl Physiol 1993;75:1019–1023.

68. Kleins B, Raben AB, Valeur AK, etc al. Benefit of simple carbohydrates on the early post-exercise muscle glycogen repletion in male athletes. Med Sci Sports Exerc 1990;22:88.

69. Coyle EF. Timing and method of increased carbohydrate intake to cope with heavy training, competition and recovery. J Sports Sci 1991;9:29–52.

70. Maughan RJ, Poole DC. The effects of a glycogen-loading regimen on the capacity to perform anaerobic exercise. Eur J Appl Physiol 1981;46:211–219.

71. Pizza FX, Flynn MG, Duscha BD, et al. A carbohydrate loading regimen improves high intensity, short duration exercise performance. Int J Sports Nutr 1995;5:110–116.

72. Rehunen S, Littsola S. Modification of the muscle-glycogen level of ice-hockey players through a drink with high carbohydrate content. Z Sportsmed 1978;2:15.

73. Pascoe DD, Gladden LB. Muscle glycogen resynthesis after short-term, high intensity exercise and resistance exercise. Sports Med 1996;21:98.

74. Roy BD, Tarnopolsky MA, MacDougall JD, et al. Effect of glucose supplement timing on protein metabolism after resistance training. J Appl Physiol 1997;82:1882–1888.

75. Roy, B., et al. The effect of oral glucose supplements on muscle protein synthesis following resistance training. Med Sci Sports Exerc 1996;28(5S):S769.

76. Food and Nutrition Board, Recommended Dietary Allowances, 10th ed., National Academy of Sciences, Washington DC, 1989;30.

77. Dohm GL, Kasperek GJ, Tapscott EG, Barakat H. Protein metabolism during endurance exercise. Fed Proc 1985;44:348–352.

78. Lemon PWR, Nagle FJ. Effects of exercise on protein and amino acid metabolism. Med Sci Sports Exerc 1981;13:141–149.

79. Friedman JE, Lemon PWR. Effect of protein intake and endurance exercise on daily protein requirements. Med Sci Sports Exerc 1985;17:231.

80. Celajowa I, Homa M. Food intake, nitrogen, and energy balance in Polish weightlifters during training camp. Nutr Metab 1970; 12:259–274.

81. Lemon PWR, Mullin JP. Effect of initial muscle glycogen levels on protein catabolism during exercise. J Appl Physiol 1980;48:624–629.

82. Stone MH, Keith R, Kearney JT, et al. Overtraining: A review of the signs and symptoms of overtraining. J Appl Sports Sci Res 1991; 5(1):35–50.

83. Tarnopolsky MA, MacDougall JD, Atkinson SA. Influence of protein intake and training status on nitrogen balance and lean body mass. J Appl Physiol 1988;64(1):187–193.

84. Lemon PWR. Protein and amino acid needs of the strength athlete. Int J Sports Nutr 1991;1:127–145.

85. Tarnopolsky MA, MacDougall JD, Atkinson SA, et al. Evaluation of protein requirements for trained strength athletes. J Appl Physiol 1992;73(5):1986–1995.

86. Tarnopolsky M, MacDougall D, Atkinson S, et al. Dietary protein requirements for body builders vs. sedentary controls. Med Sci Sports Exerc 1986;18(2):S64.

87. Lemon P, Tarnopolsky M, MacDougall J, Atkinson, S. Protein requirements and muscle mass/strength changes during intensive training in novice bodybuilders. J Appl Physiol 1992;73:767.

88. Butterfield GE. Whole body protein utilization in humans. Med Sci Sports Exerc 1987;19(Suppl):S157–S165.

89. Walberg JL, Leidy MK, Sturgill DJ, et al. Macronutrient needs in weight lifters during caloric restriction. Med Sci Sports Exerc 1987;19(2):S70.

90. Walberg JL, Leidy MK, Sturgill DJ, et al. Macronutrient content of a hypoenergy diet affects nitrogen retention and muscle function in weight lifters. Int J Sports Med 1988;9:261–266.

91. Conlee RK, Hammer RL, Winder WW, et al. Glycogen repletion and exercise endurance in rats adapted to a high fat diet. Metabolism 1990; 39:289–294.

92. Helge JW, Richter EA, Kiens B. Interaction of training and diet on metabolism and endurance during exercise in man. J Physiol 1996;492:293–306.

93. Lapachet RAB, Miller WC, Arnall DA. Body fat and exercise endurance in trained rats adapted to high-fat and/or high-carbohydrate diet. J Appl Physiol 1996;80:1173–1179.

94. Saitoh S, Matsuo T, Tagami K, et al. Effects of short-term dietary change from high fat to high carbohydrate diets on the storage and utilization of glycogen and triacylglycerol in untrained rats. Eur J Appl Physiol 1996;74:13–22.

95. Lambert EV, Speechly DP, Dennis SC, Noakes TD. Enhanced endurance in trained cyclists during moderate intensity exercise following two weeks adaptation to a high fat diet. Eur J Appl Physiol 1994;69:287–293.

96. Johannessen A, Hagen C, Galbo H. Prolactin, growth hormone, thyrotropin, 3,5,3'-triiodothyronine, and thyroxine responses to exercise after fat- and carbohydrate-enriched-diet. J Clin Endocrinol Metab 1981;52:56–61.

97. Lukaski HC, Bolonchuk WW, Klevay LM, et al. Influence of type and amount of dietary lipid on plasma lipid concentrations in endurance athletes. Am J Clin Nutr 1984;39:35–44.

98. Thompson PD, Cullinane EM, Eshelman R, et al. The effects of high-carbohydrate and high-fat diets on the serum lipid and lipoprotein concentrations of endurance athletes. Metabolism 1984;33:1003–1010.

99. Sherman WM, Leenders N. Fat loading: The next big magic bullet? Int J Sports Nutr 1995;5(Suppl):S1–S12.

100. Kiens B, Helge JW. Effect of high-fat diets on exercise performance. Proc Nutr Soc 1998;57:73–75.

101. Smith AP, Leekam S, Ralph A, McNeil G. The influence of meal composition on postlunch changes in performance efficiency and mood. Appetite 1988;10:195–203.

102. Smith AP, Miles C. Effects of lunch on selective and sustained attention. Neuropsychobiology 1986;16:117–120.

103. Lloyd HM, Green MW, Rogers PJ. Mood and cognitive performance effects of isocaloric lunches differing in fat and carbohydrate content. Physiol Behav 1994;56:51–57.

104. Wells AS, Read NW, Craig A. Influences of dietary and intraduodenal lipid on alertness, mood, and sustained concentration. Br J Nutr 1995;74:115–123.

105. Wells AS, Read NW. Influences of fat, energy, and time of day on mood and performance. Physiol Behav 1996;59(6):1069–1076.

106. Paz A, Berry EM. Effect of meal composition on alertness and performance of hospital night-shift workers. Ann Nutr Metab 1997;41:291–298.

107. Verger P, Lagarde D, Batejat D, Maitre JF. Influence of the composition of a meal taken after physical exercise on mood, vigilance, performance. Physiol Behav 1998;64(3):317–322.

108. Scott CB, Carpenter R, Taylor A, Gordon NF. Effect of macronutrient composition of an energy-restrictive diet on maximal physical performance. Med Sci Sports Exerc 1992;24(7):814–818.

109. Greenhaff PL, Gleeson M, Maughan RJ. The effects of dietary manipulation on blood acid-base status and the performance of high-intensity exercise. Eur J Appl Physiol 1987;56:331–337.

110. Kraemer WJ, Volek JS, Bush JA, et al. Hormonal responses to consecutive days of heavy-resistance exercise with or without nutritional supplementation. J Appl Physiol 1998;85(4):1544–1555.

111. Florini JR. Hormonal control of muscle cell growth. J Anim Sci 1985;61:21–37.

112. Forbes GB, Brown MR, Welle SL, Underwood LE. Hormonal response to overfeeding. Am J Clin Nutr 1989;49:608–611.

113. Thissen JP, Ketelslegers JM, Underwood LE. Nutritional regulation of the insulin-like growth factors. Endocr Rev 1994;15:80–101.

114. Hamalainen EH, Aldercreutz P, Pietinen P. Diet and serum sex hormones in healthy men. J Steroid Biochem 1984;20:459–464.

115. Chandler RM, Byrne HK, Patterson JG, Ivy JL. Dietary supplements affect the anabolic hormones after weight-training exercise. J Appl Physiol 1994;76:839–845.

116. Fahey TD, Hoffman K, Colvin W, Lauten G. The effects of intermittent liquid meal feeding on selected hormones and substrates during intense weight training. Int J Sports Nutr 1993;3:67–75.

117. Volek JS, Kraemer WJ, Bush JA, et al. Testosterone and cortisol in relationship to dietary nutrients and resistance exercise. J Appl Physiol 1997;82(1):49–54.

118. McCargar LJ, Clandinin MT, Belcastro AN, Walker K. Dietary carbohydrate-to-fat ratio: influence on whole-body nitrogen retention, substrate utilization, and hormone response in healthy male subjects. Am J Clin Nutr 1989;49:1169–1178.

119. Raben A, Kiens B, Richter EA, et al. Serum sex hormones and endurance performance after a lacto-ovo vegetarian and a mixed diet. Med Sci Sports Exerc 1992;24:1290–1297.

120. Aloi JA, Bergendahl M, Iranmanesh A, et al. Pulsatile intravenous gonadotropin-releasing hormone administration averts fasting-induced hypogonadotropism and hypoandrogenemia in healthy, normal weight men. J Clin Endocrinol Metab 1997;82(5):1543–1548.

121. Marniemi J, Vuori I, Kinnunen V, et al. Metabolic changes induced by combined prolonged exercise and low-calorie intake in man. Eur J Appl Physiol Occup Physiol 1984;53(2):121–127.

122. Yost TJ, Jensen DR, Haugen BR, Eckel RH. Effect of dietary macronutrient composition on tissue-specific lipoprotein lipase activity and insulin action in normal-weight subjects. Am J Clin Nutr 1998;68:296–302.

123. Lovejoy J, DiGirolamo M. Habitual dietary intake and insulin sensitivity in lean and obese adults. Am J Clin Nutr 1992;55:1174–1179.

124. Chen M, Bergman RN, Porte D. Insulin resistance and B-cell dysfunction in aging: The importance of dietary carbohydrate. J Clin Endocrinol Metab 1988;67:951–957.

125. Keim NL, Van Loan MD, Horn WF, et al. Weight loss is greater with consumption of large morning meals and fat-free mass is preserved with large evening meals in women on a controlled weight reduction regimen. J Nutr 1997;127(1):75–82.

126. Forslund AH, El-Khoury AE, Olsson RM, et al. Effect of protein intake and physical activity on 24-h pattern and rate of macronutrient utilization. Am J Physiol 1999;276:E964–E976.

127. Alford BB, Blankenship AC, Hagen RD. The effects of variations in carbohydrate, protein, and fat content of the diet upon weight loss, blood values, and nutrient intake of adult obese women. J Am Diet Assoc 1990;90(4):534–540.

128. Golay A, Allaz AF, Morel Y, et al. Similar weight loss with low- or high-carbohydrate diets. Am J Clin Nutr 1996;63(2):174–178.

129. Tremblay A, Buemann B. Exercise-training, macronutrient balance and body weight control. Int J Obes 1995;19:79–86.

130. Harvey-Berino J. The efficacy of dietary fat vs. total energy restriction for weight loss. Obes Res 1998;6:202–207.

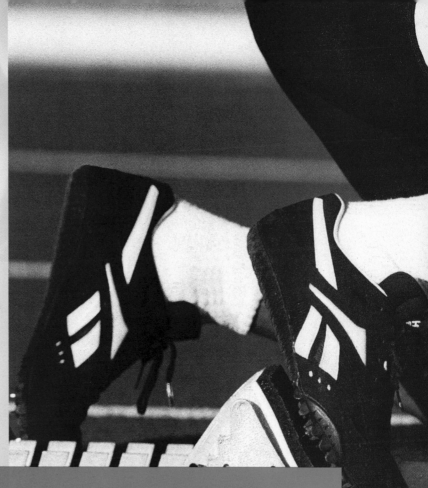

CHAPTER

3

Skeletal Muscle Mass, Strength, and Speed

Conrad P. Earnest and Chris Street

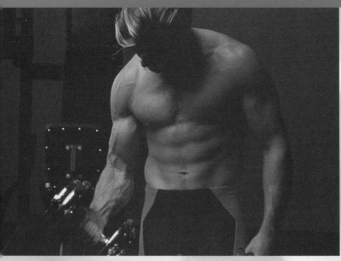

Research Review

Creatine Ingestion Augments Intramuscular Creatine Levels

The present study was undertaken to test whether creatine given as a supplement to normal subjects was absorbed, and if continued, increased the total creatine pool in muscle. An additional effect of exercise upon uptake into muscle was also investigated.

Low doses (≤1 g of creatine monohydrate in water) produced only a modest rise in the plasma creatine concentration, whereas 5 g resulted in a mean peak after 1 hour of 795 (SD, 104) μmol/L in three subjects weighing 76 to 87 kg. Repeated dosing with 5 g every 2 hours sustained the plasma concentration at around 1000 μmol/L. A single 5-g dose corresponds to the creatine content of 1.1 kg of fresh, uncooked steak.

Supplementation with 5 g of creatine monohydrate, four or six times a day for 2 or more days resulted in a significant increase in the total creatine content of the quadriceps femoris muscle measured in 17 subjects. This was greatest in subjects with a low initial total creatine content and the effect was to raise the content in these subjects closer to the upper limit of the normal range. In some, the increase was as much as 50%.

Uptake into muscle was greatest during the first 2 days of supplementation, accounting for 32% of the dose administered in three subjects receiving 6 × 5 g of creatine monohydrate/day. In these subjects renal excretion was 40, 61, and 68% of the creatine dose over the first 3 days. Approximately 20% or more of the creatine absorbed was measured as phosphocreatine. No changes were apparent in the muscle ATP content.

Harris RC, Soderlund K. Elevation of creatine in resting and exercised muscle of normal subjects by creatine supplementation. Hultman E Clin Sci (Colch) 1992;83:367–374.

Creatine

To increase muscle mass, strength, and power, one of the goals of training is to manipulate and increase the training stimulus or the physical work that is performed. At its essence, physical training depends on the coordinated balance between an imposed physical stressor, the manipulation of training variables (volume, intensity, and frequency), adequate rest intervals, and recovery between training sessions. Recovery is perhaps the most difficult to manipulate and gauge owing to the amount of time necessary to achieve it. Furthermore, barring the use of anabolic steroids for muscle repair and growth,[1] nutritional interventions are often necessary to promote a more efficient recovery following training. Although many supplements have been extolled for their *anabolic* and *ergogenic* effects, to date, only a few have withstood the rigors of science. The most notable of these is creatine monohydrate (creatine). Though most other supplements do not elicit as powerful an effect as creatine, a few are worthy of notation and future research efforts.

Bioenergetics: A Rationale for Creatine Supplementation

To fully understand the use of creatine as an ergogenic aid, one must appreciate its role in energy metabolism. In this regard, a primary objective for students to understand is that skeletal muscle performs mechanical work through the hydrolysis of adenosine triphosphate (ATP). Commonly referred to as the *energy currency* of a cell, the quantity of ATP present in skeletal muscle is approximately 3 to 5 μmol/g or 6 mmol/kg of fresh muscle.[2,3] The continuation of physical work is based on the maintenance of ATP at a rate equal to the rate of its use. Energy reserves consist of intramuscular phosphagen stores (ATP, phosphocreatine [PCr]) and muscle and liver glycogen and adipose stores. The rate and the extent to which these energy sources are used depends on the intensity and/or duration of exercise. To this end, high-intensity anaerobic exercise is supplied almost exclusively by ATP, PCr, and intramuscular glycogen stores (FIG. 3-1).

In a classic series demonstrating the shift of energy usage in skeletal muscle, Hirvonen et al.[4,5] examined the changes in the intramuscular concentrations of muscle ATP, PCr, and blood lactic acid concentration in sprinters running distances of 40 to 400 meters lasting approximately 4.5 to 50 seconds (FIG. 3-2). Blood lactic acid is a reflection of muscle glycogen usage or glycolysis. Even on casual observation it is interesting to note that despite the increase in running distance, ATP stores initially decline but appear to reach a minimal or *critical* level after which no further decrease is observed. In contrast, PCr continually and rapidly decreases while the appearance of blood lactic acid or muscle glycogen usage increases. At this point, the reader should embrace two key points. One is to recognize the immediate contribution of all energy systems simultaneously and cooperatively to facilitate energy needs. These energy contributions do not occur sequentially (i.e., one after the other), but instead are time and intensity dependent as to which system dominates. This continued energy production has been conceptualized as a *metabolic flux*[2] or *energy currency*[6] that transforms stored energy into muscle contraction.

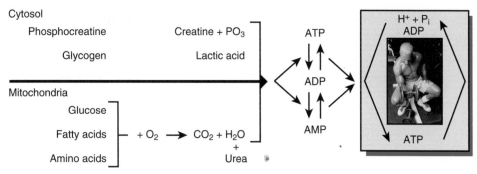

Figure 3-1. Schematic of cellular energetics reflecting the ongoing process of maintaining cellular ATP concentrations to allow the continuation of physical work.

The maximum work attainable from any energy source can be characterized as both ATP capacity (amount of ATP produced per mole of available substrate) and ATP power (the rate of ATP produced per substrate storage depot). Despite the low intramuscular stores of ATP and PCr within skeletal muscle, their energy production capabilities are exceptional (TABLE 3-1). A review by Sahlin[7] provides an excellent consensus of research findings elaborating on the available energy capacity (mol ATP), maximal ATP power produced from each source (per mmol ATP/kg of dry muscle), as well as the exercise intensity supported and duration of activity allowed per endogenous energy source. It should become readily apparent that events of shorter duration and higher intensity necessitate physical training and nutritional support aimed toward the enhancement of ATP, PCr, and muscle glycogen as opposed to alternative energy sources such as liver glycogen and adipose stores. These sources serve as less adequate sources of ATP power.

Research has shown an improvement in endogenous energy stores of glycogen, PCr, and ATP following 5 months of heavy resistance training (FIG. 3-3),[8] although

this correlation has not been universally shown.[9] Although changes in resting PCr concentrations might enhance performance during anaerobic activities (e.g., sprinting, weightlifting, etc.), increases in skeletal muscle glycogen may not confer a similar advantage in these types of activities. Strong evidence shows that the dietary manipulation of glycogen stores does not improve various anaerobic performance indices.[10–12] Also, oral ATP administration does not appear to be prudent owing to the presence of phosphatase enzymes in the blood and gut. These enzymes readily cleave the phosphate portions of ATP. Thus, it appears that oral ATP does not present itself as a suitable ergogenic aid. The same point may be argued for PCr as well. Thus, it is plausible that creatine ingestion may be the best way of augmenting athletic performance vis-à-vis changes in the phosphagen energy system.

One study that examined PCr supplementation[13] showed a performance benefit, albeit to a smaller degree than creatine supplementation. However, any effect of orally ingested PCr would be expected to be mediated by creatine alone because gut phosphatase enzymes would readily cleave off the phosphate portion of the molecule,

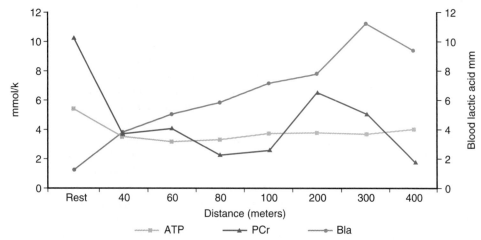

Figure 3-2. Energy contribution from ATP, phosphocreatine, and muscle glycogen, as represented by the appearance of blood lactic acid during various sprinting distances. Data from Hirvonen J, Rehunen S, Rusko H, Harkonen M. Breakdown of high-energy phosphate compounds and lactate accumulation during short supramaximal exercise. Eur J Appl Physiol 1987;56:253–259 and Hirvonen J, Nummela A, Rusko H, et al. Fatigue and changes of ATP, creatine phosphate, and lactate during the 400-m sprint. Can J Sport Sci 1992;17:141–144.

Table 3-1 **Endogenous Energy Stores and their ATP Capacity, ATP Power, Exercise Intensity Supported, and the Length of Time that Exercise is Aided for Each Depot**

	ATP produced per mol dm	mmol ATP produced per kg dm	Exercise intensity supported	Length of time work is supported
ATP	0.02	11.2	Very high	1–2 sec
Phosphocreatine	0.34	8.6	Very high	30 sec
Muscle Glycogen	5.2	5.2	High	7 min
Liver Glycogen	70	2.7	Moderate	90 min
Adipose Stores	8000	1.4	Low	350 theoretical

liberating free creatine in a smaller quantity than when taking the monohydrate form. To date, no human studies have evaluated PCr's oral absorption and intramuscular uptake. Additionally, blood serum also possesses high phosphatase activity, leading to rapid breakdown of intravenously administered PCr to creatine and phosphate.[14] A study by Peeters et al. determined that PCr-supplemented subjects exhibited a performance response that was approximately 50% less than than that of a creatine monohydrate group.[13] Given that the creatine portion of the monohydrate form makes up about 92% of the molecule and only 50% of the PCr molecule, these results are not surprising. Similarly, although glycolysis is initiated at muscle contraction, increasing glycogen stores may be more advantageous to longer, high-intensity work efforts (>400 m) because of its lower ATP power.[7] These same objectives do not appear to apply to the use of creatine supplementation because both early and more recent studies involving creatine show that it is readily found in food, is absorbed intact, appears rapidly in the blood, and increases intramuscular stores of total creatine and PCr.[15–27]

Effect of PCr on Energetics and Fatigue

PCr's major cellular function is to maintain metabolic flux during the early onset of exercise and high-intensity work performance. Given the observed greater ATP production associated with PCr,[7] and coupled with the

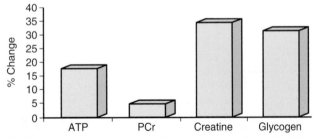

Figure 3-3. Percent changes of endogenous energy depots in skeletal muscle following 5 months of weight training. Data from MacDougall JD, Ward GR, Sale DG, Sutton JR. Biochemical adaptation of human skeletal muscle to heavy resistance training and immobilization. J Appl Physiol 1977;43:700–703.

increase in PCr associated with creatine supplementation,[23] the potential for an increase in anaerobic work output is fully justifiable. Moreover, the maintenance of PCr concentrations appears to correlate well with the development of fatigue in that its decrease is associated with a decline in muscular force.[28] Infante et al.[29] showed a direct relationship between external work and PCr breakdown in the frog rectus abdominis muscle. Spande and Schottelius[30] also showed a direct relationship between force production and PCr stores in isolated mouse soleus muscle that was tetanically stimulated. In this model, they observed a decline in PCr that was directly proportional to the development and maintenance of isometric tetanic force.

In humans, Hirvonen et al.[4,5] concluded that the slowing of running speed during maximal work efforts is related to a decline in the energy production brought forth from ATP and PCr. This effect may be a result of muscle fiber type differences in the endogenous stores of each substrate. This premise is supported by the observations of others who have noted that type II muscle fibers possess higher initial levels of PCr and, consequently, greater rates of PCr usage than do type I muscle fibers during high-intensity exercise.[31–34] PCr and glycogen recovery also appears to be slower in type II fibers following high-intensity exercise.[35] Moreover, PCr resynthesis during recovery has been shown to be an oxygen-dependent process that exhibits a two-component or biphasic pattern. The first (fast component) has a half-time of approximately 22 seconds, whereas the second (slow component) is longer than 170 seconds.[36] During continuous or intermittent high-intensity exercise, the resynthesis rate of PCr plays an important role in the force capabilities that active muscle can generate owing to the heavy reliance on PCr and ATP.

When PCr levels are not given adequate recovery time, performance is impaired and power output is decreased.[37–40] Conversely, when recovery is prolonged, increased PCr concentration is correlated with greater power output during consecutive-cycle ergometer sprints when rest periods of either 90 or 180 seconds are allowed.[39] Thus, the possibility of creatine supplementation increasing PCr recovery is important because it is the recovery of PCr following high-intensity exercise that allows athletes to continue high-intensity activity more effectively. If it is possible to increase the rate of resynthesis and PCr storage capacity through supplementation, then the use of creatine has a valid physiological base from which to assess utility.

Endogenous Synthesis, Dietary Ingestion, and Total Body Pool

During the early 20th century it was first observed that not all of the creatine ingested by animals and humans could be recovered in the urine as creatinine. This suggested that some of the creatine was retained in the body. Folin and Denis[20–22,41,42] were among the first to determine that the creatine content of the muscles in cats increased up to 70% after creatine ingestion. Creatine in humans was soon discovered to be present in skeletal and cardiac muscle, uterine and intestinal tissue, the testes, brain, kidney, nervous tissue, and sperm, as well as in adipose stores.[18–22,24,43,44] Ninety-five percent of the total creatine pool is found in skeletal muscle tissue, with the remaining 5% stored in the heart, brain, neural tissues, and testes. Normal intramuscular values for total creatine are approximately 124.4 mmol/kg (free creatine, 49.0 mmol/kg; PCr, 75.5 mmol/kg). In 1927, Fiske and Subbarow reported the discovery of a *labile phosphorus* in the resting muscle of cats, which was subsequently called phosphorylcreatine or, simply, PCr.[45] This group further observed that, during the electrical stimulation of skeletal muscle, PCr diminished only to *reappear* during recovery.

Three amino acids are involved in the synthesis of creatine: arginine, glycine, and methionine. The synthesis of creatine begins with the transfer of the amidine group from arginine to glycine, forming guanidinoacetate and ornithine. This reaction is reversibly catalyzed by the enzyme transamidinase. Creatine is then formed by a nonreversible reaction involving the addition of a methyl group from S-adenosylmethionine, with a methyl transferase being required for this process. This step is known as transmethylation. In humans, *de novo* synthesis (pathway synthesizing a biomolecule from simple precursor molecules) of creatine takes place via enzymes located in the liver, pancreas, and kidneys and involves the transport to skeletal muscle by the bloodstream after formation. The total creatine pool in humans is dictated by the combined content of creatine found in both its free and phosphorylated (PCr) form. Of the 95% of the total creatine pool found in skeletal muscle, approximately 40% is free creatine and 60% is PCr.

Once in skeletal muscle, creatine and PCr are effectively trapped and cannot exit the cell until creatine and PCr are degraded to creatinine via a nonreversible, nonenzymatic process.[46–48] Creatinine is thus filtered in the kidneys and ultimately excreted in the urine.[49] In the absence of dietary intake, normal creatine turnover to creatine is estimated to be about 1.6% per day.[48] Therefore, in a 70-kg person, the total creatine pool is approximately 120 g, with a total daily turnover of 2 g/day. The body's creatine pool is maintained via endogenous synthesis and dietary intake (e.g., meat). Although synthesized endogenously, vegetarians or those partaking in a creatine-*free* diet typically have low intramuscular levels compared with meat consumers.[23,50,51] Like all bodily functions, creatine metabolism is elegantly regulated by feedback and feedforward mechanisms.[52,53]

When ingested in the diet, creatine is obtained primarily from muscle tissues (meat or fish), with only trace amounts found in plants. For example, there are about 1.4 to 2.3 g of creatine per pound of meat (beef, pork) or fish (tuna, salmon, cod). Herring contains about 3 to 4.5 g of creatine per pound.[54] The average intake of creatine in a mixed diet is approximately 1.5 to 2.0 g/day in meat consumers. The daily needs of vegetarians are met almost exclusively through endogenous pathways.[55] Although it could be speculated that creatine could be sufficiently ingested in a diet heavy in meat products, it has recently been noted that the creatine content in meat decreases with cooking.[56] When dietary availability of creatine is low, endogenous synthesis of creatine is increased to maintain normal levels. On the other hand, when dietary availability of creatine is increased, endogenous creatine synthesis is temporarily suppressed.[44,54] Whether produced in the body or ingested, creatine is transported to its primary target tissue (i.e., skeletal muscle) via the circulation, in which uptake takes place through a concentration gradient and/or a specific creatine transporter.

The structural and functional characteristics of creatine transport to muscle have only recently been described. Creatine appears to enter several types of cells by sodium-dependent neurotransmitter transport family related to the taurine transporter and members of the subfamily of the γ-aminobutyrate/betaine transporters.[57–59] Furthermore, creatine uptake appears to be enhanced in the presence of insulin[25,60] and triiodothyronine,[61] but depressed in the presence of the drugs ouabain or digoxin[57] and vitamin E deficiency.[62] It has also been shown that creatine uptake does not appear to be influenced by PCr, creatinine, ornithine, glycine, glutamic acid, histidine, alanine, arginine, leucine, methionine, or cysteine concentrations.[63,64]

The saturable active transport of creatine is highly specific regarding sodium dependence and extracellular creatine concentration.[65–67] During uptake, two sodium ions are transported into the cell for every creatine molecule, with the K_m (Michaelis constant) for sodium being 55 mM. The K_m for creatine uptake ranges from 40 to 90 μm in the rat brain.[64] In humans, normal K_m in monocytes and macrophages appears to be approximately 30 μM.[63] Human red blood cell creatine uptake appears to be unaffected by an extracellular pH range of 6.9 to 7.9.[68]

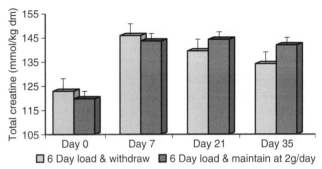

Figure 3-4. Tissue saturation effects demonstrating 6 days of creatine loading at 20 g/day followed by complete withdrawal (*shaded bars*) or continued supplementation at 2 g/day (*solid bars*). Data from Hultman E, Soderlund K. Muscle creatine loading in men. J Appl Physiol 1996;81:232–237.

In myoblasts (precursors of skeletal muscle cells), the sodium-dependent uptake of creatine *in vitro* is sensitive to extracellular creatine concentrations.[69] In this study, cultured myoblasts, maintained for 24 hours in a medium containing creatine, exhibited one-third of the uptake activity of cells bathed for the same duration in a medium lacking creatine. Under normal physiological conditions, the maximum intracellular total creatine pool proposed is about 150 mmol/kg.[23,70] Creatine supplementation data by Harris et al.[23] showed that the maximal total creatine pool (creatine and PCr) in creatine-supplemented participants ranged between 140 and 160 mmol/kg. Once maximized via supplementation, the total creatine pool appears to remain elevated for approximately 21 days without further supplementation. Intramuscular creatine concentration can be maintained beyond 21 days with small amounts (3 g/day or 0.03 g/kg) of creatine (orally ingested) (FIG. 3-4).[71] In support of these observations, one study to date has demonstrated that following a 5-day *loading* period (typifying the supplemental saturation protocol), performance measures remain elevated for 21 days even without continued supplementation (FIG. 3-5).[72]

Typically, the loading phase is divided into four equal servings per day that consist of approximately 5 g daily for

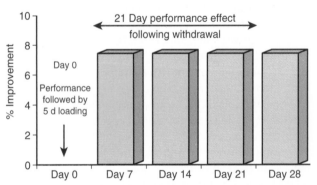

Figure 3-5. Data showing performance benefits following a 5-day creatine loading procedure followed by 28 days of withdrawal. Data from Ziegenfuss T, Gales D, Felix S, et al. Performance benefits following a 5-day creatine loading procedure persist for at least 4 weeks. Med Sci Sports Exerc 1998;30(Suppl):S265.

1 week (0.30 g/kg). Furthermore, Green et al.[25,73] have shown that creatine plus 75 or more grams of simple carbohydrate increase creatine uptake over taking creatine alone. Recent data from Stout et al.[74] show that this effect might also occur with lower quantities of carbohydrate (35 g); however, the addition of caffeine might hinder the effects of creatine.[75] Nonetheless, if an athlete can increase the amount of intramuscular creatine, and more importantly PCr, he or she should experience an improvement in anaerobic power and capacity. As previously stated, the availability of PCr is generally accepted to be one of the primary limitations to muscle performance during high-intensity, short-duration exercise.[41,76,77]

Anaerobic Performance Lasting Less Than 30 Seconds

In the first performance-related study using creatine, Greenhaff et al.[78] showed an improvement in muscle torque during repeated bouts of isokinetic work with creatine supplementation. These responses were attributed to an increased capacity for ATP resynthesis from ADP and PCr. This rationale is further supported by data that show that plasma ammonia levels are lower and thus point to a more efficient use of adenine nucleotide stores (ATP, adenosine 5'-diphosphate [ADP], adenosine monophosphate [AMP]) in the creatine group. Plasma ammonia concentration is associated with the use of total adenine nucleotide stores and is most prominent during high-intensity work efforts when adenosine monophosphate is degraded to inosine 5' monophosphate and adenosine is broken down to inosine.[79] Thus, decreased plasma ammonia concentrations reflect the intracellular maintenance of ATP.

In a replicative study of Gaitanos et al.,[80] Balsom et al.[81] further showed that creatine administration could improve power output during intermittent bouts of high-intensity cycling. In subjects who performed 10 repeated 6-second bouts of intense cycling interspersed with 30 seconds of rest, Gaitanos et al.[80] determined that the energy required to sustain mean power output during the first 6-second bout was provided equally from PCr degradation and anaerobic glycolysis. These conclusions were deduced from the observation that PCr stores fell by 57%, whereas muscle lactic acid concentrations increased to 28.6 mmol/kg of dry weight. During the tenth sprint, however, there was no change in muscle lactate concentration, and the mean power output was reduced to 73% of that generated by the first sprint. In contrast, the contribution of PCr to ATP production was calculated at nearly 80% in the final sprint and was subsequently reduced to the same extent as that of the first sprint. Because of the observed reduction in power output and contribution of anaerobic glycolysis, it was postulated that ATP resynthesis was mainly derived from PCr and oxidative metabolism.

To examine these observations in the accompaniment of creatine supplementation, Balsom et al.[81] studied subjects performing the same cycling sequence as did the subjects in the study by Gaitanos et al.,[80] using workloads of approximately 820 watts and 880 watts. Using a double-blind protocol, subjects were randomly assigned to either creatine or placebo. The results of this study demonstrated both a decrease in blood lactic acid concentration and the accumulation of hypoxanthine at both power outputs in the creatine-supplemented group. Hypoxanthine is a blood-borne marker of adenine nucleotide breakdown during high-intensity activity and is the intermediate step when inosine is further degraded into xanthine and uric acid.[79] Despite the experimental group's ability to maintain a higher work output for a longer period of time, a small, yet significant decrease in VO_2 was recognized in the creatine group during the 820-watt trial. Therefore, the lower levels of blood lactate concentration, coupled with lower hypoxanthine, suggest the preferential use of PCr versus ATP power generated from anaerobic glycolysis. This study also showed that creatine induced a significant increase in body mass after only 6 days of supplementation. The greater body mass was speculated to be a result, in part, of an increased type II muscle fiber size. Type II muscle fiber hypertrophy has been previously observed in patients with gyrate atrophy.[82] This combination of increased body mass and lower oxygen consumption demonstrates that creatine has a role in skeletal muscle hypertrophy and a bioenergetic role as a spacial (cytosolic) energy shuttle between the mitochondria and working musculature.[83–88]

In a follow-up study, Soderlund et al.[89] investigated whether changes in muscle metabolism occurred with creatine supplementation. They used a protocol that consisted of five 6-second work bouts on a cycle ergometer, interspersed with 30-second rest periods. Then, after the fifth 6-second bout, an additional 10-second bout was performed as subjects tried to maintain a pedal frequency of 140 rpm. Post-test trials were performed after each participant consumed 20 g (4×5 g/day^{-1}) of creatine for 6 days. Data analysis from this study revealed higher PCr concentration, lower blood lactate concentration, and a greater maintenance of intensity in 10-second work bouts in the creatine group.

Birch et al.[90] also used a protocol consisting of three 30-second bouts of isokinetic cycling interspersed with 4 minutes of rest to examine peak and mean power output, total work output, plasma ammonia concentration, and blood lactic acid concentration following creatine supplementation. Peak power increased by 8% in bout 1, and mean power output increased by 6% for bouts 1 and 2. In contrast to similar study results, no differences were noted for blood lactic acid concentration, although the peak plasma ammonia concentration was lower after creatine ingestion.[89]

Creatine supplementation appears to facilitate muscle PCr resynthesis during recovery from maximal exercise in individuals who demonstrate a 20-mmol/kg (2.62-mg/kg) dry muscle or greater increase in muscle creatine accumulation with supplementation.[42] Recent studies have demonstrated that the extent of PCr resynthesis during recovery following a single bout of maximal exercise is positively correlated with exercise performance during a subsequent bout of exercise.[39,41] Thus, these studies show that creatine occupies a pivotal role in the regulation and homeostasis of skeletal muscle energy metabolism and fatigue. Recent data indicate that the positive effect of creatine supplementation on maximal performance is mediated by increasing PCr availability, principally in fast-contracting muscle (type II) fibers[41]; thus, this supports the notion that PCr depletion in fast muscle fibers limits exercise performance under these conditions.[41,76] Recent investigations have also shown creatine to have an effect on singular, continuous bouts of exercise from 130 to 250 seconds,[91–93] thus challenging the *traditional* time constraints bestowed on PCr muscle energetics.

Creatine supplementation has variable effects in individuals with different levels of athletic participation. Harris et al.[94] used both trained and untrained participants and showed that a greater percentage of creatine uptake was demonstrated in the untrained cohort. Therefore, it appears that in well-trained athletes with high levels of intramuscular adenine nucleotide and phosphagen stores, supplementation may have little effect. Moreover, it is generally accepted that untrained athletes who participate in high-intensity, short-duration activities will increase intramuscular ATP, PCr, and glycogen stores through training.[8,95] Therefore, a population that both taxes and increases its phosphagen stores through training may exhibit little or no response to supplementation because endogenous stores may already be at maximal levels.

In light of research data suggesting that maximal creatine accumulation is attained within 3 to 5 days after the loading phase,[23] it is of interest to explore the effects of long-term (chronic) supplementation. The first study to investigate chronic creatine use examined the effects of 28 days of creatine supplementation (5 g taken 4 times daily) in experienced (mean = 10 yrs) resistance-trained males.[96] After 14 days of creatine use, subjects were able to perform significantly greater work on a series of three maximal anaerobic sprint bouts (stationary bicycle). After 28 days of creatine supplementation, dynamic muscular strength as well as the maximum number of complete repetitions performed using a weight 70% of the 1-repetition maximum (RM) amount (total lifting volume [TLV]) improved.

In a longer study, untrained sedentary females received creatine supplements at 5 g taken 4 times daily for 4 days, followed by 2.5 g taken twice daily for 70 days.[97] During the latter *maintenance* period, the women underwent a resistance-training program (1-hour sessions 3 times weekly). After the 4-day creatine-loading period no significant improvement in arm (biceps) endurance was seen; however, after 5 and 10 weeks of low-dose creatine, arm torque was significantly greater. Similarly, measurements of 1-RM strength with leg press, leg extension, and squat were significantly greater in the creatine group, with less striking increases in bench press and leg curl, and no difference in the shoulder press movement. After stopping the resistance-training program, a smaller group of subjects (7 of the original group who had received creatine) continued to take 5 g of creatine daily for an additional 10 weeks. Although continued creatine usage did not prevent arm torque from declining to pre-training values, it appeared to delay the decrease in strength compared with the placebo group.

Chronic creatine supplementation in NCAA Division I football players during off-season training produced significant increases in several performance variables.[98] Subjects taking a creatine mixture (5.25 g of creatine taken 3 times daily for 28 days) displayed increases in TLV for the bench press, but not for squat or power clean movements. Muscular work performed during a series of 12 maximal cycle sprints was significantly greater during only the first 5 bouts, with a trend for increased average total accumulated work in the creatine group. Similar results have also been noted in training groups following a protocol of similar length.[74,99,100]

Influence on Performance Variables Greater Than 30 Seconds

Harris et al.[101] further demonstrated that oral creatine supplementation improved cumulative repeated running times following 300 m (4×300 m; -1.5 sec; $p < 0.05$) and 1000 m (4×1000 m; -13.0 sec; $p < 0.05$). Individual running times for the final measured repeat run times improved as well. Final 300-m running time decreased by 0.7 second and 1000-m running time decreased by 5.5 seconds. However, one criticism of this study is that all subjects were asked to run at 90–95% of their maximal effort. Each running pace was therefore dictated by the subjective opinion of each runner. Although a threat to the study's internal validity, these are intriguing findings because traditionally, PCr's primary contribution to ATP maintenance takes place within approximately the first 10 seconds of intense physical exertion. Because PCr may aid ATP resynthesis for up to 3 minutes[102] (albeit in a decreasing role with time and intensity of work) and may also act as an energy shuttle between the mitochondria and myofibrils,[86–88] the efficacy of creatine as an ergogenic aid during longer anaerobic work bouts may be warranted.

In an early study, Balsom et al.[103] investigated the effects of creatine supplementation on endurance exercise performance. Performed in a double-blind manner,[18] habitually active to well-trained male subjects were evenly divided into treatment and placebo groups. After completing a standard VO_{2max} test, each subject performed pre- and post-test runs as follows: a) a treadmill run to exhaustion at 120% of VO_{2max} designed to elicit fatigue between 3 and 6 minutes, and b) a terrain run of ~6 km on a forest track. Following 6 days of creatine supplementation, no significant differences in time to exhaustion, terrain runs, or VO_{2max} were noted between groups and it was thus concluded that creatine supplementation clearly had no effect on endurance performance. However, other reports of anaerobic running performance suggest that creatine may or may not improve exhaustive work bouts that last between 40 and 240 seconds.

A study by Earnest et al.[91] sought to determine if creatine supplementation would improve intermediate-length anaerobic treadmill running. In this study,[11] male subjects randomly and blindly received a creatine or glucose placebo at 20 g/day $\times$ 4 days and 10 g/day $\times$ 6 days. Following 2 weeks of rehearsal, subjects performed two exhaustive runs, separated by 8 minutes of recovery, at individually prescribed grades. Time to exhaustion for independent runs, for both runs combined (total time to exhaustion), and blood lactic acid concentration were examined for each run. Significant treatment effects on group estimates of total time to exhaustion were noted. Overall, running times in the creatine group improved more during the second run (3.2 sec; $p = 0.07$), were negligible for the first run (1.5 sec), yet were significantly greater for total time to exhaustion (4.7 sec; $p < 0.05$).

In a follow-up to this investigation, Smith et al.[93] examined the effect of creatine ingestion on a) time to exhaustion during intense exercise bouts used to establish the work rate-time relationship, and b) the estimates of anaerobic capacity and critical power in a larger population. Fifteen (eight male and seven female) recreationally active university students were randomly assigned and completed three phases of cycle ergometer testing, including the following: 1) familiarization—three learning trials to establish subsequent work rates; 2) four baseline trials that elicited fatigue within 1 to 10 min (pre); and 3) four experimental trials (post) after 5 days of either creatine (4×5 g/day) or placebo (PL; 4×6 g/day) ingestion given in a double-blind manner. ANCOVA revealed a significant effect for creatine on anaerobic capacity ($p = 0.03$) but not critical power ($p = 0.051$). Within-group time to exhaustion was also significantly different for creatine at the two highest work rates. Effect sizes for W3 and W4 were 0.86 and 0.87, respectively. At work bouts of 357 and 268 watts, time to exhaustion increased from 93 seconds to 103 seconds ($p = 0.04$) and 236 seconds to 253 seconds ($p = 0.02$), respectively. Furthermore, anaerobic capacity increased from 17.6 to 20.2 kJ ($p = 0.03$).

The results of these last two studies suggest that creatine supplementation will improve shorter bouts of anaerobic work as well as longer exercise bouts lasting up to approximately 4 minutes. Although these results appear to remain consistent on a cycle ergometer, similar results obtained on the treadmill yield a conflict in the results. Creatine's efficacy during longer anaerobic work tasks is

Creatine Supplementation in Athletes

Richard Kreider, PhD, FACSM

Over the years, numerous nutritional supplements have been purported to affect physiological responses to exercise, enhance training adaptations, and/or improve exercise performance. Although research has generally indicated that many of these nutrients do not affect performance, creatine has consistently proven to be one of the most effective nutritional supplements available to athletes. To date, over 200 research studies have evaluated the safety and effectiveness of short- and/or long-term creatine supplementation in various untrained, trained, and diseased populations. The majority of these studies indicate that short-term creatine supplementation (0.3 g/kg/day for 5 to 7 days) increases muscle creatine and phosphocreatine content by 10–30%, has the ability to improve the ability to maintain high-intensity single effort and/or repetitive sprint performance, and may improve work output during repeated sets of muscle contractions. There is also evidence that creatine supplementation may affect exercise bouts involving anaerobic glycolysis (30 to 150 sec) and high-intensity endurance exercise (150 to 600 sec). The improved exercise capacity has been attributed to a creatine-stimulated enhancement of the phosphagen energy system, the buffering of acidity, and the shuttling of mitochondrial ATP by phosphocreatine into the cytoplasm. Additionally, long-term creatine supplementation during training (e.g., 0.3 g/kg/day for 5–7 days followed by 0.03 to 0.3 g/kg/day) has been reported to increase strength, sprint performance, and training volume, and promote greater gains in fat-free mass and muscle fiber diameter. These findings suggest that creatine supplementation may improve the quality of training, leading to greater training adaptations. Although not all studies report ergogenic benefit, it is my view that, with the exception of carbohydrate, creatine is the most effective nutritional supplement for athletes involved in high-intensity exercise bouts that rely on anaerobic energy systems.

Although creatine has been reported to be an effective ergogenic aid, there have been some concerns regarding the medical safety of creatine supplementation. Some reports, primarily in the popular media, suggest that creatine supplementation may adversely affect renal and liver function, cause long-term suppression of creatine synthesis, alter fluid and electrolyte status—promoting dehydration and muscle cramping, and/or increase the incidence of musculoskeletal injury in athletes. Additionally, some have expressed concern regarding possible side effects of long-term creatine use. Note that there is no evidence from well-controlled short- and/or long-term clinical studies (up to 5 yrs) to support any of these concerns. Furthermore, a number of recent studies that have attempted to evaluate the validity of these concerns have found no adverse effects of short- or long-term creatine supplementation on markers of clinical status.

This said, the question still remains as to whether athletes should take creatine to enhance performance. After extensively evaluating the literature, Williams et al. (1999) concluded the following in their book, *Creatine: The Power Supplement* (available at http://www.humankinetics.com). Individuals contemplating creatine supplementation should also be fully aware of the potential benefits and risks of taking the supplement so that an informed decision can be made. Adolescent athletes involved in serious training should consider creatine supplementation only with the approval and supervision of parents, trainers, coaches, and qualified health professionals. If the athlete plans to take creatine, quality supplements should be purchased from reputable vendors. Athletic administrators in organized sports who want to establish policies on creatine supplementation for teams should base such policies on the scientific literature. Any formal administration policy should be supervised by a qualified health professional. Although more research is needed, available studies indicate that creatine supplementation does not appear to pose a health risk when taken at recommended doses and may provide therapeutic benefits for various medical populations.

Williams MH, Kreider RB, Branch JD. Creatine: The Power Supplement. Champaign, IL: Human Kinetics Publishers, 1999.

---

not easily conceded in that, although improvement may be present, standardized laboratory procedures yield different results than those typically seen in practice and application. However, continued justification for this argument is provided by Jacobs et al.,[92] who demonstrated that creatine ingestion increased maximally accumulated oxygen deficit (MAOD) during treadmill work bouts at 120% of VO_{2max} lasting approximately 120 seconds. Although most studies do show a performance benefit with creatine supplementation, several studies show no response to creatine supplementation.[104–116] These results should be interpreted judiciously, however, because protocols of some studies deviated from the 5-day loading protocol shown to be effective for increasing performance. Furthermore, performance enhancement appears to be strongly related to the extent of creatine uptake into muscle with supplementation.[78] Therefore, studies that do not measure creatine uptake by the muscle cannot rule out study participants that are *nonresponders* who, for one reason or another, do not absorb creatine into the muscle.

Age and Sex Differences

Two of the most intriguing parameters that have yet to be fully addressed are the influence of age and sex on creatine's effectiveness. Each of these two groups has different physiological characteristics that may lead to varied responses in each population. For example, similar concentrations of creatine are found relative to the total creatine pool in an aging population (52–79 yrs); however, PCr levels are typically lower, and free creatine is higher.[64,117] PCr and free creatine measurements could be confounded by inactivity. In fact, a recent training study showed that free creatine and PCr levels attain concentrations similar to younger participants with no changes in the creatine pool.[117] These observations may be pertinent to future research efforts given the current activity patterns of the aged and the relative decline in the number of type II muscle fibers observed during aging. Creatine stores are found to be greatest in type II muscle fibers; therefore, supplementation with creatine in older individuals may be particularly effective in maintaining strength levels over time.

Smith[118] compared young (30 ± 5 yrs) and middle-aged (58 ± 4 yrs) men and women performing single-leg knee-extension exercise inside a whole body magnetic resonance system. Two trials were performed 7 days apart and consisted of two 2-minute bouts and a third bout continued to exhaustion. Three minutes of recovery were given between each work bout. [31P]Nuclear magnetic resonance imaging (NMR) spectra were used to determine pH and relative concentrations of inorganic phosphate, PCr, and beta-ATP every 10 seconds. After consuming 0.3 g/kg per day for 5 days, it was found that during the placebo trial, the middle-aged group do have a lower resting PCr in comparison to the young group (35.0 ± 5.2 versus 39.5 ± 5.1 mmol/kg; $p < 0.05$). This was coupled with a lower mean initial PCr resynthesis rate (18.1 ± 3.5 versus 23.2 ± 6.0 mmol/kg/min; $p < 0.05$). After creatine supplementation, resting PCr increased 15% ($p < 0.05$) in the young group and 30% ($p < 0.05$) in the middle-aged group to 45.7 ± 7.5 versus 45.7 ± 5.5 mmol/kg, respectively. Mean initial PCr resynthesis rate also increased in the middle-aged group ($p < 0.05$) to a level not different from the young group (24.3 ± 3.8 versus 24.2 ± 3.2 mmol/kg/min). Time to exhaustion was increased in both groups combined after creatine supplementation (118 ± 34 versus 154 ± 70 sec; $p < 0.05$). Therefore, it appears that creatine supplementation has a positive effect on PCr availability and resynthesis rate in middle-aged adults compared with younger persons.

In contrast, Bermon et al.[119] also sought to investigate the effects of oral creatine supplementation in 32 older adults (67–80 yrs; 16 men and 16 women). The subjects were randomly assigned to four equivalent subgroups (control-creatine; control-placebo; trained-creatine; trained-placebo). These treatments were based on whether they took part in an 8-week strength-training creatine supplementation program. The strength-training program consisted of three sets of eight repetitions at 80% of 1-repetition maximum for leg press, leg extension, and chest press, performed 3 days a week. The 52-day supplementation program consisted of 20 g of creatine (or glucose) and 8 g of glucose per day for the initial 5 days followed by 3 g of creatine (or glucose) and 2 g of glucose per day. Before and after the training and supplementation periods, body mass, body fat, lower limb muscular volume, 1- and 12-repetition maximums, and isometric intermittent endurance tests for the leg press, leg extension, and chest press were determined. In all groups, no significant changes in anthropometric parameters were observed. For all movements, the increases in 1- and 12-repetition maximums were greater ($p < 0.02$) in trained than in control subjects. No significant interactions (supplementation/training/time) were observed for the 1- and 12-repetition maximum and isometric intermittent endurance.

Although there is continued favorable evidence supporting the use of creatine as an ergogenic aid in men, the results are less clear regarding the effectiveness of creatine in women.[120] Forsberg et al.[119] examined three groups of healthy women and men (n = 50) to determine potential sex differences in muscle composition. The three groups in this study were comprised of men and women between the ages of 19 and 40 years (n = 29), 41 and 60 years (n = 11), and 61 and 85 years (n = 10). In an analysis of the vastus lateralis of men (n = 18) and women (n = 23) using muscle biopsies, they observed a greater quantity of total creatine in women relative to tissue weight. These values were 132 mmol/kg and 145 mmol/kg for men and women, respectively, with no further differences noted for the percentage of slow and fast twitch muscle tissue in each sex.

A study conducted by Earnest[26] provided a comparison of the magnitude of responses for anaerobic power and plasma ammonia concentration in women versus men. Anaerobic performance increased by 8.9% and 14.6% for men, and 4.2% and 8.8% for women during Wingate tests one and two, respectively. When comparing the relative percentage of increase for these two tests in the male and female groups, these data reflect an approximate twofold (men = 8.9%; women = 4.2%) and 1.7-fold (men = 14.6%; women = 8.8%) difference in the extent of response for Wingate tests one and two, respectively. Moreover, the appearance of plasma ammonia is attenuated by 64% and 30% for the male and female groups, respectively. This reflects a nearly twofold differential in the male-versus-female decrease in plasma ammonia concentrations and demonstrates a possible order of magnitude response characteristic between the male and female subjects. However, further research in this area is needed to help clarify these issues.

This discrepancy between sexes may be influenced by regulatory functions within the cell that have not been fully examined. Researchers have discovered that the saturable active transport of creatine is highly specific regarding sodium dependence and extracellular creatine concentration levels.[63,69,121] Therefore, following cellular saturation, excess creatine may down-regulate creatine transport owing to a combination of both elevated intracellular and extracellular creatine concentrations. Although each sex demonstrated an increase in muscle power output, differences seem to exist regarding the magnitude of response between men and women. Owing to the observation of a higher total intracellular creatine content per kilogram of dry muscle in women versus men,[122] it is hypothesized that this may reduce the relative intramuscular uptake of creatine. If an upper limit of intramuscular creatine exists, this could attenuate both the relative intramuscular uptake of creatine and changes in PCr and plasma ammonia concentrations, thereby reducing the magnitude of response for anaerobic power in response to creatine administration in men and women.

Body Composition

Many of the studies performed to date indicate that short-term creatine supplementation increases total body mass by approximately 0.7 to 1.6 kg.[27,75,120,123–125] This increase in body weight has been theorized to be a result of a creatine-stimulated water retention and/or protein synthesis.[83,85,103,124,125] In support of this hypothesis, Ziegenfuss et al.[125] reported that 5 days of creatine supplementation increased nitrogen status either by enhancing protein synthesis or reducing protein degradation. The increase in body mass was accompanied by a 7% increase in thigh muscle volume determined by magnetic resonance imaging (MRI) and a 2–3% increase in intracellular and extracellular fluid volume. Longer-duration studies (7–140 days) investigating the effects of creatine or creatine-containing supplements on body composition have also reported significantly greater gains in total body mass and fat-free mass.[74,96,97,99,126–128] These gains were associated with enhanced sprinting capacity and/or gains in strength[74,96–99] with no change in total body water expressed as a percentage of total body weight.[97,98,116,127,128]

These results appear to be consistent in women: Vandenberghe et al.[97] reported greater gains in fat-free mass in creatine-supplemented women compared with

Creatine and Skeletal Muscle Fiber Hypertrophy

Jeff Volek, PhD

Several studies have been published indicating that creatine ingestion greater than 20 g/day for 5 to 7 days increases total muscle creatine concentrations and improves performance during short-duration, high-intensity activities such as resistance training. More recent studies also indicate that creatine supplementation in conjunction with resistance exercise training from 4 to 12 weeks enhances the physiological adaptations to weight training in both men and women. Studies examining the influence of creatine supplementation (5–30 g/day) during weight training (4–12 wks) generally indicate enhanced body mass, including an increase in fat-free mass (FFM), an increase in muscular strength, and the ability to train at higher intensities. We now move towards a discussion as to the mechanisms by which creatine elicits these responses.

Several lines of research suggest that creatine could play a role in augmenting skeletal muscle fiber hypertrophy. Gyrate atrophy patients who consumed 1.5 g creatine per day for 1 year showed significant increases in type II muscle fiber diameter. Creatine supplementation has also been shown to facilitate muscle rehabilitation following disuse atrophy. In fact, our laboratory recently published data showing that muscle fiber hypertrophy was enhanced in men who consumed 25 g of creatine per day for 7 days followed by a daily 5-gram dose for the remainder of a 12-week resistance training program. In addition, creatine-supplemented subjects showed significantly greater improvements in maximal strength, fat-free mass, and creatine accumulation compared with placebo subjects. The percentage increases in cross-sectional area for all fiber types in creatine subjects ranged from 29–35%, more than twice the increase observed in placebo subjects (6–15%). Greater muscle fiber hypertrophy implies enhanced myofibrillar protein synthesis and/or reduced degradation. Creatine may play a direct role in myosin and actin synthesis *in vitro,* which may be mediated via cell swelling. A more likely scenario to explain the augmented skeletal muscle fiber cross-sectional areas observed with creatine supplementation is that the intensity of individual resistance training sessions is enhanced (i.e., heavier loads can be lifted), leading to a greater stimulus for muscle fiber hypertrophy.

The direct or indirect nature of this *anabolic* effect of creatine has not been elucidated; however, most researchers agree that endocrine mechanisms are most likely not involved. Furthermore, there is still uncertainty regarding the optimal amount of creatine required to maximize the ergogenic potential of creatine. An ideal dose may be dependent on individual differences in diet composition, fiber type distribution, sex, age, and initial total muscle creatine concentrations. Creatine requirements may be altered depending on the specific training regimen and exercise configurations. The ability to exercise more intensely with creatine supplementation and thus augment training adaptations has wide application for a large number of athletes who participate in resistance training as a part of their overall training program.

Kreider RB, Ferreira M, Wilson M, et al. Effects of creatine supplementation on body composition, strength, and sprint performance. Med Sci Sports Exerc 1998;30:73–82.

Vandenberghe KM, Goris P, Van Hecke M, et al. Long-term creatine is beneficial to muscle performance during resistance training. J Appl Physiol 1997;83:2055–2063.

Volek JS, Duncan ND, Mazzetti SA, et al. Performance and muscle fiber adaptations to creatine supplementation and heavy resistance training. Med Sci Sports Exerc 1999;31:1147–1156.

those given a placebo. Interestingly, these gains were maintained during a subsequent 70-day detraining period with continued supplementation (5 g/day) and maintained for 28 days after cessation of supplementation despite muscle PCr levels returning toward pre-supplementation values. Whether creatine-stimulated fluid retention can account for all of the gain in fat-free mass observed in these studies is consistent across short- and long-term studies is a question that still needs to be ascertained.

Blood Lipid Metabolism

Recent studies indicate that in male and female subjects who have total cholesterol concentrations exceeding 200 mg/dL, creatine supplementation reduced blood lipid parameters over a 56-day supplementation period.[129] During this investigation, measurements were performed at baseline, at week 4 and week 8 of treatment, and at 4 weeks following cessation of treatment (week 12). The results revealed significant reductions in total cholesterol after week 4 (−6%) and week 8 (−5%), before returning to baseline at week 12. Interestingly, baseline triglycerides and very low density lipoprotein (VLDL) cholesterol were reduced by 23% at week 4 and 22% at week 8, and remained attenuated by 26% at week 12. These results remained consistent when data were separated by sex and corrected for estrogen status despite the well-known hypertriglyceridemic effects of exogenous estrogens.[130] No significant differences were noted for low density lipoprotein (LDL) and high density lipoprotein (HDL), total cholesterol/HDL ratio, glucose, creatinine, body mass, body mass index (BMI), or physical activity within or between the experimental and placebo groups. However, a trend toward reduced blood glucose levels was present in creatine males (p = 0.051). More recent studies have reported similar findings in college-age male athletes. In this group, HDL cholesterol was significantly increased (13%), with some evidence of reduced VLDL cholesterol (−13%) and total cholesterol/HDL ratio (−7%).[98]

Serum creatinine levels were also measured and results revealed no elevations in values at any time during the study. Following creatine loading (20–30 g/day for 5–7 days) only transient elevations in serum creatinine have been described. However, urinary creatinine excretion increases in parallel with intramuscular creatine concentrations and is likely a result of the increased release and cyclization of intramuscular creatine as a normal consequence of myofibrillar protein turnover.[50]

Neuromuscular Disease

Despite the observation that 95% of the total creatine pool is found in muscle tissue, the remaining 5% is found in the heart, brain, neural tissue, and testes. These observations have pointed some early research efforts towards the effects of creatine in patients with neural and myocardial

disorders. In a randomized, controlled trial of creatine supplementation in patients with mitochondrial cytopathies, Tarnopolsky et al.[131] measured fatigue in patients with mitochondrial cytopathies, an abnormality associated with decreased basal and postactivity muscle PCr. Measurements included the following: activities of daily living (visual analog scale), ischemic isometric handgrip strength (1 minute), basal and postischemic exercise lactate, evoked and voluntary contraction strength of the dorsiflexors, nonischemic isometric and dorsiflexion torque (NIDFT, 2 minutes), and aerobic cycle ergometry with pre- and postlactate measurements. Creatine treatment resulted in a significantly (p < 0.05) increased handgrip strength, NIDFT, and postexercise lactate, with no changes in the other measured variables. The authors concluded that creatine increased the strength of high-intensity anaerobic- and aerobic-type activities in patients with mitochondrial cytopathies but had no apparent effects on lower-intensity aerobic activities. In another investigation, Tarnopolsky and Martin[132] administered creatine to neuromuscular disease patients at 10 g daily for 5 days and 5 g daily for 5 days in a pilot study (Study 1; n = 81), followed by a single-blinded study (Study 2; n = 21). The researchers found a significant increase in high-intensity strength in patients with neuromuscular disease.

Myocardial Disease

Creatine supplementation has also been shown to have a positive effect on exercise tolerance in chronic heart failure patients.[133,134] Reduced creatine availability has been implicated in the metabolic abnormalities of failing myocardial tissue, and creatine supplementation has been shown to attenuate pharmacologically induced metabolic stress in rat myocardium,[135] although the contribution of PCr to energy delivery in myocardial tissue is normally negligible. However, no research to date indicates whether creatine exerts its effects in cardiac patients via improving heart or skeletal muscle energetics. Alternatively, PCr has been proposed to stabilize membranes under conditions of cellular damage,[136] and the creatine-like compound, cyclocreatine, has been suggested to maintain ATP production in heart and skeletal muscle long after PCr stores have been depleted,[137] which may be more fruitful areas of future research. Two early studies have begun this examination with what appear to be favorable preliminary results.

To assess the effects of dietary creatine supplementation on skeletal muscle metabolism and endurance in patients suffering from chronic heart failure, Andrews et al.[133] used a forearm model of muscle metabolism. Maximal voluntary contractions were measured using handgrip dynamometry as subjects performed handgrip exercise of 5-seconds' contraction followed by 5 seconds of rest for 5 minutes at 25%, 50%, and 75% of maximum voluntary contraction or until exhaustion. Blood was sampled at rest and 0 and 2 minutes after exercise for measurement of lactate and ammonia.

After 30 minutes, the procedure was repeated with fixed workloads of 7 kg, 14 kg, and 21 kg. Patients were assigned to creatine at 20 g daily or matching placebo for 5 days and returned after 6 days for repeat study. During post-testing, contractions until exhaustion at 75% of maximum voluntary contraction increased after creatine treatment with no significant placebo effect. Ammonia and lactate per contraction at 75% maximum voluntary contraction fell significantly after creatine but not after placebo.

In a complementary study, Gordon et al.[134] noted that cardiac creatine levels are depressed in chronic heart failure and thus evaluated the effects of creatine supplementation on ejection fraction, symptom-limited physical endurance, and skeletal muscle strength in patients with chronic heart failure. In a double-blind, placebo-controlled design, 17 patients (age, 43–70 yrs; ejection fraction <40) were supplemented with creatine, 20 g daily for 10 days. Before and on the last day of supplementation ejection fraction was determined by radionuclide angiography, as was symptom-limited 1-legged knee extensor and 2-legged exercise performance on the cycle ergometer. Muscle strength as unilateral concentric knee extensor performance (peak torque, Nm at 180 degrees/sec) was

also evaluated. Skeletal muscle biopsies were performed to determine the amount of energy-rich phosphagens. Although no change in ejection fraction was seen in either group compared with baseline, creatine supplementation increased skeletal muscle total creatine and PCr by 17% and 12%, respectively. More specifically, however, increments were seen only in patients with less than 140 mmol total creatine/kg. Additionally, 1-legged performance (21%), 2-legged performance (10%), and peak torque (5%) also increased. Both peak torque and 1-legged performance increased linearly with increased skeletal muscle PCr (p < 0.05). The increments in 1-legged, 2-legged, and peak torque were significant compared with the placebo group. One week of creatine supplementation to patients who suffered from chronic heart failure did not increase ejection fraction but increased skeletal muscle energy-rich phosphagens and performance regarding both strength and endurance. Therefore, it appears that creatine supplementation in chronic heart failure may favorably augment skeletal muscle endurance; it attenuates the abnormal skeletal muscle metabolic response to exercise and thus provides a new and novel therapeutic approach to treatment that merits further attention.

Use of Creatine in Neuromuscular Disease

Mark Tarnopolsky, MD, PhD

Creatine is a guanidino compound that is found in meat-containing products and produced endogenously by the liver and pancreas. Creatine is transported into a variety of tissues via a sodium-dependent transporter. The major stores for creatine include brain, heart, and skeletal muscle. Creatine functions as an energy buffer during periods of increased metabolic demand, and as an energy shuttle between mitochondria and cytosol, and may have a role in protein synthesis. Studies in young, healthy males have shown an increase in muscle creatine content by 10–20% following a creatine loading protocol (approximately 20 g/day × 5 days). This has resulted in an increase in high-intensity exercise performance and an increase in fat-free mass after 3 to 7 days of *loading*. The performance effects are greatest in those who have the lowest intramuscular creatine concentrations. Patients with muscular dystrophy, inflammatory myopathies, and mitochondrial cytopathies have been shown to have low total creatine and phosphocreatine concentrations. Muscle weakness and fatigue are common symptoms in these patients. Studies have shown an increase in high-intensity exercise performance and total body weight in patients who have mitochondrial cytopathy and neuromuscular disorders following creatine loading. Longer-term studies are required to measure the impact of this on functional activities of daily living. Two recent animal studies have provided fascinating insight to the potential for creatine to attenuate neurodegenerative disorder progression. In one study, rats were poisoned with 3-nitro-proprionic (NP) acid (complex 2 inhibitor), which resulted in degeneration of the corpus striatum (Huntington's

disease model). In those rats treated with creatine and 3NP, there was an attenuation of neural drop-out and lesser oxidative stress compared with those receiving only 3NP. This research group later showed a neuroprotective effect and survival benefit from creatine administration to mice with the *G93A FALS* mutation (a model of amyotrophic lateral sclerosis [ALS]).

The aforementioned study suggests that creatine may be a useful adjunctive treatment in neuromuscular and neurometabolic disorders. However, long-term studies with objective outcome measures and functional measures are required to explore the therapeutic potential of this compound.

Juhn MS, Tarnopolsky MA. Oral creatine supplementation and athletic performance: A critical review. Clin J Sports Med 1998;8(4):286–297.

Klivenyi P, Ferrante RJ, Matthews RT, et al. Neuroprotective effects of creatine in a transgenic animal model of amyotrophic lateral sclerosis. Nature Medicine 1999;5:347–350.

Matthews RT, Yang L, Jenkins BG, et al. Neuroprotective effects of creatine and cyclocreatine in animal models of Huntington's disease. J Neurosci 1998;18(1):156–163.

Tarnopolsky MA, Parise G. Direct measurement of high-energy phosphate compounds in patients with neuromuscular disease. Muscle Nerve 1999;22(9).

Tarnopolsky MA, Martin J. Creatine monohydrate increases strength in patients with neuromuscular disease. Neurology 1999;52:854–857.

Tarnopolsky MA, MacDonald J, Roy B. A randomized, double blind trial of creatine monohydrate in patients with mitochondrial cytopathies. Muscle Nerve 1997;20:1502–1509.

Diabetes

Early research has indicated that creatine shares a similar insulin-facilitating effect as observed with other guanidine compounds.[138,139] Creatine has also been shown to have a direct suppressive effect on the insulin binding of post-dialyzed plasma from individuals with chronic kidney disease.[140] These data suggest that creatine may have a possible role in the regulation of insulin receptor binding on peripheral target cells. Creatine has also been shown to reduce circulating blood sugar concentrations 60 and 120 minutes after a single 3-gram oral dose in insulin-dependent (type I) diabetics.[141] These changes were observed without alterations in serum insulin or C-peptide concentrations, or changes in blood sugar in age-matched nondiabetic controls.[141] These data suggest that creatine can acutely enhance glucose disposal and/or reduce liver glucose production (gluconeogenesis) in hyperglycemic type I diabetics. Furthermore, the addition of creatine to carbohydrate supplementation in healthy, nondiabetic males has been shown to be effective in augmenting the release of insulin.[25] However, previous studies examining blood lipid alterations associated with creatine have noted strong trends toward reduced blood glucose levels in creatine males (p = 0.051).[134]

Renal Effects

One of the most controversial concerns involving creatine supplementation is its effect on renal function. Creatine supplementation can cause an increase in urinary creatinine excretion, which is often used as an indicator of kidney function. However, this increase correlates well with the increase in muscle creatine that is observed during supplementation and reflects the increased rate of muscle creatine degradation to creatinine rather than any abnormality of renal function.[71,142–145] Pritchard[143] recently reported on adverse effects associated with creatine supplementation in an isolated case involving presence of kidney disease. However, other studies have shown normal kidney function in creatine-supplemented healthy individuals. Normally, creatine does not exit muscle cells until it has degraded to creatinine in an irreversible reaction involving the loss of a water molecule from the creatine molecule itself. Following its formation, creatinine diffuses from skeletal muscle and is excreted by the kidneys.[53]

Poortmans[144] recently reported on five healthy men ingesting either a placebo or 20 g of creatine per day for 5 consecutive days. In their study, blood samples and urine collections were analyzed for creatine and creatinine concentrations after each experimental session. Total protein and albumin urine excretion rates were also determined. Oral creatine supplementation had a significant incremental impact on arterial content (3.7-fold) and urine excretion rate (90-fold) of this compound. In contrast, arterial and urine creatinine values were not affected by creatine ingestion. The glomerular filtration rate (creatinine clearance) and the total protein and albumin excretion rates remained within the normal range.

In one of the most recent studies, Poortmans et al.[146] examined creatinine, urea, and plasma albumin clearances in individuals supplemented with creatine as well as placebo from 10 months to 5 years. During this trial, no statistical differences were found between the control group and the creatine group in plasma concentration and urine excretion rates for creatinine, urea, or albumin. Glomerular filtration rate, tubular reabsorption, and glomerular membrane permeability were normal in both groups. Therefore, it is becoming increasingly apparent that neither short-term, medium-term, nor long-term oral creatine supplementation induces detrimental effects on kidney function in healthy individuals. Whether creatine is safe for patients who suffer from renal dysfunction has yet to be determined, indicating the need for more research in this area.

Safety and Toxicity

Several studies have evaluated the effects of short- and long-term creatine supplementation on hematological profiles and have found that creatine supplementation does not significantly affect the following variables: carbon dioxide, uric acid, total protein, albumin, alkaline phosphatase, sodium, potassium, chloride, calcium, ionized calcium, phosphorus, leukocytes, neutrophils, lymphocytes, monocytes, eosinophils, basophils, hemoglobin, hematocrit, total bilirubin, total iron, platelets, red blood cells, red blood cell distribution width, mean corpuscular volume, or mean platelet volume.[98,147,148] Studies have shown an elevation in creatine kinase, which normally rises dramatically (>1000 U/L) in the blood in response to intense exercise alone.[128] The clinical significance (if any) of these findings is difficult to discern.

Almada et al.[147] examined possible serum enzyme changes associated with creatine supplementation. After analysis, no changes were noted for AST, ALP, GGT, LDH, or pooled (male and female) CPK. However, there was a significant increase in CPK in males and group total protein at week 8 (p < 0.05). To this end, CPK values for males were 118.8, 138.3, 181.3, and 122.3 U/L for baseline, week 4, week 8, and week 12, respectively. Many studies have documented the intracellular accumulation of creatine and PCr in skeletal muscle following creatine supplementation. This is true especially of males. During this study, the authors observed an increase in total serum CPK activity only among males receiving creatine (week 8). Note, however, that muscle damage resulting from exercise is commonly associated with increases in CPK levels that may remain elevated for up to 48 hours.[149]

Overall, these data suggest that creatine supplementation may increase several markers of organ function.

However, each of the enzymes that were significantly elevated can be released from damaged skeletal muscle and are sometimes used as indicators of training intensity (e.g., creatine kinase, lactate dehydrogenase). Given the increased capacity for muscular work output following creatine loading, it is plausible that an increase in contractile forces was generated during the normal exercise regimens of these subjects. In turn, this may contribute to increased disruptions in muscle membrane integrity and thus, consequential leakage of cellular enzymes into the surrounding tissue.

Data collected by Almada et al.[147] suggest that total protein may be transiently elevated during creatine supplementation. However, note that these elevations do not exceed normal reference ranges in adults (6.4–8.3 g/dL). Also, these elevations may reflect increases in dietary protein intake, which may cause minor, yet statistically significant increases in total protein levels.[150] Additionally, estrogen status and timing of menstrual activity may also account for changes in females. However, when the data were separated by sex, no significant differences were noted.

Current Controversy: Creatine Supplementation

Although several anecdotal adverse effects have been attributed to creatine supplementation, only a few minor scientific studies have been documented. Some of these have linked creatine supplementation to gastrointestinal upset. This is attributed to osmotic distress if the crystalline creatine is not adequately dissolved into a solution before ingestion. Another common reported side effect is body weight gain due to increased creatine storage and the associated gain in fat-free mass. However, many athletes do not consider body weight gain to be a negative effect of creatine supplementation. Also interesting to note is that recent studies in infants between 2 to 4 years of age who have genetic disturbances in creatine synthesis have shown remarkable clinical, biochemical, and functional improvements following creatine supplementation in doses ranging from 136.4 to 227.3 mg/lb body weight (350 to 500 mg/kg body weight) that were maintained for over 25 months. This dose is up to 1.67 times the recommended loading dose. No adverse effects were reported, including no aggravation of seizures in one infant who presented with intractable seizures (including rare grand mal seizures) before being treated with creatine.

Muscle Strains/Pulls

Anecdotal reports from some athletic trainers and coaches suggest that creatine supplementation may promote a greater incidence of muscle strains or pulls. Because creatine supplementation may promote relatively rapid gains in strength and body mass, additional stress may be placed on bone, joints, and ligaments, leading to injury. To date, no study has documented an increased rate of injury following creatine supplementation, even though many of these studies evaluated highly trained athletes during heavy training periods.

Muscle Cramping

Some anecdotal claims have suggested that athletes training intensely in hot or humid conditions might experience severe muscle cramps while taking creatine. Proponents of this theory suggest that creatine supplementation may cause large fluid shifts in the muscle, serving to alter electrolyte status, promote dehydration, and/or increase thermal stress. No study has reported that creatine supplementation causes cramping, dehydration, or changes in electrolyte concentrations, although one study evaluated highly trained athletes undergoing intense training in hot and humid environments. Furthermore, the causes of muscle cramping are not fully understood so it is premature to suggest that creatine supplementation may elicit such an effect.

Dehydration

Numerous reports in the media suggest that creatine supplementation can produce dehydration even though there are no published studies supporting this assertion. No studies to date have demonstrated an increase or decrease in whole body hydration as determined via bioelectric impedance analysis. Recently, Ziegenfuss et al. addressed these issues in ten cross-trained and aerobically trained men. At a dose of 0.16 g/day (approximately 32 g/day for a 200 lb.-person), coupled with a multifrequency bioelectrical impedance analyzer, they found that total body water increased by 2% and paralleled the increase in total body mass associated with the 5-day loading sequence. Interestingly, extracellular water content did not change significantly, but intracellular water content changed by 3%. Kreider et al. also calculated plasma volume from the ratio of blood hemoglobin/hematocrit from available published data and found no alterations in blood volume.

Death

One of the most shameful and poorly researched press reports suggested that creatine supplementation may have been involved in the sudden deaths of three wrestlers. These athletes died suddenly while exercising in the heat in rubber suits in an attempt to cut weight before competition. Based on these reports, the Centers for Disease Control and Prevention (CDCP) and the Food and Drug Administration (FDA) launched investigations to determine whether creatine was involved in these deaths. Results of this investigation conducted by the CDCP revealed two of the wrestlers had not taken creatine and one of the athletes had stopped taking creatine at least 3 months before his death. The deaths of the wrestlers were officially attributed to hyperthermia, heart failure, and heat exhaustion/dehydration.

Grindstaff PD, Kreider R, Bishop R, et al. Effects of creatine supplementation on repetitive sprint performance and body composition in competitive swimmers. Int J Sports Nutr 1997; 7:330–346.

Kreider RB, Ferreira M, Wilson M, et al. Effects of creatine supplementation on body composition, strength, and sprint performance. Med Sci Sports Exerc 1998;30:73–82.

Mujika I, Chatard JC, Lacoste L, et al. Creatine supplementation does not improve sprint performance in competitive swimmers. Med Sci Sports Exerc 1996;28:1435–1441.

Schulze A, Hess T, Wevers R, et al. Creatine deficiency syndrome caused by guanidinoacetate methyltransferase deficiency: diagnostic tools for a new inborn error of metabolism [see comments]. J Pediatr 1997;131(4):626–631.

Stockler S, Hanefeld F. Guanidinoacetate methyltransferase deficiency: a newly recognized inborn error of creatine biosynthesis. Wien Klin Wochenschr 1997;109:86–88.

Stockler S, Hanefeld F, Frahm J. Creatine replacement therapy in guanidinoacetate methyltransferase deficiency, a novel inborn error of metabolism. Lancet 1996;348:789–790.

Stockler S, Holzbach U, Hanefeld F, et al. Creatine deficiency in the brain: a new, treatable inborn error of metabolism. Pediatr Res 1994;36:409–413.

Stockler S, Isbrandt D, Hanefeld F, et al. Guanidinoacetate methyltransferase deficiency: the first inborn error of creatine metabolism in man. Am J Hum Genet 1996;58:914–922.

Stockler S, Marescau B, De Deyn PP, et al. Guanidino compounds in guanidinoacetate methyltransferase deficiency, a new inborn error of creatine synthesis. Metabolism 1997;46:1189–1193.

Ziegenfuss T, Gales D, Felix S, et al. Performance benefits following a 5 day creatine loading procedure persist for at least four weeks. Med Sci Sports Exerc 1998;30(5 Suppl):S265.

HMB (beta-hydroxy-beta-methyl butyrate)

HMB is a metabolite of the branched-chain amino acid leucine and is found naturally in small quantities in catfish, various citrus fruits, and breast milk. Leucine, an essential amino acid, is used for protein synthesis, with the residue being transaminated to alpha-ketoisocaproate (KIC) and then partially oxidized to form HMB. The HMB derived from leucine is converted to beta-hydroxy-beta-methylglutaryl CoA (HMG-CoA) in some tissues and serves as a key carbon source for cholesterol synthesis in various cell types.

This *de novo* cholesterol synthesis is believed to be behind HMB's performance-enhancing effects. During periods of cell growth and/or differentiation, HMG-CoA may be a rate-limiting step for cholesterol synthesis, which appears to be a restrictive factor for both cell function and growth. HMB feedings are believed to saturate cells with a source of HMG-CoA, thus providing the tools for cells to undergo a maximal growth response (for strength/power athletes that would be a hypertrophic and/or hyperplastic response with regard to skeletal muscle fibers).

In Vitro Studies

Studies conducted on HMB's actions at the cellular level have been done in both animal and human cell types.[151–155] The effect of HMB on skeletal muscle metabolism was investigated by Kostiuk et al.[152] using isolated muscle strips from rats and chicks. Tissues were exposed to different concentrations of HMB and the rates of protein degradation and protein synthesis were measured. This investigation demonstrated HMB inhibited proteolysis by an average of 80% while at the same time increased protein synthesis in both muscle tissues.[152] Cheng et al.[153] also investigated the muscle protein effects of HMB in two cell lines, H9C2 (heart cells) and C2C12 (skeletal muscle cells). Samples were differentiated in culture to myotubes and exposed 2 to 4 days to 0 to 6 mM HMB. Scientists observed increased beta oxidation of palmitate by 30% ($p < 0.001$), decreased lactate dehydrogenase from myotubes by 25% ($p < 0.05$), and an increased cellular expression of creatine kinase (CK) by 25% ($p < 0.01$). These results suggest HMB may alter muscle cell metabolism by increasing cellular oxidative capacity and enhancing the expression of muscle-specific proteins—proven by the increased cellular expression of CK.[153]

HMB may also play a part in the immune response to exercise. This effect could apply to preventing overtraining syndrome in strength-power and endurance athletes in whom the immune system is compromised as well as in various medical conditions. *In vitro* studies investigating the effects of HMB in this regard have demonstrated a positive effect on lymphocytes. Nonnecke and colleagues[154] demonstrated that HMB in high concentrations affected DNA synthesis of bovine lymphocytes in a cell culture medium with adequate amounts of leucine. In another *in vitro* study, HMB was added to chicken-macrophage cultures in various concentrations (range, 100 to 1000 mM). Macrophages are important to immunity because they are involved in producing antibodies and in the mediation of cellular immune responses. In addition, they also participate in the presentation of antigens to lymphocytes. With the addition of HMB, the number of macrophages increased by 20% (p < 0.003) and nitrite production increased by 29% (p < 0.06). In chicks receiving HMB the number of Sephadex-elicited macrophages from peritoneal fluid increased two- to threefold (p < 0.05). These data demonstrate HMB exposure induces the generation of macrophages in culture and increases nitrite production and the phagocytic capabilities of macrophages.[155]

Animal Studies

Animal data regarding the beneficial effects of HMB on performance and growth parameters are equivocal and much less intriguing than the human data.[151,152] Although *in vitro* data from Kostiuk et al. demonstrated an antiproteolytic and anabolic effect in skeletal muscle, work from Papet et al.[151,152] showed that high-dose HMB supplementation in lambs had no effect on whole-body protein turnover or skeletal muscle protein synthesis.

Human Studies

Recent human studies suggest HMB displays anticatabolic and anabolic activity in skeletal muscle. Nissen et al.[156] conducted a two-part study to determine whether the administration of HMB to subjects undergoing a weight-training program would elicit any positive effects when compared against those training without supplementation. In part one, 41 untrained subjects randomly received three differing dosages of HMB (0, 1.5, or 3.0 g/day), and two different protein diets (117 or 175 g/day). The training protocol worked each muscle group once or twice weekly with either free weights or machines. Sessions alternated emphasis between upper and lower body exercises with at least 1 day of rest between workouts. The protocol lasted 3 weeks, with each subject getting 10 total workouts (5 upper and 5 lower body). Each exercise included two warm-up sets with 10 repetitions at 30–60% of the subjects' 1-RM. Work sets were performed with three sets of 3 to 5 repetitions at 90% of the 1-RM. The exercises consisted of the following: (upper body) free-weight bench press, machine latissimus dorsi pull-downs, machine seated row, machine pectoral fly, free-weight preacher biceps curl, and machine triceps push-down; (lower body) leg press machine, standing calf raise machine, leg flexion machine, leg extension machine, 45-degree inclined sit-up, inclined leg lift, and back extension. An advanced lifting protocol was used in part two of the study. Twenty-eight subjects were supplemented with either 0 or 3.0 g of HMB per day and trained 2 to 3 hours per day 6 days a week for 7 weeks.

In part one of the study, HMB supplementation significantly lowered training-induced muscle proteolysis as measured by urinary 3-methylhistidine excretion during the first 2 weeks of the study. A reduction in plasma creatine kinase was also observed with HMB administration. In subjects receiving HMB, strength increases were greater than those observed in control subjects. When looking at this study critically, a few important issues must be addressed. This was a short-term study and untrained subjects were used. Therefore, although gains in strength were observed, it is impossible to attribute those improvements to the HMB supplement only. Initial improvements in strength in untrained individuals could be a result of increased voluntary activation of muscle (neural adaptation), rather than the accretion of protein.[157] Staron et al.[158] showed that approximately 16 resistance training sessions are required to induce increases in lean body mass or muscle mass. Thus, using untrained subjects during a short-term trial severely limits drawing any conclusions to the benefit of HMB in terms of increasing muscle mass and strength.

In the second study, fat-free mass increased in the HMB-supplemented group at various intervals throughout the study, but not at the conclusion of the study. After the seventh week, strength improved in the bench press, but not the squat or hang clean exercises in the HMB-supplemented group. Thus, over time it is apparent that the effects of HMB may actually diminish. In this phase of the investigation, trained subjects were used, but the control group was stronger at the onset of the study. Therefore, these subjects did not attain the same percentage gains as the two groups receiving HMB.

Although the majority of research is conducted in male subjects, using female subjects is important as well. This research proves valuable from a scientific standpoint because of the differing hormonal milieu in women as well as from a health standpoint (i.e. weight control, prevention of osteoporosis, as well as possible safety concerns for pregnant females). With the increasing involvement of women in strength training and their interest in altering body composition, science should address the female organism's response to nutritional ergogenic aids. To determine if the same antiproteolytic effects occur in women as in their male counterparts undergoing vigorous strength training, scientists from Iowa State University, in Ames, Iowa investigated the effects of HMB (3 g/day) on 36 nonexercising females, and a second study investigated HMB supplementation (3 g/day) or a placebo given to 37 women undergoing a 3 day-per-week resistance training program. Body composition was measured via total body electrical conductivity (TOBEC) in the first part of the study and underwater weighing in the second. In contrast to the study conducted by Nissen et al., these researchers determined that HMB supplementation, combined with weight training, increased gains in lean body mass and strength. Untrained sedentary subjects receiving HMB showed no changes in lean or fat mass.[159]

Vukovich et al.[160] studied the effect of calcium HMB on maximal oxygen consumption (VO_{2peak}) and maximal blood lactate concentration in endurance-trained cyclists. During this trial, eight cyclists randomly completed three separate supplementation periods. Each supplement was administered for 2 weeks followed by a 2-week washout period. Supplements administered to the subjects were HMB (3 g/day), leucine (3 g/day), and a placebo (3 g/day). Before and after each supplementation period, subjects completed a VO_{2peak} test with blood samples obtained immediately following exercise to determine the maximal appearance of blood lactic acid. After 2 weeks of HMB supplementation, a significant increase in VO_{2peak} (pre 4.57 ± 0.14; post 4.75 ± 0.15 L/min) was noted for the calcium HMB group. VO_{2peak} was unaffected by leucine (pre 4.70 ± 0.17; post 4.61 ± 0.14 L/min) and placebo (pre 4.71 ± 0.16; post 4.60 ± 0.23 L/min) supplementation. The HMB group also showed a significantly greater time to reach VO_{2peak}, whereas leucine and placebo elicited no effect on this variable (HMB: pre 21.9 ± 0.9, post 22.7 ± 1.1 min; leucine: pre 22.2 ± 1.1, post 21.6 ± 0.9 min; placebo: pre 22.4 ± 0.9, post 21.6 ± 1.4 min). Maximal blood lactic acid concentrations were unaffected by supplementation but tended to be higher following HMB supplementation (HMB: pre 7.6 ± 1.1, post 8.1 ± 1.1 mM ($p < 0.06$); leucine: pre 6.3 ± 0.9, post 6.2 ± 0.8 mM; placebo: pre 7.9 ± 1.1, post 7.5 ± 1.3 mM). Thus, the authors concluded that HMB supplementation could have positive effects on performance by increasing VO_{2peak}.[160] Although these results may not appear to be of importance to the strength athlete *per se,* it may be beneficial to those athletes participating in running events between 400 and 1600 meters.

Whereas HMB alone appears to have limited effects in an otherwise healthy population, some researchers[161] have examined the effects of ingesting a calcium HMB/glucose supplement combined with or without creatine during sprint and strength-training exercises. In a double-blind and randomized manner, 41 NCAA Division IA football players were match-paired and assigned to supplement their diets for 28 days with either 1) a placebo containing 99 g/day of glucose, 3 g/day of taurine, 1.1 g/day of disodium phosphate, and 1.2 g/day of potassium phosphate (PotPh); 2) the PotPh mixture with 3 g/day of calcium HMB (HMB); or 3) the PotPh/HMB mixture with 15.75 g/day of HPCD pure creatine monohydrate (HMB/creatine). In this study, subjects participated in a resistance-training program (5 hrs/wk) and an agility/sprint training program (3 hrs/wk). On days 0 and 28, subjects performed 12 6-second sprints on a computerized cycle ergometer with 30-second rest periods between sprints. Subjects also performed maximal repetition tests at 70% of estimated 1-RM on the isotonic bench press, upright squat, and power clean. Using ANCOVA and ANOVA statistical techniques, this group showed that work output tended to be greater in the HMB and HMB/creatine trials ($p = 0.06$). Mean change in work tended to also be greater in the HMB and HMB/creatine groups (4442 ± 1996; 6252 ± 1318; 7533 ± 2144 J; 7.9 ± 3.8; 13.6 ± 3.1; 13.2 ± 4.3%). Gains in lifting volume tended to be greater in the HMB/creatine group for the bench press (NS; $p = 0.37$), squat (NS; ($p = 0.08$), and clean ($p = 0.008$). Results revealed that adding creatine to HMB could enhance strength and/or anaerobic capacity. However, additional research is necessary because this investigation did not control for creatine effects by using a creatine-only group.[161]

Because of the possible effects of HMB in decreasing proteolysis and increasing protein synthesis in skeletal muscle, this compound may be effective in the medical treatment of certain conditions such as certain muscle wasting diseases or in postsurgical recovery. Both practitioners and patients find it particularly interesting that HMB may have beneficial effects in preventing the profound decrease in muscle tissue and immune system function observed in the late stages of AIDS. In certain conditions L-arginine and L-glutamine have been shown to increase immune function in humans and to have beneficial effects on skeletal muscle. In an interesting study presented at the XII World AIDS Conference in June of 1998, Clark et al.[162] investigated the possibility that an amino acid combination administered with HMB could result in a synergistic action positively affecting muscle metabolism and immune function. Subjects were recruited from HIV clinics to participate in a randomized, double-blind, placebo-controlled 8-week study in which they received an amino acid mixture containing 14 g arginine, 14 g glutamine, and 3 g HMB daily. Lean body mass and fat mass were measured by an air displacement plethysmography at 0, 4, and 8 weeks. The abstract presented data from 16 subjects and results showed subjects who consumed the amino acid/HMB mixture gained 3.00 ± 0.50 kg ($p < 0.01$), whereas the placebo group gained 0.37 ± 0.84 kg. Weight gain with the experimental group was predominately lean tissue (2.55 ± 0.75 kg [$p < 0.005$]) and fat (1.60 ± 1.70 kg). The placebo group did not gain any lean tissue, but did accrue fat (1.60 ± 1.70 kg). Measures of immune system integrity demonstrated that the amino acid/HMB mixture increased absolute CD4 numbers by 17.3 ± 28.2 cells/mm^3 versus 49.0 ± 27.4 ($p < 0.10$) and absolute lymphocytes by 0.29 ± 0.14 1000/mm^3 versus −0.31 ± 0.15. Although it appears that HMB might provide a useful tool to those treating HIV-associated wasting syndrome, it would have been informative to have one group of subjects ingesting L-arginine and L-glutamine alone and in combination with creatine. As was previously demonstrated at the XI International Conference on AIDS, Daniel et al.[163] showed that a formula containing creatine was effective in increasing total body mass (−1.25 to +11.00 lbs) in HIV-positive patients and, therefore, this presents an interesting avenue of future investigation for individuals afflicted with this disease.

HMB May Decrease Cardiovascular Risk

The *Journal of Nutrition* reported safety data collected from nine studies in which humans were fed 3 g/day of HMB. In these studies ranging from 3 to 8 weeks of men and women, young and old, exercising and nonexercising, HMB had no adverse effects on a variety of measures. Organ and tissue function as determined via blood chemistries was normal. Additionally, a 7.3% decrease in LDL cholesterol, a 5.8% decrease in total cholesterol, and a 4.4 mmHg decrease in systolic blood pressure would suggest a lowering of cardiovascular risk. Thus, the utility of HMB may be in the realm of health and athletic performance.

Nissen S, Sharp RL, Panton L, et al. Beta-hydroxy-beta-methylbutyrate (HMB) supplementation in humans is safe and may decrease cardiovascular risk. J Nutr 2000;130:1937–1945.

Safety and Toxicity

According to existing human data, HMB appears to be safe and well tolerated. Studies ranging in length from 1 to 8 weeks have shown that up to 3 g/day of HMB is safe in male and female subjects; this is supported by the lack of adverse physical effects determined by blood chemistry analysis.[164]

Boron

In 1987, a study was published showing that boron (a nonessential mineral found naturally in applesauce, prunes, almonds, and wine) increased plasma testosterone concentrations.[165] Although this sounds intriguing, especially to those athletes interested in augmenting muscle mass and strength, the study was done in mineral-deficient, postmenopausal women—not in athletes.[165] Unfortunately, soon after publication, supplement companies started sales campaigns in several magazines marketed towards a bodybuilding audience. Ads boldly claimed boron could increase testosterone levels with minimal dosage.

Human Studies

In 1993, in the only investigation performed in male bodybuilders, scientists observed no increases in muscle mass or strength.[166] Subjects ranged in age from 20 to 27 years and were given 2.5 mg of boron or a placebo for 7 weeks (n = 19). Plasma total and free testosterone, plasma boron, lean body mass, and strength measurements were measured on day 1 and day 49 of the protocol. Plasma boron values were significantly elevated compared

with controls (p < 0.05). Statistical analysis showed no significant effect of supplementation on any of the performance variables tested. Despite the negative scientific evidence showing boron has no performance-enhancing effects in bodybuilders, some companies continue to this day to market boron as a supplement capable of increasing muscle mass and strength.

Safety and Toxicity

Toxicity is a possibility when consuming high dosages of certain minerals. Although low doses of boron appear quite safe, doses of 50 mg and above could be dangerous and could decrease performance by disturbing appetite and various digestive processes.

Chromium Picolinate

Chromium is a trace mineral required for normal carbohydrate and lipid metabolism.[167] Chromium is said to potentiate the effects of insulin, a peptide hormone, which plays a major role in glucose regulation, muscle growth, and fat deposition. The primary function of insulin is to facilitate the uptake of glucose and amino acids into cells for energy production and growth. Recently, athletes have become interested in insulin because of its ability to decrease protein breakdown, increase protein synthesis, and increase the intracellular availability of glucose. Thus, the rationale for chromium supplementation in bodybuilding and other sports requiring muscle size, strength, and power is related to its insulin-potentiating effects.[168] When insulin is released from the pancreas, chromium is then discharged from body stores in the liver, spleen, soft tissues, and bone. In total, about 4 to 6 mg of chromium are stored at these various sites. Some have theorized chromium's role is to help insulin bind to the receptor and possibly assist in its internalization into cells. Still, the exact mechanism of action remains unknown.

It appears, however, that the biologic action of chromium occurs via an oligopeptide, which has been named low-molecular-weight chromium-binding substance.[169] Results from *in vitro* studies using animal cells suggest low-molecular-weight chromium-binding substance functions by helping insulin after the insulin molecule binds to the external side of the insulin receptor which, in turn, activates insulin receptor kinase activity.[9,169] Thus, it seems that low-molecular-weight chromium-binding substance may function in a manner resembling the calcium-binding signal calmodulin.[169]

Animal Studies

One study conducted by researchers at the University of Kentucky demonstrated that chromium treatment in pigs resulted in an increase in muscle and a decrease in adipose tissue.[170] Seven littermate sets of Yorkshire-Hampshire barrows were fed a fortified, corn-soybean diet supplemented with either 0 or 200 μg/kg of chromium picolinate. After dissection, the pigs that were supplemented with chromium showed an increase in their percentage of muscle ($p < 0.02$), a decrease in their percentage of fat ($p < 0.06$), and no difference in the total weight of dissected bone and skin. Upon further analysis, chromium-fed pigs showed greater rates of muscle and bone accretion ($p < 0.05$) and a decrease in the daily rate of fat accretion ($p < 0.05$).

Human Studies

Dr. Gary Evans first conducted human performance studies on chromium at Bemidji State University.[171] Football players were given chromium picolinate (200 μg/day) for 6 weeks during their normal off-season weight-training program. After 42 days the supplement group lost about 7.5 pounds of fat and gained approximately 6 pounds of lean body mass. Although the study received much attention in the press, the scientific community didn't think highly of the work because, according to other scientists, the correct statistical analysis and an accurate portrayal of skeletal muscle mass measurements were not used.

These criticisms are continually being substantiated by other studies also showing that chromium has no effect on increasing muscle mass and strength in athletes. Most have used a similar protocol used by Evans et al. Recent studies have used more precise instruments to detect changes in body composition. In addition, many display better statistical analysis of the data. Today, the scientific community is in agreement that taking excess chromium above the Estimated Safe and Adequate Daily Dietary Allowance (ESADDI) of 50 to 200 μg is unnecessary and has no ergogenic effects.[172]

After Evans's work was published in 1989, six abstracts and 10 full studies clearly demonstrated that chromium has no beneficial effects on either muscle mass or strength in normal, healthy subjects.[173–177] In 1992, in a double-blind, placebo-controlled study, scientists from the Louisiana State University Department of Kinesiology administered 200 μg/day of chromium picolinate or a placebo to both male and female college students participating in a 12-week strength-training program.[174] The results of this study showed no effect of chromium on strength as measured by the one-repetition maximum (1-RM) for the squat and bench press. However, a significant treatment effect was found in chromium-supplemented female subjects, who gained more body weight compared with all other groups. Therefore, researchers concluded chromium supplementation has a greater effect on females than on males. These data have yet to be replicated by other laboratories and one must question the accuracy of such findings given that lean body mass was not assessed, nor were diet records taken to determine the chromium intake of the subjects before and during the investigation.

Like Evans, Clancy et al.[175] also examined the effects of 200 μg of chromium picolinate supplementation in male football players during spring training. The following measurements were taken at the beginning, middle, and end of the supplementation period: urinary chromium excretion, limb girth and skinfold measures, percent body fat, fat-free (*lean*) body mass, and isometric and dynamic strength. At the conclusion of this trial, no changes in body composition or strength were noted; however, urinary chromium excretion was five times greater in those receiving the supplement versus those who were given the placebo.

In another study conducted in competitive athletes, chromium was again shown to be of no benefit for increasing strength or altering body composition.[176] During this trial, 20 wrestlers from the University of Oklahoma were assigned to either a treatment group (200 μg/day of chromium picolinate), a placebo group, or control group (no supplementation). The study lasted 14 weeks and was conducted while athletes were participating in an off-season strength and conditioning program (no severe, acute weight loss practices are used during this period). Body composition, neuromuscular performance, metabolic performance, and serum insulin and glucose were measured before and immediately following the supplementation and training periods. After the trial, repeated measures ANOVA indicated no significant alterations in any of the performance variables of the group receiving chromium, while aerobic performance increased in all groups. As has rapidly become a consistent finding in chromium research, there was no benefit to chromium supplementation regarding strength testing. Researchers concluded that chromium picolinate supplementation in addition to a strength and conditioning program offers no benefits for enhancing body composition or performance beyond training alone.

Another negative report on chromium was a study conducted in older men (56–69 yrs).[177] Scientists from the Department of Geriatrics at the University of Arkansas initiated a double-blind study that randomly assigned 18 subjects to groups that received either 924 μg/day of chromium picolinate or a low-chromium placebo for a 12-week period. Subjects participated in a bi-weekly, high-intensity, resistance-training program involving three sets of 8 to 12 repetitions at 80% of their 1-RM. Chromium alone was shown to have no effect on strength, power, cross-sectional area, lean body mass, or fat mass in these subjects. However, resistance training alone resulted in significant improvements in all of these variables.

Thus, the preponderance of evidence would suggest that chromium supplementation has little to no effect on body composition or exercise performance in adult humans.[172,173]

Chromium Absorption and Excretion: A Major Consideration in Supplementation

The biologic effects of nutrients are often discussed in advertisements and in product-driven articles commonly seen in popular bodybuilding and fitness magazines.[178] However, it is unclear whether these products can be adequately absorbed by the body. Regardless of nutrient effects, if it is not assimilated into the body, any supposed effect will be negated. This is true especially of chromium and is particularly relevant when discussing chromium's biologic properties for use in physique augmentation as well as its application in medicine.

Two forms of chromium are found in food, inorganic and organic. They have different absorption rates ranging from 0.4–2% and 10–25%, respectively. Data in humans are sparse, with most of the information on absorption coming from animal studies.[179] In this regard, only organically complexed chromium is active. Inorganic chromium entering the general circulation must be changed into the organic form to be used by the body. Chromium appears to be transported in the body bound to transferrin, albumin, globulins, and lipoproteins. Although data are lacking, the liver is hypothesized to be a major site for the synthesis of organic chromium (active) from the inorganic (inactive) form of the mineral. To date, its precise transport mechanism(s) have yet to be clearly defined. Furthermore, no research studies have established how chromium moves from the digestive tract to sites of synthesis or to various storage depots throughout the body. This void in the literature becomes important when discussing oral dosing.

Three chromium supplements are commercially available: chromium picolinate (organic), chromium nicotinate (organic), and chromium chloride (inorganic). Absorption of these three compounds differ, as do their biologic effects. Chromium chloride is believed to be poorly absorbed and not well used by the body, in supplements available to the public, or in laboratory settings.

Chromium picolinate, the most widely used chromium salt, increases receptor-bound and internalized insulin in cultured cells, whereas nicotinate and chloride salts have different actions on the glucose/insulin system.[180] These differences indicate a fertile area of research, and future efforts in the laboratory should look into a) establishing how the different forms of chromium act on insulin tissue responsive and b) defining the exact mechanism by which chromium is processed and transported within the body.

Another important aspect to consider when discussing chromium usage is the pattern of excretion in athletic populations. Exercise increases chromium loss, but as with other physiological adaptations to stress, the form or type of stress (i.e., the mode of exercise) plays a large role in how the body responds. The effects of stress on urinary chromium loss are correlated directly with cortisol (TABLE 3-2).[181] Most of the data collected to date have been reported on aerobic athletes and have shown an increase in urinary excretion after training.[182,183] Those interested in the effects of aerobic exercise and chromium loss should read the articles by Anderson et al.,[182,183] because this chapter will touch on only those studies associated with resistance training.

Currently, not much research has been done on the effects of weight training and chromium excretion. What has been published indicates that those individuals who are involved in high-intensity resistance training may display altered chromium status owing to increased excretion. Despite this finding it is more than likely that these individuals are easily replacing lost chromium because of the typical high-calorie and nutrient-intake patterns associated with these athletes. Also note that a chromium deficiency is unlikely in strength athletes because the majority of these individuals are ingesting supplements (e.g., meal replacements, protein powders, multivitamins/minerals, and various *thermogenic* supplements) that contain 200 μg or more of the mineral.

Effect of Chromium on Glucose Regulation: Possible Roles in Treating The Diabetic Athlete

Another potential area to investigate is the effect of combined weight training and chromium supplementation on insulin sensitivity[184–186] and the treatment of diabetes. Because chromium functions in maintaining normal glucose tolerance by assisting in the regulation of insulin action, the presence of biologically active chromium may lower the amount of insulin required to initiate uptake of glucose and amino acids into cells.[179]

Chromium contained in the body pool (approximately 4–6 mg in adults) is believed to have release patterns similar to hormones discharged into the general circulation in response to certain physiological stimuli. In this case, the stimulus is the digestion of food and the

Table 3-2 Stress Effects on Urinary Chromium Losses of Humans (Chromium)

Stress	Urinary Chromium, μg/day	
	Mean	SEM
Basal	0.16	0.02
High Sugar Diet	0.28	0.01
Acute Exercise	0.30	0.07
Lactation	0.37	0.02
Physical Trauma	10.80	2.10

Data from Anderson RA. Chromium as an essential nutrient for humans. Regul Toxicol Pharmacol 1997; 26:S35–S41.

subsequent release of insulin.[187] Although chromium's effect in normal individuals appears to be insignificant, this mineral may prove to be valuable in treating type I, type II, and gestational diabetic athletes, particularly those engaged in strength training. Although more research is warranted, the literature shows that when chromium is given to subjects with impaired glucose tolerance, supplementation can lead to improved blood glucose, insulin, and lipid concentrations in some individuals.[188] For the clinician treating patients with chromium, it should be noted that changes in glucose and insulin are usually seen in less than 28 days. However, alterations in the lipid profile may take several months to be seen in the patient's blood profile.[189]

Regarding type II diabetics, Anderson and colleagues[190] have demonstrated that supplemental chromium has beneficial and statistically significant effects. During their investigation, the following variables were affected by the supplement regimen: HbA1c, glucose, insulin, and cholesterol. Subjects (n = 180) were randomly divided into three groups: 1) placebo, 2) 100 μg of chromium picolinate twice daily, and 3) 500 μg of chromium picolinate twice daily. Testing during this trial took place at 2- and 4-month intervals while participants maintained their usual living habits including medication, diet, and daily activities. After 4 months of treatment, both low- and high-dose chromium groups experienced significant improvements in HbA1c values. Two-hour glucose concentrations were also significantly lower in subjects receiving 500 μg at both the 2- and 4-month intervals. Additionally, plasma total cholesterol concentration decreased after 4 months of treatment in subjects receiving the lower chromium dose. Researchers concluded that the beneficial effects of chromium in individuals with type II diabetes were observed at levels higher than the upper limit of the ESADDI.

Another investigation studying chromium's action on glucose regulation was conducted by Cefalu et al.,[191] who examined subjects (14 men and 15 women) at high risk for type II diabetes determined by family history and obesity. In a randomized, double-blind study, subjects received either placebo or 1000 μg of chromium picolinate for an 8-month period. Clinical and metabolic evaluations consisted of insulin sensitivity and glucose effectiveness, measurements of glucose tolerance, insulin response to an oral glucose load, and a 24-hour glucose and insulin profile. Anthropometric measurements and magnetic resonance imaging were used to evaluate abdominal fat distribution. In addition, fasting plasma glucose, insulin, glycated hemoglobin, and frucosamine were also assessed. To date, this is the most complete study done on chromium's effects in humans in that it used highly sensitive techniques to collect data. For example, results demonstrated a significant increase in insulin sensitivity in chromium-supplemented subjects at the study's midpoint (p < 0.05) and at the end of the study (p < 0.005) when compared with the placebo. However, chromium supplementation had no effect on glucose effectiveness, body weight, abdominal fat distribution, or body mass index. Chromium significantly improved insulin sensitivity in obese subjects with a family history of type II diabetes. Thus, these findings suggest that, in diabetics, chromium may have direct effects on skeletal muscle via alteration of insulin sensitivity without interaction in adipose tissue. Insulin has profound effects in adipose through the dephosphorylation of hormone-sensitive lipase; therefore, this enzyme is converted into the inactive form and results in an increase in glucose uptake. Because body fat plays a major role in diabetes and is an important consideration when treating individual patients, additional work should be done looking at the insulin/chromium interaction in adipose tissue as well as in diabetic patients who have body fat levels ranging from normal to obese. The findings of these studies must be confirmed to fully evaluate the effects of chromium on insulin action and control of blood glucose.

Gestational Diabetes

Gestational diabetes is a condition that sometimes manifests itself during pregnancy as a result of a shift in the hormonal milieu. Some physicians may find themselves in the precarious position of having to treat pregnant recreational athletes with this condition. Because of drug testing in athletic competitions, as well as concern for the developing fetus, nutritional therapy with chromium may be a suitable alternative to the normal pharmacological measures typically used as treatment.

Jovanovic and colleagues[192] evaluated the effectiveness of chromium supplementation as a treatment for gestational diabetes in 30 women (20–24th gestational wk). Twenty subjects were randomized into two groups: 10 received 4 μg/kg/day of chromium picolinate, and 10 received a placebo. Ten additional subjects were matched for glucose intolerance and body mass index to the placebo group and received 8 μg/kg/day of chromium picolinate. Blood testing and glucose load testing (100 g) were done at the beginning of the investigation and after 8 weeks of supplementation. Results showed that the low-dose group (4 μg of chromium) had decreased levels of HbA1c compared against baseline and, after 8 weeks of study, both groups receiving chromium had significantly lower glucose and insulin levels compared with their baseline values and values of the placebo group. Chromium picolinate for gestational diabetic women appears to mitigate glucose intolerance and lowers hyperinsulinemia.

Safety and Toxicity

Despite being marketed as a safe and effective alternative to anabolic steroids, the data available suggest that chromium picolinate has the potential to be toxic in some individuals. Pharmacokinetic models have shown that chromium

Chromium—Weight-loss, Weight-gain, or Waste of Time?

Priscilla M. Clarkson, PhD

Chromium, a trace mineral essential for life, is purported to increase muscle mass and decrease fat. The estimated safe and adequate daily dietary intake (ESADDI) is 50 to 200 µg. Chromium potentiates insulin action and stimulates amino acid uptake by cells. Based on evidence that chromium supplements increase muscle mass and growth in animals, stimulating amino acid uptake with chromium is thought to increase protein synthesis and muscle mass in humans. The reason that chromium is thought to enhance fat loss is that insulin also plays a significant role in fat metabolism. Supplemental chromium is commercially available in the form of chromium picolinate, chromium nicotinate, or chromium chloride, with chromium picolinate being the most popular.

Evans first reported that chromium picolinate increased lean body mass in young men during a resistance-training program. Untrained college students and trained football players ingested 200 µg/day of chromium picolinate or a placebo for 40 to 42 days. The group who took the chromium supplement gained significantly more lean body mass compared with the placebo group. However, lean body mass was estimated from anthropometric measures, which are not highly reliable, and the observed changes were small. Thus, measurement error may have influenced the results. Several studies have failed to confirm the results of Evans's studies.

Hasten and colleagues found that males participating in a weight-training program and taking 200 µg of chromium picolinate did not show a greater increase in body mass compared with those taking placebo. However, females who took the chromium supplement gained more body weight than did the females on the placebo, but lean body mass was not assessed so it is not known if the increase in body weight was a result of increased muscle mass. Campbell et al. examined the effect of a chromium picolinate supplement or placebo in 56- to 69-year-old men during a weight-training program and found no benefit to lean body mass, muscle size, strength, or power in subjects taking the chromium. Clancy et al. found that chromium picolinate (200 µg/day) was not effective in enhancing strength or muscle gain, but that urinary chromium excretion for the chromium-supplemented group was significantly increased. Chromium stores were probably adequate and the excess chromium was excreted into the urine. In a well-controlled study, Lukaski and colleagues examined the effect of 8 weeks of chromium chloride, chromium picolinate, or a placebo supplement in untrained men who started a resistance-training program. The two types of chromium supplements similarly increased urinary chromium excretion and had no effect on body composition assessed by anthropometry and dual X-ray absorptiometry (DEXA), a reliable measure of body composition.

Trent and Thieding-Cancel investigated the effects of 400 µg/day of chromium picolinate or placebo for 16 weeks in subjects who were participating in an aerobic exercise program. Navy personnel consisting of 79 men and 16 women who exceeded the body fat standards of 22% for men and 30% for women participated as subjects. Only minimal changes in total body weight or percent fat (estimated by circumference measures) over the course of the study were found, with no significant differences between the supplemented and placebo groups. However, use of circumference measures to estimate body composition may not provide a reliable body fat assessment. Kaats et al. administered 200 and 400 µg/day of chromium picolinate or a placebo for 72 days to 154 overweight subjects, mostly women. The chromium supplement resulted in significantly greater fat loss (assessed by underwater weighing). The chromium-supplemented group lost 1.89 kg of fat compared with 0.18 kg for the placebo. Differences between groups could be influenced by differences in diet and exercise that were not controlled or assessed. In a follow-up study, Kaats et al. administered 400 µg of chromium picolinate or a placebo to 122 subjects, mostly women, for 90 days. In this study, caloric intake and expenditure were monitored and subjects maintained a daily physical activity log. DEXA was used to assess fat loss. This study confirmed results of the prior study in that the chromium group in comparison to the placebo group lost significantly more body weight (7.79 kg versus 1.81 kg, respectively) and fat (6.3% and 1.2%, respectively). The combined effect of chromium supplements and exercise was examined by Grant et al. in a study in which 400 µg of chromium picolinate, 400 µg of chromium nicotinate, or a placebo was given to 43 overweight women for 9 weeks. Subjects were placed into an exercise or nonexercise group. The nonexercising group taking the chromium picolinate supplement gained about 1 kg of fat, whereas those who exercised and ingested the chromium picolinate supplement lost about 0.4 kg of fat (assessed by underwater weighing). Subjects who exercised and ingested chromium nicotinate lost about 1.3 kg of fat. This study provides some evidence that chromium nicotinate when combined with exercise may produce a small decrease in fat weight. However, the group who took chromium picolinate supplements without participating in an exercise program appeared to increase body fat.

Sufficient scientific evidence is not available to support the contention that chromium is an effective weight-gain or weight-loss agent. Although some studies have found that chromium was effective in reducing fat in overweight subjects, the data are equivocal. Differences in chromium status among individuals may contribute to some of the variability in findings between studies because chromium supplements may only be effective in altering body composition when compensating for a deficiency. However, valid data are not available for chromium content in foods, and there are no easy means to accurately determine the body's stores—so at present it is difficult to determine normal chromium status. If chromium did induce weight loss, there is no reason to suspect that weight loss would be maintained when the supplement period ended. Thus, side effects associated with long-term use are important to consider, and at present there is not sufficient information on the safety of taking greater than 200 µg/day for an extended period of time (longer that

4 months). Although chromium could play some role in weight loss, the effects are small compared with the effects of proper exercise and diet interventions.

Campbell WW, Joseph LJ, Davey SL, et al. Effects of resistance training and chromium picolinate on body composition and skeletal muscle in older men. J Appl Physiol 1999;86:29–39.

Clancy SP, Clarkson PM, DeCheke ME, et al. Effects of chromium picolinate supplementation on body composition, strength, and urinary chromium loss in football players. Int J Sports Nutr 1994;4:142–153.

Evans, GW. The effect of chromium picolinate on insulin controlled parameters in humans. Int J Biosoc Med Res 1989;11:163–180.

Grant KE, Chandler RM, Castle AL, Ivy JL. Chromium and exercise training: effect on obese women. Med Sci Sports Exerc 1997;29:992–998.

Hallmark MA, Reynolds TH, DeSouza CA, et al. Effects of chromium and resistive training on muscle strength and body composition. Med Sci Sports Exerc 1996;28:139–144.

Hasten DL, Rome EP, Franks BD, Hegsted M. Effects of chromium picolinate on beginning weight training students. Int J Sports Nutr 1992;2:343–350.

Kaats GR, Blum K, Fisher JA, Adelman, JA. Effects of chromium picolinate supplementation on body composition—A randomized, double-masked, placebo-controlled study. Curr Ther Res: Clin Exper 1996;57:747–756.

Kaats GR, Blum K, Pullin D. et al. A randomized, double-masked, placebo-controlled study of the effects of chromium picolinate supplementation on body-composition—A replication and extension of a previous study. Curr Ther Res: Clin Exper 1998;59:379–388.

Lukaski HC, Bolonchuk WW, Siders WA, Milne DB. Chromium supplementation and resistance training: effects of body composition, strength, and trace element status of men. Am J Clin Nutr 1996;63:954–965.

Trent LK, Thieding-Cancel D. Effects of chromium picolinate on body composition. J Sports Med Phys Fit 1995;35:273–280.

Walker LS, Bemben MG, Bemben DA, Knehans AW. Chromium picolinate effects on body composition and muscle performance in wrestlers. Med Sci Sports Exerc 1998;30:1730–1737.

picolinate taken in excessive dosages or for prolonged periods of time could result in the accumulation of toxic levels of the substance in various human tissues.[193–196] For most normal nonathletic individuals, toxicity through the oral ingestion of chromium is not a concern. However, because certain athletes (especially bodybuilders) operate under the guise that more is better, excessive consumption should be a consideration for physicians, athletic trainers, strength coaches, dieticians, personal trainers, and others dealing with supplement users. Athletes may be unknowingly ingesting high amounts of chromium because the mineral is now added to many supplements currently on the market owing to its popularity. For example, an athlete takes a manufacturer's suggested use of two to three meal replacements, containing chromium, per day (examples include Met-RX, Iso-Pure, Metaform, Lean Body), plus a multivitamin/mineral supplement, in addition to a separate chromium supplement (e.g., TwinLab Bio-Formed GTF Chromium 200 μg). This would give the individual a daily total dose of over 400 μg/day. This is clearly above the ESADDI and should be a serious consideration in smaller athletes who might consume more chromium relative to body mass.

In a recent study receiving a large amount of media attention, Dr. Diane Stearns from the Department of Chemistry, Dartmouth College, examined the effect of chromium on Chinese hamster ovary cells to determine if chromium supplements could cause chromosomal aberrations. During the study, cells saturated with chromium had no ability to rid themselves of the compound. Although this may not be relevant when looking at an entire organism versus a specific cell line, chromium picolinate was found to produce chromosomal damage 3- to 18-fold greater than control levels for soluble doses of 0.050, 0.10, 0.50, and 1.0 mM after 24 hours of treatment. Particulate chromium picolinate in doses of 8.0 μg/cm^2 and 40 μg/cm^2 produced aberrations 4-fold and 16-fold

above control levels. This study suggests that long-term chromium supplementation may be carcinogenic. Further research is needed to establish safe and appropriate doses of chromium in humans. The conclusions of this study should be noted, but their applicability to athletes may be limited.[196]

Chromium supplementation in high dosages may also cause serious renal impairment. In a case study published recently in the *Annals of Pharmacology*, a 33-year-old Caucasian female presented with weight loss, anemia, thrombocytopenia, hemolysis, liver dysfunction (aminotransferase enzymes 15 to 20 times normal, total bilirubin three times normal), and renal failure (serum creatinine 5.3 mg/dL; blood urea nitrogen 152 mg/dL).[197] After a personal history was taken, it was discovered she had ingested 1200 to 2400 μg/day of chromium picolinate for the previous 4 to 5 months before experiencing health problems. The woman received blood product transfusions and hemodialysis and stabilized after 6 days. In addition, her liver and renal function returned to normal by 12 days of treatment. Although this represents only one case of chromium overuse, it does suggest that chromium picolinate can have toxic effects.

The mechanisms responsible for the purported effects of chromium have not been thoroughly investigated and studies indicate that biochemical, physiological, and behavioral actions of chromium picolinate may be a result of the effects of picolinic acid on the central nervous system. Analogues of picolinic acid have been shown to induce alterations in the metabolism of serotonin, dopamine, and norepinephrine in the brain.[198] Although such effects are unlikely at low dosages (50–200 μg/day), some individuals prone to behavioral disorders or those on antidepressants may experience untoward effects from chromium picolinate supplementation. Nonetheless, one should keep in mind that the dietary intake of chromium in most adults is insufficient.[199]

Conjugated Linoleic Acid (CLA)

Conjugated linoleic acid (CLA) is found naturally in food, although the total CLA content varies.[199] CLA is a modified isomer of linoleic acid that was introduced to the supplement market in late 1995 as one of the newer supplements available to enhance muscular development. Chemically, linoleic acid is an 18-carbon unsaturated fatty acid with two double bonds in positions 9 and 12, respectively. Both of these bonds lie in the *cis* configuration, thus giving it its own unique chemical name—c9, c12-octadecadienoic acid. CLA differs only modestly in confirmation in that the two double bonds in CLA are in one of three positions along the carbon chain: 9 and 11, 10 and 12, or 11 and 13. These small changes not only give CLA a unique chemical name, but because of the varied position of the double bonds, CLA also can take two different geometric positions. Therefore, CLA can take a *cis* or *trans* configuration. Although this may seem chemically insignificant, physiologically it is quite profound and gives CLA the chemical nomenclature of a conjugated diene that is a mixture of positional and geometric isomers of conjugated dienoic derivatives of linoleic acid.[200] With a few exceptions, the c9, t11-isomer is the predominant form.[201] CLA is found especially in foods high in saturated fat such as meat and dairy products. In addition, meat from ruminants (animals with four-chambered stomachs) contains more CLA than meat from nonruminants. Because foods typically high in CLA also contain high amounts of saturated fats, increasing CLA intake via food consumption may put individuals at risk for developing coronary artery disease. Nevertheless, there are intriguing data that demonstrate positive effects after CLA administration.[202]

During processing, various factors may contribute to the formation of CLA. Factors that increase CLA food content include higher temperatures, the addition of whey protein concentrate or sodium caseinate, and the presence of a hydrogen donor such as butylated hydroxytoluene, propyl gallate, or ascorbic acid.[203,204] Although some reports suggest that grilling ground beef may increase CLA content in beef fat by about four-fold,[205] other studies suggest that cooking has no effect on CLA concentrations.[206]

Owing to this unique molecular structure, CLA is believed to have unique mammalian tissue physiological effects compared with other fats. Scientists have theorized, from observations in various animal studies, that CLA enhances lean body mass, although the mechanism for action is unknown. Some scientists believe that CLA amplifies cell responsiveness to certain growth factors, hormones, and cellular messengers. It may also possess anticatabolic effects.[207,208] Therefore, CLA consumption by humans could theoretically increase muscular strength and lean body mass. Whether supplementation is advised is still a matter of debate.

Animal Studies

CLA has been suggested to also be anticarcinogenic. The incidence of various forms of cancer is high in the United States and other countries. Saturated fat has been correlated with the occurrence of cancer in several tissue sites.[209–211] Certain unsaturated fatty acids may affect carcinogenic factors. For example, linoleic acid has been implicated in the acceleration of mammary cancer development in rodents.[212–214] However, it is also clear that some fatty acids will inhibit carcinogenesis. In this regard, eicosapentaenoic acid and docosahexaenoic acid, which are representative of the ω-3 polyunsaturated fatty acids found in fish oil, have long been purported to have anticarcinogenic effects.[215] CLA may also inhibit carcinogenesis.

Although not designated as an essential fatty acid, CLA appears to have reproducible effects on various cancer indices.[202,216–241] To date, the specific sites of action include breast,[210,212–214,218,221,223,226–234,237,239,241–252] colon,[209,216,221,222,227,243,249,253–263] prostate,[219,220,224,231] kidney,[219,220,224,225] and skin tissue.[238,253,254,264–267] The reason CLA has these effects may lie in how it is deposited in tissues. One interesting finding is that the c9, t11-isomer appears to be found in the phospholipid layer, whereas other CLA isomers appear in triglycerides.[244,268] The reason why this relationship is important is not completely clear. However, the ingestion of CLA likely leads to an accumulation in triglyceride, which is stored as fat depot in adipocytes. Because CLA has an antioxidant potential[244,268] and because adipocytes are a major constituent of the mammary gland, the increased concentration of CLA in triglyceride may help protect certain cells against oxidant stress.[202]

Although the exact mechanism of action has yet to be confirmed, use of CLA as a therapeutic intervention shows promise. For example, Ip[202] has shown that, although fish oil is a class of lipid that inhibits both chemically induced and transplantable tumors, the amount of fish oil needed to elicit this response usually exceeds 10% of total dietary fat.[269–272] However, as little as 0.1% CLA in the diet is sufficient to produce a significant reduction in mammary tumor yield.

Although CLA appears to play a role in the inhibition of carcinogenesis, it also appears to have insulin-sensitizing effects as well. In this regard, CLA activates PPAR alpha* in the liver and shares functional similarities to ligands of PPAR gamma and thiazolidinediones, which are potent

---

*Peroxisome proliferation activated receptors (PPAR) are members of the nuclear receptor subfamily of ligand-activated transcription factors that include the steroid, retinoid and thyroid hormone receptors. To date, three mammalian PPAR subtypes, PPAR alpha, PPAR beta and PPAR gamma. Prostaglandin J2 and its derivatives have been reported to function as efficacious activators of PPAR alpha and PPAR gamma, suggesting that the J2 family of prostaglandins may exert their biologic effects in part through the activation of the PPAR signaling pathways. Glycation is the uncontrolled, nonenzymatic reaction of sugars with proteins. Chemical glycation is also very important in the damage done to diabetics when their sugar levels rise above normal, and in damage done to critical proteins of long-lived nerve cells in aging.

insulin sensitizers. Early evidence for the effect of CLA on insulin sensitivity was provided by Houseknecht et al.,[257] who reported that CLA was able to normalize impaired glucose tolerance and improve hyperinsulinemia in prediabetic rats. Additionally, dietary CLA in this trial also appeared to increase steady-state levels of aP2 (activator protein 2) mRNA in adipose tissue, which is consistent with the actions of PPAR gamma. The authors of this study proposed that the insulin-sensitizing effects of CLA are caused, at least in part, by activation of PPAR gamma because increasing levels of CLA induced a dose-dependent transactivation (stimulation of transcription by a transcription factor binding to DNA and activating adjacent proteins) of PPAR gamma.

In vitro data on human erythrocytes have also been presented by Inouye et al.[273] These investigators suggest that glycation reactions and antioxidant activity are enhanced by elevated glucose concentrations. Because it is unclear whether the diabetic state, *per se,* also induces an increase in the generation of oxygen-derived free radicals, there is some evidence that glycation itself may induce the formation of oxygen-derived free radicals. In this regard, oxygen-derived free radicals could cause oxidative damage to endogenous molecules. During this trial, investigators examined the relationship between the levels of lipid peroxidation and the levels of glycated hemoglobin A1c in the erythrocytes of both diabetic and healthy subjects. Lipid peroxidation was assessed in erythrocyte membrane lipids by monitoring peak height ratios of CLA, one of the products of lipid peroxidation, to linoleic acid. The peak height ratio of CLA to LA was used as a biomarker of lipid peroxidation and glycated hemoglobin A1c, an index of glycemic stress. The results of this trial showed a significant increase in the ratios of CLA to LA in diabetic erythrocytes compared with that of control erythrocytes. In addition, ratios of CLA to LA were also significantly correlated with glycated hemoglobin A1c values. These findings attest to the antioxidant qualities of CLA and suggest that glycation via chronic hyperglycemia links lipid peroxidation in the erythrocytes of both diabetic and healthy subjects. (Hemoglobin A1c is the substance of red blood cells that carries oxygen to the cells and sometimes joins with glucose.)

Although it has been shown that CLA may have anticarcinogenic effects and the ability to modulate diabetic and immune system responses, less is certain about its effect on body mass. Animal studies have shown that CLA can increase lean body mass and decrease fat.[207,208,274,275] Studies in animals also show that CLA improves feed efficiency, which means that animals given CLA gain weight without receiving more food. If validated in human studies, these results could have interesting applications in athletics as well as medicine.

Recent investigations have demonstrated that animals receiving a diet rich in CLA have a reduction in adipose tissue.[276] One such study fed mice a diet of 5.5% corn oil or a CLA-supplemented diet consisting of 5.0% corn oil

plus 0.5% CLA. Mice receiving the supplement exhibited 57% and 60% lower body fat and 5% and 14% increased lean body mass compared with controls ($p < 0.05$). Total carnitine palmitoyltransferase activity, an enzyme used in the oxidation of fatty acids, was increased in fat pad and skeletal muscle sites of the experimental animals. Cell culture experiments used adipocytes were also conducted and showed that CLA treatment significantly reduced heparin-releasable lipoprotein lipase activity (-66%) as well as the intracellular concentrations of triglycerides (-8%) and glycerol (-15%). However, CLA significantly increased free glycerol in the culture medium compared with the control ($p < 0.05$). Researchers concluded that the effects of CLA on body composition appear to be a result in part of reduced fat deposition and increased lipolysis in adipocytes, along with enhanced fatty acid oxidation in myocytes and adipocytes. Another interesting observation was the increase in the percentage of whole body protein and carcass water in mice receiving CLA supplementation. Unfortunately, because of the small sample size, it was not possible to conclude from these data alone that CLA induced a significant increase in protein accretion. However, these investigators also mention data combined from 10 other CLA studies, which indicate that CLA-fed mice do in fact exhibit increased whole body protein relative to control animals ($p = 0.04$). Their findings have led to further research examining alterations in lean body mass induced by the supplementation of CLA.

Park et al.[277] recently published a two-part experiment. In the first part, 8-week-old mice were fed a control diet or a diet supplemented with 0.5% CLA (CLA: 40.8–41.1% c-9, t-11 isomer; 43.5–44.9% t-10, c-12 isomer). Results from each feeding showed parallel, but significantly distinct responses for both absolute and relative changes in body fat mass, which was decreased in the CLA-fed mice. In addition, relative alterations in whole body protein and whole body water were both increased in the experimental group. In the second part of the experiment, weanling mice were fed a control diet or a diet with added CLA (0.5% CLA) for 4 weeks. After 4 weeks, all mice were fed the control diet (no CLA). The experimental group exhibited significantly reduced body fat and significantly enhanced whole body water relative to controls at the time of the shift in food composition. Time trends for the changes in relative body composition were described as the CLA-fed group exhibited significantly less body fat, but significantly more whole body protein, whole body water and whole body ash than controls. Tissue analyses of the animals revealed that the CLA isomer t-10, c-12 was cleared significantly faster than was the c-9, t-11 isomer. These findings confirm data showing that CLA given to mice can increase whole body protein and whole body water, and decrease fat mass. Changes in body composition were still visible 8 weeks after the cessation of supplementation. This indicates CLA can induce effects on muscle mass and adipose tissue for at least some time after the clearance of the compound.

Particularly interesting in these studies are the different effects of the various isomers. Currently, CLA available on the market today contains several different isomers and scientists are attempting to isolate the isomer(s) responsible for the beneficial effects of CLA supplementation. In an investigation conducted by researchers at the University of Wisconsin-Madison, the *trans*-10, *cis*-12 isomer of CLA was found responsible for inducing body composition changes.[277] Reduced body fat, enhanced body water, enhanced body protein, and enhanced body ash were associated with feeding the *trans*-10 *cis*-12 CLA isomer. In cell culture experiments, adipocytes had reduced lipoprotein lipase activity, intracellular triglyceride, and glycerol, and enhanced glycerol release into the medium as a result of the *trans*-10, *cis*-12 isomer. The *cis*-9, *trans*-11 and *trans*-9, *trans*-11 CLA isomers did not affect the biochemical markers that were tested. Thus, body composition changes are mediated by the *trans*-10, *cis*-12 CLA isomer—and it alone appears to be responsible for many of the biochemical effects of CLA.

Human Studies

Human data on CLA are at present limited. In one of the few trials available, Lowery et al.[278] examined the effects of CLA in novice bodybuilders. Twenty-four men (19–28 yrs) ingested 7.2 g/day of CLA or placebo (vegetable oil) while completing 6 weeks of bodybuilding exercise. After the trial was completed, gains in arm girth (corrected for skinfolds, body mass, and leg press strength [1-RM]) were greater in the CLA-supplemented group than in the placebo group.

- Skinfold-corrected arm girth
  CLA pre = 7175 ± 978, post = 7562 ± 1000 mm^2; Placebo pre = 7777 ± 1532, post = 7819 ± 1516 mm^2

- Body mass
  CLA pre = 77.6 ± 11.8, post = 79.0 ± 12.0 kg; Placebo pre = 77.8 ± 11.9, post = 77.8 ± 12.2 kg

- Leg press 1-RM
  CLA pre = 263.6 ± 163.0, post = 335 ± 75.1 kg; Placebo pre = 271.5 ± 52.9, post = 306.8 ± 70.2 kg; p < 0.04

However, no differences were noted for subcutaneous fat (skinfolds), total body fat (bioelectrical impedance analysis [BIA]), or body water distribution in either the intracellular or extracellular compartments. Further analysis of a subset of subjects revealed no difference in serum glucose, lipids, BUN, creatinine, LDH, SGOT, and SGPT enzymes.[279]

In another trial, Kreider et al.[280] further examined the effects of CLA supplementation and resistance-training on bone mineral content (BMC), bone mineral density (BMD), and markers of immune stress. In a double-blind and randomized trial, 23 experienced resistance-trained males were matched according to total body weight and training volume. Subjects were given supplements containing either 9 g/day of olive oil (placebo) or 6 g/day of CLA with 3.2 g/day of fatty acids for 28 days. Leukocytes from fasting whole blood were typed, and dual-energy x-ray absorptiometry (DEXA) determined whole body (excluding cranium) BMC and BMD on days 0 and 28 of supplementation. The results of this trial revealed a trend towards an increase in BMC in the CLA group. Some evidence suggested that CLA reduced the NeLy ratio (p = 8 ± 12; CLA = −25 ± 12%; p = 0.07), suggesting less immune stress. The results provide some support to contentions that CLA supplementation may improve bone and immune status during resistance training in humans. However, additional research is necessary.

Safety and Toxicity

Long-term use of CLA in humans has not been evaluated; however, animal data collected from CLA studies and data on other essential fatty acids would indicate that supplementation is likely safe and may be beneficial to the overall health of athletes, especially in regard to disease prevention.[200]

Octacosanol

Octacosanol is one of many compounds found in wheat germ oil.[281] Interestingly, this supplement may have indirect effects on muscle mass by acting on the central nervous system (CNS). Octacosanol is not known to have any anabolic or anticatabolic effects on muscle tissue itself, but may play a role in muscle and strength development by acting on nerve tissue. One aspect of increasing speed and strength, in addition to muscular hypertrophy, is via neural adaptation.[157] If athletes can increase the efficiency at which the nervous system acts, this may facilitate speed and strength production and influence the growth response in skeletal muscle by activating more muscle fibers during a given lift.

Scientists have theorized octacosanol may improve neuromuscular function by stabilizing nerve cell membranes and improving oxygen transport. However, there is no solid evidence that supports this notion. Some studies show increases in grip strength, reaction speed, and increased endurance performance with octacosanol supplementation. Others show no changes in performance. Interestingly, Russian scientists believe that the ability of octacosanol to facilitate oxygen transport was overemphasized by their American counterparts and that the real benefit of octacosanol supplementation is its ability to improve reaction time.[282]

Animal Studies

Animal studies involving octacosanol are inconclusive regarding a definite performance-enhancing effect with this supplement. Studies in the literature show equivocal data from swimming time tests in rodents.[283–285] However, the studies are quite old and investigations conducted today on octacosanol would benefit from advances in technology and laboratory techniques available to the modern sport scientist. Theoretically, this supplement may elicit beneficial effects in certain sports. Nonetheless, there is little evidence to establish scientific support for physique, strength, and/or speed athletes to use this compound.

Human Studies

Limited research exists demonstrating octacosanol has performance-enhancing effects in activities requiring a high degree of quickness (i.e., reaction time). Theoretically, specific instances in which reaction time may be aided by octacosanol are the explosive transition from eccentric to concentric phases of power lifting/Olympic weightlifting (i.e. squatting and pressing), getting out of the blocks for a sprint race, getting off the line quickly after the snap in football, and rapid throwing movements in baseball.

In one 8-week, double-blind study, 16 subjects were administered either 1000 µg of octacosanol or placebo per day.[286] Results showed that those receiving octacosanol had improved reaction time to visual stimuli as well as a significant increase in grip strength. There were no differences in either grip strength or endurance time as measured by cycle ergometry.

Safety and Toxicity

This substance has been widely used as a food and nutritional supplement since the 1950s. There are no reports in the literature of toxicity in animals or humans.

Tribulus terrestris

Tribulus terrestris is also known as Puncture Vine and Caltrop fruit. Proponents of its use claim the substance acts as a luteinizing hormone stimulant that can increase the body's production of testosterone, which in turn would augment protein synthesis. Claims are based on obscure case studies published in foreign journals that are not easily obtained. Still, despite this lack of evidence, Internet and magazine ads appear regularly touting its unfounded effects. To further fuel the fire, former Eastern block "experts," now residing in the United States, have begun to speak of "proprietary knowledge and expertise" regarding the use of this formerly guarded "state secret." Currently, however, there is only one peer-reviewed study available on the use of *Tribulus terrestris* in healthy resistance-trained subjects.[287] Of general interest to athletes and those sports medicine professionals dealing with these individuals is that studies used to substantiate advertising claims often deal with disease or deficiency states and are not applicable to healthy populations. This is certainly the case with the data cited by supplement manufacturers marketing *Tribulus terrestris*.

Human Studies

In one of a handful of studies, Wang et al.[288] treated patients with coronary heart disease (CHD) using *Tribulus terrestris*. According to 406 cases of clinical observation and a cross test (67 cases treated with Yufen Ningxin Pian as control) in this Chinese journal, the results showed that the total rate of remission of angina pectoris was 82.3% in patients treated with *Tribulus terrestris* versus 67.2% in the control group ($p < 0.05$). Similarly, the total effective rate of ECG improvement (52.7%) was higher than that of the control group (35.8%).

In another study examining the purported hormonal implications, Adimoelja et al.[289] used *Tribulus terrestris* in the treatment of male subfertility. With the primary aim of examining alternative therapies to hormonal treatment, these investigators examined the use of this traditional herbal medicine used for centuries all over the world. The use of *Tribulus terrestris* in Asian countries has been claimed to improve strength. To scientifically evaluate these claims, extraction of the active components in this study were performed, identified, and purified. The main active constituent identified was protodioscin, a nonhormonal agent having a steroidal chemical structure similar to dehydroepiandrosterone (DHEA). The dried powder extract was then experimentally administered in a double-blind study involving 45 subfertile men with moderate idiopathic oligozoosperms. During the trial, 36 of the men were treated with *Tribulus terrestris* dry powder extract and 9 men were administered a placebo. After 3 months, 7 men were able to conceive with their wives. This was attributed to the enhancement of sperm function after *Tribulus terrestris* consumption. Further studies involving diabetic impotent men treated with *Tribulus terrestris* dry powder extract showed a significant ($p < 0.05$) increase of DHEA-S blood levels as well as improvement of libido.

Despite these results, two observations should be noted. First, this is not a peer-reviewed study. Second, despite the apparent effect of *Tribulus terrestris* in a hormonally compromised population, its effectiveness remains to be determined in a healthy male population. To this end, Antonio et al.[287] examined the use of *Tribulus terrestris* with the express purpose of studying the effects on body composition and exercise performance in resistance-trained males. During this trial, 15 subjects were randomly assigned to a placebo or *Tribulus terrestris* (3.21 mg/kg body weight daily) group. Body weight, body composition, maximal strength, dietary intake, and mood states were determined before and after an 8-week exercise (periodized resistance training) and supplementation period. After 8 weeks, there were no changes in body weight, percent body fat, total body water, dietary intake, or mood states in either group. Muscle endurance (determined by the maximal number of repetitions at 100–200% of body weight) increased for the bench and leg press exercises in the placebo group (p < 0.05; bench press ±28.4%; leg press ±28.6%), whereas the *Tribulus terrestris* group experienced an increase in leg press strength only (bench press ±3.1% not significant; leg press ±28.6%; p < 0.05). Therefore, owing to these preliminary data, supplementation with *Tribulus terrestris* does not appear to enhance body composition or exercise performance in resistance-trained males.

Safety and Toxicity

There may be concerns about the safety of long-term, high-dose *Tribulus terrestris* supplementation in humans. *Tribulus terrestris* ingestion may cause toxic reactions in animals.[290–292] It should be noted that "natural" and "herbal" supplements are not safe for all individuals and can be harmful to the health and well-being of athletes if improper dosing or a potentially dangerous substance is used (see Chapter 1). *Tribulus terrestris* is promoted as a safe alternative to anabolic steroids despite the fact that no toxicity studies in athletes have been conducted.

Vanadyl Sulfate (Vanadium)

Vanadium is a metallic element that assumes several oxidized states (−1 to +5) and was first identified in 1831 in Sweden. Named after Vanadis, the Scandinavian goddess of beauty, youth, and luster,[299] vanadium enters the blood, regardless of oxidation state, and is converted into vanadyl-transferrin and vanadyl-ferrin complexes in plasma and body fluids. In the *reference human* the total-body pool of vanadium is approximately 100 μg and estimated daily intake ranges from 10 to 60 μg. Urine seems to be the major means of excretion for absorbed vanadium.[293] Little of the absorbed vanadium is retained under normal conditions in the body because most tissues contain less than 10 ng vanadium/g fresh weight. Of the tissues and fluids containing vanadium, the liver, kidney, bone, spleen, thyroid, brain, fat, milk, colostrum, bile, urine, lungs, and hair account for much of these stores.[293–295] The highest concentrations of vanadium are typically observed in city dwellers owing to the high airborne concentration from industrial production.[293–295]

The dietary sources of vanadium are a diverse group of foods. Particularly rich in vanadium are mushrooms, parsley, dill, and black pepper. Fresh fruits, vegetables, and beverages constitute some of the other sources for vanadium along with seafood, cereals, and liver.[296] Moreover, food processing appears to affect the vanadium content of refined products. For example, dairy milk has an average value of 1.1 μg/kg of vanadium, whereas powdered milk has a value as high as 25 μg/kg.[296] Meanwhile, wheat grain contains 3.6 μg/kg of vanadium while vanadium levels in milled flour can be as high as 40 μg/kg.[296] Each of these differences has been postulated to be directly attributable to refining processes of food and may originate from the stainless steel processing equipment used.[296]

Many studies confirm that, of the total dietary vanadium ingested, less than 5–10% is actually absorbed by the gastrointestinal tract,[296–298] with most of dietary vanadium absorbed by the upper GI tract.[299] High vanadium intakes in animal models are known to both influence and be affected by the gastrointestinal metabolism of chloride, iodide, chromium, iron, copper, ascorbic acid, cysteine, methionine, riboflavin, and some proteins.[297]

The distribution of this minute vanadium pool varies between the tissue compartments of the body. Vanadium accumulates mostly in organ tissues, with the highest concentrations seen in liver, kidney, and bone.[295,300] Although bone appears to be the long-term storage compartment for vanadium,[296,301] the storage of available or accessible vanadium is associated mainly with ferritin and transferrin. Thus, low vanadium concentrations are homeostatically regulated in the blood and fatty tissue, resulting in a more rapid transfer of vanadium to long-term storage sites (e.g., bone) or excretory pathways (e.g., bile, urine, hair).[296]

In human serum, the concentration of vanadium is 0.035 ng/mL (range, 0.014–0.939) and is apparently reduced by the presence of ascorbate, glutathione, and Nicotinamide adenine dinucleotide (NADH).[302] In plasma, vanadium exists as metavanadate (VO3 − [V]), whereas inside cells it exists as the reduced form, vanadyl (VO2 + [IV]).[303] Blood plays a pivotal role in exchanging dietary or intravenous vanadium with body tissues, the gastrointestinal tract, and the kidneys.[299] Nearly 95% of the vanadium transported in blood is bound to transferrin as the vanadyl (IV) ion. This is bound intracellularly[304,305] and therefore may compete with iron for both gastrointestinal absorption and cellular receptor sites. Similarly, there is some evidence that vanadium can form a complex with lactoferrin and be transported to suckling infants during breastfeeding.[306] Currently, the downstream metabolic effects of this phenomenon are not fully understood. Moreover, vanadium concentrations can be influenced by environmental factors via percutaneous and transpulmonary absorption routes.[296] In this regard, the major toxic effects of vanadium that have been observed are the result of vanadium dust inhalation in industrial situations.[296]

Functionally, vanadium influences NaK-ATPase, phosphoryl transferase enzymes, adenylate cyclase, and protein kinases, as well as glucose, lipid, bone, and tooth metabolism.[302] Other reports also allude to vanadium's influence on the prevention and treatment of infections, diabetes, atherosclerosis, anemia, the metabolism of lipids, and biogenic amines (affective disorders).[303,307–309] However, vanadium has gained wide interest largely owing to its inhibition of select ATPases by low concentrations of vanadate[310] and the observation that vanadate is a potent and selective inhibitor of phosphotyrosine phosphatases.[311,312] The phosphorylation of tyrosine is of interest because of its role in protein modifications and because of the association of growth factor receptors and certain oncogene proteins with tyrosine kinase activity. Epidermal growth factor (EGF), insulin, and platelet-derived growth factor (PDGF) all activate autophosphorylation of their respective receptors on tyrosine residues, and transformation of cells elevates total cell phosphotyrosine five- to ten-fold.[313] Vanadate appears to mimic certain effects of growth factors on cells. These effects are presumably dependent on the growth factor–induced increase in receptor tyrosine kinase. Among these effects are increased glucose oxidation and inhibited lipolysis in adipocytes via insulin[314]; increased Na+/H+ exchange via PDGF, EGF, or serum[315]; and increased S6 ribosomal protein phosphorylation via insulin and EGF.[316]

Animal Studies

The effects of vanadium are relative to different organ systems. One of the most consistent effects of vanadate is illustrated in the alterations in the function of mammalian kidneys. Infusion or injection of vanadium into the renal artery causes profound renal artery vasoconstriction. In cat and dog models, this reaction appears to be as intense as reactions caused by norepinephrine. Attenuation of this response occurs by reducing the ionized calcium concentration.[317] In dog models, infusion of ouabain and vanadate together into the renal artery causes significant natriuresis (i.e., excretion of Na+).[318] By contrast, vasoconstriction produced in the rat is much less intense with renal blood flow and glomerular filtration continuing in the presence of rather high plasma levels of vanadate.[309,319] Vanadate causes profound natriuresis and diuresis in certain experimental animals. For example, in rats whose blood has been slightly volume expanded, it is not rare to observe 50% or more of the filtered sodium appearing in the final urine in response to vanadate.

In plasma, vanadate enters erythrocytes and is reduced to vanadyl (IV),[320] and it inhibits the sodium pump and calcium transport system when present in micromolar concentrations in the external medium.[321] In nervous tissue, vanadate also inhibits calcium transport in dialyzed squid axons[322,323] and appears to inhibit dynein-like molecules in the lobster giant axon.[324] Plasma vanadium levels from patients with bipolar disorders and mania

have been reported to be elevated above normal.[325] Vanadate increases the hepatic vascular resistance in a dose-dependent manner,[326] and hepatic oxygen consumption and bile flow are decreased in response to high levels of vanadate. Vanadate enters hepatocytes but does not appear to have any effect on these cells, possibly because of changes in oxidation state.

In living animals vanadate also causes positive or negative cardiac inotropic (force of muscular contraction) effects depending on the concentration of the drug injected and the animal species.[327,328] However, verapamil (calcium channel blocker) appears to prevent the increase in arterial pressure and pulmonary arterial pressure caused by vanadate and attenuates the accompanying increase in cardiac output.[329] Several studies with intact heart preparations suggest that the effect of vanadate on cardiac performance is not caused by alterations in NaK-ATPase concentrations. Inasmuch as vanadate increases arterial blood pressure in living animals, it has been suggested that this compound may play a role in producing hypertension. Prolonged dietary administration of vanadate has been shown to cause a dose-dependent increase in the blood pressure of rats.[330] Still, it is not certain whether this increase is a result of the effects of vanadate on NaK-ATPase in vascular smooth muscle or some other property.

In animal models, the oral treatment of streptozotocin diabetic animals with vanadium causes a correction of hyperglycemia and prevention of subsequently induced diabetic complications.[331] Vanadium treatment in nondiabetic animals lowers plasma insulin levels by reducing insulin demand, suggesting that vanadium has direct *in vivo* insulin-mimetic or insulin-enhancing effects. This effect appears to continue following chronic treatment and subsequent vanadium withdrawal for up to 13 weeks. Several studies have shown normalized glucose concentrations and improved basal insulin levels in addition to near-normal glucose tolerance, despite an insignificant insulin response.[331,332] Because vanadium accumulates in several tissue sites when pharmacological doses are administered, these stores could be important in maintaining near-normal glucose tolerance, at least in the short-term, following withdrawal from treatment.[339,340] In recent work by Pepato and colleagues,[335] the effects of oral vanadyl sulfate treatment (1 mg/mL) in young streptozotocin diabetic rats were analyzed at 19 and 29 days to determine body weight, food and water intake, glycemia, urinary excretion of glucose and urea, and glycemia level. Tissue weight of the pancreas, soleus, extensor digitorum longus, and adipose tissue (epididymal and retroperitoneal) were also assessed. The results of this trial showed that the treatment of young diabetic rats with vanadyl sulfate promoted the reduction of hyperglycemia ($p < 0.01$), food ($p < 0.01$), water intake ($p < 0.05$), and body weight ($p < 0.05$). However, no group differences were noted for tissue weight, pancreas weight, or urinary urea concentration. In conclusion, the vanadyl treatment was able to reduce the main metabolic alterations often found in diabetes. Future research should attempt to verify the effects of vanadyl sulfate on muscle protein metabolism in diabetic rats. Other animal work shows a potential anticarcinogenic effect of vanadium[336]; however, more research is needed to confirm such an effect.

Human Studies

Although some of the results from animal studies are encouraging, there are no data to date supporting vanadium's role as an anabolic supplement in humans. Fawcett et al.[337] analyzed subjects during 12 weeks of weight training. During this trial, the effect of oral vanadyl sulfate (0.5 mg/kg/day) was investigated with regard to general anthropometry, body composition, and performance. Following a 12-week, double-blind, placebo-controlled trial involving weight-training volunteers, performance was assessed in the treatment and placebo groups using 1 and 10 repetitions maximum (RM) for the bench press and leg extension. Thirty-one subjects completed the trial, with two vanadyl sulfate subjects withdrawing because of apparent side effects. The study concluded there were no significant treatment effects for anthropometric parameters and body composition during the trial. Both groups had significant improvements in performance but the only significant effect of treatment was a Treatment × Time interaction in the 1-RM leg extension ($p = 0.002$), which may be because the vanadyl sulfate group had a lower performance level at baseline compared control. The authors thus concluded that oral vanadyl sulfate was ineffective in changing body composition in weight-training athletes and that further investigation is needed.

Safety and Toxicity

Vanadium is widely distributed in the environment and occurs in various concentrations in soil, water, air, plants, and animal tissues approximately equal to those of copper, lead, or zinc.[338] Natural sources of airborne vanadium are believed to be continental dust and marine aerosols. Toxic effects in humans and animals under natural conditions do occur, albeit infrequently, even when given orally.[308] Humans typically experience toxicity in association with industrial processes.[339,340] Absorption of vanadium may be gastrointestinal, respiratory, or percutaneous. Vanadium that is absorbed is excreted mainly in urine, but it also appears in feces.[309] The major effects of vanadium in humans after industrial exposure are primarily irritations to the mucous membranes of the eyes, nose, throat, and respiratory tract. Bronchitis and bronchospasm are characteristic symptoms, and pneumonia occasionally develops.[309] Inhalation of and exposure to vanadium can cause conjunctivitis, pharyngitis, rhinitis, chronic cough, and tightness of the chest.[294] In medical use, gastrointestinal disorders may also develop.[341] Likewise, vanadium has been shown to produce gastrointestinal distress, fatigue, cardiac palpitation, and kidney damage, as well as other physiological effects such as disturbances of the central nervous system, cardiovascular changes, and metabolic alterations in experimental animals.[342]

Chronic respiratory exposure to rats has produced hemorrhagic inflammation in the lungs, as well as hemorrhage in liver, kidneys, and heart, and vascular congestion. Continuous acute exposure at high levels has caused paralysis, respiratory failure, and death.[342] When ingested in drinking water at 5 or 50 mg/kg, vanadium caused elevated vanadium tissue levels but no effect on growth rate or maturity. However, moderate to severe effects were observed in rats given oral doses of 100 to 1000 mg/kg of diet[343,344] and the severity of toxic effects increases as the valency increases.[345] In most studies examining the insulin-like effectiveness of vanadium in diabetic rats and mice, vanadium was given orally in the drinking water. Concentrations of 0.2 to 1.1 mg/mL and greater were considered to be toxic.[341,345]

Administration of vanadium as metavanadate or orthovanadate causes developmental toxicity in rats and mice,[346,347] whereas vanadyl ions were embryotoxic and teratogenic in mice when given orally.[346] Hepatotoxicity of vanadium has also been demonstrated in isolated perfused hepatocytes.[348] In isolated perfused rat livers significant lipid peroxidation was shown. The pro-oxidant effects of vanadate were found to be mainly responsible for its cytotoxic activity. In diabetic rats, although vanadium treatment normalized blood glucose levels, some signs of toxicity have been observed. These include decreased body weight gain and increased serum concentrations of urea and creatinine.[349] The use of chelating agents to reduce vanadium toxicity and improve insulin potency is now being examined.[350]

In calves, the oral administration of 7.5 mg/kg of body weight does not appear to cause side effects. However, in larger doses of 20 mg/kg, weight loss, diarrhea, loss of appetite, emaciation, and elevated vanadium tissue levels have been noted.[351] In sheep, no effects were observed when dietary vanadium did not exceed 200 mg/kg. Still, diarrhea and loss of appetite occurred after 1 day of exposure to 400 or 800 mg/kg.[352] This pattern remains consistent for other species as well. In chicks, growth retardation has been reported at dietary levels of 20 mg/kg of diet or greater.[340,353-355]

Levels of 25 to 60 mg/kg have also been reported to affect developmental characteristics in animals and may apply to humans as well. To date, noted effects include decreased egg production,[340,353,356,357] reduced hatchability,[339,340,358] reduced egg quality,[339,340,358-360] and delayed onset of egg production.[358] Vanadium has been shown to accumulate to a large extent in the renal tissue of animals,[344] which may represent a major site of action.[360] Studies *in vivo* with chickens exposed to 25, 50, or 100 mg vanadium/kg of diet for 15 months showed that vanadium inhibited NaK-ATPase from renal tissue.[361,362] Studies involving exposure to vanadium and the mycotoxin ochratoxin A, a known nephrotoxic agent, show that body weight gain are reduced by ochratoxin A alone.

In humans, Boden et al.[363] sought to determine the safety and efficacy of vanadyl sulfate in a single-blind, placebo-controlled study. Eight patients (four men and four women) with noninsulin-dependent diabetes mellitus ingested vanadyl sulfate (50 mg 2x/day) for 4 weeks. Six of these patients (four men and two women) continued in the study and were given a placebo for an additional 4 weeks. Euglycemic-hyperinsulinemic clamps were performed before and after the vanadyl sulfate and placebo phases. Vanadyl sulfate was associated with gastrointestinal side effects in six of eight patients during the first week, but was well tolerated after this period. Vanadyl sulfate administration was associated with a 20% decrease in fasting glucose concentration (from 9.3 to 7.4 mmol/L; $p < 0.05$) and a decrease in hepatic glucose output during hyperinsulinemia (from 5.0 pre–vanadyl sulfate to 3.1 ± 0.9 μmol/kg post–vanadyl sulfate; $p < 0.02$). The improvement in fasting plasma glucose and hepatic glucose output that occurred during vanadyl sulfate treatment was maintained during the placebo phase. Vanadyl sulfate had no significant effect on rates of total-body glucose uptake, glycogen synthesis, glycolysis, carbohydrate oxidation, or lipolysis during euglycemic-hyperinsulinemic clamps. The authors concluded that the dose of vanadyl sulfate used was well tolerated and resulted in modest reductions of fasting plasma glucose and hepatic insulin resistance.[363] Similar results have been obtained in moderately obese patients with noninsulin-dependent diabetes. However, these effects are not observed in their non-diabetic counterparts.[364]

Fawcett et al.[365] also investigated the possibility that vanadium may contribute to anemia and changes in the leukocyte system. In this study, the effects of oral vanadyl sulfate (0.5 mg/kg/day) on hematological indices (red and white cell and platelet counts, red cell mean cell volume and hemoglobin level), blood viscosity (hematocrit, plasma viscosity, and blood viscosity) and biochemistry (lipids and indices of liver and kidney function) were investigated in a 12-week, double-blind, placebo-controlled trial in 31 weight-training athletes. Blood viscosity was evaluated at 0, 2, 4, 8, and 12 weeks and hematological indices and biochemistry were measured pre- and post-treatment. Both the treatment group and placebo group showed increases in hematocrit (3.3–3.6%) and blood viscosity but there were no significant effects of treatment. Similarly, there were no treatment effects on hematological indices and biochemistry.

In general, the possibility of toxicity is high when vanadium is given by injection, low per oral administration, and intermediate by the respiratory tract. Toxicity also varies considerably with the oxidation of the compound, but generally it increases as valency increases, with pentavalent vanadium being the most toxic. The manifestations of exposure to vanadium are many and diverse; however, the mechanisms of toxic action and/or interaction are not understood. Further work is required to answer these questions. Unfortunately, there are limited data on oral dosing with vanadium compounds in controlled studies. An early trial using oxytartratovanadate (75–125 ng/day) for 5 months showed a potential for lower cholesterol but also produced gastrointestinal distress in 50% of patients (6 of 12).[366] Additionally, it appears that vanadyl compounds are less toxic than vanadate in rats.[367] More recent evidence in insulin-dependent and noninsulin-dependent diabetics indicate that vanadyl sulfate at 100 mg and 125 mg/day is well tolerated—with some evidence of mild gastrointestinal distress,[368] but with no apparent complications in younger weight-lifting participants.[365]

SUMMARY

Currently, supplements marketed to athletes promise to enhance muscle mass, strength, and speed despite the dearth of scientific evidence supporting these claims. Often, many such products are promoted based on observations from *in vitro* (test tubes and tissue cultures) and animal trials, with no confirmation in humans. Should the "Animal Olympics" become popular in the future, a whole new marketing strategy may subsequently emerge. Indeed, although animal data are intriguing, lack of follow-up in human trials is akin to relegating those findings observed in animals to substantial leaps of faith for human usage.

For instance, companies selling nutritional products often take a sales-before-science outlook on product promotion and have fallen victim to the abhorrent practice of presenting their "scientific data" at trade shows long before it is thoroughly researched. To this end, magazines abound laden with colorful graphs and figures attempting to prove that the advertised product is the best, yet no references are provided citing any scientific evidence to back these claims.

As scientists, coaches, and practitioners of strength and power sports, it is tempting to laugh this off as just another chapter in the history of nutritional charlatanism; we are quick to condemn because it doesn't fit our current paradigm. We disbelieve new and novel findings because we are trained to be skeptical. And sadly, we discount an attempt at innovation because our governing organizations don't have a position statement covering the topic. Thus, we fall too easily into that habit of being sheep, instead of independent thinkers willing to challenge the marketplace and scientific arena. Unfortunately, this is a poor stance to take on the subject of supplements, especially as we are supposed to be the *enlightened* ones, owing to our years of training and practice in the field.

We hope that this chapter will help spur interest in both students and scientists in the gathering of scientific information that will justify the use and production of supplemental products in the future. Although it is tempting to take a myopic view on these types of investigations, many marvelous substances exist in nature that may facilitate both athletic performance and subsequent health outcomes in various populations of differing disease states. Our only true failure will lie in the unwillingness to examine in the fullest all that creative thinking can provide.

AUTHORS' RECOMMENDATIONS

Currently, only creatine has a substantial body of evidence to support its use as an ergogenic aid. The use of creatine as a supplement shows reproducible efficacy in events lasting from 6 seconds to 4 minutes—without side effects. However, the long-term effects (>5 yrs) of creatine use are not entirely known.

HMB has been shown to augment skeletal muscle mass and strength in some human studies, although the data to date have largely been obtained from one laboratory. Perhaps more substantial than the human performance data are the blood chemistry analyses showing a decrease in certain markers for training-induced muscle proteolysis as measured by urine 3-methylhistidine excretion and creatine kinase. Studies demonstrating improved immune function with HMB use are promising. Coupled with its possible anticatabolic effects, HMB may prove to be an important part of a supplement program for those individuals who have AIDS, other wasting syndromes, or other medical conditions in which pathologic weight loss is a concern.

Similar effects appear to be true for CLA; however, more research is needed.

What is evident at this point is that HMB and CLA do not produce consistent results in healthy, active populations. We hope that, as research continues, questions regarding the effectiveness of such products will become more clearly elucidated. An intriguing avenue of research may be the use of various supplements during recuperation. For instance, skeletal muscle atrophy occurs after casting, immobilization, or prolonged bed rest. If certain supplements could offset the deleterious effects of skeletal muscle atrophy, this would have a significant impact on how we *treat* wasting diseases.

Even though chromium and vanadyl sulfate do not demonstrate any appreciable benefit in healthy athletes, these compounds may be of benefit to those athletes who are type II diabetic or glucose intolerant. As for the status of *Tribulus terrestris* and other supplements that are marketed with great zeal, there is no solid scientific foundation to support their use.

FUTURE RESEARCH

Creatine is an effective ergogenic aid, particularly for strength-power athletes. Further work needs to be done to assess the role (if any) regarding creatine and muscle cramping, dehydration, and perhaps renal/hepatic function. With regard to HMB, additional studies are needed to support the claims that it can act as an anticatabolic agent (in skeletal muscle) and therefore be used as a *bodybuilding* supplement. Alternatively, HMB might be useful under conditions in which athletes are training heavily (e.g., long-distance runners) and are perhaps losing too much lean body mass. Could HMB perhaps ameliorate the loss of skeletal muscle protein in this circumstance?

Chromium and vanadium (vanadyl sulfate) have an abundance of data showing that neither of these has an effect on body composition or athletic performance. It is doubtful that further work in this area will produce different results. Boron also has little evidence to support manufacturer claims for an ergogenic effect; however, it might be worthwhile to examine boron further in older female populations.

With regard to CLA, the animal data are intriguing—particularly the dramatic changes in body composition. However, it is apparent that what occurs in animals does not always translate into a similar change in humans. Double-blind, placebo-controlled studies would need to be done on resistance-trained athletes supplementing with CLA to determine if body composition is favorably affected. Certainly, the dearth of information on *Tribulus terrestris* or octacosanol would necessitate further investigation. Until such research is performed, scientists (and consumers) will need to make educated "best guesses" to determine if these substances have potential ergogenic effects.

REFERENCES

1. Al-Habet SMH, Redda KK, Lee HJ. Uses and abuses of anabolic steroids by athletes. In: Redda KK, Walker CA, Barnett, eds. Cocaine, Marijuana and Designer Drugs: Chemistry, Pharmacology and Behaviour. Boca Raton: CRC Press, 1989:212–231.
2. Newsholme EA. Basic aspects of metabolic regulation and their application to provision of energy in exercise. In: Poortmans JR, ed. Principles of Exercise Biochemistry. 2nd ed. Vol. 38. Basel: Karger, 1993:52–88.
3. Newsholme EA, Leech AR. Biochemistry for the Medical Sciences Chester: Wiley Press, 1993.
4. Hirvonen J, Rehunen S, Rusko H, Harkonen M. Breakdown of high-energy phosphate compounds and lactate accumulation during short supramaximal exercise. Eur J Appl Physiol 1987; 56(3):253–259.
5. Hirvonen J, Nummela A, Rusko H, et al. Fatigue and changes of ATP, creatine phosphate, and lactate during the 400-m sprint. Can J Sport Sci 1992;17(2):141–144.
6. Atkinson DE. The energy charge of the adenylate pool as a regulatory parameter: interaction with feedback modifiers. Biochemistry 1968;7(11):4030–4034.
7. Sahlin K. Metabolic changes limiting muscle performance. In: Saltin B, ed. Biochemistry of Exercise. Vol. 6. Champaign, IL: Human Kinetics, 1986:323–343.
8. MacDougall JD, Ward GR, Sale DG, Sutton JR. Biochemical adaptation of human skeletal muscle to heavy resistance training and immobilization. J Appl Physiol 1977;43(4):700–703.
9. Tesch PA, Thorsson A, Colliander EB. Effects of eccentric and concentric resistance training on skeletal muscle substrates, enzyme activities and capillary supply. Acta Physiol Scand 1990;140:575–580.
10. Greenhaff PL, Gleeson M, Maughan RJ. The effects of a glycogen loading regimen on acid-base status and blood lactate concentration before and after a fixed period of high-intensity exercise in man. Eur J Appl Physiol 1988;57(2):254–259.
11. Sherman WM, Doyle JA, Lamb DR, Strauss RH. Dietary carbohydrate, muscle glycogen, and exercise performance during 7 d of training. Am J Clin Nutr 1993;57(1):27–31.
12. Wooton SA, Williams C. Influence of carbohydrate-status on performance during maximal exercise. Int J Sports Med 1984;5:126–127.
13. Peeters BM, Lantz CD, Mayhew JL. Effect of oral creatine monohydrate and creatine phosphate supplementation on maximal strength indices, body composition and blood pressure. J Strength Cond Res 1998;13:3–9.
14. Saks VA, Strumia E. Phosphocreatine: molecular and cellular aspects of the mechanism of cardioprotective action. Curr Ther Res 1983;53:565–598.
15. Benedict SR, Osterberg E. Studies in creatine and creatine metabolism: III. On the origin of urinary creatine. J Biol Chem 1914;18:195–214.
16. Benedict SR, Osterberg E. Studies in creatine and creatine metabolism: V. The metabolism of creatine. J Biol Chem 1923;26:229–252.
17. Folin O. On the preparation of creatine, creatinine and standard creatinine solutions. J Biol Chem 1914;17:463–468.
18. Folin O. On the determination of creatinine and creatine in urine. J Biol Chem 1914;17:469–473.
19. Folin O. On the determination of creatinine and creatine in blood, milk and tissues. J Biol Chem 1914;17:475–481.
20. Folin O, Buckman TE. On creatine content of muscle. J Biol Chem 1914;17:483–486.
21. Folin O, Denis W. On creatinine and creatine content of blood. J Biol Chem 1914;17:487–419.
22. Folin O, Denis W. Protein metabolism from the standpoint of blood and tissue analysis: an interpretation of creatine and creatinine in relation to animal metabolism. J Biol Chem 1914;17:493–502.
23. Harris RC, Soderlund K, Hultman E. Elevation of creatine in resting and exercised muscle of normal subjects by creatine supplementation. Clin Sci (Colch) 1992;83(3):367–374.
24. Myers VC, Fine MS. The influence of the administration of creatine and creatinine on the creatine content of muscle. J Biol Chem 1913;16:169–186.
25. Green AL, Simpson EJ, Littlewood JJ, et al. Carbohydrate ingestion augments creatine retention during creatine feeding in humans. Acta Physiol Scand 1996;158(2):195–202.
26. Earnest CP, Becham S, Whyte BO, Almada AL. Acute creatine monohydrate ingestion and anaerobic performance in men and women. J Strength Cond Res 1998;12.
27. Earnest CP, Beckham S, Whyte BO, Almada AL. Effect of acute creatine ingestion on anaerobic performance. Med Sci Sports Exerc 1998;30(Suppl):141.
28. Hultman E, Bergstrom J, Anderson NM. Breakdown and resynthesis of phosphorylcreatine and adenosine triphosphate in connection with muscular work in man. Scand J Clin Lab Invest 1967; 19(1):56–66.
29. Infante AA, Klaupiks D, Davies RE. Phosphorylcreatine consumption during single working contractons of isolated muscle. Biochem Biophysiol Acta 1965;94:504–515.
30. Spande JI, Schottelius BA. Chemical basis of fatigue in isolated mouse soleus muscle. Am J Physiol 1970;219(5):1490–1495.
31. Edstrom L, Hultman E, Sahlin K, Sjoholm H. The contents of high-energy phosphates in different fibre types in skeletal muscles from rat, guinea-pig and man. J Physiol (Lond) 1982;332:47–58.
32. Soderlund K, Hultman E. ATP and phosphocreatine changes in single human muscle fibers after intense electrical stimulation. Am J Physiol 1991;261(6 Pt 1):E737–741.
33. Soderlund K, Greenhaff PL, Hultman E. Energy metabolism in type I and type II human muscle fibres during short term electrical stimulation at different frequencies. Acta Physiol Scand 1992;144(1):15–22.
34. Tesch PA, Thorsson A, Fujitsuka N. Creatine phosphate in fiber types of skeletal muscle before and after exhaustive exercise. J Appl Physiol 1989;66(4):1756–1759.
35. Liebman M, Wilkinson JG. Carbohydrate metabolism and exercise. In: Wolinski I, Hickson JF, eds. Nutrition in Exercise and Sport. Boca Raton: CRC Press, 1994:15–47.
36. Harris RC, Edwards RH, Hultman E, et al. The time course of phosphorylcreatine resynthesis during recovery of the quadriceps muscle in man. Pflugers Arch 1976;367(2):137–142.
37. Balsom PD, Seger JY, Sjodin B, Ekblom B. Maximal-intensity intermittent exercise: effect of recovery duration. Int J Sports Med 1992;13(7):528–533.
38. Balsom PD, Seger JY, Sjodin B, Ekblom B. Physiological responses to maximal intensity intermittent exercise. Eur J Appl Physiol 1992;65(2):144–149.
39. Bogdanis GC, Nevill ME, Lakomy HKA, Boobis LH. Human muscle metabolism during repeated maximal sprint cycling. J Physiol (Lond) 1993;467.
40. Cheetham ME, Boobis LH, Brooks S, Williams C. Human muscle metabolism during sprint running. J Appl Physiol 1986;61(1):54–60.
41. Casey A, Constantin-Teodosiu D, Howell S, et al. Creatine ingestion favorably affects performance and muscle metabolism during maximal exercise in humans. Am J Physiol 1996;271(1 Pt 1):E31–E37.
42. Greenhaff PL, Bodin K, Soderlund K, Hultman E. Effect of oral creatine supplementation on skeletal muscle phosphocreatine resynthesis. Am J Physiol 1994;266(5 Pt 1):E725–E730.
43. Borsook H, Dubnoff JW. Creatine formation in liver and kidney. J Biol Chem 1940;134:635–639.
44. Chanutin A. The fate of creatine when administered to man. J Biol Chem 1926;67:29–41.
45. Fiske CH, Subbarow Y. The nature of the "inorganic phosphate" in voluntary muscle. Science 1927;65:401.
46. Crim MC, Calloway DH, Margen S. Creatine metabolism in men: urinary creatine and creatinine excretions with creatine feeding. J Nutr 1975;105(4):428–438.
47. Crim MC, Calloway DH, Margon S. Creatine metabolism in men: creatine pool size and turnover in relation to creatine intake. J Nutr 1976;6:371–378.
48. Hoberman HD, Sims EAH, Peters JH. Creatine and creatinine in the normal male adult studied with the aid of isotopoic nitrogen. J Biol Chem 1948;172:45–48.
49. Bjornsson TD. Use of serum creatinine concentrations to determine renal function. Clin Pharmacokinet 1979;4(3):200–222.
50. Greenhaff PL. Creatine and its application as an ergogenic aid. Int J Sports Nutr 1995;5(Suppl):100–110.
51. Delanghe J, De Slypere JP, De Buyzere M, et al. Normal reference values for creatine, creatinine, and carnitine are lower in vegetarians [letter]. Clin Chem 1989;35(8):1802–1803.

52. Walker JB. Metabolic control of creatine biosynthesis: I. Effect of dietary creatine. J Biol Chem 1960;235:2357–2361.

53. Walker JB. Creatine: biosynthesis, regulation and function. In: Meister A, ed. Advances in Enzymology and Related Areas of Molecular Biology. Vol 50. New York: Interscience, 1979:268–280.

54. Balsom PD, Soderlund K, Ekblom B. Creatine in humans with special reference to creatine supplementation. Sports Med 1994; 18(4):268–280.

55. Hoogwerf BJ, Laine DC, Greene E. Urine C-peptide and creatinine (Jaffe method) excretion in healthy young adults on varied diets: sustained effects of varied carbohydrate, protein, and meat content. Am J Clin Nutr 1986;43(3):350–360.

56. Harris RC, Lowe JA, Warnes K, Orme CE. The concentration of creatine in meat, offal and commercial dog food. Res Vet Sci 1997;62(1):58–62.

57. Bennett SE, Bevington A, Walls J. Regulation of intracellular creatine in erythrocytes and myoblasts: influence of uraemia and inhibition of Na,K-ATPase. Cell Biochem Funct 1994;12(2):99–106.

58. Guimbal C, Kilimann MW. A Na(+)-dependent creatine transporter in rabbit brain, muscle, heart, and kidney: cDNA cloning and functional expression. J Biol Chem 1993;268(12):8418–8421.

59. Schloss P, Mayser W, Betz H. The putative rat choline transporter CHOT1 transports creatine and is highly expressed in neural and muscle-rich tissues. Biochem Biophys Res Commun 1994; 198(2):637–645.

60. Haugland RB, Chang DT. Insulin effect on creatine transport in skeletal muscle. Proc Soc Exp Biol Med 1975;148(1):1–4.

61. Odoom JE, Kemp GJ, Radda GK. The regulation of total creatine content in a myoblast cell line. Mol Cell Biochem 1996;158(2):179–188.

62. Gerber GB, Gerber G, Koszalka TR, Emmel VA. Creatine metabolism in vitamin E deficiency. Am J Physiol 1962;202:453–460.

63. Loike JD, Somes M, Silverstein SC. Creatine uptake, metabolism, and efflux in human monocytes and macrophages. Am J Physiol 1986;251(1 Pt 1):C128–135.

64. Moller A, Hamprecht B. Creatine transport in cultured cells of rat and mouse brain. J Neurochem 1989;52(2):544–550.

65. Fitch CD, Moody LG. Creatine metabolism in skeletal muscle: V. An intracellular abnormality of creatine trapping in dystrophic muscle. Proc Soc Exp Biol Med 1969;132(1):219–222.

66. Fitch CD, Chevli R. Inhibition of creatine and phosphocreatine accumulation in skeletal muscle and heart. Metabolism 1980; 29(7):686–690.

67. Ku CP, Passow H. Creatine and creatinine transport in old and young human red blood cells. Biochim Biophys Acta 1980;600(1):212–227.

68. Syllm-Rapoport I, Daniel A, Rapoport S. Creatine transport into red blood cells. Acta Biol Med Ger 1980;39(7):771–779.

69. Odoom JE, Kemp GJ, Radda GK. Control of intracellular creatine concentration in a mouse myoblast cell line. Biochem Soc Trans 1993;21(4):441S.

70. Clark JE, Odoom J, Tracey I, et al. Experimental observations of creatine phosphate and creatine metabolism. In: Conway MA, Clark JE, eds. Creatine and Creatine Phosphate. London: Academic Press, 1996:33–50.

71. Hultman E, Soderlund K, Timmons JA, et al. Muscle creatine loading in men. J Appl Physiol 1996;81(1):232–237.

72. Ziegenfuss T, Gales D, Felix S, et al. Performance benefits following a five day creatine loading procedure persist for at least four weeks. Med Sci Sports Exerc 1998;30(Suppl):265.

73. Green AL, Hultman E, MacDonald IA, et al. Carbohydrate ingestion augments skeletal muscle creatine accumulation during creatine supplementation in humans. Am J Physiol 1996;271(5 Pt 1):E821–E826.

74. Stout J, Eckerson J, Noonan D, et al. Effects of 8 weeks of creatine supplementation on exercise performance and fat-free weight in football players during training. Nutr Res 1999;19(2):217–225.

75. Vandenberghe K, Gillis N, Van Leemputte M, et al. Caffeine counteracts the ergogenic action of muscle creatine loading. J Appl Physiol 1996;80(2):452–457.

76. Hultman E, Greenhaff PL. Skeletal muscle energy metabolism and fatigue during intense exercise in man. Sci Prog 1991;75(298):361–370.

77. Katz A, Sahlin K, Henriksson J. Muscle ammonia metabolism during isometric contraction in humans. Am J Physiol 1986;250(6 Pt 1):C834–840.

78. Greenhaff PL, Bodin K, Harris RC, et al. The influence of oral creatine supplementation on muscle phosphocreatine resynthesis following intense contraction in man. J Physiol (Lond) 1993;467.

79. Sahlin K, Katz A. Adenine nucleotide metabolism. In: Poortmans JR, ed. Principles of Exercise Biochemistry. 2nd ed. Vol 38. Basel: Karger, 1993:137–153.

80. Gaitanos GC, Williams C, Boobis LH, Brooks S. Human muscle metabolism during intermittent maximal exercise. J Appl Physiol 1993;75(2):712–719.

81. Balsom PD, Ekblom B, Soderlund K, et al. Creatine supplementation and dynamic intensity intermittent exercise. Scand J Med Sci Sports 1993;3:143–149.

82. Sipila I, Rapola J, Simell O, Vannas A. Supplementary creatine as a treatment for gyrate atrophy of the choroid and retina. N Engl J Med 1981;304(15):867–870.

83. Bessman SP, Carpenter CL. The creatine-creatine phosphate energy shuttle. Annu Rev Biochem 1985;54:831–862.

84. Bessman SP, Savabi F. The role of the phosphocreatine energy shuttle. In: Taylor AW, Gollnick PD, Green HJ, et al., eds. Biochemistry of Exercise. Vol. 8. Champaign, IL: Human Kinetics, 1990:167–178.

85. Bessman SP, Geiger PJ. Transport of energy in muscle: the phosphorylcreatine shuttle. Science 1981;211(4481):448–452.

86. Bessman SP. The physiological significance of the creatine phosphate shuttle. Adv Exp Med Biol 1986;194:1–11.

87. Bessman SP. The creatine phosphate energy shuttle–the molecular asymmetry of a "pool." Anal Biochem 1987;161(2):519–523.

88. Wallimann T, Wyss M, Brdiczka D, et al. Intracellular compartmentation, structure and function of creatine kinase isoenzymes in tissues with high and fluctuating energy demands: the 'phosphocreatine circuit' for cellular energy homeostasis. Biochem J 1992;281(Pt 1):21–40.

89. Soderlund K, Balsom PD, Ekblomb B. Creatine supplementation and high-intensity exercise: influence on performance and muscle metabolism. Clin Sci (Colch) 1994;87:120–121.

90. Birch R, Noble D, Greenhaff PL. The influence of dietary creatine supplementation on performance during repeated bouts of maximal isokinetic cycling in man. Eur J Appl Physiol 1994;69(3):268–276.

91. Earnest CP, Almada AL, Mitchell TL. Effects of creatine monohydrate ingestion upon intermediate length anaerobic treadmill running to exhaustion. J Strength Cond Res 1997;4:234–238.

92. Jacobs I, Bleue S, Goodman J. Creatine ingestion increases anaerobic capacity and maximum accumulated oxygen deficit. Can J Appl Physiol 1997;22(3):231–243.

93. Smith JC, Stephens DP, Hall EL, et al. Effect of oral creatine ingestion on parameters of the work rate-time relationship and time to exhaustion in high-intensity cycling. Eur J Appl Physiol 1998; 77(4):360–365.

94. Harris RC, Viru M, Greenhaff PL, Hultman E. The effect of oral creatine supplementation on running performance during maximal short term exercise in man. J Physiol (Lond) 1993;467.

95. Yakolev NN. Biochemistry of sport in the Soviet Union: beginning, development and present status. Med Sci Sports 1975;7:237–247.

96. Earnest CP, Snell PG, Rodriguez R, et al. The effect of creatine monohydrate ingestion on anaerobic power indices, muscular strength and body composition. Acta Physiol Scand 1995;153(2):207–209.

97. Vandenberghe K, Goris M, Van Hecke P, et al. Long-term creatine intake is beneficial to muscle performance during resistance training. J Appl Physiol 1997;83(6):2055–2063.

98. Kreider RB, Ferreira M, Wilson M, et al. Effects of creatine supplementation on body composition, strength, and sprint performance. Med Sci Sports Exerc 1998;30(1):73–82.

99. Stout JR, Eckerson JM, Housh TJ, Ebersole KT. The effects of supplementation on anaerobic working capacity. J Strength Cond Res 1999;13(2):135–138.

100. Volek JS, Kraemer WJ, Bush JA, et al. Creatine supplementation enhances muscular performance during high-intensity resistance exercise. J Am Diet Assoc 1997;97(7):765–770.

101. Harris RC, Viru M, Greenhaff PL, Hultman E. The effect of oral creatine supplementation on running performance during maximal short term exercise in man. J Physiol (Lond) 1993;467:74P.

102. Bangsbo J, Gollnick PD, Graham TE, et al. Anaerobic energy production and O2 deficit-debt relationship during exhaustive exercise in humans. J Physiol (Lond) 1990;422:539–559.

103. Balsom PD, Harridge SD, Soderlund K, et al. Creatine supplementation per se does not enhance endurance exercise performance. Acta Physiol Scand 1993;149(4):521–523.

104. Hamilton-Ward K, Meyers MC, Skelly WA, et al. Effect of creatine supplementation on upper extremity anaerobic response in females. Med Sci Sports Exerc 1997;29(Suppl):146.

105. Kurosawa Y, Iwane H, Hamaoka T, et al. Effects of oral creatine supplementation on high- and low-intensity grip exercise performance. Med Sci Sports Exerc 1997;29(Suppl):251.

106. Thompson CH, Kemp GJ, Sanderson AL, et al. Effect of creatine on aerobic and anaerobic metabolism in skeletal muscle in swimmers. Br J Sports Med 1996;30(3):222–225.

107. Burke LM, Pyne DB, Telford RD. Effect of oral creatine supplementation on single-effort sprint performance in elite swimmers. Int J Sport Nutr 1996;6(3):222–233.

108. Cooke WH, Grandjean PW, Barnes WS. Effect of oral creatine supplementation on power output and fatigue during bicycle ergometry. J Appl Physiol 1995;78(2):670–673.

109. Goldberg PG, Bechtel PJ. Effects of low dose creatine supplementation on strength, speed and power events by male athletes. Med Sci Sports Exerc 1997;29(Suppl):251.

110. Odland LM, MacDougall JD, Tarnopolsky MA, et al. Effect of oral creatine supplementation on muscle [PCr] and short-term maximum power output. Med Sci Sports Exerc 1997;29(2):216–219.

111. Ruden TM, Parcell AC, Ray ML, et al. Effects of oral creatine supplementation on performance and muscle metabolism during maximal exercise. Med Sci Sports Exerc 1996;28(Suppl):81.

112. Barnett C, Hinds M, Jenkins DG. Effects of oral creatine supplementation on multiple sprint cycle performance. Aust J Sci Med Sport 1996;28(1):35–39.

113. Cooke WH, Barnes WS. The influence of recovery duration on high-intensity exercise performance after oral creatine supplementation. Can J Appl Physiol 1997;22(5):454–467.

114. Mujika I, Chatard JC, Lacoste L, et al. Creatine supplementation does not improve sprint performance in competitive swimmers. Med Sci Sports Exerc 1996;28(11):1435–1441.

115. Redondo DR, Dowling EA, Graham BL, et al. The effect of oral creatine monohydrate supplementation on running velocity. Int J Sport Nutr 1996;6(3):213–221.

116. Terrillion KA, Kolkhorst FW, Dolgener FA, Joslyn SJ. The effect of creatine supplementation on two 700-m maximal running bouts. Int J Sports Nutr 1997;7(2):138–143.

117. Moller P, Brandt R. Skeletal muscle adaptation to aging and to respiratory and liver failure. Acta Med Scand 1982;S654:1–40.

118. Smith SA, Montain SJ, Matott RP, et al. Creatine supplementation and age influence muscle metabolism during exercise. J Appl Physiol 1998;85(4):1349–1356.

119. Bermon S, Venembre P, Sachet C, et al. Effects of creatine monohydrate ingestion in sedentary and weight-trained older adults. Acta Physiol Scand 1998;164(2):147–155.

120. Grindstaff PD, Kreider R, Bishop R, et al. Effects of creatine supplementation on repetitive sprint performance and body composition in competitive swimmers. Int J Sport Nutr 1997;7(4):330–346.

121. Guerrero-Ontiveros ML, Wallimann T. Creatine supplementation in health and disease. Effects of chronic creatine ingestion in vivo: down-regulation of the expression of creatine transporter isoforms in skeletal muscle. Mol Cell Biochem 1998;184(1-2):427–437.

122. Forsberg AM, Nilsson E, Werneman J, et al. Muscle composition in relation to age and sex. Clin Sci (Colch) 1991;81(2):249–256.

123. Greenhaff PL, Casey A, Short AH, et al. Influence of oral creatine supplementation of muscle torque during repeated bouts of maximal voluntary exercise in man. Clin Sci (Colch) 1993;84(5):565–571.

124. Lemon P, Boska M, Bredle D, et al. Effect of oral creatine supplementation on energetics during repeated maximal muscle contraction. Med Sci Sports Exerc 1995;27(Suppl):204.

125. Ziegenfuss TN, Lemon PWR, Rogers MR, et al. Acute creatine ingestion: effects on muscle volume, anaerobic power, fluid volumes, and protein turnover. Med Sci Sports Exerc 1997;29(Suppl):127.

126. Becque MD, Lochmann JD, Melrose D. Effect of creatine supplementation during strength training on 1RM and body composition. Med Sci Sports Exerc 1997;29(Suppl):146.

127. Kreider R. Effects of creatine loading on muscular strength and body composition. Strength Cond 1995;17:72–73.

128. Kredier R, Klesges R, Harmon K, et al. Effects of ingesting supplements designed to promote lean tissue accretion on body composition during resistance exercise. Int J Sports Nutr 1996;6:234–246.

129. Earnest CP, Almada AL, Mitchell TL. High-performance capillary electrophoresis-pure creatine monohydrate reduces blood lipids in men and women. Clin Sci (Colch) 1996;91(1):113–118.

130. Walsh BW, Schiff I, Rosner B, et al. Effects of postmenopausal estrogen replacement on the concentrations and metabolism of plasma lipoproteins. N Engl J Med 1991;325:1196–1204.

131. Tarnopolsky MA, Roy BD, MacDonald JR. A randomized, controlled trial of creatine monohydrate in patients with mitochondrial cytopathies. Muscle Nerve 1997;20(12):1502–1509.

132. Tarnopolsky M, Martin J. Creatine monohydrate increases strength in patients with neuromuscular disease. Neurology 1999;52(4):854–857.

133. Andrews R, Greenhaff P, Curtis S, et al. The effect of dietary creatine supplementation on skeletal muscle metabolism in congestive heart failure [see comments]. Eur Heart J 1998;19(4):617–622.

134. Gordon A, Hultman E, Kaijser L, et al. Creatine supplementation in chronic heart failure increases skeletal muscle creatine phosphate and muscle performance [see comments]. Cardiovasc Res 1995;30(3):413–418.

135. Constantin-Teodosiu D, Greenhaff PL, Gardiner SM, et al. Attenuation by creatine of myocardial metabolic stress in Brattleboro rats caused by chronic inhibition of nitric oxide synthase. Br J Pharmacol 1995;116(8):3288–3292.

136. Saks V, Stepanov V, Jaliashvilli I, et al. Molecular and cellular mechanisms of action for cardioprotective and therapeutic role of creatine phosphate. In: Conway M, Clark J, eds. Creatine and Creatine Phosphate: Scientific and Clinical Perspective. San Diego, CA: Academic Press, 1996:91–114.

137. Walker JB. Bioenergetic engineering with guanidino compounds: loading tissues with extended range synthetic thermodynamic buffers. In: De Deyn PP, Marescau B, Stalon V, Qureshi IA, eds. Guanidino Compounds in Biology and Medicine. John Libbey & Company, 1992:187–194.

138. Davidoff F. Guanidine derivatives in medicine. N Engl J Med 1973;289(3):141–146.

139. Davidoff F. Oral hypoglycemic agents: the pharmacological basis of their clinical use. R I Med 1973;56(10):409–414.

140. Rocic B, Turk Z, Misur I, Vucic M. Effect of creatine on glycation of albumin in vitro. Horm Metab Res 1995;27(11):511–512.

141. Rocic B, Breyer D, Granic M, Milutinovic S. The effect of guanidino substances from uremic plasma on insulin binding to erythrocyte receptors in uremia. Horm Metab Res 1991;23(10):490–494.

142. Greenhaff P. Renal dysfunction accompanying oral creatine supplements [letter; comment]. Lancet 1998;352(9123):233–234.

143. Pritchard NR, Kalra PA. Renal dysfunction accompanying oral creatine supplements. Lancet (North Am Ed) 1998;351(9111):1252–1253.

144. Poortmans JR, Auquier H, Renaut V, et al. Effect of short-term creatine supplementation on renal responses in men. Eur J Appl Physiol 1997;76(6):566–567.

145. Poortmans JR, Francaux M. Renal dysfunction accompanying oral creatine supplements [letter; comment]. Lancet 1998;352(9123):234.

146. Poortmans JR, Francaux M. Long-term oral creatine supplementation does not impair renal function in healthy athletes [In Process Citation]. Med Sci Sports Exerc 1999;31(8):1108–1110.

147. Almada A, Mitchell T, Earnest C. Impact of chronic creatine supplementation on serum enzyme concentrations. FASEB J 1996;10(3):A791.

148. Earnest C, Almada A, Mitchell T. Influence of chronic creatine supplementation on hepatorenal function. FASEB J 1996;10(3):A790.

149. Schwane JA, Johnson SR, Vandenakker CB, Armstrong RB. Delayed-onset muscular soreness and plasma CPK and LDH activities after downhill running. Med Sci Sports Exerc 1983;15(1):51–56.

150. Pagana KD. Mosby's Diagnostic and Laboratory Test References. St. Louis: Mosby, 1995.
151. Papet I, Ostaszewski P, Glomot F et al. The effect of a high-dose 3-hydroxy-3-methylbutyrate on protein metabolism in growing lambs. Br J Nutr 1997;77:885–896.
152. Kostiuk S, Balasinska B, Papet I, et al. The effect of the leucine metabolite 3-hydroxy 3-methylbutyrate (HMB) on muscle protein synthesis and protein breakdown in chick and rat muscle. J Anim Sci 1996;74 (Suppl):138.
153. Cheng W, Phillips B, Abumrad N. Effect of HMB on fuel utilization, membrane stability and creatine kinase content of cultured muscle cells. FASEB J 1998;12(5):A950.
154. Nonnecke BJ, Franklin ST, Nissen SL. Leucine and its catabolites alter mitogen-stimulated DNA synthesis by bovine lymphocytes. J Nutr 1991;121(10):1665–1672.
155. Peterson A, Qureshi MA, Ferket PR, Fuller J. Beta-hydroxy-beta-methylbutyrate is a positive modulator of chicken macrophage growth and function. Poult Sci 1996;75(Suppl):139.
156. Nissen S, Sharp R, Ray M, et al. Effect of leucine metabolite beta-hydroxy-beta-methylbutyrate on muscle metabolism during resistance-exercise training. J Appl Physiol 1996;81(5):2095–2104.
157. Kraemer WJ, Fleck SJ, Evans WJ. Strength and power training: Physiological mechanisms of adaptation. In: Holloszy JO, ed. Exercise and Sports Science Reviews. Vol 24. Baltimore: Williams & Wilkins, 1996:363–397.
158. Staron RS, Karapondo DL, Kraemer WJ, et al. Skeletal muscle adaptations during early phase of heavy-resistance training in men and women. J Appl Physiol 1994;76(3):1247–1255.
159. Nissen S, Panton L, Fuller J Jr., et al. Effect of feeding beta-hydroxy-beta-methylbutyrate (HMB) on body composition and strength of women. FASEB J 1997;11(3):A150.
160. Vukovich MD, Stubbs NB, Bohlken RM, et al. The effect of dietary beta-hydroxy-beta-methylbutyrate (HMB) on strength gains and body composition changes in older adults. FASEB J 1997;11(3):A376.
161. Almada A, Kreider R, Ferreira M, et al. Effects of calcium beta-HMB supplementation with or without creatine during training on strength and sprint capacity. FASEB J 1997;11(3):A374.
162. Clark RH, Feleke GM, Din M, et al. Effect of amino acid mixture containing beta hydroxy beta methylbuterate (HMB) in HIV related wasting. XII World AIDS Conference. Geneva, Switzerland, 1998.
163. Daniel V, Hollister AS, Almada AL. Tolerability and effects of a biochemical/nutritional supplement in HIV related wasting. XI International Conference on Aids, 1996.
164. Panton LB, Rathmacher JA, Baier S, Nissen S. Nutritional supplementation of the leucine metabolite beta-hydroxy-beta-methylbutyrate (HMB) during resistance training. Nutrition 2000;16:734–739.
165. Nielson FH, Hunt CD, Mullen LM, Hunt JR. Effect of dietary boron on mineral, estrogen and testosterone metabolism in postmenospausal women. FASEB J 1987;1:394–397.
166. Ferrando AA, Green NR. The effect of boron supplementation on lean body mass, plasma testosterone levels and strength in male body builders. Int J Sport Nutr 1993;3:140–149.
167. Mertz W. Chromium in human nutrition: a review. J Nutr 1993;123(4):626–633.
168. Wagner J. Use of chromium cobamide by athletes. Clin Pharm 1989;8:832–834.
169. Vincent JB. Mechanisms of chromium action: low-molecular-weight chromium-binding substance. J Am Coll Nutr 1999;18(1):6–12.
170. Mooney KW, Cromwell GL. Effects of dietary chromium picolinate supplementation on growth, carcass characteristics, and accretion rates of carcass tissues in growing-finishing swine. J Anim Sci 1995;73(11):3351–3357.
171. Evans GW. The effect of chromium picolinate on insulin controlled parameters in humans. Int Biosoc Med Res 1989;11:163–180.
172. Clarkson PM. Effects of exercise on chromium levels: is supplementation required? Sports Med 1997;23(6):341–349.
173. Lukaski HC, Bolonchuk WW, Siders WA, Milne DB. Chromium supplementation and resistance training: effects on body composition, strength, and trace element status of men [see comments]. Am J Clin Nutr 1996;63(6):954–965.
174. Hasten DL, Rome EP, Franks BD, Hegsted M. Effects of chromium picolinate on beginning weight training students. Int J Sports Nutr 1992;2(4):343–350.
175. Clancy SP, Clarkson PM, DeCheke ME, et al. Effects of chromium picolinate supplementation on body composition, strength, and urinary chromium loss in football players. Int J Sports Nutr 1994;4(2):142–153.
176. Walker LS, Bemben MG, Bemben DA, Knehans AW. Chromium picolinate effects on body composition and muscular performance in wrestlers. Med Sci Sports Exerc 1998;30(12):1730–1737.
177. Campbell WW, Joseph LJO, Davey SL, et al. Effects of resistance training and chromium picolinate on body composition and skeletal muscle in older men. J Appl Physiol 1999;86(1):29–39.
178. Antonio J, Street C, Kalman D, Colker C. Dietary supplements used by athletes. J Am Med Athlet Assoc 1999;13(1):6–8.
179. Groff JL, Gropper SS, Hunt SM. Advanced Nutrition and Human Metabolism. Minneapolis/St. Paul: West Publishing, 1995:385–389.
180. Evans GW, Bowman TD. Chromium picolinate increases membrane fluidity and rate of insulin internalization. J Inorgan Biochem 1992;46(4):243–250.
181. Anderson RA. Chromium as an essential nutrient for humans. Regul Toxicol Pharmacol 1997;26(1):S35–S41.
182. Anderson RA, Polansky MM, Bryden NA, et al. Effect of exercise (running) on serum glucose, insulin, glucagon, and chromium excretion. Diabetes 1982;31(3):212–216.
183. Anderson RA, Polansky MM, Bryden NA. Strenuous running and acute effects on chromium, copper, zinc, and selected clinical variables in urine and serum of male runners. Biol Trace Elem Res 1984;6:327–336.
184. Honkola A, Forsen T, Eriksson J. Resistance training improves the metabolic profile in individuals with type 2 diabetes. Acta Diabetol 1997;34(4):245–248.
185. Ishii T, Yamakita T, Sato T, et al. Resistance training improves insulin sensitivity in NIDDM subjects without altering maximal oxygen uptake. Diabetes Care 1998;21(8):1353–1355.
186. Wallberg-Henriksson H, Rincon J, Zierath JR. Exercise in the management of non-insulin-dependent diabetes mellitus [published erratum appears in Sports Med 1998;25(2):130]. Sports Med 1998;25(1):25–35.
187. Mertz W. Effects and metabolism of glucose tolerance factor. Nutr Rev 1975;33(5):129–135.
188. Lefavi RG, Wilson GD, Keith RE, et al. Lipid-lowering effect of a dietary chromium III nicotinic acid complex in male athletes. Nutr Res 1993;13(3):239–249.
189. Anderson RA. Nutritional factors influencing the glucose/insulin system: chromium. J Am Coll Nutr 1997;16(5):404–410.
190. Anderson RA, Cheng N, Bryden NA, et al. Elevated intakes of supplemental chromium improve glucose and insulin variables in individuals with type 2 diabetes. Diabetes 1997;46(11):1786–1791.
191. Cefalu WT, Bell-Farrow AD, Stegner J, et al. Effect of chromium picolinate on insulin sensitivity in vivo. J Trace Elem Exper Med 1999;12(2):71–83.
192. Jovanovic L, Gutierrez M, Peterson CM. Chromium supplementation for women with gestational diabetes mellitus. J Trace Elem Exper Med 1999;12(2):91–97.
193. Stearns DM, Wetterhahn KE. Intermediates produced in the reaction of chromium (VI) with dehydroascorbate cause single-strand breaks in plasmid DNA. Chem Res Toxicol 1997;10(3):271–278.
194. Stearns DM, Kennedy LJ, Courtney KD, et al. Reduction of chromium(VI) by ascorbate leads to chromium-DNA binding and DNA strand breaks in vitro. Biochemistry 1995;34(3):910–919.
195. Stearns DM, Belbruno JJ, Wetterhahn KE. A prediction of chromium(III) accumulation in humans from chromium dietary supplements. FASEB J 1995;9(15):1650–1657.
196. Stearns DM, Wise JP, Sr., Patierno SR, Wetterhahn KE. Chromium(III) picolinate produces chromosome damage in Chinese hamster ovary cells. FASEB J 1995;9(15):1643–1648.
197. Cerulli J, Grabe DW, Gauthier I, et al. Chromium picolinate toxicity. Ann Pharmacother 1998;32(4):428–431.
198. Reading SA. Chromium picolinate. J Fla Med Assoc 1996;83(1):29–31.
199. Kobla HV, Volpe SL. Chromium, exercise, and body composition. Crit Rev Food Sci Nutr 2000;40:291–308.

200. Pariza MW, Ha YL. Conjugated dienoic derivatives of linoleic acid: a new class of anticarcinogens. Med Oncol Tumor Pharmacother 1990;7(2–3):169–171.

201. Chin SF, Liu W, Storkson JM, et al. Dietary sources of conjugated dienoic isomers of linoleic acid: a newly recognized class of anti-carcinogens. J Food Comp Anal 1992;5(3):185–197.

202. Ip C. (National live stock and meat board.) Conjugated linoleic acid in cancer prevention research: a report of current status and issues. May, 1994.

203. Shantha NC, Decker EA. Conjugated linoleic acid concentrations in processed cheese containing hydrogen donors, iron and dairy-based additives. Food Chem 1993;47(3):257–261.

204. Shantha NC, Decker EA, Ustunol Z. Conjugated linoleic acid con-centration in processed cheese. J Am Oil Chem Soc 1992;69(5):425–428.

205. Ha YL, Grimm NK, Pariza MW. Newly recognized anticarcinogenic fatty acids: identification and quantification in natural and processed cheeses. J Agric Food Chem 1989;37:75–81.

206. Shantha NC, Crum AD, Decker EA. Evaluation of conjugated linoleic acid concentrations in cooked beef. J Agric Food Chem 1994;42(8):1757–1760.

207. Miller CC, Park Y, Pariza MW, Cook ME. Feeding conjugated linoleic acid to animals partially overcomes catabolic responses due to endotoxin injection. Biochem Biophys Res Commun 1994;198(3):1107–1112.

208. Cook ME, Miller CC, Park Y, Pariza M. Immune modulation by altered nutrient metabolism: nutritional control of immune-induced growth depression. Poult Sci 1993;72(7):1301–1305.

209. Turek JJ, Li Y, Schoenlein IA, et al. Modulation of macrophage cytokine production by conjugated linoleic acids is influenced by the dietary n-6:n-3 fatty acid ratio. J Nutr Biochem 1998;9(5):258–266.

210. Kesteloot H, Lesaffre E, Joossens JV. Dairy fat, saturated animal fat, and cancer risk. Prev Med 1991;20(2):226–236.

211. Hankin JH, Zhao LP, Wilkens LR, Kolonel LN. Attributable risk of breast, prostate, and lung cancer in Hawaii due to saturated fat. Cancer Causes Control 1992;3(1):17–23.

212. Welsch CW. Relationship between dietary fat and experimental mammary tumorigenesis: a review and critique. Cancer Res 1992;52(Suppl):2040–2048.

213. Welsch CW. Review of the effects of dietary fat on experimental mammary gland tumorigenesis: role of lipid peroxidation. Free Radic Biol Med 1995;18(4):757–773.

214. Welsch CW. Dietary fat, calories, and mammary gland tumorigen-esis. Adv Exp Med Biol 1992;322:203–222.

215. Cave WT, Jr. Dietary n-3 (omega-3) polyunsaturated fatty acid effects on animal tumorigenesis. FASEB J 1991;5(8):2160–2166.

216. Banni S, Angioni E, Casu V, et al. Decrease in linoleic acid metabo-lites as a potential mechanism in cancer risk reduction by conju-gated linoleic acid. Carcinogenesis 1999;20(6):1019–1024.

217. Cesano A, Visonneau S, Scimeca JA, et al. Opposite effects of linole-ic acid and conjugated linoleic acid on human prostatic cancer in SCID mice. Anticancer Res 1998;18(3A):1429–1434.

218. Chang FJ, Shultz TD. Lipid peroxidation in human MDA-MB-231 breast cancer cells enriched in vitro with linoleic acid and conju-gated linoleic acid. FASEB J 1994;8(4–5):A426.

219. Cornell K, Waters DJ, Watkins B, Robinson JP. Conjugated linoleic acid exhibits differential inhibition of canine prostate cancer cells in vitro. Proc Am Assoc Cancer Res Annu Meet 1998;39:590.

220. Cornell KK, Waters DJ, Coffman KT, et al. Conjugated linoleic acid inhibited the in vitro proliferation of canine prostate cancer cells. FASEB J 1997;11(3):A579.

221. Cunningham DC, Harrison LY, Shultz TD. Proliferative responses of normal human mammary and MCF-7 breast cancer cells to linoleic acid, conjugated linoleic acid and eicosanoid synthesis inhibitors in culture. Anticancer Res 1997;17(1A):197–203.

222. Decker EA. The role of phenolics, conjugated linoleic acid, carno-sine, and pyrroloquinoline quinone as nonessential dietary antiox-idants. Nutr Rev 1995;53(3):49–58.

223. Des Bordes C, Lea MA. Effects of C18 fatty acid isomers on DNA synthesis in hepatoma and breast cancer cells. Anticancer Res 1995;15(5B):2017–2021.

224. Gallagher PA, Harrell A, Howell PE, Godley P. Conjugated linoleic acid (CLA) decreases the mono-unsaturaed fatty acid content of human prostate cancer cells in a dose dependent manner. FASEB J 1999;13(4 Pt 1):A540.

225. Gallagher PA, Kohlomeier M, Miranda S, Godley P. Human adipose tissue levels of conjugated linoleic acid in a case: control study of prostate cancer. FASEB J 1998;12(8):A1377.

226. Ip C, Briggs SP, Haegele AD, et al. The efficacy of conjugated linole-ic acid in mammary cancer prevention is independent of the level or type of fat in the diet. Carcinogenesis 1996;17(5):1045–1050.

227. Ip C, Lisk DJ, Scimeca JA. Potential of food modification in cancer prevention. Cancer Res 1994;54(Suppl):1957–1959.

228. Ip C, Scimeca JA, Thompson H. Effect of timing and duration of dietary conjugated linoleic acid on mammary cancer prevention. Nutr Cancer 1995;24(3):241–247.

229. Ip C, Thompson H, Singh M, Scimeca J. Dietary intake of conju-gated linoleic acid CLA and inhibition of mammary carcinogenesis. Proc Am Assoc Cancer Res Annu Meet 1993;34:553.

230. Ip C, Zhu Z, Thompson H. Downregulation of mammary epithelial growth and proliferation by conjugated linoleic acid (CLA): impli-cation for reduction in mammary cancer risk. Proc Am Assoc Cancer Res Annu Meet 1998;39:289.

231. Jain M. Dairy foods, dairy fats, and cancer: a review of epidemio-logical evidence. Nutr Res 1998;18(5):905–937.

232. Jarvinen R, Knekt P, Seppanen R, Teppo L. Diet and breast cancer risk in a cohort of Finnish women. Cancer Lett 1997;114(1-2):251–253.

233. Knekt P, Albanes D, Seppanen R, et al. Dietary fat and risk of breast cancer. Am J Clin Nutr 1990;52(5):903–908.

234. Knekt P, Jarvinen R, Seppanen R, Pukkala E, Aromaa A. Intake of dairy products and the risk of breast cancer. Br J Cancer 1996;73(5):687–691.

235. O'Shea M, Stanton C, Devery R. Antioxidant enzyme defence responses of human MCF-7 and SW480 cancer cells to conjugated linoleic acid [In Process Citation]. Anticancer Res 1999;19(3A):1953–1959.

236. Oshea M, Lawless F, Stanton C, Devery R. Conjugated linoleic acid in bovine milk fat: a food-based approach to cancer chemopreven-tion. Trends Food Sci Technol 1998;9(5):192–196.

237. Park Y, Shultz TD, Allen KGD. Modulation of MCF-7 breast cancer cell signal transduction by linoleic acid and conjugated linoleic acid in culture. FASEB J 1998;12(4):A565.

238. Parodi PW. Milk fat components: possible chemopreventive agents for cancer and other diseases. Austr J Dairy Technol 1996;51(1):24–32.

239. Shultz TD, Chew BP, Seaman WR. Differential stimulatory and inhibitory responses of human MCF-7 breast cancer cells to linole-ic acid and conjugated linoleic acid in culture. Anticancer Res 1992;12(6B):2143–2145.

240. Shultz TD, Chew BP, Seaman WR, Luedecke LO. Inhibitory effect of conjugated dienoic derivatives of linoleic acid and beta-carotene on the in vitro growth of human cancer cells. Cancer Lett 1992;63(2):125–133.

241. Thompson H, Zhu ZJ, Banni S, et al. Morphological and biochem-ical status of the mammary gland as influenced by conjugated linoleic acid: implication for a reduction in mammary cancer risk. Cancer Res 1997;57(22):5067–5072.

242. Durgam VR, Fernandes G. Role of dietary fatty acids in breast cancer: molecular approaches. Immunol Infect Dis (Lond) 1996;6(3–4):125–131.

243. Ip C. Review of the effects of trans fatty acids, oleic acid, n-3 polyunsaturated fatty acids, and conjugated linoleic acid on mam-mary carcinogenesis in animals. Am J Clin Nutr 1997;66(Suppl):1523–1529.

244. Ip C, Chin SF, Scimeca JA, Pariza MW. Mammary cancer prevention by conjugated dienoic derivative of linoleic acid. Cancer Res 1991;51(22):6118–6124.

245. Ip C, Jiang C, Thompson HJ, Scimeca JA. Retention of conjugated linoleic acid in the mammary gland is associated with tumor inhi-bition during the post-initiation phase of carcinogenesis. Carcino-genesis (Oxford) 1997;18(4):755–759.

246. Ip C, Scimeca JA. Conjugated linoleic acid and linoleic acid are distinctive modulators of mammary carcinogenesis. Nutr Cancer 1997;27(2):131–135.

247. Ip C, Singh M, Thompson HJ, Scimeca JA. Conjugated linoleic acid suppresses mammary carcinogenesis and proliferative activity of the mammary gland in the rat. Cancer Res 1994;54(5):1212–1215.

248. Ip C, Thompson HJ, Scimeca JA. Multiple mechanisms of conjugated linoleic acid (CLA) in mammary cancer prevention. Proc Am Assoc Cancer Res Annu Meet 1996;37:279.

249. Ip MM, Masso-Welch PA, Shoemaker SF, et al. Conjugated linoleic acid inhibits proliferation and induces apoptosis of normal rat mammary epithelial cells in primary culture. Exp Cell Res 1999; 250(1):22–34.

250. Visonneau S, Cesano A, Tepper SA, et al. Conjugated linoleic acid (CLA) suppresses growth of human breast carcinoma MDA-MB468 in SCID mice. FASEB J 1995;9(4):A869.

251. Visonneau S, Cesano A, Tepper SA, et al. Conjugated linoleic acid suppresses the growth of human breast adenocarcinoma cells in SCID mice. Anticancer Res 1997;17(2A):969–973.

252. Zangani D, Masso-Welch PA, Darcy KM, et al. Conjugated linoleic acid (CLA) modulates stromal cell differentiation in the rat mammary gland: Switch from the endothelial to the adipogenic differentiation pathway. Proc Am Assoc Cancer Res Annu Meet 1999; 40:361.

253. Belury MA, Kempa-Steczko A. Conjugated linoleic acid modulates hepatic lipid composition in mice. Lipids 1997;32(2):199–204.

254. Belury MA, Moya-Camarena SY, Liu KL, Heuvel JPV. Dietary conjugated linoleic acid induces peroxisome-specific enzyme accumulation and ornithine decarboxylase activity in mouse liver. J Nutr Biochem 1997;8(10):579–584.

255. Butcher GP, Raqabah A, Jackson MJ, et al. Failure of electron paramagnetic resonance spectroscopy studies to detect elevated free radical signals in liver biopsy specimens from patients with alcoholic liver disease. Free Radic Res 1995;22(2):99–107.

256. Chin SF, Storkson JM, Liu W, et al. Conjugated linoleic acid (9, 11- and 10,12-octadecadienoic acid) is produced in conventional but not germ-free rats fed linoleic acid. J Nutr 1994;124(5): 694–701.

257. Houseknecht KL, Vanden Heuvel JP, Moya-Camarena SY, et al. Dietary conjugated linoleic acid normalizes impaired glucose tolerance in the Zucker diabetic fatty fa/fa rat [published erratum appears in Biochem Biophys Res Commun 1998 Jun 29;247(3): 911]. Biochem Biophys Res Commun 1998;244(3):678–682.

258. Huang YC, Luedecke LO, Shultz TD. Effect of cheddar cheese consumption on plasma conjugated linoleic acid concentrations in men. Nutr Res 1994;14(3):373–386.

259. Ip C, Scimeca JA, Thompson HJ. Conjugated linoleic acid: a powerful anticarcinogen from animal fat sources. Cancer 1994; 74(Suppl):1050–1054.

260. Liew C, Schut HAJ, Chin SF, et al. Protection of conjugated linoleic acids against 2-amino-3-methylimidazo(4,5-f)quinoline-induced colon carcinogenesis in the F344 rat: a study of inhibitory mechanisms. Carcinogenesis 1995;16(12):3037-3043.

261. Pariza MW. Animal studies: summary, gaps, and future research. Am J Clin Nutr 1997;66(Suppl):1539S–1540S.

262. Visoneau S, Cesano A, Tepper SA, et al. Conjugated linoleic acid suppresses the growth of human breast adenocarcinoma cells in SCID mice. Anticancer Res 1997;17(2A):969–973.

263. Yamasaki M, Mansho K, Mishima H, et al. Dietary effect of conjugated linoleic acid on lipid levels in white adipose tissue of Sprague-Dawley rats [In Process Citation]. Biosci Biotechnol Biochem 1999;63(6):1104–1106.

264. Belury MA, Nickel KP, Bird CE, Wu Y. Dietary conjugated linoleic acid modulation of phorbol ester skin tumor promotion. Nutr Cancer 1996;26(2):149–157.

265. Kavanaugh CJ, Liu KL, Belury MA. Effect of dietary conjugated linoleic acid on phorbol ester-induced PGE2 production and hyperplasia in mouse epidermis. Nutr Cancer 1999;33(2):132–138.

266. Liu KL, Belury MA. Conjugated linoleic acid reduces arachidonic acid content and PGE2 synthesis in murine keratinocytes. Cancer Lett 1998;127(1-2):15–22.

267. Parodi PW. Conjugated linoleic acid: an anticarcinogenic fatty acid present in milk fat. Austr J Dairy Technol 1994;49(2):93–97.

268. Ha YL, Storkson J, Pariza MW. Inhibition of benzo(a)pyrene-induced mouse forestomach neoplasia by conjugated dienoic derivatives of linoleic acid. Cancer Res 1990;50(4):1097–1101.

269. Cannizzo F Jr, Broitman SA. Postpromotional effects of dietary marine or safflower oils on large bowel or pulmonary implants of CT-26 in mice. Cancer Res 1989;49(15):4289–4294.

270. Karmali RA. Effect of dietary fatty acids on experimental manifestation of Salmonella-associated arthritis in rats. Prostaglandins Leukot Med 1987;29(2-3):199–204.

271. O'Connor TP, Roebuck BD, Peterson FJ, et al. Effect of dietary omega-3 and omega-6 fatty acids on development of azaserine-induced preneoplastic lesions in rat pancreas. J Natl Cancer Inst 1989;81(11):858–863.

272. Reddy BS, Burill C, Rigotty J. Effect of diets high in omega-3 and omega-6 fatty acids on initiation and postinitiation stages of colon carcinogenesis. Cancer Res 1991;51(2):487–491.

273. Inouye M, Hashimoto H, Mio T, Sumino K. Levels of lipid peroxidation product and glycated hemoglobin A1c in the erythrocytes of diabetic patients. Clin Chim Acta 1998;276(2):163–172.

274. Hayek MG, Han SN, Wu D, et al. Dietary conjugated linoleic acid influences the immune response of young and old C57BL/6NCrlBR mice. J Nutr 1999;129(1):32–38.

275. West DB, Delany JP, Camet PM, et al. Effects of conjugated linoleic acid on body fat and energy metabolism in the mouse. Am J Physiol 1998;275(3 Pt 2):R667–R672.

276. Park Y, Albright KJ, Storkson JM, et al. Changes in body composition in mice during feeding and withdrawal of conjugated linoleic acid. Lipids 1999;34(3):243–248.

277. Park Y, Storkson JM, Albright KJ, et al. Evidence that the trans-10, cis-12 isomer of conjugated linoleic acid induces body composition changes in mice. Lipids 1999;34(3):235–241.

278. Lowery LM, Appicelli PA, Lemon PWR. Conjugated linoleic acid enhances muscle size and strength gains in novice body bodybuilders. Med Sci Sports Exer 1998;30(Suppl):182.

279. Lowery LM, Appicelli PA, Lemon PWR. Conjugated linoleic acid enhances muscle size and strength gains in novice body bodybuilders. Med Sci Sports Exerc 1998;30(Suppl):182.

280. Kreider R, Ferreira M, Wilson M, Almada A. Effects of conjugated linoleic acid (CLA) supplementation during resistance-training on bone mineral content, bone mineral density and markers of immune stress. FASEB J 1998;12(4):A244.

281. Bucci L. Nutrients as Ergogenic Aids for Sports and Exercise. Boca Raton: CRC Press, 1993:94.

282. Brozek B. Soviet studies on nutrition and higher nervous activity. Ann NY Acad Sci 1963;93:665.

283. Ershoff BH, Levin E. Beneficial effect of an unidentified factor in wheat oil on the swimming performance of guinea pigs. Fed Proc Fed Am Soc Exp Biol 1955;14:341.

284. Consolazio CF, Matoush LO, Nelson RA, et al. Effect of octacosanol, wheat germ oil and vitamin E on performance of swimming rats. J Appl Physiol 1964;19:265.

285. Entenman C, Coughlin JA, Ackerman PD. Substrate utilization and maximum swimming ability in rats and guinea pigs fed wheat germ oil. Proc Soc Exp Biol Med 1972;141(1):43–46.

286. Saint-John M, McNaughton L. Octocosanol ingestion and its effects on metabolic responses to submaximal cycle ergometry, reaction time and chest and grip strength. Int Clin Nutr Rev 1986;6:81.

287. Antonio A, John Uelmen J, Rodriguez R, Earnest C. The effects of *Tribulus terrestris* on body composition and exercise performance in resistance-trained males. Int J Sports Nutr 2000;10:208–215.

288. Wang B, Ma L, Liu T. [406 cases of angina pectoris in coronary heart disease treated with saponin of Tribulus terrestris]. Chung Hsi I Chieh Ho Tsa Chih 1990;10(2):68,85–87.

289. Arif-Adimoelja FX, Tancio TD, Surjaatmaja S. Phytopharmaca: an alternative treatment for male subfertility. Int J Androl 1997; 20(Suppl):39; Abstract 153.

290. Bourke CA. Staggers in sheep associated with the ingestion of Tribulus terrestris. Aust Vet J 1984;61(11):360–363.

291. Bourke CA, Stevens GR, Carrigan MJ. Locomotor effects in sheep of alkaloids identified in Australian Tribulus terrestris. Aust Vet J 1992;69(7):163–165.

292. Tapia MO, Giordano MA, Gueper HG. An outbreak of hepatogenous photosensitization in sheep grazing Tribulus terrestris in Argentina. Vet Hum Toxicol 1994;36(4):311–313.

293. Nechay BR, Nanninga LB, Nechay PSE, et al. Role of vanadium in biology. Fed Proc 1986;45:123–132.

294. Nechay BR. Mechanisms of action of vanadium. Annu Rev Pharmacol Toxicol 1984;24:501–524.

295. Byrne AR, Kosta L. Vanadium in foods and in human body fluids and tissues. Sci Total Environ 1978;10(1):17–30.

296. French RJ, Jones PJ. Role of vanadium in nutrition: metabolism, essentiality and dietary considerations. Life Sci 1993;52(4): 339–346.

297. Nielsen FH, Uthus EO. Vanadium in biological systems: physiology and biochemstry. In: Chasteen ND, ed. London: Kluwer Academic, 1990:51–62.

298. Wiegmann TB, Day HD, Patak RV. Intestinal absorption and secretion of radioactive vanadium (48VO3-) in rats and effect of Al(OH)3. J Toxicol Environ Health 1982;10(2):233–245.

299. Patterson BW, Hansard SLD, Ammerman CB, et al. Kinetic model of whole-body vanadium metabolism: studies in sheep. Am J Physiol 1986;251(2 Pt 2):R325–332.

300. Mongold JJ, Cros GH, Vian L, et al. Toxicological aspects of vanadyl sulphate on diabetic rats: effects on vanadium levels and pancreatic B-cell morphology. Pharmacol Toxicol 1990;67(3):192–198.

301. Hansard SLd, Ammerman CB, Henry PR, Patterson BW. Vanadium metabolism in sheep: III. Influence of dietary vanadium on kinetics of 48V administered orally or intravenously and comparison of compartmental and graphical models. J Anim Sci 1986;62(3): 804–812.

302. Nielsen FH. The importance of diet composition in ultratrace element research. J Nutr 1985;115(10):1239–1247.

303. Biggs WR, Swinehart JH. Vanadium in selected biological systems. In: Sigel H, ed. Metal Ions in Biological Systems. New York: Dekker, 1976:141–196.

304. Sabbioni E, Marafante E, Amantini L, et al. Similarity in metabolic patterns of different chemical species of vanadium in the rat. Bioinorg Chem 1978;8(6):503–515.

305. Harris WR, Friedman SB, Silberman D. Behavior of vanadate and vanadyl ion in canine blood. J Inorg Biochem 1984;20(2):157–169.

306. Edel J, Sabbioni E. Vanadium transport across placenta and milk of rats to the fetus and newborn. Biol Trace Elem Res 1989;22(3): 265–275.

307. Naylor GJ. Vanadium and affective disorders. Biol Psychiatry 1983; 18(1):103–112.

308. Schroeder HA, Balassa JJ, Tipton LH. Abnormal trace minerals in man—vanadium. J Chron Dis 1963;16:1047–1071.

309. Waters MD. Toxicology of vanadium. Adv Mod Toxicol 1977;2: 147–189.

310. Josephson L, Cantley LC Jr. Isolation of a potent (Na-K)ATPase inhibitor from striated muscle. Biochemistry 1977;16(21): 4572–4578.

311. Swarup G, Cohen S, Garbers DL. Inhibition of membrane phosphotyrosyl-protein phosphatase activity by vanadate. Biochem Biophys Res Commun 1982;107(3):1104–1109.

312. Swarup G, Speeg KV Jr, Cohen S, Garbers DL. Phosphotyrosyl-protein phosphatase of TCRC-2 cells. J Biol Chem 1982;257(13): 7298–7301.

313. Sefton BM, Hunter T. Tyrosine protein kinases. Adv Cyclic Nucleotide Protein Phosphorylation Res 1984;18:195–226.

314. Degani H, Gochin M, Karlish SJ, Shechter Y. Electron paramagnetic resonance studies and insulin-like effects of vanadium in rat adipocytes. Biochemistry 1981;20(20):5795–5799.

315. Cassel D, Whiteley B, Zhuang XY, Rothenberg P. Stimulation of Na/H exchange by mitogens. J Cell Biochem 1984:252.

316. Rehder D. Vanadium and its role in life. In: Sigel H, Sigel A, eds. Metal Ions in Biological Systems. vol 31. New York: Marcel Decker, 1995:1–594.

317. Benabe JE, Cruz-Soto MA, Martinez-Maldonado M. Critical role of extracellular calcium in vanadate-induced renal vasoconstriction. Am J Physiol 1984;246(3 Pt 2):F317–322.

318. Cruz-Sato MA, Martinez-Maldonado M. Modification of the renal response to ouabain by vanadate in vivo. Clin Res 1984;32.

319. Day H, Middendorf D, Lukert B, et al. The renal response to intravenous vanadate in rats. J Lab Clin Med 1980; 96(3):382–395.

320. Heinz A, Rubinson KA, Grantham JJ. The transport and accumulation of oxyvanadium compounds in human erythrocytes in vitro. J Lab Clin Med 1982;100(4):593–612.

321. Rossi JP, Garrahan PJ, Rega AF. Vanadate inhibition of active Ca2+ transport across human red cell membranes. Biochim Biophys Acta 1981;648(2):145–150.

322. DiPolo R, Rojas HR, Beauge L. Vanadate inhibits uncoupled Ca efflux but not Na — Ca exchange in squid axons. Nature 1979; 281(5728):229–230.

323. DiPolo R, Beauge L. The effects of vanadate on calcium transport in dialyzed squid axons: sidedness of vanadate-cation interactions. Biochim Biophys Acta 1981;645(2):229–236.

324. Forman DS, Brown KJ, Livengood DR. Fast axonal transport in permeabilized lobster giant axons is inhibited by vanadate. J Neurosci 1983;3(6):1279–1288.

325. Dick DA, Naylor GJ, Dick EG. Plasma vanadium concentration in manic-depressive illness. Psychol Med 1982;12(3):533–537.

326. Thomsen OO, Larsen JA. Comparison of vanadate and ouabain effects on liver hemodynamics and bile production in the perfused rat liver. J Pharmacol Exp Ther 1982;221(1):197–205.

327. Inciarte DJ, Steffen RP, Dobbins DE, et al. Cardiovascular effects of vanadate in the dog. Am J Physiol 1980;239(1):H47–56.

328. Takeda K, Akera T, Yamamoto S, Shieh IS. Possible mechanisms for inotropic actions of vanadate in isolated guinea pig and rat heart preparations. Naunyn Schmiedebergs Arch Pharmacol 1980; 314(2):161–170.

329. Sundet WD, Wang BC, Hakumaki MO, Goetz KL. Cardiovascular and renin responses to vanadate in the conscious dog: attenuation after calcium channel blockade. Proc Soc Exp Biol Med 1984; 175(2):185–190.

330. Steffen RP, Pamnani MB, Clough DL, et al. Effect of prolonged dietary administration of vanadate on blood pressure in the rat. Hypertension 1981;3(3 Pt 2):I173–I178.

331. Bhanot S, McNeill JH. Vanadyl sulfate lowers plasma insulin and blood pressure in spontaneously hypertensive rats. Hypertension 1994;24(5):625–632.

332. Dai S, Thompson KH, Vera E, McNeill JH. Toxicity studies on one-year treatment of non-diabetic and streptozotocin-diabetic rats with vanadyl sulphate. Pharmacol Toxicol 1994;75(5):265–273.

333. Cros GH, Cam MC, Serrano JJ, et al. Long-term antidiabetic activity of vanadyl after treatment withdrawal: restoration of insulin secretion? Mol Cell Biochem 1995;153(1–2):191–195.

334. Cros G, Mongold JJ, Serrano JJ, et al. Effects of vanadyl derivatives on animal models of diabetes. Mol Cell Biochem 1992;109(2): 163–166.

335. Pepato MT, Magnani MRT, Kettelhut IDC, Brunetti IL. Effects of oral vanadyl sulfate treatment in young diabetic rats. Revista de Ciencias Farmaceuticas 1998;19(1):93–108.

336. Liasko R, Kabanos TA, Karkabounas S, et al. Beneficial effects of a vanadium complex with cysteine, administered at low doses on benzo(alpha)pyrene-induced leiomyosarcomas in Wistar rats. Anticancer Res 1998;18(5A):3609–3613.

337. Fawcett JP, Farquhar SJ, Walker RJ, et al. The effect of oral vanadyl sulfate on body composition and performance in weight-training athletes. Int J Sports Nutr 1996;6(4):382–390.

338. (Nat Acad Sci). National Research Council Committee on Biologic Effects of Atmospheric Pollutants: Vanadium 1974.

339. Berg LR. Evidence of vanadium toxicity resulting from the use of certain commercial phosphorous supplements in chick rations. Poult Sci 1963;42:760–769.

340. Berg LR, Bearse GE, Merrill LH. Vanadium toxicity in laying hens. Poult Sci 1963;42:1407–1411.

341. Domingo JL, Llobet JM, Tomas JM, Corbella J. Short-term toxicity studies of vanadium in rats. J Appl Toxicol 1985;5(6):418–421.

342. Roshchin V. (Atomic Energy Commission). Toxicology of Rare Metals 1967.

343. Parker RD, Sharma RP. Accumulation and depletion of vanadium in selected tissues of rats treated with vanadyl sulfate and sodium orthovanadate. J Environ Pathol Toxicol 1978;2(2):235–245.

344. Schroeder HA, Mitchener M, Nason AP. Zirconium, niobium, antimony, vanadium and lead in rats: life term studies. J Nutr 1970;100(1):59–68.

345. Llobet JM, Domingo JL. Acute toxicity of vanadium compounds in rats and mice. Toxicol Lett 1984;23(2):227–231.

346. Paternain JL, Domingo JL, Llobet JM, Corbella J. Embryotoxic effects of sodium metavanadate administered to rats during organogenesis. Rev Esp Fisiol 1987;43(2):223–227.

347. Sanchez D, Ortega A, Domingo JL, Corbella J. Developmental toxicity evaluation of orthovanadate in the mouse. Biol Trace Elem Res 1991;30(3):219–226.

348. Younes M, Strubelt O. Vanadate-induced toxicity towards isolated perfused rat livers: the role of lipid peroxidation. Toxicology 1991; 66(1):63–74.

349. Domingo JL, Gomez M, Llobet JM, et al. Oral vanadium administration to streptozotocin-diabetic rats has marked negative side-effects which are independent of the form of vanadium used. Toxicology 1991;66(3):279–287.
350. Gomez M, Domingo JL, Llobet JM, Corbella J. Effectiveness of some chelating agents on distribution and excretion of vanadium in rats after prolonged oral administration. J Appl Toxicol 1991;11(3):195–198.
351. Platanow N, Abbery HK. Toxicity of vanadium in calves. Vet Res 1968;82:292–293.
352. Hansard SL, II, Ammerman CB, Fick KR, Miller SM. Performance and vanadium content of tissues in sheep as influenced by dietary vanadium. J Anim Sci 1978;46(4):1091–1095.
353. Hathcock JN, Hill CH, Matrone G. Vanadium toxicity and distribution in chicks and rats. J Nutr 1964;82:106–110.
354. Nelson TS, Gillis MB, Peeler HT. Studies on the effect of vanadium of chick growth. Poult Sci 1962;41:519–522.
355. Romoser GL, Dudley WA, Machlis LJ, Loveless L. Toxicity of vanadium and chromium for the growing chick. Poult Sci 1961;40:52–60.
356. Kubena LF, Phillips TD. Toxicity of vanadium in female Leghorn chickens. Poult Sci 1983;62(1):47–50.
357. Kubena LF, Phillips TD, Creger CR, et al. Toxicity of ochratoxin A and tannic acid to growing chicks. Poult Sci 1983;62(9):1786–1792.
358. Kubena LF, Phillips TD, Witzel DA, Heidelbaugh ND. Influence of various tissue levels of vanadium on female laying strain chicks. Poult Sci 1980;59:1628–1629.
359. Eyal A, Moran ET. Egg changes associated with reduced interior quality because of dietary vanadium toxicity in lien. Poult Sci 1984;63:1378–1385.
360. Grantham JJ. The renal sodium pump and vanadate. Am J Physiol 1980;239(2):F97–F106.
361. Phillips TD, Nechay BR, Neldon SL, et al. Vanadium-induced inhibition of renal Na+, K+-adenosinetriphosphatase in the chicken after chronic dietary exposure. J Toxicol Environ Health 1982;9(4):651–661.
362. Phillips TD, Nechay BR, Heidelbaugh ND. Vanadium: chemistry and the kidney. Fed Proc 1983;42(13):2969–2973.
363. Boden G, Chen X, Ruiz J, et al. Effects of vanadyl sulfate on carbohydrate and lipid metabolism in patients with non-insulin-dependent diabetes mellitus. Metabolism 1996;45(9):1130–1135.
364. Halberstam M, Cohen N, Shlimovich P, et al. Oral vanadyl sulfate improves insulin sensitivity in NIDDM but not in obese nondiabetic subjects [published erratum appears in Diabetes 1996 Sep;45(9):1285]. Diabetes 1996;45(5):659–666.
365. Fawcett JP, Farquhar SJ, Thou T, Shand BI. Oral vanadyl sulphate does not affect blood cells, viscosity or biochemistry in humans. Pharmacol Toxicol 1997;80(4):202–206.
366. Schroeder HA, Balassa JJ. Arsenic, germanium, tin and vanadium in mice: effects on growth, survival and tissue levels. J Nutr 1967;92(2):245–252.
367. Brichard SM, Henquin JC. The role of vanadium in the management of diabetes. Trends Pharmacol Sci 1995;16(8):265–270.
368. Goldfine AB, Simonson DC, Folli F, et al. Metabolic effects of sodium metavanadate in humans with insulin-dependent and noninsulin-dependent diabetes mellitus in vivo and in vitro studies. J Clin Endocrinol Metabol 1995;80(11):3311–3320.

Fat Reduction

Matthew Vukovich

Research Review

Effect of Chromium Supplementation on Body Composition, and Strength in Men

Chromium picolinate is one of the most common ingredients in fat loss products. However, as this study demonstrates, it does not appear to produce any benefits. The purpose of this study was to determine whether chromium supplementation in conjunction with an exercise program resulted in a greater rate of fat loss than exercise alone.

Thirty-six men were divided into three groups: placebo, chromium chloride, and chromium picolinate. The study was double-blinded so neither investigators nor the subjects knew what supplement was assigned to whom. Before and after the 8-week treatment period, body composition was assessed by dual x-ray absorptiometry (DEXA). DEXA is a form of body composition measurement that uses x-rays to determine body density and then body composition. Bone, fat, and muscle possess different densities and will thus absorb x-rays at different amounts. This allows researchers then to quantify body composition. During the 8-week treatment period, subjects were supervised during a 5-day-per-week exercise program, which consisted of a general warm-up, stretching, and resistance training.

Fat-free mass increased in all three groups an equal amount. Body fat, expressed in absolute (kg) or relative (%) terms did not change during the 8-week treatment period in any of the three groups. Furthermore, Lukaski and coworkers reported that chromium supplementation resulted in an adverse interaction between chromium and iron. The elevated chromium reduced the binding of iron and transferrin. This could possibly result in iron deficiency, depending on the dose and duration of supplementation.

Thus, the results of this study indicate that chromium supplementation does not result in accelerated fat loss as is commonly advertised. In addition, prolonged chromium supplementation could result in iron deficiency and possibly suboptimal oxygen carrying capacity of the blood.

REFERENCE
Lukaski HL, et al. Chromium supplementation and resistance training: Effects on body composition, strength, and trace element status of men. Am J Clin Nutr 1996;63:954–965.

Introduction

Walk into any dietary supplement store and you will notice that more products fall into the category of diet or fat loss aids than any other product category. A recent search of an online dietary supplement store indicated that there are close to 400 products that are marketed for fat loss. Fifty-five products contain the dietary supplement, chromium.

This chapter will focus on supplements that are designed to promote fat loss. The term *fat loss* will be used rather than *weight loss* because the latter term does not differentiate between muscle mass and fat mass. Supplements designed to promote fat loss can function on one of a number of different principles. These principles as well as the most commonly used fat loss supplements will be discussed in detail.

Over the last 20 years, there has been about a 10% increase in the prevalence of overweight individuals.[1] Furthermore, one in five adolescents are considered obese, which is a 45% increase.[2] Because of societal pressures, it seems that everyone has used or at least has thought of using a fat loss product at one time or another. This includes adolescents as well as older adults. Just because these supplements are sold in health food and vitamin stores does not guarantee their safety. Some of these supplements may have cross-reactivity with some prescription medications and alcoholic beverages.

Mechanism of Action for Fat Loss Supplements

Supplements marketed to promote fat loss can theoretically function on one of a number of principles, from increasing adipose tissue lipolysis or fat breakdown, to suppressing the appetite or the desire for food to reducing the amount of fat absorbed from food during the digestive process. To better understand how fat loss supplements function, their potential mechanisms of action should first be understood.

Increase in Fat Oxidation

Several factors are involved in the use of lipids as fuel. For muscles to oxidize fatty acids, fat (triacylglycerol) must first be mobilized from the adipose tissue. This is referred to as lipolysis. Once the free fatty acids are lysed and released from adipose tissue, they must be transported by albumin in the blood to the muscle, where uptake occurs via a specific transporter protein called the *fatty acid binding protein* (FABP).[3,4] When the free fatty acid (FFA) enters the muscle it is activated, after which the activated fatty acid is transported into the mitochondria where β-oxidation occurs.

Theoretically, an increase in fatty acid oxidation could be achieved at any one of seven sites. However, the mobilization of free fatty acids from the adipose tissue appears to be the best site because the uptake of FFA by the muscle is dependent on the arterial blood concentration of FFA.[5–8] The more FFA released by the adipose tissue, the higher the concentration of FFA in the circulation. Therefore, any product that increases lipolysis should increase fatty acid oxidation at the muscle.

Reducing Lipid Absorption

Dietary lipid (predominately fat) is digested by specific enzymes including lipases, phospholipids, and cholesterol esterase. Most of the lipid digestion occurs in the duodenum of the small intestine in which lipids are emulsified by the detergent action of bile salts. Lipids and bile salts spontaneously form micelles. The micelles contain fatty acids and cholesterol, and serve as transporters. Micelles migrate to the brush border where lipids diffuse out of the micelles into mucosal cells.

Agents that can prevent lipid digestion and/or absorption appear an attractive approach as a fat loss mechanism or, more importantly, reducing blood cholesterol levels. In fact, there are some prescriptions and fat substitutes that function to reduce fat absorption. However, a reduction in lipid absorption has potentially negative side effects, including gastrointestinal discomfort, diarrhea, and a reduction in the absorption of fat soluble vitamins.

Suppressing the Appetite

The hypothalamus is the neural center for the regulation of food intake. One area of the hypothalamus consisting of the lateral nuclei, controls hunger, or the craving for food. Another area consisting of the ventromedial nuclei, controls satiety, or the feeling of fulfillment. Therefore, drugs or supplements that act on the hypothalamus can act as an anorectic (appetite reducing) agent. Prescription drugs like amphetamine and fenfluramine function by increasing the level of brain catecholamines and 5-hydroxytryptamine (serotonin), which causes a feeling of fullness and suppresses the appetite, respectively.[9] Some dietary supplements could alter the levels of neurotransmitters in the hypothalamic region and regulate food intake.

The body may also produce its own satiety chemical or hormone that suppresses the appetite. The Set-Point Theory suggests that fat cells prefer to maintain a certain size. FIGURE 4-1 shows a model of how the Set-Point Theory

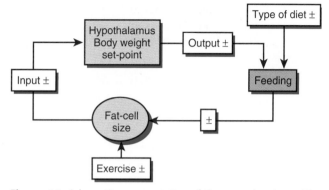

Figure 4-1. Schematic representation of the set point theory. The input signal to the hypothalamus from the adipocyte regulates feeding behavior. In animal modes, the protein hormone leptin appears to act as the input signal. Both exercise and type of diet can modify feeding behavior and fat cell size. (*Data reprinted with permission from* Booth DA. Acquired behavior controlling energy intake and output: In: Stunkard AJ, ed. Obesity. Philadelphia: WB Saunders. 1980: 101–143.)

may work.[10] When there is a reduction in the size of the adipocyte due to dieting, a signal is sent to the hypothalamus resulting in an increase in appetite. As the fat cell regains its size, another signal is sent to the hypothalamus, which instructs the hypothalamus to reduce or stop the desire to eat.

The maintenance of an adequate body weight is a survival mechanism for higher organisms including mammals. Furthermore, the maintenance of body weight requires both the maintenance of energy and nutrient balance. This means that the diet must contain both adequate amounts of calories, macronutrients (carbohydrate, protein, and fat), and micronutrients (vitamins and minerals).

Research using rodents may have discovered the signal for the Set-Point Theory. The signal is called leptin, and it appears to have a dual role: it decreases food intake and increases energy expenditure resulting in an increase in fat oxidation. When rats are bred to be deficient in this hormone, it causes them to overeat and become obese. When this hormone is administered to rats, it causes them to stop eating and increases fat oxidation, resulting in fat loss but not a loss in lean tissue (i.e., muscle). However, human research indicates that the hormone is not the problem, but rather the transporter. Obese individuals appear to develop a resistance to leptin that is similar to insulin resistance. Therefore, it may be impractical to expect leptin administration to humans to be a viable means of controlling obesity. If the transporters are already saturated or downregulated from excessive endogenous leptin, it does not make sense to provide more. Therefore, research has begun to focus on the leptin transporter and binding site in hopes of discovering the post-binding signaling cascade and any potential defects in this system. Leptin research is interesting and may one day provide a drug to control obesity, but this probably won't happen for many years. For more information on leptin, read the excellent reviews by Hwang et al.[11] and by Jequier and Tappy.[12]

Although several mechanisms could be used as a target for fat loss, most of the dietary supplements targeted as a fat loss agent do not have scientific research to support their claims.

Caffeine

Caffeine is one of the most commonly used ingredients in fat loss supplements. It occurs naturally in the leaves, seeds, or fruits of more than 60 different plants including cola nuts, mate leaves, and guarana paste. It is commonly found in coffee and chocolate, and is often used as a flavoring agent in cola beverages.

Caffeine exerts effects through a number of different mechanisms. The primary actions of caffeine are it stimulates the central nervous system and amplifies lipolysis. Lipolysis is controlled by an enzyme called hormone-sensitive lipase (HSL). This enzyme exists in an inactive and active form. To activate HSL, another enzyme, adenylate cyclase, converts ATP into cyclic-3',5'-AMP (cAMP) (FIG. 4-2). Cyclic-AMP then activates cAMP-dependent protein kinase which in turn phosphorylates HSL, thus activating the enzyme. The active form of the enzyme is responsible for cleaving the FFA off of the glycerol backbone of the triacylglycerol molecule. The FFA is then released into the bloodstream. Lipolysis ceases when cAMP is degraded to 5'AMP by phosphodiesterase, thus becoming inactivated. Therefore, it stands to reason that any process which maintains cAMP levels will prolong the life of the active form of HSL and consequently lipolysis.

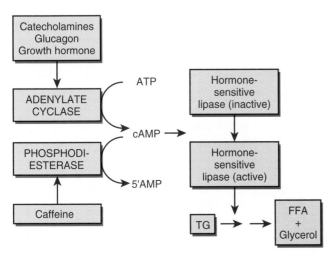

Figure 4-2. Control of adipocyte lipolysis. Various hormones are responsible for stimulating adenylate cyclase, thus forming cyclic AMP from ATP. Cyclic-AMP activates the cAMP-dependent protein kinase, which activates the hormone-sensitive lipase (HSL). HSL is responsible for cleaving the fatty acids off of the glycerol backbone of the triacylglycerol molecule. cAMP is inactivated by phosphodiesterase. When cAMP is broken down to 5'-AMP, HSL is inactivated by the removal of the phosphate group. However, caffeine can inhibit phosphodiesterase, which allows lipolysis to be prolonged.

Caffeine and other methylxanthines inhibit phosphodiesterase activity.[13] Caffeine is thus able to prolong the responses of cAMP by slowing the degradation of this messenger. Therefore, lipolysis continues for a longer period of time resulting in more FFAs being released to the bloodstream. Several studies have been conducted in animals and humans regarding the effectiveness of caffeine. In many of those studies, caffeine has been combined with other agents that will be discussed later.

In Vitro Studies

In vitro studies allow scientists to determine the possible mechanism of action of a particular substance on metabolism. Research on caffeine, as discussed previously, shows us that caffeine inhibits phosphodiesterase activity and that this leads to an increase in adipose tissue lipolysis, a catabolic process. For a cell to carry on both catabolic and anabolic processes at the same time is difficult. The purpose of adipocytes is to store fat. The adipocyte can use fatty acids or glucose for triacylglycerol synthesis. In the case of glucose, the cell must first convert the glucose into fat through a process called lipogenesis. However, if lipolysis is going on, it is not possible for the cell to perform lipogenesis. Steinfelder and Petho-Schramm[14] have demonstrated that caffeine inhibits glucose transport into rat adipocytes.

In addition to affecting adipose tissue, caffeine also affects brain tissue. Some of its effects in the brain will be discussed in the section on adverse reactions; however, other effects of caffeine in the brain may aid in the stimulation of lipolysis. The anterior pituitary gland is responsible for growth hormone (GH) production and secretion. Growth hormone, in addition to stimulating glucose and amino acid uptake, also stimulates lipolysis. Therefore, GH can increase fatty acid oxidation. *In vitro* research in cultured rat pituitary cells suggests that caffeine stimulates growth hormone secretion.[15] This increase is more than likely caused by the inhibition of phosphodiesterase. As in many cells, cAMP acts as a second messenger, which stimulates a number of metabolic pathways inside a cell. In this case, caffeine's effect on phosphodiesterase results in an increase in GH secretion. It remains to be determined whether the oral consumption of caffeine stimulates GH secretion in humans, and if it does, whether the increase in GH is significant enough to alter lipolysis. Some insight into this question will be provided when animal and human research is discussed.

When the HSL is working at cleaving the fatty acids off of the glycerol backbone of the triacylglycerol molecule, glycerol is released into the circulation along with the three FFAs. Although not related to lipid oxidation at the muscle, the body needs to do something with the glycerol, which may enter glycolysis for oxidation or gluconeogenesis. In addition to stimulating lipolysis, caffeine also stimulates gluconeogenesis, or the making of glucose in the liver. Caffeine added to the suspensions of rat hepatocytes resulted in a two-fold increase in gluconeogenesis.[16] The resulting increase in glucose produced by this pathway would then be used to maintain blood glucose levels or act as a precursor for liver glycogen. The increase in gluconeogenesis is likely due to the increase in the intracellular calcium concentration associated with caffeine.[17]

Animal Studies

The affect of caffeine on growth hormone secretion in animals is not as clear as the *in vitro* work. Work from two different laboratories has produced conflicting results. One lab has reported that caffeine injection results in a lowering of GH and thyroid hormones.[18] Another lab[19] reported that GH levels were increased following a single injection of caffeine. Following 10 days of caffeine injection, GH levels were still elevated but not to the extents that were observed following the initial injection. The differences between the two studies could be attributed to the age of the rats used. Clozel et al.[18] used 5-day-old rats while Spindel et al.[19] used older rats. This lends support to human research showing an age effect of caffeine, which will be discussed in the Human Studies section.

In addition to affecting GH, caffeine influences catecholamine release from chromaffin granules in the adrenal medulla. Catecholamines can also stimulate lipolysis. Catecholamine biosynthesis begins with the amino acid tyrosine. Tyrosine is hydroxylated to dopa by tyrosine hydroxylase, which is the rate-limiting enzyme in catecholamine biosynthesis. Tyrosine hydroxylase appears to be regulated by cAMP-dependent protein kinase. Therefore, caffeine may have the same effect on catecholamine biosynthesis as it does on lipolysis. That is, caffeine may prolong the activity of tyrosine hydroxylase by inhibiting phosphodiesterase. Furthermore, the release of catecholamines is calcium dependent and, as discussed above, caffeine is able to increase intracellular calcium levels through the release of calcium from intracellular stores and by increasing the entry of calcium from extracellular stores.[20]

Though the effect of caffeine on hormones in animals is not all that clear, caffeine's effect on lipolysis is clear. Numerous studies have reported that caffeine increases lipolysis in laboratory animals. Furthermore, research indicates that caffeine results in a more rapid loss in fat mass in exercised rats compared to rats that did not receive caffeine but still exercised.[21]

Human Studies

Caffeine research in humans has produced some mixed results with positive results probably depending on the age, sex, and weight of the subject, and also the prior use of caffeine by the subject.

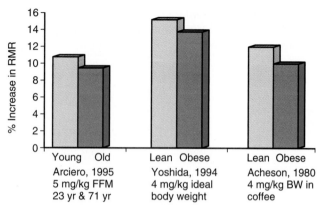

Figure 4-3. Effect of caffeine supplementation on resting metabolic rate. (*Data from* Arciero PJ, Gardner AW, Calles-Escandon J, et al. Effects of caffeine ingestion on NE kinetics, fat oxidation, and energy expenditure in younger and older men. Am J Physiol 1995;268: E1192–E1198; Yoshida T, Sakane N, Umekawa T, Kondo M. Relationships between basal metabolic rate, thermogenic response to caffeine, and body weight loss following combined low calorie and exercise treatment in obese women. Int J Obes Relat Metab Disord 1994;18:345–350; and Acheson KJ, Zahorska-Markiewicz B, Pittet P, et al. Caffeine and coffee: their influence on metabolic rate and substrate utilization in normal weight and obese individuals. Am J Clin Nutr 1980;33:989–997.)

The effect of caffeine supplementation on resting metabolic rate and thermogenesis has been studied in the lean, obese, post-obese (following weight loss), and young and old (FIG. 4-3). Metabolic rate and/or thermogenesis increases with caffeine consumption in all populations and is dose dependent[22]; but, fat oxidation appears to increase only in lean individuals.[23–25] Obese and older adults appear to have a blunted response to caffeine in regard to an increase in fat oxidation (FIG. 4-4).[24,25] There could be a number of reasons why the lean and obese respond differently to caffeine. One reason could be the way caffeine is metabolized by the body. However, Caraco[26] reported that obesity minimally alters caffeine pharmacokinetics and that this small alteration should not necessitate any significant dosage modifications.

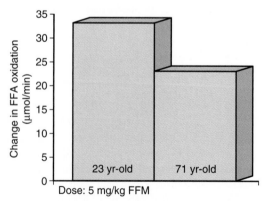

Figure 4-4. Caffeine and fat oxidation. (*Data from* Arciero PJ, Gardner AW, Calles-Escandon J, et al. Effects of caffeine ingestion on NE kinetics, fat oxidation, and energy expenditure in younger and older men. Am J Physiol 1995;268:E1192–E1198.)

The differences among the populations may be due to the form in which caffeine was consumed. The studies that reported a difference between lean and obese individuals used coffee as the form of delivery. Research by Graham et al.[27] has reported that there is a blunted catecholamine response during exercise following coffee consumption when compared with pure caffeine consumption. This will be discussed in more detail in the next chapter. The study by Arciero[24] that compares young and old men used pure caffeine. The other factor that could have influenced the results was the varying amount of caffeine used.

As in animals, caffeine also alters the plasma levels of certain hormones. Caffeine has repeatedly been shown to increase catecholamine levels.[28] Furthermore, the increase in catecholamines appears to be dose dependent.[29]

Additional research indicates that a single dose of caffeine (500 mg) may also elevate growth hormone and triiodothyronine (T_3) in men, but not women.[30] As discussed above, the caffeine-associated increase in growth hormone could further increase lipolysis and fat oxidation. Triiodothyronine is a thyroid hormone that increases resting metabolic rate and amplifies physiological signals responsible for stimulating lipolysis and fat mobilization.

Safety and Toxicity

Although it would appear that caffeine works well as a fat loss supplement, it has negative side effects. Caffeine has been reported to elevate arterial blood pressure and heart rate.[31] Furthermore, it results in diuresis and increased gastric secretion, the latter of which can lead to loose bowels and possibly diarrhea at higher dosages.[32]

Chronic caffeine ingestion is associated with a decrease in cerebral blood flow and an increase in mean arterial pressure.[31] Six days of chronic caffeine use resulted in the loss of the acute effects on mean arterial blood pressure, but not on blood flow. This indicates that there may be a development in peripheral tolerance but not central tolerance. The headaches associated with caffeine withdrawal, experienced by some people, would be difficult to explain based on this research. The physiological effects of caffeine appear to last about 4 days.[33]

Acute toxicity is characterized by hematemesis, tachycardia, hyperventilation, hyperglycemia, ketonuria, hypokalemia, and metabolic acidosis. Although deaths have been associated with excessive caffeine intake, the overdose of caffeine is rare because of the spontaneous and recurrent vomiting associated with the intake of toxic levels of caffeine. The LD_{50} (the lethal dose for half the subjects) of caffeine has been estimated to be between 150 and 200 mg/kg. A dose of caffeine that results in blood levels that exceed 100 $\mu g/mL$ is considered lethal, although acute toxicity begins at blood levels of 30 to 50 $\mu g/mL$.[34,35] A typical cup of coffee contains roughly 100 mg of caffeine and can increase blood caffeine levels to 1–2 $\mu g/mL$. Several deaths have been associated with too much caffeine consumption; the most recent was a 22-year-old female who overdosed on diet pills. A serum toxicology report indicated that her blood levels were in the range of 1500 $\mu g/mL$.[34]

L-Carnitine

Carnitine is synthesized from the amino acids lysine and methionine in liver and kidney, and is particularly abundant in heart and skeletal muscle. The role of L-carnitine is to facilitate the oxidation of long-chain fatty acids (LCFA) by assisting in their transfer across the inner mitochondrial membrane. When LCFA enter the cell they become activated and are directed toward the mitochondria. The activated fatty acid, now known as acyl-CoA, is unable to traverse the mitochondrial membrane and requires a transport system. As can be seen in FIGURE 4-5, carnitine assists in that transfer.

Supplement companies and manufacturers have hypothesized that if one were to increase the amount of carnitine within the muscle, more acyl-CoAs could be transported into the mitochondria and thus increase β-oxidation (a catabolic process in which fatty acids are used to make energy). This theory was initially based on research performed with carnitine-deficient patients who were unable to properly use fatty acids as fuel.[36,37] Carnitine supplementation in these patients restored their ability to oxidize fatty acids.[38] However, as we will see, it isn't that simple when it comes to fat loss.

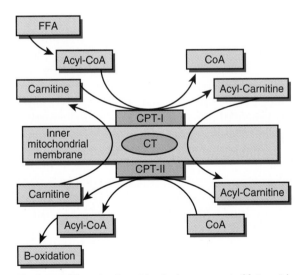

Figure 4-5. The role of carnitine in the transport of fatty acids through the mitochondrial membrane. The transport process involves the coordinated action of three enzymes, carnitine palmitoyltransferases I and II (CPT-I, CPT-II), and carnitine-acylcarnitine translocase (CT). The activated fatty acid (acyl-CoA) is transferred into the mitochondria by replacing the CoA with carnitine. Once inside the mitochondria, the CoA is replaced and the carnitine is recycled to be used again.

In Vitro Studies

In 1955, Fritz[39] first demonstrated that carnitine added to liver homogenates stimulated fatty acid oxidation. Subsequent research by Fritz[40,41] included other tissue preparations and indicated heart tissue responds to carnitine to the greatest degree.

In cell incubation, carnitine has been shown to be actively transported into rat skeletal muscle.[42] The process is saturable and energy dependent, and uptake is greater in slow-twitch muscle compared with fast-twitch muscle.[42]

In vitro studies have provided ample evidence about carnitine and its function in fatty acid oxidation. However, the major obstacle with carnitine—or any dietary supplement for that matter—is increasing its concentration within the tissue where it is to be active. Although *in vitro* studies provide evidence that cells can actively uptake carnitine, *in vivo* studies in animals and humans are less convincing.

Animal Studies

As with human studies, most of the research investigating carnitine supplementation has been conducted under exercise conditions. The research on animals has produced equivocal results. Some carnitine supplementation studies have shown that carnitine is taken up by the muscle, reducing fat stores and plasma fatty acid levels presumably by increasing fatty acid oxidation.[43,44] However, other researchers report that endogenous levels of muscle carnitine are adequate to support fatty acid oxidation.[45,46]

Human Studies

Carnitine has never been investigated as a mechanism to promote fat loss in humans. The majority of research in humans has investigated carnitine's effect on fatty acid oxidation during exercise, with these studies focusing primarily on fatty acid oxidation and performance. Carnitine could be beneficial during fat-loss exercise and nutrition programs if it can show that carnitine can increase human muscle carnitine content and therefore increase fatty acid oxidation during exercise. However, there is no evidence to suggest that muscle carnitine content is the rate-limiting step in the oxidation of fatty acids.[47] At this moment, carnitine's ability to increase fatty acid oxidation during exercise is lacking scientific support.

Safety and Toxicity

Carnitine is one of the safest dietary supplements on the market. It is found in baby formula because some premature infants are unable to endogenously produce their own carnitine. No negative side effects have been reported from carnitine supplementation. However, some companies have included DL-carnitine in their weight loss formulations. DL-carnitine may be toxic, as it may lead to L-carnitine deficiency.

Chitosan

One method of reducing fat weight may be decreasing the amount of fat absorbed following digestion. Chitosan is a fiber supplement that is a form of chitin (a homopolymer of modified glucose) and is extracted from the shells of crustaceans. It has been marketed as an inhibitor of fat absorption. Chitosan can function in one of two ways: 1) by binding bile acids and reducing their recycling, or 2) by delaying the digestion and blocking absorption of fat by binding to the fat in the intestine.

Animal Studies

Most of the studies on Chitosan have been performed on animals. In those studies, Chitosan was primarily investigated as a hypocholesterolemic agent. Because Chitosan is supposed to reduce fat absorption, it would stand to reason that cholesterol levels would also be affected. Seven studies have been conducted in rats, and all seven report that Chitosan is effective in reducing blood cholesterol levels, especially when the rats consumed a high-fat diet.[48–54] Whether a reduction in fat absorption results in a decrease in body fat has yet to be determined.

Human Studies

Only one study has investigated the effect of Chitosan in humans as a weight-reducing agent.[54] Obese subjects were divided into one of three groups: placebo and two treatment groups. The treatment contained 240 mg of Chitosan, 55 mg of Garcinia cambogia (contains HCA), and 19 mg of chromium. The treatment groups received either one or two capsules. All three groups were required to consume a hypocaloric diet, about 100 kcals. The authors reported that the dietary supplement containing Chitosan and HCA in conjunction with a hypocaloric diet can achieve a greater reduction in weight that is dose dependent.[54] Furthermore, subjects experienced a significant reduction in total cholesterol and LDL and triglycerides, and a significant elevation in HDL.[54]

Although this study shows positive results, Chitosan alone has not been determined to be effective as a fat-loss product. However, when combined with HCA, it appears to promote fat loss. Additional research should be conducted to verify these results and to determine any effects of these substances in isolation.

Safety and Toxicity

Chitosan seems to be effective in reducing lipid digestion and absorption. However, when fat absorption is inhibited, the fat is eliminated in the feces. The most common side effect associated with products inhibiting fat absorption is diarrhea. Other documented side effects include a reduction in calcium absorption[55] and a reduction in the absorption of fat-soluble vitamins,[56] especially vitamin E.[55] Deuchi et al.[55] reported that the decrease in calcium absorption was enough to reduce bone mineral content of rats in just 2 weeks of treatment. Animal studies also indicate that Chitosan may decrease *Bifidobacterium* and *lactobacillus*. These are bacteria that are normally found in the intestinal tract, which have important roles including the regulation of digestion and vitamin manufacture and release. Therefore, it would be necessary for vitamin and mineral supplementation during the consumption of Chitosan supplements.

Chromium

Chromium is one of the most used ingredients in weight loss products. It is probably an active ingredient in well over 55 dietary supplements. However, as the research will show, there is little evidence to suggest that chromium enhances fat loss.

In the 1970s, chromium deficiency was recognized in humans on long-term total parenteral nutrition[57] and was characterized by insulin resistance and hypercholesterolemia. Subsequent research reported that chromium acts as part of the glucose tolerance factor (GTF) by enhancing the effectiveness of insulin. In type II diabetics, chromium supplementation improved fasting blood glucose and insulin levels after 2 and 4 months of treatment.[58,59] This is important because chromium may improve insulin sensitivity in this population. Chromium appears to act by increasing the rate of insulin internalization, which could be due to an increase in membrane fluidity.[60]

Human Studies

Because chromium may increase the muscle cell's sensitivity to insulin and thus increase amino acid transport into the muscle, researchers theorized that chromium supplementation during strength training programs would result in greater gains in muscle mass and concurrent losses in fat weight than training alone.[61,62] In the beginning, chromium was thought of and researched as an aid to increase muscle mass during training; it was not researched as a fat-loss supplement. The fat loss, if any, would be subsequent to the gains in muscle mass and the increase in resting metabolic rate associated with the gain in muscle. Therefore, it would stand to reason, if chromium did indeed *work,* it would only be under conditions of exercise training, and fat-loss would be a secondary benefit. Furthermore, it would also suggest that chromium would be ineffective as a fat loss product without exercise. This further supports the fact that fat loss can be achieved only through reduced caloric intake and increased caloric expenditure.

Initial studies did report an increase in body weight during a 40-day and 12-week training program.[61,62] However, in the Hasten study (1992), an increase in body weight was reported only in females; the results of this study[62] are questionable. Though the authors reported an increase in FFM, there was no increase in strength associated with the increase in FFM. Also, body composition was determined by skinfold measurements, and body weight was measured with the subjects wearing shorts, T-shirt, and tennis shoes. No mention was made as to whether the researchers required the subjects to wear the same clothing and shoes for each of the 3-week measurements. The subjects in Evans's study[61] were poorly controlled during the training program, and there was no standardization regarding prior weight training experience.

The majority of research in healthy, active humans suggests that chromium is ineffective as a fat-loss supplement.[63–69] These studies have reported that 8 to 14 weeks of a training with chromium supplementation program did not provide any additional benefits over training alone. Grant and coworkers[70] reported that chromium supplementation without training may result in an increase in body weight. Grant and colleagues[70] reported that a nonexercising group of obese women gained almost 2.0 kg of body weight over a 9-week period. However, they reported that a chromium nicotinate supplement in conjunction with a 9-week exercise training program with obese women did result in about a 1-kg decrease in body weight. An exercising placebo group and an exercising group consuming a chromium picolinate supplement did not experience any change in body weight, FFM, or fat mass during the 9-week period. This was the first study to report a statistically significant weight-loss effect with chromium nicotinate, and it is not known why the chromium nicotinate group responded better than the chromium picolinate group. Although this study did report a significant effect from chromium supplementation, it is in the minority. It is safe to say that the majority of research does not support the use of chromium as a weight-loss supplement.

Safety and Toxicity

In addition to questioning the effectiveness of chromium, some researchers have questioned the safety of chromium. The National Research Council claims that toxicity from chromium occurring in the diet is so low that there is a wide range between the amount normally consumed and the amount that has harmful effects.[71] However, the National Research council did not consider the effects of supplemental chromium. Chromium is a metal and must be chelated to another compound to increase absorption.

The most popular compound for chelation of chromium is picolinic acid. Chromium picolinate is stable in the body. However, this stability could lead to an accumulation in cells, which could result in cell damage. Chromium picolinate has been associated with a 24% decrease in transferrin saturation of iron.[64] Transferrin is the iron-transporting protein in the plasma. Because chromium competes with iron for transferrin, an increase in blood chromium levels could reduce the iron transport and distribution, which could ultimately affect oxygen-binding capacity of the blood. Additional studies have reported that picolinic acid may prevent the availability of minerals for metabolism and tissue function by increasing mineral excretion.[72] In vitro studies have reported that picolinic acid alters cell size, shape, and function.[66] In addition, chromium supplementation has been associated with kidney failure and rhabdomyolysis.[73,74] In both case reports, the individuals were consuming chromium above the recommended dosage. A study was presented at the 1999 Annual Meeting of the American Chemical Society. Dr. Vincent from the University of Alabama reported that chromium picolinate, at 100 times less than the concentration found in human body tissue after long-term use, reacts to form chromium II, which interacts with oxygen to produce hydroxyl radicals. These molecules are known to alter the DNA structure. Furthermore, Dr. Vincent reported that when vitamin C is combined with chromium picolinate the potential for damage is even greater. As Lefavi and coworkers[66] pointed out in their review of chromium, the potential safety concerns associated with chromium challenge its effectiveness as a dietary supplement, and more research should be conducted on the potential adverse reactions that have been reported from in vitro studies.

Conjugated Linoleic Acid

Conjugated linoleic acid (CLA) is a collective term for a group of isomers of linoleic acid. There are eight major CLA isomers, but the cis-9,trans-11 isomer appears to be the most biologically active or relevant form.[75] Conjugated linoleic acid is a fatty acid that is found primarily in meat and dairy products (FIG. 4-6).

Initial research on CLA indicated that it had potential anticarcinogenic properties.[76,77] In addition to its anticarcinogenic properties, CLA has been reported to protect against atherosclerosis in rabbits[78] and overcome the cata-

bolic response of endotoxin injection.[79] This anticatabolic action of CLA led to additional studies investigating its effect on body composition.

In Vitro Studies

The way a fatty acid can alter body composition remains to be determined. However, some preliminary research may provide some insight as to the mechanism of CLA. Park and coworkers[80] reported that CLA added to the culture medium of differentiated 3T3-L1 adipocytes significantly reduced intracellular triacylglycerol and glycerol concentrations while significantly increasing glycerol in the culture medium. This indicates that CLA somehow stimulates lipolysis. What is lacking from the study is the measurement of FFA in the incubation medium. If triacylglycerol breakdown is occurring, not only will extracellular glycerol increase, but extracellular FFA would also increase. The reason why FFA was not measured is unclear.

Animal Studies

In the same study by Park et al.,[80] CLA supplementation was also investigated in mice. The investigators reported CLA-fed mice exhibited an enhanced norepinephrine-induced lipolysis and HSL activity in isolated epididymal adipocytes. The authors concluded that CLA decreases fat deposition, while increasing lipolysis that could lead to an increase in fatty acid oxidation in muscle cells. Subsequent studies have confirmed that CLA reduces body fat in mice. West and colleagues[81] investigated the effect of CLA supplementation in mice on either a low-fat (15% of total kcals) or high-fat diet (45% of total kcals). In both the high- and low-fat diet groups, CLA supplementation resulted in a reduction in energy intake, which was associated with a reduction in fat stores. However, a negative consequence of CLA supplementation was a reduction in growth rate and total body protein. On the other hand, Delany and coworkers[82] reported that CLA supplementation in mice resulted in a marked reduction in fat accumulation and an increase in protein accumulation. In both studies, the mice were of the same breed line (AKR/J) and CLA was provided at a dose of 1.0% to 1.2% body weight. Therefore, the only other factor to consider for the differences would be the type of diet provided. Further research needs to address the effects of CLA supplementation on growth retardation and protein accretion.

Human Studies

Whether CLA has any effect in humans is difficult to determine. A few studies have been conducted investigating the effects of CLA on body composition. However, these studies are not published in peer-reviewed journals, and only two have been presented in abstract form. Before

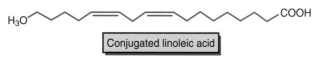

H₃O — COOH

Conjugated linoleic acid

Figure 4-6. Structure of the polyunsaturated fatty acid–conjugated linoleic acid.

discussing these investigations, note that they are preliminary studies and some potential flaws exist in the methodology, analysis, or interpretation of the data by the authors, which will be pointed out. However, they will help in aiding other researchers to develop more sound protocols for CLA research in humans.

Supplementation of CLA was investigated in college-aged males with resistance-training experience. The researchers tested the subjects for changes in strength and body composition by dual-energy x-ray absorptiometry (DEXA) following 28 days of CLA supplementation.[83,84] The researchers reported the group consuming CLA had slightly greater gains in strength, but there was no change in fat-free mass or fat mass. Because FFM did not increase, where did the increase in strength come from? In general, when resistance-trained individuals are used as subjects, it is unlikely that any changes in strength will be due to neural adaptations, as seen in untrained individuals. Therefore, the increase in strength observed in this study is more than likely due to testing procedures or the subjects not putting forth their best effort. In conclusion, the results of this preliminary study show body fat did not change when subjects consumed CLA.

Interestingly, one researcher did report that the CLA-supplemented group did experience an increase (25 ± 14 g or $1.1 \pm 0.6\%$) in bone mineral content in only 28 days[83]; although not significant, it did approach a level of significance ($P = 0.08$). An increase in bone mineral content of only 1.1% is within the coefficient of variation of measurement of DEXA analysis for bone mineral content, which ranges from 0.8% to 1.5%.[85,86] Furthermore, a control group was not included in the study design to rule out the possibility of such an error occurring. Finally, how quickly can bone density change? Most studies that have investigated changes in bone density during resistance training have been conducted over months (4 to 18 months) to detect changes in bone density (see Layne and Nelson[87] for a review). Even then, there is some conflicting evidence on whether resistance training can increase bone density. Therefore, it seems unlikely that bone mineral content or density would change in that short period of time. Although bone density is not part of fat reduction, the results of the study indicate that testing or interpretation errors can occur when testing subjects and analyzing data.

A 6-week study investigating CLA supplementation was performed in novice bodybuilders.[88] The treatment group received 7.2 g of CLA, and the placebo group received vegetable oil. The authors reported that skinfold-corrected arm girth and body mass increased to a greater extent in the CLA group.[88] The methodology used to measure arm girth is questionable. It is subject to error and the authors did not report the reproducibility of the procedure. A more sensitive method, like MRI or CT scan, for assessing muscle growth, may have been a more appropriate method of measurement.

An unpublished study used in press releases reports that "CLA preferentially produces deposition of lean body mass rather than fat mass" (Pharmanutrients press release). This study investigated the effects of CLA supplementation during a 6-month treatment program with 80 obese subjects. The study was poorly controlled. The subjects were asked to reduce their energy intake by about 500 kcal/day, and were asked to exercise at least three times per week for a minimum of 30 minutes. Of the 71 subjects who finished, there were no differences in body composition; following the treatment period, both the CLA group and the placebo group lost the same amount of weight. The weight loss was a combination of fat mass and fat-free mass. On average, the CLA group lost 3.0 lbs of FFM, while the placebo group lost 2.5 lbs of FFM. Of the 71 subjects, the author finds that only 15 gained FFM, and 10 of these subjects were in the CLA group. Based on this observation, the authors conclude that CLA is able to preferentially increase FFM rather than fat mass during an anabolic state. The interpretation of the data in this manner is not appropriate. In a sense, the authors are digging for something that is not there. The appropriate conclusion that can be drawn from the data presented in the abstract is that during an unsupervised diet and exercise program, CLA does not result in an increase in FFM. Furthermore, CLA was unable to prevent the loss in FFM that occurred during the treatment and exercise program.

Though the CLA research in mice seems promising, more well-controlled research is needed in humans to determine whether CLA works in preserving or enhancing FFM while promoting fat loss during periods of dieting.

Safety and Toxicity

In the animal studies that have been performed, and the few human studies, there have been no reports of adverse health incidences or toxicity. It is unlikely that CLA would result in any problems when consumed in the recommended amount. The usual dose is about 2 to 3 g. A person normally consumes ten times that amount of fat during a normal meal. Potential problems, if any, could exist from altering fatty acid content of the phospholipids in cell membranes. Research suggests that diet can influence membrane fluidity by altering the structure of the phospholipids. Furthermore, membrane fluidity can influence the activity of membrane-bound enzymes. Whether CLA affects the activity of membrane enzymes is only theoretical, but deserves attention.

Cyclo-HisPro (CHP)

Histidyl-proline diketopiperazine is a cyclic dipeptide otherwise known as cyclo (His-Pro) or CHP. CHP is a cyclic structure formed from the amino acids histidine and proline, and is a major metabolite of thyrotropin-releasing hormone (TRH).[89] In addition to being a metabolite of TRH, it appears that CHP may be derived from sources other than TRH.[90,91] Thus, CHP is found throughout the human body. More specifically, CHP is found in the central nervous system, gastrointestinal tract, and a variety of body fluids including milk, blood, cerebrospinal fluid, and urine.[92] CHP is also found in many foods including tuna, shrimp, and ham.[93] Some dietary supplements that contain casein or soy protein may also contain relatively large amounts of CHP.[94]

Research indicates that CHP exhibits a variety of biological functions including appetite suppression, a reduction of ethanol narcosis (CNS depression), a decrease in cholesterol synthesis, and an inhibition of insulin secretion.[95] CHP is not yet a dietary supplement but does show promise in animal studies.

Animal Studies

As discussed above, a supplement that can increase satiety is probably altering the chemical signals within the hypothalamus because that is where the hunger center appears to be located. Studies have shown that CHP exhibits a neuromodulatory mechanism, which appears to be responsible for its satiety effect.[96]

The first study reporting the anorectic role of CHP was conducted by Morley et al.[97] Rats who received CHP ate 50–80% less food than control rats. The researchers postulated that the CHP was inhibiting dopamine uptake in nerve terminals thought to be responsible for feeding behavior.[97] The anorectic role of CHP has been supported by subsequent research. In two separate studies, CHP has been reported to reduce food intake by 20–50% in rats.[98,99]

Although the exact mechanism of action for CHP is unknown, CHP has been hypothesized to act through a number of mechanisms such as dopamine, norepinephrine, and serotonin metabolism or even their transporters.[95,100] In addition, CHP may act like gut peptides. Food in the GI tract may stimulate the release peptide hormones that reduce food intake. Circulating CHP has been shown to change following a glucose load.[101] Plasma CHP showed a rise followed by a fall below baseline and then a recovery toward normal after an oral glucose load, but not after intravenous administration of glucose.[101] This pattern is similar to that reported in humans.[102]

Human Studies

Descriptive research of CHP in humans indicates that endogenous CHP is distributed throughout the body and responds similarly to the CHP in rats.[102,103] The role of CHP administration in humans is unknown due to the lack of research studies and to ethical considerations. More research is needed to investigate the safety of CHP

before it can be administered to humans. However, a few investigations have focused on the changes in endogenous CHP levels following the consumption of food by humans and in different human diseases as they related to food consumption. Steiner and coworkers[104] investigated the relationship of endogenous CHP levels in patients with anorexia nervosa and bulimia. Anorexia is accompanied by an absence of hunger, which results in malnutrition. Bulimia, on the other hand, is associated with an inability to feel satiety even after massive food consumption. Steiner[104] reported that as anorexics lost weight their CHP levels actually increased. In fact, a 2-kg weight loss was associated with a 42% increase in CHP levels. This negative correlation between weight loss and CHP levels indicates that anorexics had less desire to eat with the more weight they lost. On the other hand, bulimics responded in just the opposite manner. As bulimics lost weight, CHP levels dropped as well, suggesting that bulimics experience an absence of satiety, increasing the likelihood of the binge eating and purging that is characteristic of this disease.

Currently, there are some plans to conduct fat-loss studies in adults. However, one of the problems the researchers are having is finding a manufacturer for CHP. Small amounts can be purchased for animal studies, but the cost of this dipeptide makes it cost prohibitive to give to humans.

Another important item is that while a reduction in energy intake will result in weight loss, the weight loss may not be permanent. During a reduction in energy intake, metabolic rate will often decrease to compensate for this reduction in intake. This reduction in metabolic rate may be linked to a decrease in thyroid hormones. The decrease in metabolic rate will result in the negative caloric balance being offset, and may possibly result in a positive caloric balance, leading to an increase in body weight. This is why long-term weight loss cannot be achieved without exercise. Exercise helps maintain and even increase the metabolic rate.

Safety and Toxicity

The studies investigating the physiological effects of CHP administration have been careful to document any adverse reactions. Peters et al.[105] administered 400 μg of CHP intravenously to humans and reported that throughout the study there were no subjective or objective side effects of CHP administration. Animal studies have also verified that CHP administration has minimal or no negative side effects. Nevertheless, more human studies need to be performed. Exogenous CHP may alter a variety of endocrine and CNS-related activities including thermoregulation, pain responsiveness, inhibition of insulin release, and inhibition of prolactin.

Prolactin is a hormone released by the anterior pituitary gland. Many studies have reported that CHP may inhibit basal levels of prolactin and the amount secreted during suckling in women.[106-110] In women, prolactin is responsible for milk production and let-down. Therefore, a decrease in prolactin may decrease milk production. If CHP reaches the market as a dietary supplement, it should not be consumed by women who are breast feeding because it will appear in breast milk. Also, prolactin enhances testosterone production by a direct interaction with receptors on Leydig cells. Therefore, a decrease in prolactin may result in a decrease in testosterone production, which could alter protein synthesis and muscle mass, leading to a change in metabolic rate.

Since CHP may also decrease insulin release,[111] athletes may find that both glycogen resynthesis and protein synthesis may be decreased. In male athletes, coupled with the possible decrease in testosterone, CHP may not be a supplement to consume because of the potential negative effects on muscle mass.

DHEA or Dehydroepiandrosterone

Dehydroepiandrosterone (DHEA) is a precursor to testosterone. In the biochemical pathway to testosterone, it lies two steps away (FIG. 4-7). DHEA was one of the first prohormones to enter the dietary supplement market after the 1994 DSHEA (see Chapter 1). It is found in wild yams and in the pollen or seeds of the Austrian pine.

Because DHEA is a precursor to testosterone it was thought that it would increase testosterone production if supplemented in the diet. However, research has shown that DHEA may have biological activity itself. DHEA exists in two forms within the body: free-DHEA and the sulfated form, DHEAS. The exact physiological role of DHEAS and its parent compound DHEA are not entirely known; however, research is beginning to provide us with more information about its function. It is known that DHEA decreases with age. Because aging is associated with an increase in obesity, insulin resistance, and atherosclerosis, some researchers are investigating the interaction of DHEA supplementation with obesity and related physiological problems.

Animal Studies

Numerous animal studies have reported that DHEA supplementation is able to lower body fat stores even during periods of high fat intake in rats.[112-120] In young rodents DHEA inhibits fat accumulation[113,115] whereas in adult rats, supplementation of DHEA decreases body fat.[117] Furthermore, DHEA supplementation has been reported to lower cholesterol and triacylglycerol levels, as well as improve insulin sensitivity in old and obese rats.[119,120]

After knowing where DHEA falls in the metabolic pathway of testosterone biosynthesis, one would assume that the anti-obesity effect of DHEA could have been brought about by an increase in downstream androgen levels. However, if one reviews the literature, it is not clear whether DHEA influences androgen production. This could mean that DHEA is producing the effect itself or through other mechanisms. It appears that DHEA prevents the accumulation or storage of body fat by increasing resting metabolic rate and heat production through futile cycling and/or by increasing the flux of fatty acids through β-oxidation in peroxisomes.[115,116] The increase in fatty acid oxidation may be caused by an increase in mitochondrial protein, which may include an increase in carnitine palmitoyltransferase, an enzyme that shuttles activated fatty acids from the cytosol into the mitochondrial matrix.[121]

Another mechanism through which DHEA may alter fat stores is by decreasing food intake and creating a negative caloric balance.[122-124] If you remember, one possible mechanism by which fat loss may be promoted is through a decrease in food intake. Neurotransmitters within the brain control satiety and hunger. A few researchers have reported that exogenous DHEA can alter levels of serotonin and dopamine causing a feeling of fullness or satiety.[122-124] Furthermore, the decrease in food intake may be primarily fat intake, based on research in Zucker rats.[118]

One question that has not been answered is whether the physiological effects described are originating from DHEA or a metabolite of DHEA. Two metabolites of DHEA are 3α-hydroxyetiocholanolone and 3β-hydroxyetiocholanolone. In one research study, researchers have reported that an effective dose of these etiocholanolones is 25% of the effective dose for DHEA.[125] What were once thought to be inert end products of steroid metabolism could possess beneficial physiological effects. More research should investigate the actions of these etiocholanolones.

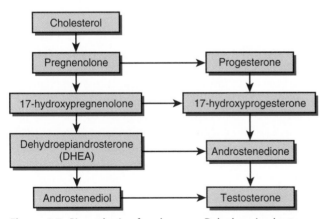

Figure 4-7. Biosynthesis of androgrens. Dehydroepiandrosterone (DHEA) can be converted to testosterone via two pathways; one is through the conversion of androstenedione, the other through androstenediol.

Human Studies

An important physiological difference between rats and humans is that the adrenal gland in rats does not produce DHEA. However, as discussed above, rat tissues are able to respond to DHEA when it is supplemented in the animals' diets. Because of this important physiological difference between rats and humans, humans may respond differently to DHEA supplementation.

The positive outcomes of DHEA supplementation in rats has led to a number of studies investigating the relationship of DHEA to obesity in humans.[126–131] Research indicates that a positive relationship exists in women for endogenous DHEA and the amount of fat located on the trunk,[126–128] suggesting that higher levels of endogenous DHEA are associated with abdominal obesity and insulin resistance in women. In men, there does not appear to be a relationship between endogenous DHEA and abdominal obesity.

Studies that have investigated the effects of exogenous DHEA on body composition in humans have produced mixed results and the positive results cannot necessarily be linked to dosage, sex, weight, or age. Based on the relationship between endogenous DHEA and body fat, it would appear that DHEA would not be advisable for women, because higher levels of DHEA are associated with abdominal obesity.[126–128] Before we actually decide whether DHEA supplementation is beneficial or not, we should review the literature.

One study in young men (mean age, 24 years) reported that 1600 mg/day for 28 days resulted in a significant reduction in percent body fat (31%) with no change in total body weight.[129] However, another study, also using young men (mean age, 26 years) and supplementing DHEA at 1600 mg/day reported no changes in body weight, fat-free mass (total body water and total body potassium), resting metabolic rate, or protein metabolism.[130] The second study reported that DHEA does not affect resting metabolic rate; therefore, it is difficult to speculate why the subjects in the first study experienced a decline of almost 4 pounds of body fat over the 4-week period.

In older individuals, there appears to be possible dosing and sex effects. In 1994, Morales and colleagues[131] reported that a 50-mg dose of DHEA for 6 months did not result in changes in percent body fat or BMI in either men or women. However, a follow-up study by the same group[132] reported that older men experienced a significant reduction in body fat mass following 6 months of DHEA supplementation at 100 mg/day. Older women experienced a significant increase in body weight, but no change in composition.

And finally, in obese individuals there does not seem to be an effect of DHEA supplementation. Adult males who had a mean BMI of 31.5 ± 2.9 kg/m^2 had no change reported in body weight or fat mass following 28 days of supplementation at 1600 mg/day. Furthermore, neither did obese teenagers who received 80 mg/day for 8 weeks experience any change in body weight, fat mass, and lean body mass.[133]

While research in animals supports the use of DHEA as an anti-obesity agent, research in humans does not support the same conclusions. The differences are more than likely caused by the constant level of DHEA that is always circulating in humans, but not in rodents.

Safety and Toxicity

Supplementation of DHEA in men does not seem to pose a health risk. In fact, there is some research that reports that DHEA reduced serum total and LDL cholesterol in men.[129] However, in women, DHEA supplementation has been associated with increases in androgen levels, decreases in HDL, and a decline in insulin sensitivity.[131, 134, 135] Two of these studies investigated the effects of DHEA in postmenopausal women. Recent research has indicated that postmenopausal women have an increased risk for heart disease.[136] If this population of women were consuming DHEA, it would appear that their risk for heart disease would increase further because of the decline in HDL and insulin sensitivity, both part of the *deadly quartet*.[137]

Ephedrine

Ephedrine is a stimulant acting as β_2-agonist, which means it mimics norepinephrine.[22] An increase in sympathetic activity is associated with increased lipolysis, heart rate, heart contractility, and glycolysis. Again, the increase in lipolysis will result in a higher level of circulating FFA, which will likely increase β-oxidation. Ephedrine also possesses thermogenic properties. Thermogenesis is an increase in heat production and resting metabolic rate, which increases caloric expenditure. Because ephedrine mimics norepinephrine it may be able to suppress hunger.

In most dietary fat-loss supplements, ephedrine appears as an extract from one of two herbs: ephedra or Ma Huang. The amount of ephedrine in these herbs is usually standardized to about 6% ephedrine. Furthermore, ephedrine does not appear in fat-loss supplements by itself; it is usually found at least with caffeine. Ephedrine by itself can easily be altered by underground drug labs to make methamphetamine (*speed, crank, meth, crystal*); thus its sale alone is prohibited. Research indicates that ephedrine is more effective as a fat-loss product when combined with caffeine,[138] and most of the research has used ephedrine in combination with caffeine at a standard dose of 20 mg of ephedrine and 200 mg of caffeine, two to three times per day. Therefore, we will focus on ephedrine and the combination of ephedrine and caffeine as a fat-loss product in this section.

Animal Studies

The administration of ephedrine to rats has been shown to increase thermogenesis by 32% as measured by oxygen consumption.[139] However, the addition of caffeine resulted in a 50% increase in oxygen consumption.[139] Dulloo and Miller[140] reported that the addition of ephedrine to the diets of mice increased energy expenditure by 10% which led to a 42% reduction in body fat stores over a 6-week period. The effects of ephedrine were amplified with the addition of caffeine, which resulted in a further 10% increase in energy expenditure and a 75% reduction in body fat.[140]

Energy-restricted diets are usually associated with a reduction in metabolic rate. The supplementation of ephedrine and caffeine during food-restricted diets may prevent the decrease in metabolic rate. In genetically obese Zucker rats, an ephedrine/caffeine combination resulted in a fourfold reduction in body fat during a food-restricted diet.[141] The rats whose diet was food restricted experienced only a twofold decrease in body fat and a 50% reduction in total body protein. Furthermore, energy expenditure in the food-restricted group was about 30% lower than in the food-restricted group, which received the ephedrine/caffeine combination.[141]

Human Studies

Research in humans indicates that the effect of the ephedrine/caffeine combination has been just as effective as in rats. Most research on the ephedrine/caffeine combination has been conducted by Dr. Astrup at the University of Copenhagen in the Research Department of Human Nutrition. His and other research reports that the ephedrine/caffeine combination is effective in increasing fat loss, especially when combined with a diet and exercise program (FIG. 4-8).

During a 24-week study investigating the effects of an ephedrine/caffeine combination, obese patients were required to consume about 1000 calories a day.[138] They were divided into four groups: caffeine, ephedrine, caffeine + ephedrine, and placebo. Following 24 weeks of treatment, the caffeine + ephedrine group lost almost 17 kg of weight, while the other three groups lost from 11 to 14 kg.

In one 8-week study, the group consuming the ephedrine/caffeine combination lost 4.5 kg more fat and 2.8 kg less muscle mass than the placebo group, when both groups were on a calorically restricted diet.[142] Furthermore, the drop in energy expenditure was significantly less in the ephedrine/caffeine group compared with the placebo group. In another 8-week study, the ephedrine/caffeine group lost almost 3 kg more weight than the placebo group.[143]

Because dietary supplements are sold over the counter, some people believe that they are not as effective as pre-

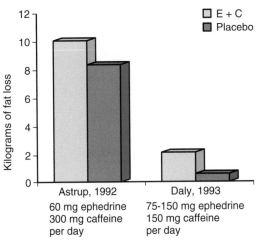

Figure 4-8. Human studies on the effect of ephedrine/caffeine combination in increasing fat loss. (*Data from* Astrup A, Breum L, Toubro S, et al. The effect of safety of an ephedrine/caffeine compound compared to ephedrine, caffeine and placebo in obese subjects on an energy restricted diet: a double blind trial. Int J Obes 1992;16:269–277; and Daly PA, Krieger DR, Dulloo AG, et al. Ephedrine, caffeine and aspirin: safety and efficacy for treatment of human obesity. Int J Obes 1993;17: S73–S78.)

scription medications. One research group compared the effectiveness of an ephedrine/caffeine combination with the prescription drug dexfenfluramine. Dexfenfluramine is a serotonin agonist and has been shown to be successful at promoting weight loss in obese patients[144] and was prescribed frequently in the last few years until heart complications surfaced in patients. During a 15-week study, patients consuming the ephedrine/caffeine combination lost about 8 kg, while the dexfenfluramine group lost about 7 kg.[144] In a subgroup of patients with a BMI over 30 kg/m[2], the ephedrine/caffeine combination resulted in a significantly greater amount of weight loss compared to the dexfenfluramine group (9.0 kg vs. 7.0 kg).[144]

Based on the research, the combination of ephedrine and caffeine appears to be one of the most effective dietary supplements for weight loss. However, the supplement does pose health risks if used improperly.

Safety and Toxicity

Side effects during ephedrine/caffeine consumption appear to be minimal. In one study, the caffeine + ephedrine group did experience more negative side effects (tremor, dizziness, insomnia). But, these effects appeared to be transient, and after 8 weeks of treatment the frequency of side effects had reached the level of the placebo group.[138] Other side effects may include arrhythmias and headaches.[145]

The FDA reports that well over 800 adverse incidents have occurred as well as a significant number of deaths associated with ephedrine-based products. Some states have banned the sale of ephedrine-based products. However, all of those who died in association with the products consumed well above the recommended dose for stimulant purposes. Based on the research evidence, if the product is consumed according to label directions, and the individual does not have a medical condition, which would warrant against consuming the product, it appears that the combination of both ingredients are safe and effective for fat-loss procedures.

Enterostatin

A peptide that acts similar to Cyclo (His-Pro) is enterostatin. Enterostatin is a pentapeptide that has been shown to be selective in inhibiting fat intake.[146–166] It is formed following the cleavage of the enzyme procolipase by trypsin in the gastric juice of the intestinal lumen. Procolipase is an enzyme essential for fat digestion. Following the cleavage of procolipase, enterostatin and colipase are produced. Colipase is an obligatory cofactor for pancreatic lipase digestion of fat. Enterostatin appears to act as a fat satiety factor that is believed to inhibit fat intake via receptors in the gut and brain. However, there may be a limitation to enterostatin administration, which will be discussed below. Most of the research so far has investigated exogenously administered enterostatin in animals; only one study has administered it to humans. Therefore, it is difficult to know whether enterostatin will be functionally effective in humans.

Animal Studies

Several studies have shown that peripherally or centrally administered enterostatin inhibits the intake of dietary fat.[146–166] Two mechanisms appear to be of action, depending on the location of administration. Peripherally, enterostatin reduces gastric emptying.[148] The slow rate of gastric emptying could result in greater gastric distension increasing satiety.[155] Furthermore, enterostatin may also interact with gut receptors, regulating motility and satiety.[150] Centrally, enterostatin appears to interact with an opioid pathway for modulating selection and consumption of diets high in fat.[157] Enterostatin does not delay the onset of feeding but appears to shorten the time spent eating.[158]

An interesting aspect of enterostatin function in rats is that it appears to reduce fat intake only in animals that have been adapted to diets which are high in fat before testing.[146,149,159,160] In animals that have been adapted to a standard diet or a high-carbohydrate diet, there appears to be no effect of enterostatin in reducing fat intake.[161,162]

Human Studies

Enterostatin response to feeding in humans is similar to that in rats. Serum enterostatin increased in response to a large meal.[163] However, some sensitivity and detection problems have been associated with the immunoreactive assay for measuring enterostatin.[156]

Intravenous administration of enterostatin in obese men resulted in no significant effect on feeding behavior.[164] However, other researchers have reported that the intravenous administration is not the most efficient method of administration.[156] Animal studies have reported that intravenous administration results in a prolonged response delay.[156] No other studies have been published which have orally administered enterostatin to humans.

Safety and Toxicity

Animal studies have not reported any adverse reactions associated with enterostatin administration, either peripherally or centrally. The only human study to administer enterostatin reported no adverse reactions. The only potential problem that could be found with enterostatin relates to the dosage. The dose-response to enterostatin is U-shaped, exhibiting an inhibition of fat intake at lower doses, but stimulation of food intake at higher doses.[147,148,165,166] Because of this dose response curve, there could be a range of functional dosages which could depend on a number of physiological factors.

Gugglesterone

The most common method of dieting is to reduce caloric intake. However, as we discussed above, this will ultimately result in a reduction in metabolic rate. The most likely explanation for the reduction in metabolic rate is a reduction in thyroxine (T4) and triiodothyronine (T3), the thyroid hormones.[167–170] These hormones are responsible for maintaining metabolic rate.

Gugglesterone is reported to be the active ingredient of Guggulu, a resin product isolated from *Commiphora mukul*, a plant native to India.[171] Many studies have reported that guggulsterone has hypocholesterolemic activity.[172–175] However, gugglesterone may also increase thyroid hormone levels.[176]

Animal Studies

A study investigating the potential thyroid-stimulating effects of gugglesterone administered gugglesterone (10 mg/kg body weight/day) or a placebo to carbimazole-treated rats. Carbimazole is a hypothyroid agent. Administration of gugglesterone for 6 days restored thyroid function and resulted in a significant elevation in both T3 and T4.[176]

Human Studies

Studies investigating the effects of gugglesterone in humans have focused on its hypolipidemic properties. No specific studies have investigated its thyroid-stimulating potential in humans. However, that does not mean that the supplement is worthless. Hypercholesterolemia and hypertriglyceridemia are common in overweight individuals. Therefore, gugglesterone may provide some benefit to overweight individuals who have high levels of serum cholesterol and triglyceride levels.

The administration of gugglesterone for 4–24 weeks at a dose of 75 mg–1 g per day has been effective in lowering serum cholesterol and triglyceride levels by 18–30%.[172–175] Furthermore, LDL and HDL have also been affected by gugglesterone supplementation, with a typical drop of approximately 12–19% in LDL and an increase of about 20% in HDL.[172,175]

The exact mechanism of action is not known, but animal studies suggest that gugglesterone increases LDL binding sites within the liver membrane, resulting in a significant uptake of LDL by the liver.[172] Therefore, serum cholesterol appears to be reduced by increasing the rate of lipoprotein catabolism.

Safety and Toxicity

Of the studies investigating the effect of gugglesterone as a hypolipidemic agent, just one study has included additional tests to determine its safety.[173] The authors reported that gugglesterone administration was completely safe and devoid of any effect on liver, kidney, or cardiovascular function. However, caution should be given to individuals who are taking prescription medications for hyperlipidemia who intend on taking gugglesterone. Research suggests that gugglesterone may lead to a diminished effectiveness and even nonresponsiveness of certain prescription drugs, such as propranolol or diltiazem.[177] Gugglesterone administration may alter the absorption of these drugs by nearly 35%. As with any drug or even any dietary supplement, if you are taking prescription medications, you should be monitored by your physician.

Hydroxycitric Acid (HCA)

The conversion of carbohydrate to fat requires that pyruvate be oxidized to acetyl-CoA. This oxidative process occurs within the mitochondria. However, fatty acid synthesis occurs predominately in the cytosol. Therefore, the acetyl group, which is the intermediate substrate for fatty acid synthesis, must be transported from inside the mitochondria to the cytosol before it can be incorporated into fatty acids. The acetyl group is transported out of the mitochondria as citrate. Once outside, an enzyme, ATP-citrate lyase, catalyzes the reaction, which cleaves citrate into acetyl-CoA and oxaloacetate.[178] The acetyl group then enters the biosynthetic pathway of fatty acid synthesis.

Hydroxycitric acid (HCA) is an inhibitor of the enzyme ATP-citrate lyase. Therefore, it prevents the conversion of carbohydrates into fatty acids by preventing the breakdown of citrate in the cytosol.[178,179] Many products are currently on the market that contain HCA among other ingredients. HCA is obtained from the extracts of the herbs *Garcinia cambogia* and *Garcinia indica,* both native to India.

Animal studies have shown HCA to be effective in reducing fatty acid synthesis. However, there is a lack of well-controlled human studies.

Animal Studies

Several well-controlled animal studies have investigated HCA's effect on fatty acid synthesis.[180–184] In general, they have all shown that HCA—administered orally, intravenously, or by intraperitoneal injection—inhibits fatty acid biosynthesis in the liver[180–184] and adipose tissue.[180,182,183] The degree of inhibition depends on the dosage and can range from 20% to 80%.[183,184] The decrease in fatty acid biosynthesis resulted in significant reductions in epididymal fat stores and total body fat.[180,182,183]

Another interesting aspect of HCA was the reduction in food intake during HCA administration.[180,182] Curiously, the reduction in food intake could not completely account for the decrease in body weight. Also, cholesterol and triglyceride levels were lower following HCA administration.[180,184]

Human Studies

As mentioned above, well-controlled human studies investigating the fat-loss potential of HCA are lacking. Most of the studies that have investigated HCA's effect on body composition have been performed using products containing other ingredients, which could also be active ingredients. Of the seven studies reviewed by Heymsfield et al.[185] only two have been published in peer-reviewed journals. Heymsfield and coworkers are the only ones to use HCA by itself.[185] The other studies have appeared only in abstract form and have investigated HCA in combination with other components that may also be considered to promote fat loss.

All but one of the studies have reported that HCA, combined with other fat-loss supplements, produced significantly greater losses in fat than a placebo.[185] The single study to investigate HCA by itself as the active ingredient reported that HCA failed to produce weight loss and fat mass loss beyond that observed with a placebo in overweight men and women.[185]

Based on the limited research, HCA could promote fat loss, but only when used in combination with other components of fat loss supplements. Further research needs to investigate HCA supplementation alone and when used in combination with other ingredients. The discrepancies between the animal and human studies are interesting. But, as we are learning from leptin research, the regulation of fat metabolism in rats appears to be much different than that in humans.

Safety and Toxicity

Neither animal nor human studies have reported any treatment-related adverse events. A few animal studies have included tests specifically to look at liver function. The human studies have simply used an adverse incident reporting form and have reported that adverse events were not significantly different between the treatment group and placebo group.

β-hydroxy-β-methylbutyrate (HMB)

One of the newest dietary supplements on the market is β-hydroxy-β-methylbutyrate (HMB). HMB has been reported to increase fat-free mass gains during resistance training. In addition to affecting protein synthesis, HMB may also stimulate fat oxidation. Even though HMB is relatively new to the market, more research has been conducted on its physiological effects than many other supplements. However, because it is relatively new to the market, more research is still needed in humans.*

In Vitro Studies

To further elucidate the mechanisms of HMB, Cheng et al.[186,187] investigated the effects of HMB on fatty acid uptake and oxidation in two different muscle cell lines, derived from heart and skeletal muscle. Their research indicated that beta-oxidation increased about 30% following the incubation of muscle cells in a medium containing HMB. The exact mechanism as to how HMB influences fat oxidation is unknown. Also what is unknown is whether the in vitro research will be verified in animals and humans.

Human Studies

A single human study investigating the effects of HMB on body composition has been published in a peer-reviewed journal.[188] In this study, they reported a significant increase in fat-free mass, but not a significant drop in body fat compared with the placebo. In the same reference, the authors reported that another group of subjects did not experience a decline in fat mass during a 7-week treatment with HMB. Although research is limited, it seems unlikely that HMB affects lipid oxidation in humans.

*Recently published data further showed the effectiveness of HMB. Panton, et al. (Nutrition 2000;16(9):734–739) demonstrated that 3 grams of HMB daily for 4 weeks resulted in an increase in fat-free mass (+1.4 kg) and a decreased percentage body fat (−1.1%) whereas the placebo group experienced more modest changes in fat-free mass (+0.9 kg) and percentage body fat (−0.5%). Also, Nissen, et al. (J Nutr 2000;130(8):1937–1945) found that compared to a placebo, a daily dose of 3 grams of HMB for a 3–8 week duration resulted in a net decrease in plasma total cholesterol, LDL-cholesterol, and systolic blood pressure in comparison to the placebo. Thus, "HMB can be taken safely as an ergogenic aid for exercise and that the objective measures of health and perception of well-being are generally enhanced (Nissen et al., 2000)."

Safety and Toxicity

The safety data for HMB are impressive. Every HMB study that has been funded by either Metabolic Technologies, Inc. or by Experimental and Applied Sciences, Inc. has included safety data. Although the longest human study to date is 8 weeks long, it appears that HMB has no adverse reactions. Animal studies report that dosages greater than 100 times the normal human dose do not result in any changes in blood chemistry and hematology measurement in pigs.[189] Furthermore, there were no effects of HMB on gross organ pathology and histology.[189] Longer-term studies are needed to determine how the body responds to chronic consumption of HMB over a period of a year or more. But for now one can confidently say that HMB is one of the safest dietary supplements on the market.

Medium-Chain Triglycerides (MCT)

Triglycerides are composed of a glycerol backbone with three free fatty acids attached. In the case of medium-chain triglycerides (MCTs) these fatty acids are made up of a mixture of C6 to C12 medium-chain fatty acids. Unlike long-chain triglycerides, the MCTs are liquid at room temperature and are relatively soluble in water. For example, the water solubility of a C8 saturated fatty acid is 68 mg/100 mL at 20°C versus 0.72 mg/100 mL for a C16 saturated fatty acid. Also, as discussed above, long-chain fatty acids require the carnitine transport system to enter the mitochondria. Medium-chain fatty acids (MCFAs) cross the mitochondrial membrane rapidly through a diffusion process[190] and therefore can be oxidized into CO_2 at a faster rate than long-chain fatty acids.[191] The liver is capable of producing ten times more CO_2 from a C8:0 fatty acid than from a C16:0 fatty acid.[191] However, when MCTs are consumed, there is an increase in ketone body production. Because of the increased rate of oxidation of MCFA, there is an excess of acetyl-CoA, and Krebs cycle intermediates will be in short supply, resulting in a large part of the MCFA being directed toward ketone body production.

The reason MCTs have been used in the treatment of obesity is of interest because the research does not necessarily support its use as a weight-loss product, especially in humans. Furthermore, a mechanism as to why fat intake would result in fat loss has not been provided.

Animal Studies

Several studies have investigated the potential use of MCTs in weight reduction.[192–197] However, the results are equivocal and many of them have not reported a significant effect from MCT supplementation. One possible mechanism by which MCT may function is through enhanced thermogenesis induced by MCT.[198] However, this study has only appeared in abstract form and has not been verified.

Human Studies

Of the few human studies to be conducted that have investigated the use of MCTs as a fat-loss supplement, none have reported a significant effect.[199–201] These studies have primarily used obese subjects on a restricted caloric intake (500 to 1200 calories per day). One study, however, reported that MCTs decreased food intake during the day when the MCT was consumed with breakfast.[200] In general, the results of these studies have failed to provide any evidence in favor of MCTs providing any benefit during dieting. For example, one study reported that obese women consuming a 550-kcal diet containing 30 g of MCTs lost the same amount of weight as when MCTs were replaced by sugars.[201]

Safety and Toxicity

For some populations, there is some concern regarding MCT supplementation. MCTs are ketogenic in the normal individual and even more so in a diabetic. A ketogenic state (ketosis) can result in acidosis. In this condition, homeostasis is compromised, leading to dehydration, hypovolemia, and hypotension caused by an increase in Na^+ and K^+ excretion in the urine. Furthermore, the acidosis and dehydration can lead to a state of unconsciousness, and in severe cases, coma. For the normal, healthy individual, there appears to be no risk in consuming MCTs.

Phosphates

Most individuals are familiar with phosphates as being part of adenosine triphosphate (ATP). As we know, phosphates (inorganic) can control the rate of enzymes, especially in glycolysis. Some evidence suggests that phosphate supplementation may provide some benefits during periods of dieting. Minimal, if any, animal research has been reported investigating the potential use of phosphate as a fat-loss agent. Therefore, this discussion will focus on the few studies that have examined humans.

Human Studies

The supplementation of phosphate in the form of potassium-phosphate and magnesium-phosphate has been shown to increase postprandial thermogenesis in obese women but not in lean women.[202,203] The increase in energy expenditure ranged between 6–16%. The mechanism as to how a single dose of phosphate can increase energy expenditure may be related to futile cycling, but this is speculative.

Phosphate supplementation during a period of caloric restriction has not been shown to promote a more rapid rate of fat loss.[204] Obese women consuming about 1000 kcal/day, in addition to 4 g/day of phosphate salts, experienced a 4.5-kg loss of body mass, while the placebo group experienced about a 5-kg loss of body mass over a 28-day period.[204] However, resting metabolic rate (RMR) significantly increased in the phosphate group, but the placebo group did not experience a change in RMR. An increase in RMR is associated with an increase in caloric expenditure. However, the increased RMR associated with phosphate supplementation did not result in greater rate of fat loss.

A follow-up study by the same group provides an explanation for the effect phosphates have on RMR. They reported that phosphate supplementation (about 4 g/day) prevented a decrease in triiodothyronine (T3) during caloric restriction, while the RMR increased approximately 12–19% during the treatment periods.[205] Even though RMR was significantly elevated during the treatment phase, weight loss was not affected by phosphate supplementation.

Although phosphate supplementation does not appear to accelerate fat loss during periods of reduced caloric intake, phosphates may help prevent a decline in RMR that is common during dieting. Further research needs to verify this finding.

Safety and Toxicity

Adverse side effects do not appear to be associated with phosphate supplementation. However, an excess of phosphorus (a calcium-to-phosphorus ratio lower than 1:2) has been shown to lower the blood calcium level, which may result in the loss of bone.

Pyruvate

Another fairly new supplement to the market is pyruvate. If you have had a biochemistry class or are familiar with biochemistry, you know that pyruvate is the end product of glycolysis. Some people consider lactate the end product of glycolysis, but that is only under anaerobic conditions. Glycolysis is always running and during resting conditions or low-intensity exercise pyruvate is the end product. Pyruvate is taken up by the mitochondria, and in the process is converted to acetyl-CoA and carbon dioxide by the enzyme complex pyruvate dehydrogenase (PDH). During high-intensity exercise, the mitochondria's ability to use pyruvate cannot keep up with the production of pyruvate via glycolysis; therefore, pyruvate is reduced to lactic acid via lactate dehydrogenase (LDH). The lactic acid that is formed dissociates into lactate and a hydrogen ion. This allows glycolysis to continue for a few more moments, until the accumulation of hydrogen ions exceeds the buffering capacity of the muscle and blood, and fatigue sets in.

How pyruvate results in fat reduction is unknown. It may increase thermogenesis or decrease lipogenesis. Furthermore, once we review the studies, and you read the section Current Controversy, you will question why it is being sold as a supplement and more importantly, why people are buying the product.

Animal Studies

In the early 1980s, it was reported that a mixture of pyruvate and dihydroxyacetone (PYR-DHA) supplemented to a nutritionally balanced diet prevented fat accumulation associated with ethanol consumption in rats.[206] Subsequent studies reported that this same mixture reduced triglyceride synthesis in the liver.[207] A collateral observation in these studies was that treated rats had less abdominal fat than control rats. This led to a study to specifically investigate the effects of PYR-DHA on body composition in the rat, with the hypothesis that the mixture would have a generalized inhibitory effect on lipid synthesis. The authors of this study reported that the rats receiving the PYR-DHA diet had 32% less body fat than the control rats.[208] Furthermore, rats consuming PYR-DHA had lower rates of lipid synthesis and a higher rate of energy expenditure.[208]

Contrary to these findings a study investigating pyruvate supplementation with and without the co-administration of dihydroxyacetone reported that muscle weights and fat pad weights were not different across treatments when total body weight was accounted.[209] Overall, rats fed pyruvate, dihydroxyacetone, or both experienced a slower rate of growth development leading to smaller weight gains.[209] In addition, liver glycogen content was 40–50% lower in the experimental groups compared with the control groups.[209] A subsequent study from the same laboratory[210] reported that pyruvate supplementation lowered respiratory exchange ratio, indicating a greater reliance on fat for energy. However, the rats receiving pyruvate also experienced lower muscle weights than the control group.[210]

Based on the above studies, it would be logical to conclude that the effect of pyruvate supplementation on body composition changes is equivocal. In the first study, pyruvate was used in conjunction with dihydroxyacetone. In the second study pyruvate was investigated with and without co-administration of dihydroxyacetone. Only the last study used pyruvate in the form found in dietary supplements. What about the human studies? Is the evidence any more compelling for humans?

Human Studies

Human studies have reported that pyruvate supplementation will result in an increased weight and fat loss (FIG. 4-9).[211–214] However, before we decide unequivocally

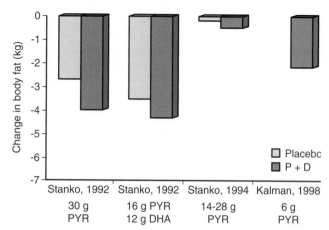

Figure 4-9. Human studies on pyruvate supplementation resulting in increased fat loss. (*Data from* Stanko RT, Tietze DL, Arch JE. Body composition, energy utilization, and nitrogen metabolism with a severely restricted diet supplemented with dihydroxyacetone and pyruvate. Am J Clin Nutr 1992;55:771–776; Stanko RT, Arch JE. Inhibition of regain in body weight and fat with addition of 3-carbon compounds to the diet with hyperenergetic refeeding after weight reduction. Int J Obes Relat Metab Disord 1996;20:925–930; Stanko RT, Reynolds HR, Hoyson R, et al. Pyruvate supplementation of a low-cholesterol, low-fat diet: effects of plasma lipid concentrations and body composition in hyperlipidemic patients. Am J Clin Nutr 1994;59:423–427; and Kalman D, Colker CM, Stark R, et al. Effect of pyruvate supplementation on body composition and mood. Curr Ther Res 1998;59:793–802.)

that pyruvate is effective, we should first evaluate the research.

Five studies have been published in peer-reviewed journals investigating pyruvate supplementation in humans.[211–215] Four of those studies have been published by Stanko and colleagues.[211–213,215] These studies by Stanko et al. have focused on the effect of pyruvate in promoting fat loss during caloric-restricted diets.[211,213,215] One study investigated the effect of pyruvate in preventing re-accumulation of fat with re-feeding following weight loss.[212] Although all three studies reported that the pyruvate group experienced significantly more fat loss than the placebo group, the changes were not that great. One study reported a difference of 0.8 kg between the two groups,[211] while the other two studies reported a difference of 1.3 kg and 0.4 kg, respectively.[213,215] In addition to fat loss, the subjects in all three studies also lost lean tissue mass, suggesting the pyruvate supplementation does not help spare tissue protein during periods of severe caloric restriction. During the re-feeding study, the group receiving pyruvate (plus DHA) gained 0.8 kg, and the placebo group gained 1.8 kg.[212]

A few issues need to be addressed in the above studies. First, the amount of pyruvate that the subjects consumed was relatively large. In all but one study, the amount of pyruvate administered ranged from 15 g to 44 g. In one study 75 g of dihydroxyacetone was also administered.[211–213,215] Only one study provided a dose of 6 g/day.[214] This issue is important because on labels of pyruvate products, the recommended dose is 3–5 g. If the research reports that an effective dose is in the range of 15–44 g/day, it seems almost impossible to expect the same results from a dose that is anywhere from three to fifteen times lower than the effective dose reported in the literature. Although the Kalman study[214] did report a significant effect from 6 g, this study needs to be verified. Furthermore, there are some methodological problems with this study as well. In the study by Kalman and coworkers, subjects received either 6 g/day of pyruvate or placebo, and a control group also participated. During the 6-week training program, subjects exercised 3 days per week, for 30 minutes per session. Exercise consisted of a circuit resistance-training program. Subjects in the pyruvate group experienced a 2.1-kg decline in fat mass, and the control and placebo groups did not experience any change in body composition. This latter observation is unusual. One would expect that a group of individuals who were exercising, and who were allowed to consume a limited amount of calories (about 2000 kcals) would experience some decline in weight. Furthermore, males and females were not equally distributed among groups. There were twice as many males in the placebo group as females (12 vs. 6), while the control group had half as many males as females (5 vs. 10). The pyruvate group had two fewer males than females (8 vs. 10). The reason this could be a problem is that males and females may respond to supplementation and training at different rates.

The research on pyruvate supplementation and its effect on body composition in rats and humans is highly equivocal. Based on the research that has been published, we don't know why or how pyruvate works. Furthermore, the product you buy may not contain dihydroxyacetone, yet most of the animal research and some of the human research used dihydroxyacetone in conjunction with pyruvate. And finally, the effective dose reported in the literature would require a person to consume an amount of pyruvate that is equal to about half-a-cup of the product per day, a large and expensive amount. Until further research provides a mechanism as to how this product functions, it is not a product that is recommended to be highly effective.

Safety and Toxicity

No adverse side effects appear to be associated with pyruvate supplementation.

Yohimbe

Yohimbe is an herbal extract from the bark of the African tree *Pausinystalia yohimbe,* which contains yohimbine, the active ingredient. In most dietary supplements, yohimbe is standardized to 3% yohimbine. Yohimbine is an α_2-antagonist.[216] Human fat cells possess both alpha- and beta-adrenergic receptors. Catecholamines are able to stimulate lipolysis through beta-receptors, whereas they inhibit lipolysis through alpha$_2$-receptors. The balance between these receptors controls the rate of lipolysis. Therefore, an increase in thermogenesis for fat-loss purposes could be achieved by either stimulating beta-receptors or by blocking alpha$_2$-receptors. Because yohimbine has alpha$_2$-antagonistic properties, this supplement could be used during fat-loss procedures to further increase the rate of lipolysis. This discussion will focus on the lipolytic effect of yohimbine. However, it should be noted that yohimbine is a prescription drug. No specific studies have been done on yohimbe.

Animal Studies

Oral or intravenous administration of yohimbine in dogs has resulted in a significant elevation in plasma free fatty acids and an increase in sympathetic nervous system activity. Norepinephrine was significantly elevated following yohimbine administration.[217,218] Furthermore, chronic oral administration resulted in a reduction in body weight and in food intake, suggesting that alpha$_2$-antagonists may influence satiety.[218] The lipolytic effect of yohimbine may result either from a direct action of yohimbine or from an activation of the sympathetic nervous system.

Human Studies

As mentioned above, the interplay of beta-receptors and alpha$_2$-receptors regulates the lipolytic response of adipose tissue to the catecholamines.[219] A supplement which would inhibit the alpha$_2$-receptors would theoretically increase the action of catecholamines on lipolysis. Yohimbine has been shown to effectively increase lipolysis.

An abundance of studies have been done investigating the lipolytic action of yohimbine in humans.[220–225] *In vitro* studies using human adipocytes have indicated stimulatory effects of yohimbine on lipolysis when catecholamines are present.[220]

Oral administration of yohimbine to humans has been shown to significantly elevate plasma glycerol and free-fatty acids.[221] Furthermore, the effect of yohimbine was further enhanced during physical exercise when the levels of catecholamines are further elevated.[221] Yohimbine also appears to stimulate norepinephrine levels by increasing sympathetic nerve activity.[222]

When yohimbine was administered during a low-energy diet, patients lost significantly more weight than patients receiving a placebo.[223] Energy expenditure did not decline in the patients consuming yohimbine, while the placebo group experienced a 15% reduction in energy expenditure.[223]

Safety and Toxicity

Alpha$_2$-receptors are present in a number of tissues including heart, arteries, lung, and adipose tissue. Therefore, yohimbine could react with any of these receptors and influence those tissues. However, both animal and human studies indicate that cardiovascular changes are either nonexistent or minimal following yohimbine administration.

Some side effects associated with yohimbine include feelings of panic, clumsiness, and confusion.[225] There have also been reports of chills, nausea, and tremors.[225] The prescription form of yohimbine is normally prescribed for impotence problems; therefore, individuals may experience heightened sexual arousal. Furthermore, there have been reports of mood disturbances and anxiety.

Another concern regarding yohimbe is the purity of the dietary supplement. As mentioned above, yohimbine is the major alkaloid of the plant and the active ingredient. The bark of the tree has been reported to contain 6% total alkaloids, 10–15% of which are yohimbine. Most dietary supplements have been standardized to 3% yohimbine. Therefore, a 100-mg dose of yohimbe will contain only 3 mg of yohimbine. In research studies, yohimbine is usually administered at a dose of about 0.2 mg/kg of body weight.

SUMMARY

Several agents have been discussed that have been promoted to increase fat loss. However, as you have read, minimal scientific data are actually available to support many of these products. The products, which have been shown to be beneficial in aiding fat loss, from a scientific point of view, include caffeine with or without ephedrine. Although caffeine alone or in combination with ephedrine appears to be the most effective, there is some controversy surrounding the use of these ingredients. When abused, ephedrine has been associated with adverse reactions including death. The use of caffeine also produces some unwanted side effects. However, if a caffeine and/or ephedrine product is used according to the manufacturer's recommendations and if used alone, it is unlikely that any life-threatening events would occur with the use of the product. Nevertheless, appropriate supervision by a physician is always recommended.

If you have read the chapter and/or the literature presented in the chapter carefully, you will realize that in most of the studies, an exercise intervention program was used in conjunction with the dietary supplement. The supplement, in most cases, did not produce a great effect, if any. The key to fat loss, as mentioned at the beginning of the chapter, is that caloric expenditure must be greater than caloric intake. If it is not, fat loss will not occur.

Although new fat reduction supplements will appear on the market, the main physiological mechanism of body weight regulation, energy balance, is reflected by energy intake and energy expenditure. Excess energy intake without a concomitant rise in energy expenditure will result mainly in the deposition of fat into adipocytes. This excess energy may be in the form of carbohydrates, fat, and protein. A balanced diet with energy expenditure exceeding energy intake is the best form of fat reduction—guaranteed.

Current Controversy: Supplement Warning

Several dietary supplements have been granted patents. As we all know, the patent protects the inventor from unscrupulous people or businesses practices. In most cases, the patent holder is the researcher who discovered the product or the use for the product. Patents have been issued for the following products/ingredients: chromium, CLA, HMB, and pyruvate. The inventor of a specific product has shown in published and/or unpublished studies that the product produces an effect. In the case of the products listed above, the effect is an alteration in body composition: either an increase in muscle mass or a decrease in fat mass.

Once a chemical, product, or ingredient has been shown to alter body composition, other scientists conduct research to verify the reported claims. However, in the case of chromium, the majority of the research finds that chromium supplementation is ineffective as an agent to alter body composition. Of the few studies that have shown a positive effect, the majority are from the inventor's laboratory. The authors and editors of this book are not suggesting that the researchers/ inventors are biased in reporting their findings. Many of the inventors are well-respected scientists. However, to remove the potential for biased reporting, financially independent scientists are encouraged to validate their findings.

Another item of concern is the purity and bioavailability of the active agent. A number of the products discussed in this chapter and others are herbs. During the manufacturing process, the active ingredient is standardized to a certain percentage. Because ingredients are not monitored by a regulatory agency, manufacturers can deviate from the effective percentage. Furthermore, when manufacturers do not control the manufacturing process, a number of impurities can contaminate the product, leading to an ineffective and potentially dangerous ingredient.

FUTURE RESEARCH

Products that promote fat loss are probably the most sought after products by both consumers and researchers. Obesity is a major health problem in the United States, and over the last 20 years the prevalence of obesity has increased. Furthermore, the weight-loss industry produces an astounding amount of revenue. This revenue potential is seen by both supplement and pharmaceutical companies. For example, the biotechnology company Amgen Inc. reportedly paid nearly 20 million dollars for the exclusive rights to leptin. This was before human studies were conducted. Because of this large potential to generate revenue, there are many unscrupulous, fly-by-night companies that market ineffective and/or unsafe fat-loss products. The FDA has issued numerous warnings regarding deaths or the potential for serious adverse reactions associated with many of the fat-loss supplements.

I believe that as future research unfolds, we will find out that there is not one cause for obesity and thus, one product will not work for everyone. Some individuals may experience metabolic problems, while others experience satiety problems. Several supplements or potential supplements are currently being investigated as fat-loss supplements. I was unable to include these substances in this chapter due to length considerations. These include 7-oxo-DHEA, arginine-a-ketoglutarate, and many others. When looking for a fat-loss supplement, make sure there is research to support the claims that the company makes. But remember, for fat loss to occur, caloric expenditure must be greater than caloric intake, and the best way to achieve that is through exercise.

REFERENCES

1. Kuczmarski RJ, Flegal KM, Campbell SM, Johnson CL. Increasing prevalence of overweight among US adults. The National Health and Nutrition Examination Surveys, 1960 to 1991. JAMA 1994; 272:205–211.
2. Must A, Jacques PF, Dallal GE, et al. Long-term morbidity and mortality of overweight adolescents. A follow-up of the Harvard Growth Study of 1922 to 1935. N Engl J Med 1992;327:1350–1355.
3. Potter BJ, Sorrentino D, Berk PD. Mechanisms of cellular uptake of free fatty acids. Ann Rev Nutr 1989;9:253–270.
4. Calles-Escandon J, Sweet L, Ljungqvist O, Hirshman MF. The membrane associated 40kD fatty acid binding protein (Berk's protein), a putative fatty acid transporter, is present in skeletal muscle. Life Sci 1996;58:19–28.
5. Romihn JA, Coyle EF, Sidossis LS, et al. Regulation of endogenous fat and carbohydrate metabolism in relation to exercise intensity and duration. Am J Physiol 1993;265:E380–E391.
6. Gollnick PD, Saltin B. Fuel for muscular exercise: role of fat. In: Exercise, nutrition and energy metabolism. New York: Macmillan, 1988:71–88.
7. Armstrong DT, Steele R, Altszuler N, et al. Regulation of plasma free fatty acid turnover. Am J Physiol 1961;201:9–15.
8. Hagenfeldt L, Wahren J. Metabolism of free fatty acids and ketone bodies in skeletal muscle. In: Muscle metabolism during exercise. New York: Plenum Press, 1971:153–163.
9. Bray GA. Use and abuse of appetite-suppressant drugs in the treatment of obesity. Ann Intern Med 1993;119:707–713.
10. Booth DA. Acquired behavior controlling energy intake and output. In: Stunkard AJ, ed. Obesity. Philadelphia: WB Saunders, 1980:10–143.
11. Hwang CS, Loftus TM, Mandrup S, Lane MD. Adipocyte differentiation and leptin expression. Annu Rev Cell Dev Biol 1997;13:231–259.
12. Jequier E, Tappy L. Regulation of body weight in humans. Physiol Rev 1999;79:451–480.
13. Butcher RW, Baird CE, Sutherland EW. Effects of lipolytic and antilipolytic substances on adenosine $3',5'$-monophosphate levels in isolated fat cells. J Biol Chem 1968;2430:1705–1712.
14. Steinfelder HJ, Petho-Schramm S. Methylxanthines inhibit glucose transport in rat adipocytes by two independent mechanisms. Biochem Pharmacol 1990;40:1154–1157.
15. Hochberg A, Hertz P, Benderly A. Caffeine stimulates growth hormone secretion by cultured rat pituitary cells. J Endocrinol Invest 1984;7:59–60.
16. Kashiwagura T, Kagaya T, Takeguchi N. Effects of caffeine on gluconeogenesis and urea synthesis induced by alpha-adrenergic stimulation in suspensions of rat hepatocytes. Jpn J Physiol 1987;37: 979–993.
17. Kieke M, Kashwwagura T, Takeguchi N. Gluconeogenesis stimulated by extracellular ATP is triggered by the initial increase in the intracellular Ca^{++} concentration of the periphery of hepatocytes. Biochem J 1992;283:265–272.
18. Spindel E, Arnold M, Cusack B, Wurtman RJ. Effects of caffeine on anterior pituitary and thyroid function in the rat. J Pharmacol Exp Ther 1980;214:58–62.

19. Clozel M, Branchaud CL, Tannenbaum GS, et al. Effect of caffeine on thyroid and pituitary function in newborn rats. Pediatr Res 1983;17:592–595.
20. Xu Y, Forsberg EJ. Effects of caffeine on cholinergic agonist- and K(+)-induced cytosolic Ca++ signals and secretion in porcine adrenal chromaffin cells. J. Pharmacol Exp Ther 1993;264:770–775.
21. Wilcox AR. The effects of caffeine and exercise on body weight, fat-pad weight, and fat-cell size. Med Sci Sports Exerc 1982;14:317–321.
22. Astrup A, Toubro S, Christensen NJ, Quaade F. Pharmacology of thermogenic drugs. Am J Clin Nutr 1992;55:246S–248S.
23. Bracco D, Ferrarrra JM, Arnaud MJ, et al. Effects of caffeine on energy metabolism, heart rate, and methylxanthine metabolism in lean and obese women. Am J Physiol 1995;269:E671–E678.
24. Arciero PJ, Gardner AW, Calles-Escandon J, et al. Effects of caffeine ingestion on NE kinetics, fat oxidation, and energy expenditure in younger and older men. Am J Physiol 1995;268:E1192–E1198.
25. Acheson KJ, Zahorska-Markiewicz B, Pittet P, et al. Caffeine and coffee: their influence on metabolic rate and substrate utilization in normal weight and obese individuals. Am J Clin Nutr 1980; 33:989–997.
26. Caraco Y, Zylber-Katz E, Berry EM, Levy M. Caffeine pharmacokinetics in obesity and following significant weight reduction. Int J Obes Relat Metab Disord 1995;19:234–239.
27. Robertson D, Frolich JC, Carr RK, et al. Effects of caffeine on plasma renin activity, catecholamines and blood pressure. N Engl J Med 1978;298:181–186.
28. Graham TE, Spriet LL. Metabolic, catecholamine, and exercise performance responses to various doses of caffeine. J Appl Physiol 1995;78:867–874.
29. Graham TE, Hibbert E, Sathasivam P. Metabolic and exercise endurance effects of coffee and caffeine ingestion. J Appl Physiol 1998;85:883–889.
30. Spindel ER, Wurtman RJ, McCall A, et al. Neuroendocrine effects of caffeine in normal subjects. Clin Pharmacol Ther 1984;36: 402–407.
31. Debrah K, Haigh R, Sherwin R, et al. Effect of acute and chronic caffeine use on the cerebrovascular, cardiovascular and hormonal responses to orthostasis in healthy volunteers. Clin Sci 1995; 89:475–480.
32. Wald A, Back C, Bayless TM. Effect of caffeine on the human small intestine. Gastroenterology 1976;71:738–742.
33. Fisher SM, McMurray RG, Berry M, et al. Influence of caffeine on exercise performance in habitual caffeine users. Int J Sports Med 1986;7:276–280.
34. Mrvos RM, Reilly PE, Dean BS, Krenzelok EP. Massive caffeine ingestion resulting in death. Vet Hum Toxicol 1989;31:571–572.
35. Stavric B. Methylxanthines: Toxicity to humans. 2. Caffeine. Food Chem Toxicol 1988;26:645–662.
36. Engel AG, Angelini C. Carnitine deficiency of human skeletal muscle with associated lipid storage myopathy: a new syndrome. Science 1973;316:124–135.
37. Schwenk WF, Hale DE, Haymond MW. Decreased fasting free fatty acids with L-carnitine in children with carnitine deficiency. Pediatr Res 1988;23:491–494.
38. Levitan MD, Murphy JT, Sherwood WG, et al. Adult onset carnitine deficiency: favorable response to L-carnitine supplementation. Can J Neurol Sci 1987;14:50–54.
39. Fritz IB. The effects of muscle extracts on the oxidation of palmitic acid by liver slices and homogenates. Acta Physiol Scand 1955;34:367–385.
40. Fritz IB. Carnitine and its role in fatty acid metabolism. Advances Lipid Res 1963;1:285–334.
41. Fritz IB, Yue KTN. Long-chain carnitine acetyltransferase and the role of acylcarnitine derivatives in the catalytic increase of fatty acid oxidation induced by carnitine. J Lipid Res 1963;4:279–288.
42. Willner JH, Ginsburg S, Dimauro S. Active transport of carnitine into skeletal muscle. Neurology 1978;28:721–724.
43. Clouet P, Sempore G, Tsoko M, et al. Effect of short- and long-term treatments by a low levels of dietary L-carnitine on parameters related to fatty acid oxidation in Wistar rat. Biochim Biophys Acta 1996;1299:191–197.
44. Maccari F, Arseni A, Chiodi P, et al. L-carnitine effect on plasma lipoproteins of hyperlipidemic fat-loaded rats. Lipids 1987; 22:1005–1008.
45. Askew EW, Dohm GL, Weiser PC, et al. Supplementation dietary carnitine and lipid metabolism in exercising rats. Nutr Metab 1980;24:32–42.
46. Meijer GW, Beynen AC. Influence of dietary carnitine on lipid and carbohydrate metabolism in rats. Z Ernahrungswiss 1988;27: 77–83.
47. Brass EP, Hiatt WR. The role of carnitine and carnitine supplementation during exercise in man and in individual with special needs. J Am Coll Nutr 1998;17:207–215.
48. Sugano M, Fujikawa T, Hiratsuji Y, et al. A novel use of Chitosan as a hypocholesterolemic agent in rats. Am J Clin Nutr 1980;33: 787–793.
49. Sugano M, Watanabe S, Kishi A, et al. Hypocholesterolemic action of chitosans with different viscosity in rats. Lipids 1988;23: 187–191.
50. Ebihara K, Schneeman BO. Interaction of bile acids, phospholipids, cholesterol and triglyceride with dietary fibers in the small intestine of rats. J Nutr 1989;119:1100–1106.
51. Ikeda I, Tomari Y, Sugano M. Interrelated effects of dietary fiber and fat on lymphatic cholesterol and triglyceride absorption in rats. J Nutr 1989;119:1383–1387.
52. LeHouz JG, Grondin F. Some effects of Chitosan on liver function in the rat. Endocrinology 1993;132:1078–1084.
53. Deuchi K, Kanauchi O, Imasato Y, Kobayashi E. Effect of the viscosity or deacetylation degree of chitosan on fecal fat excreted from rats fed on a high-fat diet. Biosci Biotechnol Biochem 1995;59: 781–785.
54. Girola M, De Bernardi M, Contos S, et al. Dose effect in lipid-lowering activity of a new dietary integrator (Chitosan, Garcinia cambogia extract and chrome). Acta Toxicol Ther 1996;17:25–40.
55. Deuchi K, Kanauchi O, Shizukuishi M, Kobayashi E. Continuous and massive intake of chitosan affects mineral and fat-soluble vitamin status in rats fed on a high-fat diet. Biosci Biotechnol Biochem 1995;59:1211–1216.
56. Thomson AB, De Pover A, Keelan M, et al. Inhibition of lipid absorption as an approach to the treatment of obesity. Methods Enzymol 1997;286:3–44.
57. Jeejeebhoy KN, Chu RC, Marliss EB, et al. Chromium deficiency, glucose intolerance, and neuropathy reversed by chromium supplementation, in a patient receiving long-term total parenteral nutrition. Am J Clin Nutr 1977;30:531–538.
58. Anderson RA. Nutritional factors influencing the glucose/insulin system: chromium. J Am Coll Nutr 1997;16:404–410.
59. Anderson RA, Cheng N, Bryden NA, et al. Elevated intakes of supplemental chromium improve glucose and insulin variables in individuals with type 2 diabetes. Diabetes 1997;46:1786–1791.
60. Evans GW, Bowman TD. Chromium picolinate increases membrane fluidity and rate of insulin internalization. J Inorg Biochem 1992;46:243–250.
61. Evans GW. The effect of chromium picolinate on insulin controlled parameters in humans. Int J Biosoc Med Res 1989;11:163–180.
62. Hasten DL, Rome EP, Franks BD, Hegsted M. Effects of chromium picolinate on beginning weight training students. Int J Sports Nutr 1992;2:343–350.
63. Trent LK, Thieding-Cancel D. Effects of chromium picolinate on body composition. J Sports Med Phys Fitness 1995;35: 273–280.
64. Lukaski HC, Bolonchuk WW, Siders WA, Milne DB. Chromium supplementation and resistance training: effects on body composition, strength, and trace element status of men. Am J Clin Nutr 1996;63:954–965.
65. Walker LS, Bemben MG, Bemben DA, Knehans AW. Chromium picolinate effects on body composition and muscular performance in wrestlers. Med Sci Sports Exerc 1998;30:1730–1737.
66. Lefavi RG, Anderson RA, Keith RE, et al. Efficacy of chromium supplementation in athletes: emphasis on anabolism. Int J Sports Nutr 1992;2:111–122.
67. Hallmark MA, Reynolds TH, DeSouza CA, et al. Effects of chromium and resistive training on muscle strength and body composition. Med Sci Sports Exerc 1996;28:139–144.
68. Campbell WW, Joseph LJO, Davey SL, et al. Effects of resistance training and chromium picolinate on body composition and skeletal muscle in older men. J Appl Physiol 1999;86:29–39.
69. Clancy SP, Clarkson PM, DeCheke ME, et al. Effects of chromium picolinate supplementation on body composition, strength, and

urinary chromium loss in football players. Int J Sports Nutr 1994;4:142–153.

70. Grant KE, Chandler RM, Castle AL, Ivy JL. Chromium and exercise training: effect on obese women. Med Sci Sports Exerc 1997;29:992–998.

71. National Research Council. Trace elements. In: Recommended Dietary Allowances, 10th ed. Washington DC: National Academy Press, 1989:195–246.

72. Seal CJ. Influence of dietary picolinic acid on mineral metabolism in the rat. Ann Nutr Metab 1988;32:186–191.

73. Cerulli J, Grabe DW, Gauthier I, et al. Chromium picolinate toxicity. Ann Pharmacother 1998;32:428–431.

74. Martin WR, Fuller RE. Suspected chromium picolinate-induced rhabdomyolysis. Pharmacotherapy 1998;18:860–862.

75. Pariza MW, Ha YL, Benjamin H, et al. Formation and action of anti-carcinogenic fatty acids. Adv Exp Med Biol 1991;289:269–272.

76. Ip C, Singh M, Thompson HJ, Scimeca JA. Conjugated linoleic acid suppresses mammary carcinogenesis and proliferative activity of the mammary gland in the rat. Cancer Res 1994;54:1212–1215.

77. Ip C, Scimeca JA, Thompson HJ. Conjugated linoleic acid: a powerful anticarcinogen from animal fat sources. Cancer 1994;74:1050–1054.

78. Lee KN, Kritchevsky D, Pariza MW. Conjugated linoleic acid and atherosclerosis in rabbits. Atherosclerosis 1994;108:19–25.

79. Miller CC, Park Y, Pariza MW, Cook ME. Feeding conjugated linoleic acid to animals partially overcomes catabolic response due to endotoxin injection. Biochem Biophys Res Commun 1994;198:1107–1112.

80. Park Y, Albright KJ, Liu W, et al. Effect of conjugated linoleic acid on body composition in mice. Lipids 1997;32:853–858.

81. West DB, Delany JP, Camet PM, et al. Effects of conjugated linoleic acid on body fat and energy metabolism in the mouse. Am J Physiol 1998;275:R667–R672.

82. Delany JP, Blohm F, Truett AA, et al. Conjugated linoleic acid (CLA) rapidly reduces body fat content in the mouse without affecting energy intake. Am J Physiol 1999; 276:R1172–R1179.

83. Kreider R, Ferreira M, Wilson M, Almada A. Effects of conjugated linoleic acid (CLA) supplementation during resistance training on bone mineral content, bone mineral density, and markers of immune stress [Abstract]. FASEB J 1998;12:A244.

84. Ferreira M, Kreider R, Wilson M, Almada A. Effects of CLA supplementation during resistance training on body composition and strength [Abstract]. J Strength Conditioning Res 1998;11:280.

85. Kohrt WM, Birge SJ Jr. Differential effects of estrogen treatment on bone mineral density of the spine, hip, wrist and total body in late postmenopausal women. Osteoporos Int 1995;5:150–155

86. Kohrt WM. Preliminary evidence that DEXA provides an accurate assessment of body composition. J Appl Physiol 1998;84:372–377.

87. Layne JE, Nelson ME. The effects of progressive resistance training on bone density: a review. Med Sci Sports Exerc 1999;31:25–30.

88. Lowery LM, Appicelli PA, Lemon PWR. Conjugated linoleic acid enhances muscle size and strength gains in novice bodybuilders [Abstract]. Med Sci Sports Exerc 1998;30:S182.

89. Prasad C, Peterkofsky A. Demonstration of pyroglutamyl-peptidase and amidase activities towards thyrotropin-releasing hormone in hamster hypothalamic extracts. J Biol Chem 1976;251:3229–3234.

90. Prasad C, Jayaraman A, Robertson HJ, Rao JK. Is all cyclo(His-Pro) derived from thyrotropin-releasing hormone? Neurochem Res 1987;12:767–774.

91. Yamada M, Shibusawa N, Hashida T, et al. Abundance of cyclo (His-Pro)-like immunoreactivity in the brain of TRH-deficient mice. Endocrinology 1999;140:538–541.

92. Prasad C, Kumar S, Adkinson W, McGregor JU. Hormones in foods: abundance of authentic cyclo (His-Pro)-like immunoreactivity in milk and yogurt. Nutr Res 1995;15:1623–1635.

93. Hilton CW, Prasad C, Vo P, Mouton C. Food contains the bioactive peptide, cyclo (His-Pro). J Clin Endocrinol Metab 1992;75:375–378.

94. Prasad C, Hilton CW, Svec F, et al. Could dietary proteins serve as cyclo (His-Pro) precursors? Neuropeptides 1991;19:17–21.

95. Prasad C. Bioactive cyclic dipeptides. Peptides 1995;16:151–164.

96. Kow LM, Pfaff DW. Neuropeptides TRH and cyclo (His-Pro) share neuromodulatory, but not stimulatory, action on hypothalamic neurons in vitro: implication for the regulation of feeding. Exp Brain Res 1987;67:93–99.

97. Morley JR, Levine AS, Prasad C. Histidyl-proline diketopiperazine decreases food intake in rats. Brain Res 1981;210:475–478.

98. Wilber JF, Rogers D, Iriuchijima T, Prasad C. Histidyl-proline diketopiperazine: a potent and chronic appetite-inhibiting neuropeptide. Trans Assoc Am Physicians 1986;99:245–249.

99. Kow LM, Pfaff DW. The effects of the TRH metabolite cyclo (His-Pro) and its analogs on feeding. Pharmacol Biochem Behav 1991;28:359–364.

100. Yamada M, Izumi SI, Makino T, Mori M. Lack of effect of histidyl-proline diketopiperazine on basal level and TRH-induced response of cytosolic calcium concentration in rat lactotrophs. Endocr J 1991;38:239–244.

101. Hilton CW, Reddy S, Prasad C, Wilber JF. Change in circulating cyclo (His-Pro) concentrations in rats after ingestion of oral glucose compared to intravenous glucose and controls. Endocr Res 1990;16:139–150.

102. Hilton CW, Prasad C, Wilber JF. Acute alterations of cyclo (His-Pro) levels after oral ingestion of glucose. Neuropeptides 1990;15:55–59.

103. Herminghuysen D, Cook C, Thompson H, et al. The gut-brain peptide cyclo (His-Pro) is secreted in a pulsatile fashion in fasting humans. Neuropeptides 1994;26:273–280.

104. Steiner H, Wilber JF, Prasad C, et al. Histidyl-proline diketopiperazine (cyclo [His-Pro]) in eating disorders. Neuropeptides 1989;14:185–189.

105. Peters J, Foord S, Dieguez C, et al. Lack of effect of the TRH related dipeptide histidyl-proline diketopiperazine on TSH and PRL secretion in normal subjects, in patients with microprolactinomas and in primary hypothyroidism. Clin Endocrinol 1985;23:289–293.

106. Bauer K, Graf KJ, Faivre-Bauman A, et al. Inhibition of prolactin secretion by histidyl-proline-diketopiperazine. Nature 1978;274:174–175.

107. Prasad C, Wilber JF, Akerstrom V, et al: a selective inhibitor of rat prolactin secretion in vitro. Life Sci 1980;27:1979–1983.

108. Brabant G, Wickings EJ, Nieschlag E. The TRH-metabolic histidyl-proline-diketopiperazine (DKP) inhibits prolactin secretion in male rhesus monkeys. Acta Endocrinol 1981;98:189–194.

109. Melmed S, Carlson HE, Hershman JM. Histidyl-proline diketopiperazine suppresses prolactin secretion in human pituitary tumour cell cultures. Clin Endocrinol 1982;16:97–100.

110. Lamberts SW, Visser TJ. The effects of histidyl-proline-diketopiperazine, a metabolite of TRH, on prolactin release by the rat pituitary gland in vitro. Eur J Pharmacol 1981;71:337–341.

111. Wilber JF, Mori M, Kandarakis ED, et al. Histidyl-proline diketopiperazine [cyclo(His-Pro)]: a new neuropeptide modulator of insulin and glucagon secretion. Trans Assoc Am Physicians 1984;97:88–94.

112. Cleary MP, Billheimer J, Finan A, et al. Metabolic consequences of dehydroepiandrosterone in lean and obese adult Zucker rats. Horm Metab Res 1984;16:43–46.

113. Cleary MP, Shepaherd A, Jenks B. Effect of dehydroepiandrosterone on growth in lean and obese Zucker rats. J Nutr 1984;114:1242–1251.

114. Muller S, Cleary MP. Glucose metabolism in isolated adipocytes from lean and obese Zucker rats following treatment with dehydroepiandrosterone. Metabolism 1985;24:278–284.

115. Tagliaferro AR, Davis JR, Truchon S, Van Hamont N. Effects of dehydroepiandrosterone acetate on metabolism, body weight and composition of male and female rats. J Nutr 1986;116:1977–1983.

116. Mohan PF, Cleary MP. Effect of short-term DHEA administration on liver metabolism of lean and obese rats. Am J Physiol 1988;255:E1–E8.

117. Mohan PF, Ihnen JS, Levin BE, Cleary MP. Effects of dehydroepiandrosterone treatment in rats with diet-induced obesity. J Nutr 1990;120:1103–1114.

118. Svec F, Porter J. Effect of DHEA on macronutrient selection Zucker rats. Physiol Behav 1996;59:721–727.

119. Hansen PA, Han DH, Nolte LA, et al. DHEA protects against visceral obesity and muscle insulin resistance in rats fed a high-fat diet. Am J Physiol 1997;273:R1704–R1708.

120. Han DH, Hansen PA, Chen MM, Holloszy JO. DHEA treatment reduces fat accumulation and protects against insulin resistance in male rats. J Gerontol A Biol Sci Med Sci 1998;53:B19–B24.

121. Brady LJ, Ramsay RR, Brady PS. Regulation of carnitine acyltransferase synthesis in lean and obese rats by dehydroepiandrosterone and clofibrate. J Nutr 1999;121:525–531.

122. Porter JR, Abadie JM, Wright BE, et al. The effect of discontinuing dehydroepiandrosterone supplementation on Zucker rat food intake and hypothalamic neurotransmitters. Int J Obes Relat Metab Disord 1995;19:480–488.

123. Abadie JM, Wright B, Correa G, et al. Effect of dehydroepiandrosterone on neurotransmitter levels and appetite regulation of the obese Zucker rat. The obesity research program. Diabetes 1993; 42:662–669.

124. Wright BE, Svec F, Porter JR. Central effects of dehydroepiandrosterone in Zucker rats. Int J Obes Relat Metab Disord 1995;19: 887–892.

125. Coleman DL. Antiobesity effects of eitocholanolones in diabetes (db), viable yellow (Avy), and normal mice. Endocrinology 1985; 117:2279–2283.

126. Williams DP, Boyden TW, Pamenter RW, et al. Relationship of body fat percentage and fat distribution with dehydroepiandrosterone sulfate in premenopausal females. J Clin Endocrinol Metab 1993; 77:80–85.

127. Mantzoros CS, Georgiadis EI, Evangelopoulou K, et al. Dehydroepiandrosterone sulfate and testosterone are independently associated with body fat distribution in premenopausal women. Epidemiology 1996;7:513–516.

128. Ebeling P, Koivisto VA. Physiological importance of dehydroepiandrosterone. Lancet 1994;343:1479–1481.

129. Nestler JE, Barlascini CO, Clore JN, Blackard WG. Dehydroepiandrosterone reduces serum low density lipoprotein levels and body fat but does not alter insulin sensitivity in normal men. J Clin Endocrinol Metab 1988;66:57–61.

130. Welle S, Jozefowicz R, Statt M. Failure of dehydroepiandrosterone to influence energy and protein metabolism in humans. J Clin Endocrinol Metab 1990;71:1259–1264.

131. Morales AJ, Nolan JJ, Nelson JC, Yen SSC. Effects of replacement dose of dehydroepiandrosterone in men and women of advancing age. J Clin Endocrinol Metab 1994;78:1360–1367.

132. Morales AJ, Jaubrich RH, Hwang JY, et al. The effect of six months treatment with a 100 mg daily dose of dehydroepiandrosterone (DHEA) on circulating sex steroids, body composition and muscle strength in age-advanced men and women. Clin Endrocrinol 1998; 49:421–432.

133. Vogiatzi MG, Boeck MA, Vlachopapadopoulou E, et al. Dehydroepiandrosterone in morbidly obese adolescents: effects on weight, body composition, lipids and insulin resistance. Metabolism 1996;45:1011–1015.

134. Mortola JF, Yen SCC. The effects of oral dehyroepiandrosterone on endocrine-metabolic parameters in postmenopausal women. J Clin Endocrinol Metab 1990;71:696–704.

135. Yen SCC, Morales AJ, Khorram O. Replacement of DHEA in aging men and women: potential remedial effects. Ann NY Acad Sci 1995;774:128–142.

136. Tchernof A, Calles-Escandon J, Sites CK, Poehlman ET. Menopause, central body fatness, and insulin resistance: effects of hormone-replacement therapy. Coron Artery Dis 1998;9: 503–511.

137. Despres JP. Abdominal obesity as important component of insulin-resistance syndrome. Nutrition 1993;9:452–459.

138. Astrup A, Breum L, Toubro S, et al. The effect of safety of an ephedrine/caffeine compound compared to ephedrine, caffeine and placebo in obese subjects on an energy restricted diet: a double blind trial. Int J Obes 1992;16:269–277.

139. Tulp OL, Buck CL. Caffeine and ephedrine stimulated thermogenesis in LA-corpulent rats. Comp Biochem Physiol C 1986;85: 17–19.

140. Dulloo AG, Miller DS. The thermogenic properties of ephedrine/methylxanthine mixtures: animal studies. Am J Clin Nutr 1986; 43:388–394.

141. Dulloo AG, Miller DS. Reversal of obesity in the genetically obese fa/fa Zucker rat with an ephedrine/methylxanthines thermogenic mixture. J Nutr 1987;117:383–389.

142. Astrup A, Buemann B, Christensen NJ, et al. The effect of ephedrine/caffeine mixture on energy expenditure and body composition in obese women. Metabolism 1992;41:686–688.

143. Daly PA, Krieger DR, Dulloo AG, et al. Ephedrine, caffeine and aspirin: safety and efficacy for treatment of human obesity. Int J Obes 1993;17:S73–S78.

144. Guy-Grand B, Apfelbaum M, Crepaldi G, et al. International trial of long-term dexfenfluramine in obesity. Lancet 1989;2: 1142–1145.

145. Breum L, Pedersen JK, Ahlstrom F, Frimodt-Moller J. Comparison of an ephedrine/caffeine combination and dexfenfluramine in the treatment of obesity: a double-blind multicentre trial in general practice. Int J Obes 1994;18:99–103.

146. Okada S, York DA, Bray GA, Erlanson-Albertsson C. Enterostatin (Val-Pro-Asp-Pro-Arg) the activation peptide of procolipase selectively reduces fat intake. Physiol Behav 1991;49:1185–1189.

147. Sorhede M, Mei J, Erlanson-Albertsson C. Enterostatin—a gut-brain peptide-regulating fat intake in rat. J Physiol Paris 1993;87: 273–275.

148. Lin L, Okada S, York DA, Bray GA. Structural requirements for the biological activity of enterostatin. Peptides 1994;15:849–854.

149. Mei J, Erlanson-Albertsson C. Role of intraduodenally administered enterostatin in rats: inhibition of food. Obes Res 1996; 4:161–165.

150. Erlanson-Albertsson C, Mei J, Okada S, et al. Pancreatic procolipase propeptide, enterostatin, specifically inhibits fat intake. Phsyiol Behav 1991;49:1191–1194.

151. Okada S, York DA, Bray GA, et al. Differential inhibition of fat intake in two strains of rat by the peptide enterostatin. Am J Physiol 1992;262:R1111–R1116.

152. Okada S, Lin L, York DA, Bray GA. Chronic effects of intracerebral ventricular enterostatin in Osborne-Mendel Rats fed a high fat diet. Physiol Behav 1993;54:325–329.

153. Okada S, Onai T, Kilroy G, et al. Adrenalectomy of the obese Zucker rat: effects on the feeding response to enterostatin and specific mRNA levels. Am J Physiol 1993;265:R21–R27.

154. Lin L, York DA. Comparisons of the effects of enterostatin on food intake and gastric emptying in rats. Brain Res 1997;745:205–209.

155. Deutseh JA, Gonzalez MF, Young WG. Two factors control meal size. Brain Res Bull 1997;5:55–57.

156. Erlanson-Albertsson C, York D. Enterostatin—a peptide regulating fat intake. Obes Res 1997;5:360–372.

157. Ookuma K, Barton C, York DA, Bray GA. Effect of enterostatin and kappa-opiods on macronutrient selection and consumption. Peptides 1997;18:785–791.

158. Lin L, McClanahan S, York DA, Bray GA. The peptide enterostatin may produce early satiety. Physiol Behav 1993; 53:789–794.

159. Mei J, Cheng Y, Erlanson-Albertsson C. Enterostatin—its ability to inhibit insulin secretion and to decrease high-fat food intake. Int J Obes Relat Metab Disord 1993;17:701–714.

160. Mei J, Erlanson-Albertsson C. Effect of enterostatin given intravenously and intracerebroventricularly on high-fat feeding in rats. Regul Pept 1992; 41:209–218.

161. Corwin RL, Rice HB. Effects of enterostatin in non-food-deprived rats with limited or continuous access to oil or sucrose. Physiol Behav 1998;65:1–10.

162. Lin L, York DA. Chronic ingestion of dietary fat is a prerequisite for inhibition of feeding by enterostatin. Am J Physiol 1998;275: R619–R623.

163. Bowyer RC, Rowston WM, Jehanli AM, et al. Effect of a satiating meal on the concentrations of procolipase propeptide in the serum and urine of normal and morbidly obese subjects. Gut 1993;34: 1520–1525.

164. Rossner S, Barkeling B, Erlanson-Albertsson C, et al. Intravenous enterostatin does not affect single meal food intake in man. Appetite 1995;24:37–42.

165. Erlanson-Albertsson C, Larsson A. A possible physiological function of pancreatic pro-colipase activation peptide in appetite regulation. Biochimie 1988;70:1245–1250.

166. Shargill NS, Tsujii S, Bray GA, Erlanson-Albertsson C. Enterostatin suppresses food intake following injection into the third ventricle of rats. Brain Res 1991;544:137–140.

167. Wilson JH, Lamberts SW. The effect of obesity and drastic caloric restriction on serum prolactin and thyroid stimulating hormone. Int J Obes 1981;5:275–278.

168. van der Heyden JT, Docter R, van Toor H, et al. Effects of caloric deprivation on thyroid hormone tissue uptake and generation of low-T3 syndrome. Am J Physiol 1986;251:E156–163.

169. Visser TJ, Lamberts SW, Wilson JH, et al. Serum thyroid hormone concentrations during prolonged reduction of dietary intake. Metabolism 1978;27:405–409.

170. Katzeff HL, Selgrad C. Maintenance of thyroid hormone production during exercise-induced weight loss. Am J Physiol 1991;261: E382–E388.

171. Singh V, Kaul S, Chander R, Kapoor NK. Stimulation of low density lipoprotein receptor activity in liver membrane of guggulsterone treated rats. Pharmacol Res 1990;22:37–44.

172. Singh RB, Niaz MA, Ghosh S. Hypolipidemic and antioxidant effects of Commiphora mukul as an adjunct to dietary therapy in patients with hypercholesterolemia. Cardiovasc Drugs Ther 1994; 8:659–664.

173. Agarwal RC, Singh SP, Saran RK, et al. Clinical trial of gugulipid— a new hypolipidemic agent of plant origin in primary hyperlipidemia. Indian J Med Res 1986;84:626–634.

174. Gopal K, Saran RK, Nityanand S, et al. Clinical trial of ethyl acetate extract of gum gugulu (gugulipid) in primary hyperlipidemia. J Assoc Physician India 1986;34:249–251.

175. Beg M, Singhal KC, Afzaal S. A study of effect of guggulsterone on hyperlipidemia of secondary glomerulopathy. Indian J Physiol Pharmacol 1996;40:237–240.

176. Tripathi YB, Tripathi P, Malhotra OP, Tripathi SN. Thyroid stimulatory action of (Z)-guggulsterone: mechanism of action. Planta Med 1988;54:271–277.

177. Dalvi SS, Nayak VK, Pohujani SM, et al. Effect of gugulipid on bioavailability of diltiazem and propranolol. J Assoc Physicians India 1994;42:454–455.

178. Watson JA, Fang M, Lowenstein JM. Tricarballylate and hydroxycitrate: substrate and inhibitor of ATP:citrate oxaloacetate lyase. Arch Biochem Biophys 1969;135:209–217.

179. Watson JA, Lowenstein JM. Citrate and the conversion of carbohydrate into fat. J Biol Chem 1970;245:5993–6002.

180. Rao RN, Sakariah KK. Lipid lowering and antiobesity effect of (-)hydroxycitric acid. Nutr Res 1988;8:209–212.

181. Lowenstein JM. Effect of (-)-Hydroxycitrate on fatty acid synthesis by rat liver in vivo. J Biol Chem 1971;246:629–632.

182. Sullivan AC, Triscari J, Hamilton JG, Miller ON. Effect of (-)hydroxycitrate upon the accumulation of lipid in the rat: II. Appetite. Lipids 1973;9:129–134.

183. Sullivan AC, Triscari J, Hamilton JG, Miller ON. Effect of (-)hydroxycitrate upon the accumulation of lipid in the rat: I. Lipogenesis. Lipids 1973;9:121–128.

184. Sullivan AC, Hamilton JG, Miller ON, Wheatley VR. Inhibition of lipogenesis in rat liver by (-)-hydroxycitrate. Arch Biochem Biophys 1972;150:183–190.

185. Heymsfield SB, Allison DB, Vasselli JR, et al. Garcinia cambogia (hydroxycitric acid) as a potential antiobesity agent. JAMA 1998; 280:1596–1600.

186. Cheng W, Phillips B, Abumrad N. Beta-hydroxy-beta-methylbutyrate increases fatty acid oxidation by muscle cells [Abstract]. FASEB J 1997;11:A381.

187. Cheng W, Phillips B, Abumrad N. Effect of HMB on fuel utilization, membrane stability and creatine kinase content of cultured muscle cells [Abstract]. FASEB J 1998;12:A950.

188. Nissen S, Sharp R, Ray M, et al. Effect of leucine metabolite β-hydroxy-β-methylbutyrate on muscle metabolism during resistance-exercise training. J Appl Physiol 1996;81:2095–2104.

189. Nissen S, Abumrad NN. Nutritional role of the leucine metabolite β-hydroxy-β-methylbutyrate (HMB). Nutr Biochem 1997;8:300–311.

190. Bach AC, Babayan VK. Medium-chain triglycerides: an update. Am J Clin Nutr 1982;36:950–962.

191. Scheig R. Hepatic metabolism of medium chain fatty acids. In: Senior JR, ed. Medium chain triglycerides. Philadelphia: University of Pennsylvania Press, 1968:39–49.

192. Allee GL, Romsos DR, Leveille GA, Baker DH. Metabolic consequences of dietary medium chain triglycerides in the pig. Proc Soc Exp Biol Med 1972;139:422–427.

193. Lavau MM, Hashim SA. Effect of medium chain triglyceride on lipogenesis and body fat in the rat. J Nutr 1978;108:613–620.

194. Wiley JH, Leveille GA. Metabolic consequences of dietary medium-chain triglycerides in the rat. J Nutr 1973;103:829–835.

195. Bray GA, Lee M, Bray TL. Weight gain of rats fed medium chain triglycerides is less than rats fed long-chain triglycerides. Int J Obes 1980;4:27–32.

196. Lau HC, Flaim E, Ritchey SJ. Body weight and depot fat changes as influenced by exercise and dietary fat sources in adult BHE rats. J Nutr 1979;109:495–500.

197. Bach A, Schirardin H, Chanussot F, et al. Effects of medium and long-chain triglyceride diets in the genetically obese Zucker rat. J Nutr 1980;110:686–696.

198. Travis D, Minenna A, Frier H. Effects of medium chain triglyceride on energy metabolism and body composition in the rat. Fed Proc 1979;38:561.

199. Kaunitz H, Slanetz CA, Johnson RE, et al. Relation of saturate, medium- and long-chain triglycerides to growth, appetite, thirst and weight maintenance requirements. J Nutr 1958;64:513–524.

200. Van Wymelbeke V, Himaya A, Louis-Sylvestre J, Fantino M. Influence of medium-chain and long-chain triacylglycerols on the control of food intake in men. Am J Clin Nutr 1998;68:226–234.

201. Rath F, Skala, I, Nathova E. Metabolic aspects of the use of medium chain triglycerides in the treatment of obesity. Z Ernahrungswiss 1972;13:116–124.

202. Jaedig S, Henningsen NC. Increased metabolic rate in obese women after ingestion of potassium, magnesium- and phosphate-enriched orange juice or injection of ephedrine. Int J Obes 191;15: 429–436.

203. Jaedig S, Lindgarde F, Arborelius M. Increased postprandial energy expenditure in obese women after peroral K- and Mg-phosphate. Miner Electrolyte Metab 1994;20:147–152.

204. Kaciuba-Uscilko H. Nazar, K. Chwalbinska-Moneta, J, et al. Effect of phosphate supplementation on metabolic and neuroendocrine responses to exercise and oral glucose load in obese women during weight reduction. J Physiol Pharmacol 1993;44:425–440.

205. Nazar K, Kaciuba-Uscilko H, Szczepanik J, et al. Phosphate supplementation prevents a decrease of triiodothyronine and increases resting metabolic rate during low energy diet. J Physiol Pharmacol 1996;47:373–383.

206. Stanko RT, Mendelow H, Shinozuka H, et al. Prevention of alcohol-induced fatty liver by natural metabolites and riboflavin. J Lab Clin Med 1978;91:228–235.

207. Stanko RT, King D, Adibi SA. Inhibition of lipid synthesis and stimulation of energy expenditure by addition of pyruvate, dihydroxyacetone and riboflavin to the diet [Abstract]. Clin Res 1983;31: 526A.

208. Stanko RT, Adibi SA. Inhibition of lipid accumulation and enhancement of energy expenditure by the addition of pyruvate and dihydroxyacetone to a rat diet. Metabolism 1986;35:182–186.

209. Cortez MY, Torgan CE, Brozinick Jr JT, et al. Effects of pyruvate and dihydroxyacetone consumption on the growth and metabolic state of obese Zucker rats. Am J Clin Nutr 1991;53:847–853.

210. Ivy JL, Cortez MY, Chandler RM, et al. Effects of pyruvate on the metabolism and insulin resistance of obese Zucker rats. Am J Clin Nutr 1994;59:331–337.

211. Stanko RT, Tietze DL, Arch JE. Body composition, energy utilization, and nitrogen metabolism with a severely restricted diet supplemented with dihydroxyacetone and pyruvate. Am J Clin Nutr 1992;55:771–776.

212. Stanko RT, Arch JE. Inhibition of regain in body weight and fat with addition of 3-carbon compounds to the diet with hyperenergetic refeeding after weight reduction. Int J Obes Relat Metab Disord 1996;20:925–930.

213. Stanko RT, Reynolds HR, Hoyson R, et al. Pyruvate supplementation of a low-cholesterol, low-fat diet: effects of plasma lipid concentrations and body composition in hyperlipidemic patients. Am J Clin Nutr 1994;59:423–427.

214. Kalman D, Colker CM, Stark R, et al. Effect of pyruvate supplementation on body composition and mood. Curr Ther Res 1998; 59:793–802.

215. Stanko RT, Tietze DL, Arch JE. Body composition, energy utilization, and nitrogen metabolism with a 4.25 MJ/d low-energy diet supplemented with pyruvate. Am J Clin Nutr 1992;56:630–635.

216. Berlan M, Le Verge R, Galitzky J, Le Corre P. Alpha 2-adrenoceptor antagonist potencies of two hydroxylated metabolites of yohimbine. Br J Pharmacol 1993;108:927–932.

217. Valet P, Taouis M, Tran MA, et al. Lipomobilizing effects of procatrol and yohimbine in the conscious dog: comparison of endocrinological, metabolic and cardiovascular effects. Br J Pharmacol 1989;97:229–239.

218. Berlan M, Galitzky J, Tran MA, Montastruc P. Anorectic effect of alpha 2-antagonists in dog: effect of acute and chronic treatment. Pharmacol Biochem Behav 1991;39:313–320.

219. Berlan M, Lafontan M. Evidence that epinephrine acts preferentially as an antilipolytic agent in abdominal human subcutaneous fat cells: assessment by analysis of beta and alpha 2 adrenoceptor properties. Eur J Clin Invest 1985;15:341–348.

220. Richelsen B, Pedersen SB, Moler-Pedersen T, Bak JF. Regional differences in triglyceride breakdown in human adipose tissue: effects of catecholamines, insulin, and prostaglandin E2. Metabolism 1991;40:990–996.

221. Galitzky J, Taouis M, Berlan M, et al. Alpha 2-antagonist compounds and lipid mobilization: evidence for a lipid mobilizing effect of oral yohimbine in healthy male volunteers. Eur J Clin Invest 1988;18:587–594.

222. Lafontan M, Berlan M, Galitzky J, Montastruc JL. Alpha-2 adrenoceptors in lipolysis: alpha 2 antagonists and lipid-mobilizing strategies. Am J Clin Nutr 1992;55:219S–227S.

223. Kucio C, Jonderko K, Piskorska D. Does Yohimbine act as a slimming drug? Isr J Med Sci 1991;27:550–556.

224. Berlan M, Galitzky J, Riviere D, et al. Plasma catecholamine levels and lipid mobilization induced by yohimbine in obese and nonobese women. Int J Obes 1991;15:305–315.

225. Mattila M, Seppala T, Mattila MJ. Anziogenic effect of yohimbine in healthy subjects: comparison with caffeine and antagonism by clonidine and diazepam. Int Clin Psychopharmacol 1988;3: 215–229.

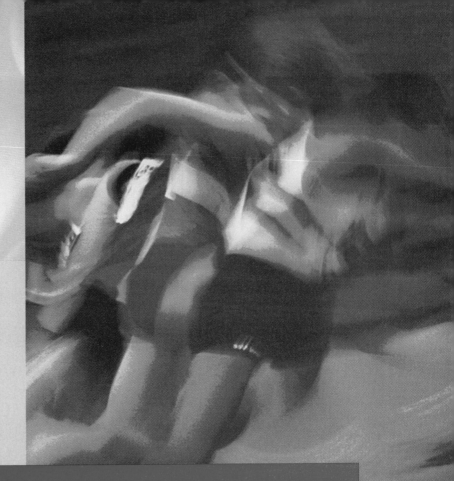

CHAPTER

5

The Anticatabolics

Thomas Incledon and Jose Antonio

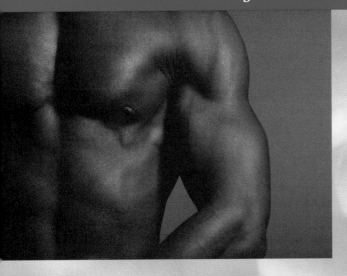

Research Review

Glutamine Promotes Muscle Glycogen Storage

In this study, seven male subjects of average physical fitness took part in three different trials. First, subjects performed bicycle exercise designed to deplete their fast and slow-twitch fibers of muscle glycogen. Then they received either a) an 18.5% solution of glucose polymer, b) 8 g of glutamine, or c) an 18.5% solution of glucose polymer plus 8 g of glutamine. During the three trials, they also received a continuous infusion of glucose for 2 hours. Plasma glutamine concentration increased dramatically after the ingestion of glutamine alone or with the glucose polymer. Glutamine concentrations were approximately 70% higher than baseline 30–45 minutes after glutamine ingestion. Moreover, glutamine ingestion had no effect on insulin levels. As expected glucose polymer ingestion (with or without glutamine) produced a substantive rise in insulin that lasted 30–90 minutes. Glutamine was as effective as the glucose polymer solution in increasing muscle glycogen after the glycogen-depleting exercise bout (see FIGURE).

According to the investigators, "Oral glutamine alone promoted storage of muscle glycogen to an extent

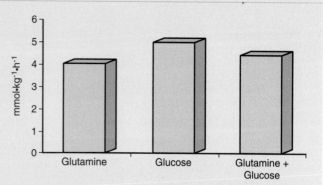

Research Review Figure. Average rate of muscle glycogen storage during 2 hours of recovery (no difference between groups. Effect of glutamine on the net rate of skeletal muscle glycogen storage. Note that during 2 hours of recovery, the amino acid glutamine is just as effective as glucose with regard to the rate of glycogen resynthesis. (Data from Bowtell et al., 1999.)

similar to oral glucose polymer. Ingestion of glutamine and glucose polymer together promoted the storage of carbohydrate outside of skeletal muscle, the most feasible site being the liver."

Bowtell JL, et al. Effect of oral glutamine on whole body carbohydrate storage during recovery from exhaustive exercise. J Appl Physiol 1999;86:1770–1777.

Introduction

An adequate supply of macronutrients and micronutrients are required for survival, growth, and development, and for the maintenance of health and well-being throughout life. Regarding skeletal muscle growth, the accretion of protein (primarily contractile) represents one of the primary goals that a select group of athletes (e.g., bodybuilders, powerlifters, Olympic-style weightlifters) aspire towards. Rates of protein accretion (and loss) are a function of the balance between protein synthesis and degradation. An increase in skeletal muscle mass can occur via an increase in synthesis, a decrease in degradation, or a combination of the two. Note that each process is mechanistically distinct. That is, one can occur in the absence of changes in the other.[1,2]

Nutritional status and the hormonal milieu present in the body have a profound impact on how protein is used (i.e., oxidized, used to make additional contractile or noncontractile protein, etc.). Various supplements have been touted as "muscle-builders" based on the notion that they impact protein metabolism, specifically, via an inhibition of protein degradation. Some of these supplements, it is clear, do in fact ameliorate the decline in protein synthesis seen under certain stressful states; however, protein synthesis may also be affected when these supplements are consumed.

A couple factors must be taken into account regarding the degradation of cellular protein.[3] The half-lives of different proteins vary tremendously between and within cells. Also, proteins do not exist within solution intracellularly but are part of distinct structures (e.g., contractile protein, cytoskeleton, etc.) within the cell. If the integrity of each cell is to be maintained, the degradation of various proteins within a cell must be regulated smoothly. Regarding skeletal muscle, there is evidence that myofibrillar and nonmyofibrillar protein are independently regulated.[4] Thus, when examining the existing data on how various dietary supplements affect protein synthesis and degradation, one must remain cognizant of the fact that whole-body protein synthesis and degradation may (or may not) reflect changes in skeletal muscle protein synthesis and degradation.

The supplements that this chapter will cover are those that have been touted as *anticatabolic*. It would seem plausible that a decrease in protein degradation with no change in protein synthesis should result in the accumulation of extra protein. This of course would be particularly important for athletes involved in the strength-power sports (i.e., bodybuilding, powerlifting, Olympic-style weightlifting, shot put, discus, etc.).

Glutamine

Perhaps the most popular of the *anticatabolic* supplements, glutamine is the amide of the amino acid glutamate. Glutamine is synthesized from glutamate by the action of glutamine synthetase.[5] Glutamate is formed from alpha-ketoglutarate, an intermediate of the Krebs cycle, and ammonia.

Glutamine is the most abundant amino acid in plasma and skeletal muscle[6] and accounts for greater than 60% of the total intramuscular free amino acid pool.[7] Furthermore, skeletal muscle is quantitatively the most important site of glutamine synthesis even though glutamine synthetase activity is relatively low per unit mass in skeletal muscle.[8] Adipose tissue may also represent a site of glutamine synthesis similar in magnitude to skeletal muscle.[9] In addition, the lungs, liver, and brain are other sites of glutamine synthesis.

Glutamine is one of the major fuels of the gut, particularly during fasting. In fact, the GI tract accounts for approximately 40% of the total glutamine that is used by the body.[10] Glutamine metabolism in the GI tract is similar whether one has fasted or has recently consumed a meal.

The use of glutamine (and other amino acids) by the GI tract is partly due to high turnover of intestinal mucosal cells and the need for continual provision of amino acids to sustain high protein synthetic rates. The health of these cells is critical not only for normal uptake of nutrients, but also because these cells serve as a barrier or protection against invading bacteria from the lumen of the gut. Thus, cells of the GI tract may be preferentially supplied amino acids for oxidation and protein synthesis at the expense of skeletal muscle protein. We speculate that by providing extra exogenous glutamine (via dietary supplementation), you can *spare* intramuscular glutamine while feeding the GI tract. Thus, you would avoid muscle proteolysis secondary to lower concentrations of glutamine.

Besides the small intestine (i.e., enterocytes), cells of the immune system (i.e., neutrophils, thymocytes, lymphocytes, and macrophages) and hair follicles use glutamine as fuel.[7,8,11] Glutamine is used for glucose and urea synthesis in the liver, whereas the brain uses glutamine as a precursor for neurotransmitter substances.[8] In the normal fed state, and to an even greater extent during fasting and metabolic acidosis, glutamine is used as fuel by the kidneys (i.e., kidneys use glutamine to support renal ammoniagenesis).[12,13] During metabolic acidosis, glutamine is converted to α-ketoglutarate, thus generating ammonium ions (NH_4^+). The excretion of ammonium ions helps buffer the acidotic condition.

Evidence indicates that glutamine is important for the maintenance of skeletal muscle protein levels. The reclassification of glutamine as a *conditionally essential* amino acid[6,14] is based on the notion that under certain stressful conditions, the body's need for glutamine exceeds its ability to synthesize glutamine endogenously. But with the provision of exogenous glutamine, the loss of skeletal muscle protein during stressful states may be alleviated.

Because skeletal muscle accounts for most of the protein pool in the body, the regulation of protein metabolism in skeletal muscle is important for whole-body protein homeostasis. Skeletal muscle and adipose tissue represent the most important source of glutamine.[9] However, skeletal muscle accounts for a much larger fraction of the body's total mass and is therefore more important than adipose tissue as a source of glutamine. According to Wagenmakers,[15] the liver can oxidize most of the 20 amino acids, whereas skeletal muscle can oxidize 6 amino acids (i.e., the branched-chain amino acids, aspartate, asparagine, and glutamate). This is important for the oxidation of these amino acids and for the conversion of these amino acids into glutamine and alanine.

Animal Studies

The effect of glutamine on protein synthesis and degradation in cultured rat skeletal muscle myotubes (developing skeletal muscle cell) under normal and heat-stressed conditions was assessed by Zhou and Thompson.[16] They found that glutamine augments protein synthesis in myotubes that are under heat-stressed conditions; however, there was no effect on myotubes under normal conditions. A similar study from the University of Alberta found a positive relationship between intracellular concentrations of glutamine and the rate of muscle protein synthesis in isolated chick extensor digitorum communis muscle.[17] That is, the greater the glutamine concentration, the greater the anabolic effect on these skeletal muscles.

The regulation of cellular volume is intimately associated with protein synthesis and degradation. An increase in cellular volume or hydration status acts as an anabolic signal, whereas a decrease in cellular volume promotes catabolic processes.[18,19] Evidence suggests that glutamine may exert an anticatabolic effect by mediating increases in cellular volume.[20] Using an isolated rat skeletal muscle preparation, changes in the osmolarity of the surrounding medium affected the rates of glutamine and alanine release from skeletal muscle.[21]

MacLennan[22] found that increasing the concentration of glutamine significantly increased intracellular glutamine and protein synthesis in the absence of insulin in perfused rat skeletal muscle. Further, glutamine has an anticatabolic effect on the noncontractile protein constituent of rat skeletal muscle.[23]

The depletion of intramuscular glutamine is associated with increased muscle catabolism. Thus, it is important that these stores are maintained to prevent the loss of muscle protein. The infusion of the dipeptide, alanyl-glutamine, can lessen muscle atrophy and glutamine synthetase production in rats given hydrocortisone 21-acetate (a type of glucocorticoid, a catabolic steroid with respect to skeletal muscle).[24] The mechanisms by which glutamine decreases glucocorticoid-induced muscle atrophy are not associated with changes in plasma levels of insulin-like growth factor 1 (IGF-1) or insulin-like growth factor binding proteins.[25] Although at the molecular level, glutamine prevents the down-regulation of myosin-heavy chain synthesis that is seen in glucocorticoid-induced muscle atrophy.[26]

In dogs that had undergone a laparotomy (an abdominal operation), the effects of a saline or an amino acid solution (with or without glutamine) on skeletal muscle nitrogen was determined before and 24 hours after surgery.[27] Skeletal muscle nitrogen declined in the placebo-treated animals as well as those that received only 2 g/kg of an amino acid solution (with or without glutamine). However, both intracellular nitrogen and glutamine were maintained in animals that received 4 g/kg of solution regardless of whether glutamine was present. In this case, providing sufficient amino acid nutrition may preserve intramuscular glutamine levels and may be needed for preservation of muscle protein. Roth et al.[28] found that the infusion of the dipeptide alanylglutamine reduced nitrogen release from the hindlimb of anesthetized postoperative dogs.

In septic rats, the rate of glutamine production in skeletal muscle is markedly elevated,[29] although increasing the intramuscular concentrations of glutamine in septic rats did not alter muscle protein synthesis.[30,31] On the other hand, the infusion of an alanyl-glutamine dipeptide increased protein synthesis in liver and skeletal muscle of rats that were infected with *Escherichia coli*.[32]

The effects of L-glutamine provision (20 g/kg) and swim training (3 hrs/day) on tumor growth in rats was examined by Shewchuk et al.[33,34] After 14 days of glutamine treatment, the average tumor weight of the glutamine-treated rats was less than in the untreated group. Exercise had no effect on tumor growth whether the animal received glutamine or not.[33,34] However, Austgen et al.[35] found that the provision of 20% of total parenteral nutrition (TPN) protein as glutamine had no effect on tumor growth in rats implanted with methylcholanthrene-induced fibrosarcoma.

Human Studies

Several clinical studies in humans have, for the most part, confirmed the effectiveness of glutamine in the prevention or lessening of muscle mass or protein during times of stress or illness. In a human study comparing the effects of glutamine versus glycine, investigators found that the enteral (direct feeding into the intestine) infusion of glutamine increased protein synthesis.[36] Conversely, an isonitrogenous amount of the amino acid glycine did not affect protein synthesis but did slightly decrease proteolysis. Thus, the mere provision of amino acid nitrogen does not produce the anticatabolic effects seen with glutamine.

Hammarqvist et al.[37] examined the role of glutamine as part of TPN in patients who had undergone elective abdominal surgery. TPN provides the caloric needs of patients via a catheter into the neck vein (subclavian vein). Patients received a conventional amino acid solution with or without glutamine. The glutamine group received 0.285 g/kg body weight per day. This is about 21 g of glutamine for a 75-kg individual. They found that the addition of glutamine to TPN improved nitrogen balance and lessened the decrease in protein synthesis. In patients who had undergone surgical removal of the gallbladder, the addition of an alanyl-glutamine dipeptide improved nitrogen balance and prevented a decline in muscle protein synthesis.[38,39]

The use of another glutamine-containing dipeptide, glycyl-glutamine, preserved free glutamine levels in skeletal muscle after surgery, but when treatment was discontinued, skeletal muscle levels of free glutamine dropped in spite of normal enteral nutrition.[40] However, in patients who had undergone heart surgery, the administration of large doses of glutamine did not prevent endotoxemia during or after surgery.[41]

Perhaps another mechanism by which glutamine could exert anticatabolic effects is via an enhancement of plasma growth hormone concentration.[42] Nine healthy subjects consumed 2 g of glutamine dissolved in a cola drink and investigators found an increase in plasma growth hormone 90 minutes post-ingestion. Whether chronic ingestion of glutamine results in a consistent daily increase is not known.

There is a scarcity of data regarding glutamine supplementation as a mode of altering body composition (see Research Review). Rosene et al.[43] examined the effects of 14 days of high-dose (0.35 g/kg body weight per day) glutamine supplementation in wrestlers consuming a hypocaloric diet. These investigators found that the glutamine group maintained positive nitrogen balance while the placebo group was in negative nitrogen balance after the 14-day treatment.

Furthermore, glutamine may have an ergogenic effect based on its ability to elevate plasma bicarbonate concentrations.[44] Increasing blood pH may elicit improvements in exercise performance.[45] Haub et al.[46] examined the effects of acute glutamine ingestion on exercise performance. The ingestion of 0.03 g/kg of glutamine had no effect on cycle ergometer exercise at 100% of VO_{2peak}. These investigators found that the oral glutamine load given to these subjects had no effect on plasma pH or bicarbonate concentration; thus, the low doses used in this study may have been inadequate to elicit an alkalinizing effect. Without a change in pH status, it is unlikely that glutamine could improve anaerobic exercise performance.

Glucose Regulation

The role of glutamine regarding glucose regulation may be important in exercise-trained individuals. Its function in gluconeogenesis (formation of glucose) and glycogen repletion may serve as a useful function during and after exercise. Gluconeogenesis from glutamine can occur without changes in plasma insulin and glucagon levels, providing evidence that glutamine itself can regulate gluconeogenesis.[47]

Nurjhan et al.[48] compared the contribution of alanine and glutamine to glucose formation in postabsorptive (fasted) normal human volunteers and found that the amount of glucose carbon that came from protein-derived glutamine was 100% greater than from alanine. Varnier et al.[49] studied the effects of glutamine, alanine plus glycine, and saline infusion on glycogen accumulation in subjects who cycled for 90 minutes. Two hours postexercise, glutamine infusion resulted in a twofold greater concentration of muscle glycogen than either saline or alanine plus glycine infusion. In postabsorptive humans, glutamine could be more important than alanine for glucose formation derived from proteolysis. Further, glutamine carbon can be directed to glycogen accumulation in skeletal muscle that had been previously glycogen depleted.

In mice that were genetically predisposed to being overweight and hyperglycemic, the administration of glutamine in conjunction with a high-fat diet resulted in a reduction of body weight and a drop in hyperglycemia and hyperinsulinemia.[50] The mechanism(s) for a glutamine-induced weight reduction is not known, though it may be related to the ability of glutamine to lessen the insulin resistance induced by a high-fat diet. Further, the administration of glutamine to lipid-based TPN can prevent glucose intolerance and insulin resistance.[51]

Safety and Toxicity

The high doses of glutamine that are needed for exerting an anticatabolic effect cannot be met via a normal diet. Thus, the safety of such high doses has often been questioned. Anecdotal reports from bodybuilders who consume up to 40–50 g of glutamine per day without any ill effects suggest that glutamine is quite safe. Work by Ziegler et al.[52] further confirm what many bodybuilders have believed from their personal experience. In an initial short-term study, oral doses of glutamine (0, 0.1, and 0.3 g/kg; 0.3 g/kg is equal to 22.5 g for a 75-kg individual) produced an acute rise in plasma glutamine as well as in amino acids known to be end products of glutamine metabolism (i.e. alanine, citrulline, arginine). However, toxicity was not evident as indicated by the lack of change in ammonia or glutamate levels. As a component of TPN (glutamine dose of 0.285 and 0.570 g/kg body weight per day), glutamine had no harmful effects after a period of

5 days of administration in normal subjects. The safety of glutamine use was confirmed in patients receiving glutamine for several weeks.[52] Glutamine infusion as a dipeptide (glycyl-glutamine) was examined in polytrauma patients. Using doses equal to 14, 21, and 28 g of glutamine (calculated for a 70-kg individual) per day, they found no ill effects of glycyl-glutamine.[53,54]

Glutamine is absorbed efficiently in the human jejunum *in vivo* and is safe—the doses used to elicit a positive effect on nitrogen balance are large (~0.2–0.6 g/kg body weight per day).[54] This would be comparable to a 70-kg individual consuming 14 to 42 g of glutamine per day. Thus, the notion that glutamine could adversely affect the health of normal, healthy, active individuals would seem ludicrous inasmuch as high doses of glutamine are directly infused into critically ill patients. For the time being, it would seem plausible that high-dose (>5 g) supplementation of glutamine is safe for athletes.

α-Ketoglutarate

α-Ketoglutarate (α-KG) is an intermediate of the Krebs cycle and is the precursor for the synthesis of glutamine, glutamate, proline, and arginine. Few data exist on the use of α-KG as an ergogenic aid. Like glutamine, however, there are some clinical data that suggest a possible anti-catabolic role. Wernerman et al.[55] state that the "addition of alpha-ketoglutarate to postoperative total parenteral nutrition prevented the decrease in muscle protein synthesis and free glutamine that usually occurs after surgery." α-KG was infused into anesthetized postoperative dogs, resulting in a net uptake by skeletal muscle predominantly, and the kidneys, liver, and gut secondarily.[56] However, α-KG infusion did not change intramuscular glutamine or glutamate concentrations. In a study from the Karolinska Institute in Stockholm, researchers found that α-KG had similar effects as glutamine.[57] In this investigation, biopsies of skeletal muscle were taken before surgery (removal of the gall bladder) and 3 days after surgery. On each day following the operation, the control group was in negative nitrogen balance but not in the α-KG–supplemented group. Blomqvist et al.[58] compared the effects of α-KG, glutamine, and glucose on protein metabolism in postoperative patients. Healthy patients that underwent total hip replacement surgery received either 2 g/kg of glucose, 0.28 g/kg of glutamine, or 0.28 g/kg of α-KG during surgery and the first 24 hours. Protein synthesis decreased in the glucose group but not in the glutamine or α-KG groups. Intramuscular glutamine concentration did not change in the α-KG or glutamine group but decreased in the control.

Based on the little evidence that exists, α-KG may exert an anticatabolic effect similar to glutamine under conditions of stress such as postsurgery. This is hardly surprising inasmuch as α-KG can be converted to glutamine.

Safety and Toxicity

No studies have specifically examined the safety of high-dose α-KG use. However, because much of the work done on α-KG is on patients postsurgery, it would seem plausible that the use of α-KG for those who are healthy should not pose an undue health risk. Doses as high as 0.28 g/kg have been used in clinical studies (comparable to 21 g for a 75-kg individual).

Ornithine-α-ketoglutarate

Also known as OKG, this compound is formed from two molecules of the amino acid ornithine and one α-KG. OKG has been shown in a variety of studies to have an anabolic/anticatabolic effect. OKG has been used successfully via enteral or parenteral administration in conditions such as burn, postsurgery, malnutrition, and wound healing. The mechanism by which OKG exerts these effects is not known; however, the secretion of hormones such as insulin and growth hormone and the conversion to other metabolites (e.g., glutamine, arginine, etc.) might play a role.

Animal Studies

Vaubourdolle et al[59] used an animal burn model to study the effects of OKG administration during a hypercatabolic state. Rats were studied after having their dorsum in water at 90°C for 10 seconds (inducing a burn injury) and then starved for 24 hours. The supplementation of OKG (5 g/kg/day) for 2 days decreased the level of muscle mass loss and increased intramuscular glutamine concentration. An isonitrogenous amount of glycine had no effect. Similar work by Le Boucher et al.[60] found that OKG inhibits myofibrillar degradation in burn-injured rats while glycine had no such effect. In an interesting study using malnourished animals, male rats were starved for 3 days, then re-fed for 7 days with an oral diet (192 kcal/kg/day; 2.25 g/kg/day of nitrogen) supplemented with either OKG, glutamine, or casein.[61] Starvation caused a drop in most tissue-amino acids except skeletal muscle leucine (+43%) and liver glutamate (+11%). The primary effect of OKG was to normalize the amino acid concentrations in the liver and small bowel while glutamine normalized glutamine and leucine concentrations in skeletal muscle. In this case, it is apparent that OKG and glutamine act on different tissues (OKG—viscera glutamine—skeletal muscle). In rats implanted with a tumor, the administration of OKG (3.4–4.0 g/kg/day) for 5 days reduced muscle proteolysis by 33% while an isonitrogenous amount of glycine had no effect.[62]

In another animal model of trauma (bilateral femur fracture in the rat), there was no difference in body weight gain per gram of nitrogen intake after the administration of ornithine, OKG, or α-KG.[63] On the other hand, a study that compared OKG with arginine-α-ketoglutarate (AKG) suggested that the effects of OKG are not due to its α-KG content nor to its nitrogen content.[64] That is, OKG produced a greater increase than AKG in muscle glutamine concentrations in burn injured rats. A decrease in intramuscular glutamine concentration is associated with skeletal muscle catabolism; thus, the action of OKG is neither solely related to its nitrogen content, nor to the presence of α-KG.

Human Studies

OKG has similarly been shown to have positive effects in humans on protein metabolism during hypercatabolic states. Vanbourdolle et al.[65] showed that the enteral (via the intestine) administration of OKG to burn patients improved glucose tolerance. In a study that compared varying doses of OKG (10, 20, and 30 g) delivered as one large bolus or via continuous infusion, investigators found that nitrogen balance improved and urinary 3-methylhistidine was reduced (an indicator of muscle protein degradation).[66] In fact, the administration of 30 g as a bolus seemed to have the greatest benefit.

TPN supplemented with 0.35 g/kg of OKG to patients after elective abdominal surgery prevented the drop in protein synthesis seen in the unsupplemented controls.[67] OKG supplementation might exert its anticatabolic effect via the maintenance of intramuscular glutamine levels.[68] However, the mere provision of extra nitrogen does not confer similar effects. In a study that compared TPN supplemented with either OKG or branched-chain amino acids ([BCAAs] valine, leucine, isoleucine), there was less of a decrease in intramuscular glutamine levels in the OKG group.[68,69] Thus, one could argue that OKG administration is more effective than the BCAAs in reducing muscle glutamine loss and therefore ameliorating skeletal muscle proteolysis.

It is unclear if OKG exerts further anabolic/anticatabolic effects via alterations in the hormonal milieu. For instance, OKG administered to burn patients had no effect on plasma insulin or growth hormone concentration.[65] On the other hand, OKG (15 g) given to growth-retarded prepubertal children produced an increase in plasma insulin-like growth factor–1 level.[70]

Safety and Toxicity

High-dose OKG administration (up to 30 g/day) in humans has not been shown to have harmful side effects. It is not known if chronic ingestion (>6–12 months) has any deleterious effects.

Branched-Chain Amino Acids

The branched-chain amino acids (BCAAs) are comprised of valine, leucine, and isoleucine. The BCAAs have been shown to have various functions such as serving as a nitrogen source for glutamine synthesis in skeletal muscle. In addition, they are the primary amino acids that are oxidized (used as fuel) in tissues other than the liver. Keep in mind, however, that all tissues can convert amino acids into Krebs cycle intermediates and vice versa.[71] This occurs via transamination reactions (e.g., alanine ↔ pyruvate, aspartate ↔ oxaloacetate, glutamate ↔ α-ketoglutarate). An abundance of animal and human studies have examined the potential utility of BCAA supplementation in various conditions (e.g., postsurgery, burns, starvation, carbohydrate depletion, exercise, etc.).

Animal Studies

In rats that were subjected to 15% full-thickness scald burns, regular TPN (21% BCAA) or BCAA-enriched TPN (45% BCAA) was administered for 48 hours after resuscitation by saline infusion for 24 hours.[72] The solutions received by the two groups of rats were isocaloric (same number of calories) and isonitrogenous (same amount of amino acid–derived nitrogen). The BCAA-enriched TPN significantly improved liver and rectus abdominus muscle RNA and protein levels more than the conventional TPN. In rats with acute liver failure, the provision of BCAA improved whole-body protein synthesis in comparison to saline, glucose, or a standard amino acid formula.[73] Kawamura et al.[74] compared amino acid solutions containing 25%, 30%, 40%, 45%, and 50% BCAAs on protein catabolism in rats that had been made septic via ligature and puncture of the cecum. They found that a solution of 45% BCAAs was most effective at influencing nitrogen balance.

On the other hand, many studies have shown no effect from BCAA administration. In rats given TPN with either low (~20% BCAA) or high (~50% BCAA) concentrations of BCAA after surgery, they found no difference in nitrogen balance or in the rate of liver protein synthesis.[75] Seventy-one burned guinea pigs were divided into six groups: 10%, 20%, 30% calories as whey protein with the remaining three groups having equivalent whey protein (10%, 20%, 30%) plus BCAA supplementation so as to increase the percentage of BCAAs to 50% of the total amino acids.[76] Interestingly, BCAA administration worsened cumulative nitrogen balance and mortality during the 14 days of administration. In protein-starved rats, the administration of BCAAs did not improve the healing of musculo-aponeurotic wounds of the abdominal wall.[77]

Human Studies

In a large-scale study of 173 surgical patients with gastric cancer, the supplementation of TPN with BCAAs

significantly improved nitrogen balance.[78] BCAA-rich TPN improved the mortality rate in septic patients.[79] Furthermore, BCAA administration has positive effects in normal individuals. The overnight infusion of BCAAs significantly reduced skeletal muscle breakdown in normal volunteers.[80] Also, the oral ingestion of BCAAs with an equal amount of essential amino acids (threonine, methionine, and histidine) was studied in normal men.[81] Direct measure of skeletal muscle protein synthesis via tracer incorporation revealed no differences between groups. However, whole-body phenylalanine flux was reduced to a greater extent by the BCAAs, thus indicating a suppression of whole-body proteolysis.

Several studies show no effect of BCAA administration. TPN supplemented with BCAAs (44.6% BCAAs) did not affect nitrogen balance differently than standard TPN (19% BCAAs) in critically ill patients.[82] In patients that had undergone elective abdominal surgery, TPN was supplemented with either glutamine, OKG, or BCAAs. Both glutamine and OKG reduced the loss of intramuscular glutamine with the BCAAs having no such effect.[83,84] In patients that were injured or septic, BCAA supplementation had no effect on nitrogen balance.[85,86] Thus, in the clinically ill population, the effects of BCAA are equivocal.

Several studies suggest an ergogenic effect of BCAA supplementation in exercising individuals. Sixteen subjects participating in a 21-day trek at an altitude of 3255 meters (10,679 feet) were age-, sex-, and fitness-matched in a double-blind, placebo-controlled study.[87] They received a placebo or BCAAs (5.76, 2.88, 2.88 g of leucine, isoleucine, valine respectively; total = 11.5 g). During the trek, the mean daily energy intake decreased by 4% in both groups compared to sea level. The BCAA and placebo groups lost 1.7% and 2.8% body mass. Fat mass decreased in the BCAA (−11.7%) and placebo (−10.3%) groups; moreover, lean body mass improved in the BCAA group (+1.5%) with no change in the placebo group. Lower limb maximal power decreased less in the BCAA than in the placebo (−2.4% versus 7.8%). Arm muscle cross-sectional area did not change in the BCAA group; on the other hand, the placebo group experienced a 6.8% decrease. Thus, BCAA supplementation has a slight anabolic effect, an anticatabolic effect, and lessens the drop in muscular power as a result of exercising in high altitudes (FIG. 5-1).

Bigard et al.[88] examined 24 highly trained subjects that participated in six consecutive sessions of ski mountaineering (6–8 hours per session; 2500–4100 meters altitude). Half of the subjects ingested BCAAs (7.8 g leucine, 3.4 g isoleucine, 11.2 g valine; total = 22.4 g) while the other half consumed a carbohydrate placebo. Further, each subject consumed a standard prepackaged diet that was isocaloric. Body weight decreased significantly in the placebo group (−2.1%); however, the weight loss in the BCAA group was not significant (−1.2%). Body composition alterations were not different between groups. Peak

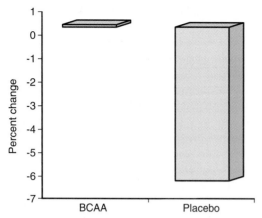

Figure 5-1. Arm muscle cross-sectional area after BCAA supplementation. Effect of BCAA supplementation during the 21-day trek at altitude. Note that BCAA supplementation had an anticatabolic effect as determined by changes in arm muscle cross-sectional area. (*Data from* Schena F, Guerrini F, Tregnaghi P, Kayser B. Branched-chain amino acid supplementation during trekking at high altitude: the effects on loss of body mass, body composition, and muscle power. Eur J Appl Physiol Occup Physiol 1992;65:394–398.)

power measured during incremental bicycle exercise decreased in the placebo but not in the BCAA group. Maximal voluntary contraction (MVC) strength (isometric) of the knee extensors was not different between groups. In this study, BCAA administration had equivocal effects (i.e., less weight loss but no differences in body composition, maintained higher peak power output on the bicycle but no differences in MVC of the knee extensors). The reasons for these discrepancies are unclear.

Thirty days of oral consumption of 14 g/day of BCAAs (50% leucine, 25% valine and isoleucine each) resulted in a slight but significant increase (+1.3%) in fat-free mass and grip strength (+8.1%) in healthy untrained male subjects.[89] It is not clear if the change in fat-free mass reflected an increase in skeletal muscle protein or other tissue protein. In a group of elite wrestlers, the effects of BCAA administration (0.9 g/kg/day) during caloric restriction was examined.[90] Twenty-five wrestlers restricted caloric intake (28 kcal/kg/day; ~2100 kcal for a 75-kg individual) for 19 days using a hypocaloric control, hypocaloric high protein, hypocaloric low protein, or a hypocaloric high BCAA diet. Using magnetic resonance imaging technology, they found the BCAA group had the greatest body weight and fat loss of the treatment groups. Of particular interest is the fact that the BCAA-supplemented group experienced the greatest abdominal visceral fat loss (−34.4%). This would suggest a reduction in cardiovascular disease risk as a result of BCAA supplementation.

The effects of BCAA administration during a 30-kilometer cross-country race and a full marathon were examined by Blomstrand and Newsholme.[91] When BCAAs (7.5–12 g) were ingested during exercise, the plasma and skeletal muscle concentration of these amino acids increased, whereas the placebo group experienced a drop in BCAA concentration in plasma with no change in skeletal muscle. Moreover, the placebo group had a 20–40% increase in the muscle concentration of tyrosine and phenylalanine and an increased plasma concentration of these amino acids. The increased concentrations of phenylalanine and tyrosine would suggest a net protein degradation during exercise inasmuch as skeletal muscle does not take up or metabolize these two amino acids. But in subjects given BCAAs, no such change in plasma phenylalanine or tyrosine was observed. Thus, BCAAs given during prolonged endurance events may have an antiproteolytic effect.

BCAAs may further reduce the protein breakdown associated with resistance-type exercises. Five men performed single-leg knee extensions for 60 minutes at 71% of maximal work capacity with or without BCAA (77 mg/kg; equal to 5.77 g of BCAA for a 75-kg individual) supplementation.[92] Intramuscular BCAA concentrations were higher for the BCAA trial and remained higher throughout the exercise bout. Furthermore, the net release of essential amino acids from skeletal muscle was higher in the control than in the BCAA group, thus suggesting an attenuation of muscle protein breakdown during exercise.

On the contrary, Blomstrand et al.[93] found that the provision of BCAA with carbohydrates was no different than carbohydrates alone with regard to decreasing proteolysis during exercise, although BCAA ingestion may have a glycogen-sparing effect.[94] In another study that investigated the effects of a 6-week endurance training program with daily BCAA (16, 2, and 2 g of leucine, isoleucine, and valine, respectively) supplementation, there were no differences (in comparison to the placebo) in the number of capillaries per fiber, muscle fiber composition, or muscle fiber cross-sectional area as a result of BCAA ingestion.[95]

Although clinical evidence is weak, data from human exercise studies suggest a potential antiproteolytic effect of BCAA ingestion. Doses ranging from 6–14 g daily may be needed to inhibit protein breakdown.

Safety and Toxicity

No toxic effects of high-dose BCAA consumption are known.

Leucine

Leucine is one of the three branched-chain amino acids, with valine and isoleucine being the other two. To maintain a positive nitrogen balance in adults is essential.

However, leucine can be synthesized from the keto acids α-ketoisovalerate, α-isopropylmalate, β-isopropylmalate, or α-ketoisocaproate (KIC). Catabolism of the amino acid results in the production of carbon dioxide along the following pathway: α-ketoisocaproate → isovaleryl-CoA, → β-methylcrotonyl-CoA, → β-methylglutoconyl-CoA, → β-hydroxy-β-methylglutaryl-CoA, → acetoacetate or acetyl-CoA. An alternative pathway for the metabolism of leucine has also been described.[96] Catabolism of leucine can take place in the liver, kidney, muscle, heart, and adipose tissue. Because of the increase in leucine catabolism that occurs in skeletal muscle during exercise, studies have linked the effects of leucine supplementation on performance. This section will review the effects of leucine supplementation on protein synthesis and protein degradation.

Animal Studies

Leucine has been shown to affect amino acid and protein metabolism.[97–100] With *in vitro* studies indicating a potential for leucine to stimulate protein synthesis via a variety of mechanisms, scientists have examined the effects of different feeding strategies on leucine metabolism, and the effects of leucine feedings on protein synthesis and nitrogen balance. After a 3-day fast in sheep, leucine arterial concentrations increased, leucine turnover in muscle decreased, hepatic use was unchanged, leucine oxidation increased, and protein synthesis decreased.[101] Fasting promoted skeletal muscle catabolism to provide precursors for hepatic protein synthesis.

As leucine in the diet is progressively increased, the rate of leucine oxidation stays low until the leucine blood concentration exceeds the amount needed for the maximal rate of weight gain.[102] Plasma concentrations of leucine in rats were low when dietary levels of leucine were low and increased with increasing dietary leucine content.[102] When leucine is administered to rats enterally, first-pass effects extract 27%.[103] Only 3% of this amount was used by the liver to synthesize new protein, while the rest was believed to represent first-pass use of leucine in intestinal protein synthesis and other metabolic pathways in the splanchnic bed. With leucine enterally administered to dogs, 31.4% was used for protein synthesis, 27.9% was deaminated, 6.0% was oxidized by the splanchnic region, and 4.8% was oxidized by the liver.[104] Leucine administered via infusion to lambs raised plasma leucine levels up to 15 times above baseline.[105] Plasma amino acid concentrations were lowered, but protein synthesis rates in skeletal muscles and the whole body did not change.[105]

The addition of glucose or sucrose can change the kinetics of leucine metabolism. Pigs fed glucose had a hindlimb uptake of leucine that was three times greater than pigs fed sucrose.[106] Preprandial protein synthesis was higher in the sucrose group whereas postprandial protein synthesis was higher in the glucose-treated group. These observations indicate that dietary carbohydrate source can influence both pre- and postprandial aspects of leucine metabolism.[106] Additional work in this area examined the effects of leucine on insulin, using the islet cells from rats with chronic renal failure.[107] In this condition there is impaired insulin secretion. Insulin secretion in response to leucine was significantly decreased in isolated islet cells.[107] Insulin release improved when the rats underwent parathyroidectomy or treatment with verapamil. Verapamil blocks the action of parathyroid hormone (PTH) on the islets. The high levels of PTH induced a secondary state of impaired leucine-induced insulin secretion.[107] The defective pathway involves abnormal leucine activation of glutamate dehydrogenase, impaired use of α-ketoglutarate, and a reduction in the maximal reaction rate of glutaminase. The interrelationships of leucine, insulin, and PTH require further study to determine if protein synthesis and insulin production are impacted.

Human Studies

The effects of leucine during fasted conditions have also been studied in humans.[108] Each subject underwent three separate 14-day fasts: 34 mM/day of leucine infused on days 1–7; 34 mM/day of α-ketoisocaproate infused on days 1–7; and a third control fast in which no infusions were given. The daily urinary urea nitrogen (UUN) excretion was similar for the control and leucine treatments, while KIC infusion significantly reduced daily urine urea nitrogen (UUN) excretion. In this study, KIC infusions decreased nitrogen wasting during starvation, whereas leucine, studied under identical conditions, did not. In another study on abdominal surgery patients, KIC and leucine were infused at 70 mmol/day.[109] KIC was found to decrease nitrogen wastage, whereas under the same conditions leucine did not.

Mendall et al.[110] administered patients with Duchenne muscular dystrophy (DMD) either a placebo or oral leucine at a dose of 0.2 g/kg/day in a randomized, double-blind, controlled trial. Although there were some transient improvements over 1 month, after 1 year, leucine failed to produce a therapeutic response. Research on the effects of leucine in cirrhotic patients indicates that it can increase oxidation without affecting protein synthesis *in vivo*.[111]

In contrast to the above studies, infusions of either leucine or leucine plus glucose were found to decrease muscle proteolysis.[112] Both leucine and glucose infusions decreased the aromatic amino acids and the basic amino acids in muscle. Glucose stimulated insulin, which decreased plasma essential amino acid concentrations. This effect was augmented by leucine. Lower amino acid levels were also found in track athletes administered 50 mg/kg/day of leucine for 10 weeks in a randomized, double-blind, placebo-controlled, crossover study.[113] Leucine concentrations had decreased significantly in the

Whey Protein Plus Glutamine and BCAAs

Whey protein plus glutamine and branched-chain amino acids augment gains in lean body mass, according to Colker et al. In this investigation, subjects consumed whey protein (40 g/day) or a combination of whey protein (40 g/day) with 5 g of glutamine and 3 g of BCAAs (leucine, valine, isoleucine). Each subject consumed 1.6 g of total protein per kg body weight per day (as per an RD's instructions). In addition, all subjects followed a body-building resistance-training regimen. After 10 weeks of treatment, the group that consumed the whey, glutamine, BCAA combination improved significantly more than the whey-only group with regard to bench press performance and body composition (see FIGURES).

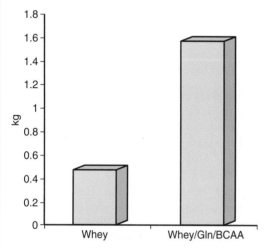

Sidebar Figure 1. Mean change in lean body mass after the consumption of a whey protein/glutamine/BCAA supplement mixture. There is approximately a 1-kg difference between the two groups. (*Data from* Colker et al. 2000.)

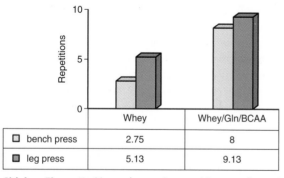

	Whey	Whey/Gln/BCAA
bench press	2.75	8
leg press	5.13	9.13

Sidebar Figure 2. Mean change in repetitions performed for the bench and leg press exercise after 10 weeks of exercise training and whey protein/glutamine/BCAA supplementation. Note the greater improvement in performance versus the whey-only group. (*Data from* Colker et al. 2000.)

Colker CM, et al. Effects of supplemental protein on body composition and muscular strength in healthy athletic male adults. Curr Ther Res 2000;61(1):19–28.

placebo group during the first 5 weeks, but not during the second 5 weeks. Leucine concentrations did not change in the treatment group. The total serum amino acid pool decreased significantly in all the subjects during the 10-week training period. Of all the amino acids, glutamine decreased the most. Net protein synthesis was not measured; therefore, it is difficult to interpret the findings. The fact that leucine and other amino acids were lower during the treatment condition may be indicative of increased protein synthesis or oxidation. Note that these subjects were ingesting 1.26 g/kg/day of protein. The effects of leucine occurred during a metabolic state in which protein intake was greater than the RDA.

Safety and Toxicity

Infusions of large amounts of leucine into rats do not cause an imbalance in plasma amino acids, even under severe catabolic conditions.[114] In addition, oral loading of a 15-month-old girl with propionic acidemia produced no ketoacidosis.[115] Infusions and oral loading of leucine appear to be well tolerated.[108,110,111,112] Toxic cases of leucine are rare in the literature and overload of leucine in young rats produced no significant changes in growth, food consumption, and hematological and immune responsiveness when the basic diet was balanced.[116] Of greater concern is lack of leucine, which can decrease nitrogen balance and decrease antitumor activity.[117]

α-Ketoisocaproate (KIC)

KIC is the branched-chain ketoacid produced from the transamination of leucine. The reaction is reversible, allowing KIC to serve as a precursor for, and a product of, leucine metabolism. The metabolism of KIC continues along the pathways previously described for leucine. KIC has been well studied *in vitro* and *in vivo*, using both animals and humans.[118–127,138] In several studies, radiolabeled KIC has been used as a marker of protein synthesis.

Animal Studies

From the *in vitro* studies previously discussed, KIC has the potential to impact protein synthesis based on its ability to serve as an acceptor or donator of amino groups with other amino acids and keto acids, and indirectly through its ability to stimulate insulin release. In animal studies the effects of KIC on protein synthesis are difficult to understand because of the various interconversions that can take place. The majority of KIC administered to dogs is converted to leucine or other keto acids.[128] However, in rats fed a leucine-deficient diet, leucine and KIC plasma concentrations did not increase in proportion to increasing dietary KIC content.[129] Additional work on rats found that KIC as a replacement for leucine had a nutritional efficiency for growth between 0.23 and 0.46.[130] After varying the dosage of KIC, no effects were found on the relative rates of use (or oxidation) of α-ketoisocaproate versus leucine. Later work found that the nutritional efficiency of KIC as a dietary substitute for leucine in individual organs, and in the whole animal, is strongly dependent on the level of protein intake.[131] The inefficiency of KIC is due to the fact that first-pass effects oxidize 9–14% when given orally.[132] In addition, KIC is 80% more susceptible to oxidation then leucine. However, in certain liver diseases, the nutritional efficiency of KIC may be increased, despite the fact that KIC use for protein synthesis may be unaffected.[133]

During fasted conditions in sheep, KIC arterial concentrations and turnover increase.[134] Skeletal muscle produces and releases KIC, which is then transported to the liver and other organs to maintain protein synthesis. Thus, hepatic and splanchnic protein synthesis is maintained at the expense of skeletal muscle during fasted conditions in sheep. Once KIC is infused, up to 12% is converted into leucine and then incorporated into protein.[135] During fed conditions, this serves to spare nitrogen and increase protein synthesis by providing additional leucine.[136] This has been demonstrated in lambs in which KIC injected intraperitonally increased weight gain and muscle growth while decreasing fat deposition.[137] KIC appears to act by slightly reducing proteolysis, resulting in a net protein deposition. However, this was not associated with an increase in muscle size or cross-sectional area. The protein deposition was most likely concentrated in the liver and splanchnic tissues.

Human Studies

In humans, KIC has been shown to spare nitrogen during fasted conditions, whereas leucine was unable to under the same conditions,[138] and affect protein metabolism.[139] The nitrogen-sparing effects were not related to changes in ketone production or insulin levels. Also, in abdominal surgery patients, infused KIC was able to spare nitrogen.[140] In contrast, however, blood ketone bodies, plasma prealbumin, and plasma retinol-binding protein concentrations at the end of the study were significantly higher after the KIC treatment. The nitrogen-sparing effects of KIC were postulated to be due to the heightened ketosis that followed its administration, the suppression of protein degradation, or an effect on liver protein turnover.[140]

In 24 patients with GI cancer, the effects of branched-chain amino acids versus ketoisocaproate on protein metabolism after surgery were compared.[141] The subjects were randomized to receive one of three nutritional treatments. All patients received a balanced amino acid solution. Group 1 (n = 8) received no further supplements, group 2 (n = 8) received 17 g day-1 α-ketoisocaproate, and group 3 (n = 8) received a branched-chain solution including leucine, isoleucine, and valine, corresponding to 3.3 g of nitrogen day-1. In all three groups, albumin and prealbumin concentrations fell after surgery. Fibronectin levels fell only in group 2 and there was also a significant increase in serum urea concentration after the operation. After 3 days there were no significant differences on cumulative nitrogen balance or protein degradation. The researchers concluded that a balanced amino acid solution with an adequate energy supply has an optimal nitrogen-sparing effect and branched-chain amino acids or α-ketoisocaproate treatments do not improve nitrogen balance or reduce protein degradation after GI cancer surgery.[141]

Safety and Toxicity

Infusion studies in humans indicate that KIC is well tolerated and no side effects have been reported. Oral studies in animals reveal that although feeding leucine may adversely affect immune function by suppressing lymphocyte activity, oral administration of KIC has a positive influence on immune function in sheep by increasing lymphocyte activity.[142,143]

In primary cultures of rat cerebral cortical astrocytes, KIC influences the metabolism of glutamate and leads to altered concentrations of other metabolites, including aspartate, lactate, and leucine.[144] As a result, energy metabolism of astrocytes may be compromised because of the diminished ability to transfer reducing equivalents. As a metabolite of KIC, several investigators have examined how HMB (hydroxy-methylbutyrate) affects various aspects of metabolism.[145–159] For a more detailed examination of HMB, the reader is referred to Chapter 3.

Whey Protein

Whey is the fluid portion of milk that is obtained by coagulating and removing the curd (casein) during cheese production.[160] After its separation from milk, whey contains almost all of the vitamins and minerals, 50% of the milk solids, and 20–24% of the milk proteins. The main protein fractions of whey are α-lactalbumin and β-lactalbumin, which comprise between 70–80% of whey.[161] Additional protein fractions include glycomacropeptides, bovine serum albumin, lactoferrin, immunoglobulins, phospholipoproteins, and other bioactive factors and enzymes.[161] Although the nutritional value of this protein was recognized and applied to animal nutrition, its application to human nutrition was delayed. Initially, the major limitation was because whey was available only in a heat-denatured form.[162] Morr et al.[163] reviewed a variety of techniques that were developed to produce undenatured whey in commercial quantities. The results after generations of developing whey separation techniques include a whey protein concentrate (WPC) with a high protein concentration and low levels of minerals, fat, and lactose.

In most protein foods the limiting amino acid is either lysine or methionine plus cystine. Whey proteins are unique in that they contain high levels of essential amino acids (EAAs), which include lysine, methionine, cystine, and the branched-chain amino acids (leucine, isoleucine, and valine). The excellent amino acid profile led to the application of whey protein to medical disorders. WPCs were exposed to different types of hydrolysis (enzymatic and pH) to create whey protein hydrolysates (WPH). The use of acid and alkali media to hydrolyze whey can cause denaturation of essential amino acids, so enzymatic hydrolysis became the method of choice. However, this method can result in incomplete hydrolysis and bitter-tasting hydrolysates. The use of different enzymatic methods (i.e., papain) can result in hydrolysates that are far less bitter tasting. The final products are high quality (providing undenatured amino acids and peptides) and have received tremendous attention from not only the scientific community, but life extensionists, athletes, and health/ fitness enthusiasts as well.

Animal Studies

To understand the mechanism(s) by which whey protein can exert its effects on protein synthesis, several areas must be investigated. These areas include the impact of whey on growth during development and recovery from stress or injury. Studies *in vitro* and in animals have investigated the effects of whey protein on growth and development,[164–168] recovery from severe burns,[171] and repair of gastric mucosa.[169] In general, WPC is better for calf growth and development than dried skim milk (DSM) when supplied as 67% or 100% of the major protein source.[166] However, if a starter formula is added to both the WPC and DSM diets, then growth rates between the two diets are similar. When studied as a replacement for colostrum in calves, WPC resulted in similar weight gain and a lower immune status for calves. From this brief summary it may be concluded that whey protein concentrate is better than dried skim milk, but not colostrum, in terms of the growth and development of calves.

Poullain et al.[169] compared the effects of different molecular forms of whey such as WPC, WPH, or amino acid mixture (AAM) on growth and nitrogen retention in rats. The male Wistar rats were divided into six groups of eight. Three groups were starved for 72 hours before being refed one of the three forms of whey ad libitum for 96 hours. The other three groups served as controls and were fed one of the three whey diets. Animals that were starved before feeding lost on average about 13% of their body weight. Although no differences were found in the control groups, the WPH-refed group regained weight much faster than the WPC- or AAM-refed groups. Urinary nitrogen excretion was much lower for both the refed and

control WPH groups, in comparison to all other groups. This suggests the mechanisms of increased nitrogen intake are not influenced by nutritional status (i.e., gut atrophy). The improved protein anabolism of the WPH diets were not associated with an increase in ureagenesis. The diets were identical in energy, nitrogen, amino acids, and nonnitrogenous nutrient content. The intakes of the rats were all the same; therefore, it is speculated that the different absorption rates and blood patterns of amino acids may be the cause of the differences in nitrogen balance between the WPH, WPC, and AAM diets. These differences may be related to the effects of blood levels of amino acids on hormone production. Thus, by ingesting a WPH, a sudden surge in blood levels of specific amino acids may induce the release of insulin or some other anabolic hormone, resulting in increased protein synthesis and greater nitrogen uptake.

Data from the previous study, published separately, examined the effects of WPH, WPC, and AAM diets on the jejunal mucosa of controls versus starved then refed rats.[170] During starvation for 72 hours, gut atrophy occurred and villus height decreased. After refeeding, all diets resulted in repair of the fasting-induced gut atrophy. The WPC diet produced the most rapid repair and growth of intestinal villi in the refed rats. The WPH and AAM diets produced better results on villus growth and disaccharidase activity in the control groups. The significance of this work is the demonstration that enteral feedings of different molecular forms of whey can alter jejunal morphology and enzyme activity. Combining the data from the two Poullain studies,[169,170] it is noted that the increased body weight and positive nitrogen balance in the WPH refed rats occurred even though the mucosal lining had not undergone the same extent of repair as that in the WPC refed rats. This provides further evidence that the mechanisms by which whey protein positively affects nitrogen balance and body weight may be independent of nutritional status.

During periods of stress, hypermetabolism may result in the excessive catabolism of protein and lean body mass. An example of such a condition is severe thermal injury, whereby the protein requirements may be much greater than normal. Because whey proteins contain high concentrations of branched-chain amino acids (BCAAs), a comparison was made between different levels of dietary whey versus different levels of BCAAs on the recovery from severe burns in guinea pigs.[171] Guinea pigs were divided into six groups. Each group received either 10%, 20%, or 30% of their calories from whey or BCAAs. Although rates of protein synthesis were not measured in this study, the cumulative effects of nitrogen balance and mortality were significantly better in the whey protein groups than the BCAA groups. This provides evidence that WPC may prove superior to BCAAs in recovery from thermal stress because it provides other EAAs in addition to the BCAAs. The availability of other amino acids may allow whey to stimulate protein synthesis in which BCAAs may be limited due to rate-limiting amino acids.

Human Studies

Research on protein synthesis in humans incorporates the use of infused radiolabeled tracers under near-steady-state conditions by the additional infusion of nasogastric or nasojejunal feedings.[172] This practical application of this approach has been questioned because feeding is not constant in normal humans and the steady state may overshadow acute initial events.[173] In addition, the plasma amino acid and hormone levels are different between single meal and constant feeding.[174,175] Given this scenario, an appropriate study would be to investigate the effects of feeding an intrinsically labeled whey protein meal (no carbohydrates or fats present) on whole-body protein synthesis. Boirie et al.[173] gave 30 g of a radiolabeled whey protein to ten male subjects (23.5 ± 3.6 years). The subjects had fasted overnight before receiving the tracer

proteins. The results demonstrated an increase in whole-body protein synthesis, with little inhibition of protein breakdown.[173] The investigators concluded that it appears dietary amino acids are geared toward protein synthesis and the formation of *new* amino acids, while *old* amino acids may be geared toward oxidation.

In a later study by the same group, the digestion and absorption of whey were compared with casein.[176] Labeled casein and whey proteins were ingested as liquid meals without any carbohydrates or fats after a 10-hour fast. Whey protein ingestion resulted in a rapid, transient elevation of the plasma levels of amino acids.[176] The sudden surge of amino acids results in an increased rate of protein synthesis and oxidation with little to no change in protein breakdown. These results were obtained after a 10-hour fast, which is not typical of normal human feeding patterns. The effects of a normal feeding pattern (i.e., three meals plus snacks or several small meals) on protein metabolism would offer tremendous insight to the mechanisms behind protein accretion.

Whey Protein as an Ergogenic Aid?

Researchers from McGill University in Montreal, Canada gave 20 young adults (10 men, 10 women) a whey protein supplement (10 g, twice daily) or a casein placebo for 3 months. Casein was used as the placebo because the investigators wanted to determine if protein itself conferred these benefits or if these benefits were specific to whey protein. Subjects were monitored for activity via questionnaires. The time spent in moderate (e.g., walking) and intense (e.g., running, cycling) exercise was calculated for each time period. Also, the percentage of awake-time spent being active was determined. In addition, the investigators performed before and after measures of lymphocyte glutathione levels, 30-second work capacity on a bicycle, and body composition.

After 3 months of consuming their respective supplements, they found that the whey protein group was superior to the casein group with regards to various measures. These included the following:

Peak cycling power–   +13.3% (whey),
                       +1.6% (placebo)

30-second cycling work capacity– +12.7% (whey),
                                  +0.9% (placebo)

Lymphocyte glutathione–   +35.5% (whey),
                          −0.9% (placebo)

Time spent in activity–   +13.7% (whey),
                          +4.7% (placebo)

Perhaps the most important change is the increase in lymphocyte glutathione activity, which is an indirect measure of tissue glutathione levels. This is important because glutathione, a compound produced from three amino acids (cysteine, glutamic acid, and glycine) is one of the most important

antioxidants in our bodies. Glutathione is located in the watery portion of the cell (known as the cytosol or cytoplasm) as opposed to vitamin E, which is in the fatty portion of each cell. So, whey protein increases cellular glutathione. This in turn improves the free-radical fighting ability of your body. This should theoretically improve muscle recovery and overall health. Additionally, within the constraints of this study, whey protein altered body composition favorably (see FIGURE). This is important for many types of athletes (e.g., bodybuilders, runners, etc.).

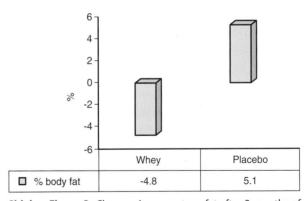

	Whey	Placebo
☐ % body fat	-4.8	5.1

Sidebar Figure 3. Changes in percentage fat after 3 months of supplementation with whey or casein protein. Note the decrease in body fat percentage in the whey group. (*Data from* Lands et al. 1999.)

Lands LC, et al. Effect of supplementation with a cysteine donor on muscular performance. J Appl Physiol 1999;87:1381–1385.

Nonetheless, it should be pointed out that there is no direct evidence in humans that shows that whey protein by itself can promote gains in lean body mass. And certainly, it would be difficult to perform a study in which whey protein could serve as the sole source of protein. However, the animal data are intriguing enough that further study on whey is warranted.

Safety and Toxicity

Research on the use of a whey protein concentrate in HIV/AIDS[177] and cancer patients reports no side effects and an improved sense of well-being.[178] Whey protein has also been used to treat cystic fibrosis in infants[179] and cirrhosis in children,[180] with positive results. However, the concern with ingestion of any type of protein concentrate or hydrolysate is the occurrence of an allergic reaction. In addition, whey protein ingested as an AAM could result in osmotic diarrhea if the oral dose is too high. This is a temporary event and can be dealt with by decreasing the dose.

Casein Protein

Casein represents a class of phosphoproteins (α, β, κ, γ) derived from bovine milk. Food scientists consider bovine casein as the fraction of milk that precipitates from raw milk at a pH of 4.6 and 20°C.[181] However, some whey protein may also precipitate under these same conditions, thereby contaminating the casein with lactalbumin and lactoferrin. Casein comprises 82% of the protein fraction of milk, compared to 18% for whey. Casein is commercially available primarily as sodium caseinate, potassium caseinate, and calcium caseinate and is used in the production of infant formulas, dried skim milk, and protein powders. It is considered a high-quality protein capable of increasing amino acid levels in man[182] as well as improving protein metabolism.[183,184]

Animal Studies

Studies in animals have examined the effects of casein on liver protein synthesis[185] and fractional synthesis rates of whole-body proteins.[186] The effects of casein and lactalbumin on radiolabeled leucine incorporation into the liver protein of Sprague-Dawley rats were compared.[185] More [14]Cleucine was incorporated into the liver of rats from the casein group, indicating higher rates of liver protein synthesis. Curiously, the wet weight and total protein content of the liver was lower for the casein group than the lactalbumin group. These contradictory effects were thought to result from increased liver catabolism or an increased secretion rate of liver proteins into circulation. The casein-induced increase in liver protein synthesis may be an advantage during times of infection or illness by allowing the liver to regenerate at a higher rate.

Insulin-like growth factor-1/somatomedin C (IGF-1) is a peptide hormone produced primarily by the liver.[187] In addition, it is also a potent stimulator of protein synthesis.[188] Male Wistar rats fed diets differing only in protein content had significantly higher levels of IGF-1 on a casein diet compared with rats fed gluten- or protein-free diets.[186,189] Casein has also been shown to increase levels of IGF-1 when infused into pregnant ewes[190] and steers[191] and affect IGF-1 receptor levels of various tissues in rats.[192] The casein-fed rats also had significantly greater rates of whole-body protein synthesis.[186] These results lend some support to the previously discussed findings of James and Treloar[185] that showed greater levels of liver protein synthesis with reduced liver weights in rats. Previous work has also shown that casein can stimulate the hepatic content of mRNA species of IGF-1.[189] By stimulating the liver to produce IGF-1, casein may exert an indirect effect on protein synthesis.

Casein may also affect IGF-1 levels by increasing IGF-1 absorption from the gastrointestinal tract.[193,194] The survival profiles of a bolus of[125]I-labelled IGF-1 (8.6 ng) *in vivo* in various ligated gut segments of fasted adult rats was investigated. IGF-1 administered orally is rapidly proteolyzed and loses its bioactivity. However, when administered with casein, IGF-1 structural integrity and receptor binding activity in both stomach and duodenum fluids were maintained. IGF-1 uptake via endocytosis by enterocytes may allow the safe transport of unaltered IGF-1 into the blood.[193] Casein has a slow gastric emptying rate and long gastrointestinal transit time,[195] and therefore may allow enterocytes to endocytized IGF-1.

From the above studies, casein may modulate IGF-1 levels by three separate pathways: by increasing (a) amino acid availability and therefore modulating skeletal muscle protein synthesis and accretion through an autocrine or paracrine IGF-1 influence,[196] (b) absorption of IGF-1 from the GI tract,[194] and (c) liver production of IGF-1.[189] There are some problems with directly applying these data. The research on animals using casein infusions[190,191,196] is based on the introduction of undegraded proteins into the GI tracts of these animals. Normally, these proteins would have undergone hydrolysis and the positive effects on IGF-1 may be lost. However, oral feeding studies on rats do demonstrate that casein can exert positive effects on IGF-1 levels.[193,194] But the positive effects of casein on IGF-1 do not steadily increase.[196] Initially, casein administration increases plasma and muscle levels of IGF-1, but levels return back to baseline after 14 days.[196] Another important point to consider is that these studies have all compared casein (an animal protein) with either a plant protein or a protein-free diet. The effects of casein on IGF-1 may also be due to the presence of additional EAAs. Future research comparing casein, whey, specific milk protein isolates, and their combinations is needed to elucidate the specific mechanisms involved. The presence of other bioactive fractions in casein may also indicate that either the individual fractions themselves or some combination mediate the indirect effects of casein on protein synthesis.

Human Studies

Earlier studies examined the effects of amino acid mixtures simulating casein and hydrolysates of casein on absorption after oral[182] or jejunal[197] administration. This work supports similar work done on whey protein, indicating that hydrolysates are absorbed better than their amino acid counterparts. Additional work examined the effects of casein on postprandial amino acid responses[198] and on insulin and glucagon.[199] The most recent research on casein focused on the delayed gastric emptying time[200] and impact on protein synthesis.[201,202]

Research on healthy men and women agrees with research on animals that casein has a slow gastric emptying time.[200,201] This delay results in elevated plasma amino acid concentrations up to 300 minutes postingestion.[201] The significance of this effect is exemplified by marked differences in protein metabolism compared with whey. Casein protein ingestion results in a slight increase in protein synthesis, moderate increase in protein oxidation, and large decrease in protein breakdown. This profile results in a more positive protein balance compared with whey.[201] This effect may be lost if casein oligopeptides are given in place of whole casein protein.[202]

Safety and Toxicity

Casein, like any protein, has the potential to induce allergic reactions in some individuals. This is more of a concern for infants receiving formulas[203,204,205] than adults. A more practical concern for adults is the potential hypercholesterolemic effects of casein[199,206–209] and data from animal studies on the potential carcinogenic effects of cooked or heated casein.[210–212] So, individuals with hypercholesterolemia or those consuming high saturated fat diets should use casein products cautiously. Long-term research demonstrates similar side effects in rats fed semi-purified diets containing either casein or soy proteins.[213]

However, a recent study demonstrated that a casein protein diet produced a dramatic drop in Lp(a) levels, thus potentially decreasing cardiovascular risk.[214] Also, if casein has deleterious effects on blood lipids and tumor formation, then one would speculate that heavy milk drinkers would suffer from a malady of health problems. Clearly, this is not the case.

Milk Protein Isolates

Milk is a food that contains numerous components. These components include proteins, fat, lactose, vitamins, minerals, enzymes, hormones, growth substances, and immunoglobulins. In addition, hydrolysis of milk proteins can produce bioactive peptides.[215] The two primary proteins are casein and whey. Casein is further subdivided into α-casein, β-casein, κ-casein, and γ-casein, whereas whey protein contains α-lactalbumin, β-lactalbumin, serum albumin, lactoferrin, and various growth factors such as IGF-1, platelet-derived growth factor (PDGF), and TGF-β (transforming growth factor-beta).[216–235] Although many of these factors were once thought to be destroyed during the processing of bovine milk, recent improvements in protein technology may also allow many of these factors into the food supply. Therefore, this section will review various isolated fractions and growth factors of bovine milk that have been identified to influence cell growth and/or protein synthesis.

Animal Studies

The use of bovine growth hormone in dairy cows received enormous attention when it was first proposed. Research indicates that it can increase the absolute amount and percentage of total milk protein of α-lactalbumin in bovine milk,[236] as well as increase levels of IGF-1.[237,238] The significance of the additional lactalbumin in milk has yet to be scientifically demonstrated. However, Campbell and Baumrucker[239] showed that increases in IGF-1 plasma levels are paralleled by increases in milk. The increase in IGF-1 bioactivity is further increased by pasteurization.[238,240] The significance of this bioactivity is demonstrated by research on rats where oral administration of IGF-1 stimulated growth.[238]

Human Studies

Debate over the significance of various components of milk has stimulated research in this area. Research on the effects of exogenous administration of albumin to hypoalbuminemic patients receiving nutrition support does not appear warranted due to lack of improved outcomes.[241] Although exogenous albumin may not be beneficial to improving nutritional status, other unrelated work demonstrates that IGF-1 levels in bovine milk are bioactive.[238] Initially it was thought that heat (121°C for 5 min) would decrease IGF-1 concentrations in bovine milk to undetectable levels for infant formula preparations or in commercially available infant formulas.[240] However, although IGF-1 may be undetectable in infant formulas, it is not destroyed by pasteurization. To put this into perspective, it is lower than concentrations reported for human milk, yet similar to those reported for human saliva.[240]

Although bovine colostrum is not typically thought of as a food supplement, it has been available to bodybuilders and athletes for many years. It is touted as capable of stimulating muscle protein synthesis due to the high concentration of growth factors. Only until recently, has scientific evidence been available in this area. Mero et al.[242] supplemented nine male sprinters with a bovine colostrum supplement (Bioenervi). Each athlete underwent three treatments in a randomized fashion in which they ingested a 125-mL drink containing 25 mL of Bioenervi, a 125-mL drink containing 125 mL of Bioenervi, or a 125-mL drink containing normal milk whey (placebo) for 8 days. The researchers found that serum immunoglobulin G, growth hormone, amino acid, and saliva immunoglobulin A responses were similar during the three treatments, whereas IGF-1 levels had increased during the supplemented periods. They concluded that a bovine colostrum supplement (Bioenervi) could increase serum IGF-1 concentration in athletes during strength and speed training.

Safety and Toxicity

Research on the side effects of all the specific growth factors present in milk is not yet available. A growth factor from bovine milk that has received attention from the scientific community is IGF-1. A great deal of concern has been expressed over the increase in IGF-1 due to hyperstimulation of dairy cows with biosynthetic bovine growth hormones and the further increase in bioactivity by pasteurization.[238,240] What effects could an increase in IGF-1 in the food supply have on humans? In rats, oral administration of IGF-1 has stimulated growth.[238] Evidence exists that because IGF-1 is absorbed from the gastrointestinal tract, as proven in rat studies, absorption is likely in humans. IGF-1 is considered a potential risk factor for both breast, prostate, and gastrointestinal cancer.[238,243,244] However, there is no clear evidence now that would indicate an increased cancer risk due to a dietary-induced increase in IGF-1.

Miscellaneous Supplements

Structured Lipids

Advances in the technology behind lipid synthesis led to the development of structured lipids (SLs). A structured lipid (SL) is a triglyceride that includes both medium (8–12 carbons) and long-chain fatty acids (14–22 carbons) within the same triglyceride. Emulsions including SL have demonstrated increased protein synthesis and increased nitrogen balance (NB) in burned animals.[245–250] The SL has also been superior to medium-chain triglyceride (MCT) and long-chain triglyceride (LCT) emulsions in stimulating muscle protein synthesis[245,246] in animal studies.

The use of SLs has been primarily limited to clinical and experimental settings whereby it has become necessary to develop medical nutrition therapies that minimize the adverse effects of high lipid feedings and maximize the positive outcomes.[251–266] Such positive outcomes include increased protein synthesis, enhanced immune function, decreased risk for cardiovascular disease, and improved

glucose homeostasis. The ability to increase protein synthesis, maintain the health of the immune system, and stabilize blood glucose are factors that can also play a role in improving athletic performance. Research on the application of this clinical technology to athletic performance is not available at this time.

Amino Acid Mixtures

Although most recent research has focused on the effects of individual amino acids such as leucine and glutamine on protein synthesis, other work has shown that mixtures of amino acids can also stimulate protein synthesis.[267–269] Dogs were subjected to treadmill running (150 minutes at 10 km/hr and 12% incline) and intravenously infused with a solution containing amino acids and glucose (AAG), amino acids (AA), glucose (G), or saline (S) in a randomized order.[267] Both AAG and AA increased leucine uptake by the gut, while G and S resulted in a net release. Moreover, AAG resulted in greater uptake of leucine versus AA. The AAG treatment was the only condition that did not result in a significant release of phenylalanine from skeletal muscle. The results indicate that AA supplementation may reduce exercise-induced proteolysis in the gut, and this effect may be enhanced by the simultaneous administration of G. Another important observation was that both AA and G might be required to prevent net protein degradation in skeletal muscle during exercise.

In another study using six healthy untrained men, an intravenous infusion of an amino acid mixture (about 0.15 g/kg-1.h-1 for 3 hours) was administered at rest and after a leg resistance exercise routine.[268] The intravenous amino acid infusion resulted in similar elevations in arterial amino acid concentrations at rest and after exercise, whereas leg blood flow was greater after exercise than at rest. The increases in amino acid transport above baseline were greater after exercise than at rest during the hyperaminoacidemia. Although muscle protein synthesis was elevated after the infusion and was greater after exercise than at rest, muscle protein breakdown was not significantly affected either at rest or after exercise. The researchers concluded that the stimulatory effect of exogenous amino acids on muscle protein synthesis might be enhanced by prior exercise because of enhanced blood flow.[268] Furthermore, the results implied that protein intake immediately after exercise may be more anabolic than when ingested at some later time.

The anabolic actions of amino acids may also be independent of exercise.[269] Research on elderly individuals (age 71 ± 2 yrs.) also used an intravenous infusion of an amino acid mixture. Muscle protein synthesis was stimulated by the increased amino acid availability whereas protein breakdown did not change. This resulted in a positive net balance of amino acids across the muscle. The researchers concluded that although muscle mass is decreased in the elderly, muscle protein anabolism might be stimulated by an increase in amino acid availability.[269]

Peptides

In an effort to provide glutamine to TPN patients in a form that can remain stable in liquid, the amino acid has been bonded with other amino acids, such as the dipeptide alanyl-glutamine.[270] This combination can preserve muscle glutamine levels and muscle protein synthesis after surgery and improve whole-body nitrogen balance.[270] This finding is supported by research on rats with peritonitis.[271] Alanyl-glutamine increased protein synthesis in the liver and skeletal muscle, protected the morphology of the intestinal mucosa, and improved survival in protracted bacterial peritonitis. The researchers concluded that alanyl-glutamine supplementation may be useful in septic patients.[271]

Soy Protein

Recent evidence regarding the cardioprotective benefits of soy isoflavones has stimulated an increase in consumption of soy protein powders. Although consumers are most likely ingesting soy powders for the isoflavones present, they will also benefit from the protein itself. Studies on nitrogen balance in man indicate that isolated soy is comparable to that of animal proteins.[272–274] The effects of a soy-based diet versus an animal protein-based diet on whole-body protein turnover was evaluated using two groups of six males.[275] The rates of protein synthesis and protein breakdown were similar in both groups. However, more recent research compared soy with casein on net protein retention in pigs.[276] Constant infusions of either casein or soy were performed with measurements taken postabsorptively and 2–6 hours after the enteral feeding. Amino acid and urea kinetics were assessed using a primed-constant infusion protocol with L-[ring-2,6-3H]phenylalanine, L-[3,4-3H]valine and [15N-15N]urea. During the meal, the appearance of amino acids into the portal vein and their uptake by the liver was lower with the casein infusion. Muscle uptake did not differ between the casein or soy infusions. The soy infusion stimulated a lower rate of gut protein synthesis and higher rate of muscle protein turnover. The casein infusion stimulated a higher rate of liver protein synthesis and degradation. In the postabsorptive condition, casein infusion did not alter liver urea production, whereas soy infusion significantly increased it. In contradiction to previous studies, the researchers concluded that the soy protein is an inferior quality in comparison to that of casein protein.

Studies indicate that soy is well tolerated and there are no adverse effects associated with its use. Soy stimulates lower rates of liver protein synthesis and degradation; therefore, future research on the combinations of soy with other proteins may prove insightful in providing a protein that not only lowers the risk for cardiovascular disease, but also maintains higher levels of protein synthesis and lower levels of protein degradation.

SUMMARY

Although there are few data that have examined the use of glutamine in athletes, it would seem plausible based on the existing clinical data that glutamine supplementation may exert a beneficial effect for individuals engaged in chronic and intense exercise training. Skeletal muscle glutamine concentration decreases in a dose-dependent manner relative to the degree of stress. Like glutamine, OKG and α-KG has potential utility as an anticatabolic agent. As a practical matter, however, the lower cost of purchasing glutamine versus OKG and α-KG would preclude the use of the latter. The BCAAs could serve as an auxiliary fuel source for an exercising individual and have a potential muscle-sparing effect under conditions of prolonged exercise. A body of evidence (though somewhat equivocal) suggests that the BCAAs are an effective ergogenic aid. Leucine has shown anticatabolic actions *in vitro*. However, its effects on *in vivo* protein synthesis in animals and humans are mixed. Some evidence indicates that metabolites of leucine (e.g., HMB, KIC) exert antiproteolytic effects.

Technological advances in the isolation and purification of whey protein have resulted in the production of a high-quality product with minimal ash, mineral, lactose, or fat content. Whey protein is digested and absorbed rapidly after a 10-hour fast, which results in the elevation of amino acids in plasma. Research on the application of these effects on lean body mass in healthy people or athletic performance is lacking at this time. Whey appears to be well tolerated, without side effects, and its use in a variety of clinical settings is increasing. Casein is a high-quality protein containing sufficient quantities of essential amino acids. It travels slower through the gastrointestinal tract compared to whey protein, resulting in sustained plasma levels of amino acids. This serves to increase net protein synthesis by slightly increasing total protein synthesis and oxidation, and dramatically decreasing protein breakdown. The decrease in protein breakdown results in a greater net protein gain.

AUTHORS' RECOMMENDATIONS

The protein-sparing effect of glutamine would certainly be important for athletes engaged in strength-power sports. We speculate that glutamine supplementation may be useful over the course of an intense competitive season. For instance, professional football is a sport that, for many teams, involves 5 months of intense training and competition. It is likely that many of these athletes are experiencing an enormous level of fatigue during the season, particularly near the end of the season. The provision of glutamine may help offset some of the lean body mass or muscle mass loss associated with a long season. And secondly, glutamine could serve to ameliorate the effects of overtraining on the immune system. Because glutamine is such an important fuel for the gastrointestinal tract and cells of the immune system, one could theorize that glutamine supplementation could in essence spare muscle protein while providing fuel for other cells and tissues. Anecdotal reports show that dosages as high as 40–50 g/day as a free-form amino acid have been taken by bodybuilders. It is not clear if this is an excess amount of glutamine; however, we would hypothesize that a reasonable dose of 5–15 g/day may be warranted.

The effect of OKG in mediating protein metabolism is partly due to maintaining intramuscular glutamine concentrations; thus, it would seem more feasible to consume glutamine rather than OKG as an *anticatabolic* supplement. The BCAAs (leucine, valine, isoleucine) have been shown to have anticatabolic and anabolic effects, though the evidence is not entirely conclusive. Doses as high as 6–14 g may be warranted to exert an ergogenic effect. However, consumption of whey protein (which has a high concentration of the BCAAs) may provide a large quantity of the BCAAs in a form that may be more palatable to some.

Despite the prodigious consumption of whey protein by bodybuilders and other athletes, there is little direct scientific evidence demonstrating ergogenic properties. The primary advantage of whey protein is the rapid availability of amino acids after its consumption. This is derived from data on fasted adults with no other nutrients in the drink. The ingestion of the typical post-workout drink, which contains protein, carbohydrates, vitamins, minerals, some fat, etc., may dramatically alter the amino acid response. It appears that carbohydrate/protein drinks elevate insulin levels more than either protein or carbohydrate by themselves. Perhaps we will find out in the future that a glucose polymer or sucrose plus whey protein drink is better for stimulating protein synthesis (and therefore muscle protein accretion), based on its ability to increase insulin.

As a source of protein that is low in fat and nutrient-dense, whey protein may provide an adjunct to the normal dietary routine of athletes. For this reason alone, it is highly recommended that athletes regularly consume a whey protein meal replacement powder (MRP).

Casein is a high-quality protein that has been consumed by athletes and patients for years. Years ago it was in vogue for bodybuilders and strongmen to drink plenty of milk for muscle growth. It would be interesting to find out that there are indeed sufficient levels of IGF-1 and other growth factors in milk that can be absorbed intact into the body, thereby promoting muscle growth. For athletes trying to maximize protein accretion, it may make more sense to take a casein-based protein at night and before training and take a whey-based protein after training and at other times of the day. This feeding strategy is based on current research that indicates that casein is absorbed quite slowly from the GI tract and can therefore help maintain high levels of plasma amino acids over a prolonged period. Many MRPs contain both casein and whey.

The use of milk protein isolated as potential ergogenic aids is intriguing. A biologically significant amount of milk proteins are hydrolyzed in the GI tract into peptides that may have distinct biological function(s). It is too early to make any recommendations in this area yet, but it appears that certain oral peptides and proteins (i.e., IGF-1) can be ingested from/with milk and cross the GI barrier in significant quantities. What effects this has on protein synthesis and muscle mass can only be extrapolated from IGF-1 research and anecdotal evidence from athletes. A concern that we would have is that these growth factors may have widespread effects in stimulating a variety of cells.

FUTURE RESEARCH

Despite the abundant clinical evidence, scientists need to venture into the realm of healthy exercising individuals for examining glutamine's various effects. First of all, short-term and long-term resistance training studies need to be done to ascertain if glutamine has an anabolic effect in individuals who are eating adequate calories, macronutrients, and micronutrients. Similar studies in exercising individuals who may be on a hypocaloric diet may be an even better approach because many scientists (and athletes) believe that the effects of glutamine are best seen in catabolic states. Also, changes at the cellular/molecular level (e.g., muscle fiber cross-sectional area, myosin heavy-chain isoforms, cytoskeletal proteins, mRNA levels, etc.) need to be examined further.

Leucine has been used in a variety of diseased populations with mixed results. Its effects on protein synthesis are varied and require further investigation to elucidate the mechanism involved. Although the effects of leucine alone and in conjunction with other amino acids have been studied in humans, there are limited data on the effects of leucine on protein synthesis rates during or after exercise. Additional research needs to examine the effects of leucine under these conditions as well as under different dietary protein intakes. It appears that higher dietary protein intakes result in metabolic environments in which amino acids are readily oxidized. Perhaps extremely high dosages of leucine are required in this condition, whereas people acclimated to lower protein intakes may need less leucine to get an anticatabolic effect.

KIC is believed to spare nitrogen under certain conditions. Most of these treatments involve the intravenous administration of KIC. The gut and liver metabolize a significant portion of KIC; therefore, additional research on the effects of oral KIC preparations on protein metabolism is needed. Animal data provide convincing evidence that even though KIC increases nitrogen content and protein deposition, it does this in other tissues, not skeletal muscle. Research on the effects of KIC on protein deposition need to address the target tissues or sites of protein accretion or decreased proteolysis. Although KIC may improve nitrogen balance in the liver and splanchnic tissues under certain conditions, there is a lack of available data on the effects of KIC on human body composition and performance. Because of the potential transamination between KIC and other amino acids and keto acids, additional work should try to elucidate the direct impact on protein metabolism by KIC as compared with its metabolites.

Currently, it is known that whey protein hydrolysates are high-quality proteins and rapidly increase blood amino acid concentrations. The interaction of other dietary nutrients, such as carbohydrates and fats with whey, require further investigation. Although whey is categorized as a fast dietary protein based on its absorption, these data are derived from fasted subjects. The effects of whey protein on the plasma amino acids levels of humans in fed states require further investigation. The logical extension of this would be to investigate the impact of whey on the protein synthesis rates of athletes. In addition, the effects of the whey amino acid response profile on anabolic hormones, like insulin, and recovery from physical exercise present exciting opportunities to investigate how a specific diet may influence muscle growth.

Research on the effects of casein in humans was done after fasting for 10 or more hours and ingesting alone[175,199] or in continuous feeding with specific amounts of lipids and carbohydrates.[199] These same results may not apply when casein is ingested with other foods yielding different levels of proteins, lipids, and carbohydrates in the meal. The combination of casein with other nutrients requires further research to determine the modifying role other nutrients may have on casein's impact on protein synthesis.

Casein's ability to decrease protein breakdown has yet to be applied to athletic performance or training. Protein synthesis is stimulated after overload-type training; therefore, casein may have a potential role in modifying the effects of recovery from this type of exercise and requires further research. An ideal comparison would be between post-workout drinks containing vitamins, minerals, and glucose polymers, yet differing only in the protein source by containing either whey or casein.

The potential application of casein as an absorption enhancer for orally administered products is interesting. The ability of casein to enhance IGF-1 absorption requires investigation in humans to see if the results of animal experiments can be duplicated. In addition, comparisons between casein and other animal proteins on the effects of IGF-1 need to be done. Most evidence at this time seems to indicate that protein in general can stimulate IGF-1, yet most of the animal research has used casein as the sole animal protein.

Furthermore, future research should examine the effects of growth factors (present in milk) on humans. In addition, with the tremendous popularity of protein supplements among athletes, research on the content of bioactive ingredients is needed as well. The links between isolated protein fractions, growth factors, and other bioactive substances from milk on stimulating protein synthesis and/or performance are currently weak. Only one paper shows an increase in IGF-1 levels in athletes[242]; however, it did not examine the effects of this particular supplement on protein synthesis or exercise performance. Future research should focus on how these growth factors could enhance lean body mass and athletic performance.

SLs are an application of bioengineered foods to the world of clinical nutrition. This category of nutrients is receiving attention because of its ability to be rapidly absorbed, spare protein, improve renal and liver function, and reduce infections and GI disturbances, while minimizing side effects in patients. The current SLs used in clinical settings include a combination of fish oils and MCTs, which are randomly transesterified (the process by which fatty acids are added to the glycerol backbone). Challenges facing developers of SL products include manufacturing specific SLs in a cost-effective fashion. Although the current production costs to manufacture SLs are high, improvements in technology will allow costs to be controlled and wide-scale production to be implemented.

The concept of custom-tailored SLs for a population based on the disease and the fatty acid requirements is an exciting one. Already SLs have been designed for cystic fibrosis patients who typically have difficulty absorbing LCTs. By incorporating a lung chain fatty acid (LCFA) with two medium chain fatty acids (MCFAs) the LCFAs can be absorbed and the risk for fatty acid deficiencies decreased. Infant formulas may also make use of this technology to increase growth and development of low birth weight and premature babies. Genetic engineering of plants will also allow the development of lipids that lower plasma triglycerides and cholesterol, thus decreasing risk factors for cardiovascular and other diseases.

The research in this area is a new frontier; however, there are still some key areas that haven't been addressed in the literature to date. The first issue is that the longest TPN and enteral studies have lasted about 1 week in humans. For most hospital patients, this time may be sufficient. However, patients in a coma, or vegetative state, or nursing home residents may require TPN and/or enteral feeding for much longer time periods. The long-term effects have yet to be established in humans, although data from acute human studies and 6-week long animal studies do appear promising. Another issue is the potential interaction either directly or indirectly (via altered production of prostaglandins or other eicosanoids) of SLs with other nutrients and/or drugs. Because this area of clinical nutrition is so young, little evidence is available on SL-nutrient and SL-drug interactions. Future research will enhance our understanding of this area and the potential complications.

REFERENCES

1. Ballard FJ. Regulation of protein accumulation in cultured cells. Biochem J 1982;208:275–287.
2. Florini JR. Hormonal control of muscle growth. Muscle Nerve 1987;10:577–598.
3. Ziegler EE, Filer LJ, eds. Present Knowledge in Nutrition. 7th ed. Washington, DC: ILSI Press, 1996.
4. Kasperek GJ, Snider RD. Total and myofibrillar protein degradation in isolated soleus muscles after exercise. Am J Physiol 1989;257(1 Pt 1):E1–5.
5. Newsholme EA, Leech AR. Biochemistry for the Medical Sciences. New York: John Wiley & Sons, 1983:423–425.
6. Lacey JM, Wilmore DW. Is glutamine a conditionally essential amino acid? Nutr Rev 1990;48:297–309.
7. Rowbottom DG, Keast D, Morton AR. The emerging role of glutamine as an indicator of exercise stress and overtraining. Sports Med 1996;21:80–97.
8. Curthoys NP, Watford M. Regulation of glutaminase activity and glutamine metabolism. Annu Rev Nutr 1995;15:133–159.
9. Frayn KN, Khan K, Coppack SW, Elia M. Amino acid metabolism in human subcutaneous adipose tissue in vivo. Clin Sci 1991;80:471–474.
10. Windmueller HG, Spaeth AE. Uptake and metabolism of plasma glutamine by the small intestine. J Biol Chem 1974;249:5070–5079.
11. Curi TC, de Melo MP, de Azevedo RB, Curi R. Glutamine utilization by rat neutrophils. Biochem Soc Trans 1997;25:249S.
12. Fine A. Effects of acute metabolic acidosis on renal, gut, liver, and muscle metabolism of glutamine and ammonia in the dog. Kidney Int 1982;21:439–444.
13. Squires EJ, Brosnan JT. Measurements of the turnover rate of glutamine in normal and acidotic rats. Biochem J 1983;210:277–280.
14. Hall, JC, Heel K, McCauley R. Glutamine. Br J Surg 1996;83:305–312.
15. Wagenmakers AJM. Muscle amino acid metabolism at rest and during exercise: role of human physiology and metabolism. Exerc Sport Sci Rev 1988;26:287–314.
16. Zhou X, Thompson JR. Regulation of protein turnover by glutamine in heat-shocked skeletal myotubes. Biochim Biophys Acta 1997;1357:234–242.
17. Wu GY, Thompson JR. The effect of glutamine on protein turnover in chick skeletal muscle in vitro. Biochem J 1990;265:593–598.
18. Haussinger D, Roth E, Lang F, Gerok W. Cellular hydration state: an important determinant of protein catabolism in health and disease. Lancet 1993;341:1330–1332.
19. Waldegger S, Busch GL, Kaba NK, et al. Effect of cellular hydration on protein metabolism. Miner Electrolyte Metab 1997;23:201–205.
20. Vom Dahl S, Haussinger D. Nutritional state and the swelling-induced inhibition of proteolysis in perfused rat liver. J Nutr 1996;126:395–402.
21. Parry-Billings M, Bevan SJ, Opara E, Newsholme EA. Effects of changes in cell volume on the rates of glutamine and alanine release from rat skeletal muscle in vitro. Biochem J 1991;276:559–561.
22. MacLennan PA, Brown RA, Rennie MJ. A positive relationship between protein synthetic rate and intracellular glutamine concentration in perfused rat skeletal muscle. FEBS Lett 1987;215:187–191.
23. MacLennan PA, Smith K, Weryk B, et al. Inhibition of protein breakdown by glutamine in perfused rat skeletal muscle. FEBS Lett 1988;237:133–136.
24. Hickson RC, Wegrzyn LE, Osborne DF, Karl IE. Alanyl-glutamine prevents muscle atrophy and glutamine synthetase induction by glucocorticoids. Am J Physiol 1996;271:R1165–R1172.
25. Hickson RC, Oehler DT, Byerly RJ, Unterman TG. Protective effect of glutamine from glucocorticoid-induced muscle atrophy occurs without alterations in circulating insulin-like growth factor (IGF-1) and IGF-binding protein levels. Proc Soc Exp Biol Med 1997;216:65–71.
26. Hickson RC, Czerwinski SM, Wegrzyn LE. Glutamine prevents downregulation of myosin heavy chain synthesis and muscle atrophy from glucocorticoids. Am J Physiol 1995;268:E730–E734.
27. Kapadia CR, Colpoys MF, Jiang ZM, et al. Maintenance of skeletal muscle intracellular glutamine during standard surgical trauma. J Parenter Enteral Nutr 1985;9:583–589.
28. Roth, E, Karner J, Ollenschlager G, et al. Alanylglutamine reduces muscle loss of alanine and glutamine in post-operative anaesthetized dogs. Clin Sci 1988;75:641–648.
29. Ardawi MS, Majzoub MF. Glutamine metabolism in skeletal muscle of septic rats. Metabolism 1991;40:155–164.
30. Wusteman M, Elia M. Effect of glutamine infusions on glutamine concentration and protein synthetic rate in rat muscle. J Parenter Enteral Nutr 1991;15:521–525.
31. Fang CH, James JH, Fischer JE, Hasselgren, PO. Is muscle protein turnover regulated by intracellular glutamine during sepsis? J Parenter Enteral Nutr 1995;19:279–285.
32. Naka S, Saito H, Hashiguchi Y, et al. Alanyl-glutamine-supplemented total parenteral nutrition improves survival and protein metabolism in rat protracted bacterial peritonitis model. J Parenter Enteral Nutr 1996;20:417–423.
33. Shewchuck, LD, Baracos VE, Field CJ. Dietary L-glutamine supplementation reduces the growth of the Morris Hepatoma 7777 in exercise-trained and sedentary rats. J Nutr 1997;A127:158–166.
34. Shewchuck LD, Baracos VE, Field CJ. Dietary L-glutamine supplementation does not improve lymphocyte metabolism or function in exercise-trained rats. Med Sci Sports Exerc 1997B;29:474–481.
35. Austgen TR, Dudrick PS, Sitren H, et al. The effects of glutamine-enriched total parenteral nutrition on tumor growth and host tissues. Ann Surg 1992;215:107–113.
36. Hankard RG, Haymond MW, Darmaun D. Effect of glutamine on leucine metabolism in humans. Am J Physiol 1996;271:E748–E754.

37. Hammarqvist F, Wernerman J, Ali R, et al. Addition of glutamine to total parenteral nutrition after elective abdominal surgery spares free glutamine in muscle, counteracts the fall in muscle protein synthesis, and improves nitrogen balance. Ann Surg 1989;209:455–461.

38. Hammarqvist F, Wernerman J, Von Der Decken A, Vinnars E. Alanyl-glutamine counteracts the depletion of free glutamine and the postoperative decline in protein synthesis in skeletal muscle. Ann Surg 1990;212(5):637–644.

39. Petersson B, Von Der Decken A, Vinnars E, Wernerman J. Long-term effects of postoperative total parenteral nutrition supplemented with glycylglutamine on subjective fatigue and muscle protein synthesis. Br J Surg 1994A;81:1520–1523.

40. Petersson B, Waller SO, Vinnars E, Wernerman J. Long-term effect of glycyl-glutamine after elective surgery on free amino acids in muscle. J Parenter Enteral Nutr 1994B;18:320–325.

41. Suojaranta-Ylinen R, Ruokonen E, Pulkki K, et al. Preoperative glutamine loading does not prevent endotoxemia in cardiac surgery. Acta Anaesthesiol Scand 1997;41:385–391.

42. Welbourne TC. Increased plasma bicarbonate and growth hormone after an oral glutamine load. Am J Clin Nutr 1995;61:1058–1061.

43. Rosene MF, Finn KJ, Antonio J, et al. Glutamine supplementation may maintain nitrogen balance in wrestlers during a weight reduction program. Med Sci Sports Exerc 1999;31(5):S123.

44. Welbourne TC, Claville W, Langford M. An oral glutamine load enhances renal acid secretion and function. Am J Clin Nutr 1998;67:660–663.

45. Potteiger J, Nickel G, Webster M, et al. Sodium citrate ingestion enhances 30km cycling time. Int J Sports Med 1996;17:7–11.

46. Haub MD, Potteiger JA, Nau KL, et al. Acute L-glutamine ingestion does not improve maximal effort exercise. J Sports Med Phys Fitness 1998;38:240–244.

47. Perriello G, Nurjhan N, Stumvoll M, et al. Regulation of gluconeogenesis by glutamine in normal post-absorptive humans. Am J Physiol 1997; 272:E437–E445.

48. Nurjhan N, Bucci A, Perriello G, et al. Glutamine: a major gluconeogenic precursor and vehicle for interorgan carbon transport in man. J Clin Invest 1995;95:272–277.

49. Varnier M, Leese GP, Thompson J, Rennie MJ. Stimulatory effect of glutamine on glycogen accumulation in human skeletal muscle. Am J Physiol 1995;269:E309–E315.

50. Opara EC, Petro A, Tevrizian A, et al. L-glutamine supplementation of a high fat diet reduces body weight and attenuates hyperglycemia and hyperinsulinemia in C57BL/6J mice. J Nutr 1996; 126:273–279.

51. Ballard TC, Farag A, Branum GD, et al. Effect of L-glutamine supplementation on impaired glucose regulation during intravenous lipid administration. Nutrition 1996;12:349–354.

52. Ziegler TR, Benfell K, Smith RJ, et al. Safety and metabolic effects of L-glutamine administration in humans. J Parenter Enteral Nutr 1990;14:137S–146S.

53. Dechelotte P, Darmaun D, Rongier M, et al. Absorption and metabolic effects of enterally administered glutamine in humans. Am J Physiol 1991;260:G677–G682.

54. Weingartmann G, Fridrich P, Mauritz W, et al. Safety and efficacy of increasing dosages of glycly-glutamine for total parenteral nutrition in polytrauma patients. Wien Klin Wochenschr 1996;108:683–688.

55. Wernerman J, Hammarqvist F, Vinnars E. Alpha-ketoglutarate and postoperative muscle catabolism. Lancet 1990;24:335(8691):701–703.

56. Roth E, Karner J, Roth-Merten A, et al. Effect of alpha-ketoglutarate infusions on organ balances of glutamine and glutamate in anaesthetized dogs in the catabolic state. Clin Sci (Colch) 1991;80:625–631.

57. Hammarqvist F, Wernerman J, von der Decken A, Vinnars E. Alpha-ketoglutarate preserves protein synthesis and free glutamine in skeletal muscle after surgery. Surgery 1991;109:28–36.

58. Blomqvist BI, Hammarqvist F, von der Decken A, Wernerman J. Glutamine and alpha-ketoglutarate prevent the decrease in muscle free glutamine concentration and influence protein synthesis after total hip replacement. Metabolism 1995;44:1215–1222.

59. Vaubourdolle M, Coudray-Lucas C, Jardel A, et al. Action of enterally administered ornithine alpha-ketoglutarate on protein breakdown in skeletal muscle and liver of the burned rat. J Parenter Enteral Nutr 1991;15:517–520.

60. Le Boucher J, Obled C, Farges MC, Cynober L. Ornithine alpha-ketoglutarate modulates tissue protein metabolism in burn-injured rats. Am J Physiol 1997;273:E557–E563.

61. Ziegler F, Coudray-Lucas C, Jardel A, et al. Ornithine alpha-ketoglutarate supplementation during refeeding of food-deprived rats. J Parenter Enteral Nutr 1992;16:505–510.

62. Le Bricon T, Cynober L, Baracos VE. Ornithine alpha-ketoglutarate limits muscle protein breakdown without stimulating tumor growth in rats bearing Yoshida ascites hepatoma. Metabolism 1994; 43:899–905.

63. Jeevanandam M, Holaday NJ, Petersen SR. Ornithine alpha-ketoglutarate (OKG) supplementation is more effective than its component salts in traumatized rats. J Nutr 1996;126:2141–2150.

64. Le Boucher J, Coudray-Lucas C, Lasnier E, et al. Enteral administration of ornithine alpha-ketoglutarate or arginine alpha-ketoglutarate: a comparative study of their effects on glutamine pools in burn-injured rats. Crit Care Med 1997b;25:293–298.

65. Vaubourdolle M, Cynober L, Lioret N, et al. Influence of enterally administered ornithine alpha-ketoglutarate on hormonal patterns in burn patients. Burns Incl Therm Inj 1987;13:349–356.

66. De Bandt JP, Coudray-Lucas C, Lioret N, et al. A randomized trial of the influence of the mode of enteral ornithine alpha-ketoglutarate administration in burn patients. J Nutr 1998;128:563–569.

67. Wernerman J, Hammarqvist F, von der Decken A, Vinnars E. Ornithine alpha-ketoglutarate improves skeletal muscle protein synthesis as assessed by ribosome analysis and nitrogen use after surgery. Ann Surg 1987;206:674–678.

68. Wernerman J, Hammarqvist F, Ali MR, Vinnars E. Glutamine and ornithine alpha-ketoglutarate but not branched-chain amino acids reduce the loss of muscle glutamine after surgical trauma. Metabolism 1989;38(suppl):63–66.

69. Hammarqvist F, Wernerman J, Ali R, Vinnars E. Effects of an amino acid solution enriched with either branched chain amino acids or ornithine alpha-ketoglutarate on the postoperative intracellular amino acid concentration of skeletal muscle. Br J Surg 1990;77:214–218.

70. Moukarzel AA, Goulet O, Salas JS, et al. Growth retardation in children receiving long-term parenteral nutrition: effects of ornithine alpha-ketoglutarate. Am J Clin Nutr 1994;60:408–413.

71. Marks DB, Marks AD, Smith CM. Basic Medical Biochemistry. Baltimore: Williams & Wilkins, 1996.

72. Mori E, Hasebe M, Kobayashi K, Suzuki H. Immediate stimulation of protein metabolism in burned rats by total parenteral nutrition enriched in branched-chain amino acids. J Parenter Enteral Nutr 1989;13:484–489.

73. Miwa Y, Kato M, Moriwaki H, et al. Effects of branched-chain amino acid infusion on protein metabolism in rats with acute hepatic failure. Hepatology 1995;22:291–296.

74. Kawamura I, Yamazaki K, Tsuchiya H, et al. Optimum branched-chain amino acids concentration for improving protein catabolism in severely stressed rats. J Parenter Enteral Nutr 1990;14:398–403.

75. Kirvela O, Takala J. Postoperative parenteral nutrition with high supply of branched-chain amino acids: effects on nitrogen balance and liver protein synthesis. J Parenter Enteral Nutr 1986;10:574–577.

76. Mochizuki H, Trocki O, Dominioni I, Alexander JW. Effect of a diet rich in branched chain amino acids on severely burned guinea pigs. J Trauma 1986;26:1077–1085.

77. McCauley R, Platell C, Hall J, McCulloch R. Influence of branched chain amino acid infusions on wound healing. Aust N Z Surg 1990; 60:471–473.

78. Okada A, Mori S, Totsuka M, et al. Branched-chain amino acids metabolic support in surgical patients: a randomized, controlled trial in patients with subtotal or total gastrectomy in 16 Japanese institutions. J Parenter Enteral Nutr 1988;12:332–337.

79. Garcia-de-Lorenzo A, Ortiz-Leyba C, Planas M, et al. Parenteral administration of different amounts of branched-chain amino acids in septic patients: clinical and metabolic aspects. Crit Care Med 1997;25:418–424.

80. Louard RJ, Barrett EJ, Gelfand RA. Overnight branched-chain amino acid infusion causes sustained suppression of muscle proteolysis. Metabolism 1995;44:424–429.

81. Ferrando AA, Williams BD, Stuart CA, et al. Oral branched-chain amino acids decrease whole-body proteolysis. J Parenter Enteral Nutr 1995;19:47–54.

82. Vander Woude P, Morgan RE, Kosta JM, et al. Addition of branched-chain amino acids to parenteral nutrition of stressed critically ill patients. Crit Care Med 1986;14:685–688.

83. Wernerman J, Hammarkvist F, Ali MR, Vinnars E. Glutamine and ornithine-alpha-ketoglutarate but not branched-chain amino acids reduce the loss of muscle glutamine after surgical trauma. Metabolism 1989;38(Suppl):63–66.

84. Hammarqvist F, Wernerman J, Ali R, Vinnars E. Effects of an amino acid solution enriched with either branched chain amino acids or ornithine-alpha-ketoglutarate on the postoperative intracellular amino acid concentration of skeletal muscle. Br J Surg 1990;77:214–218.

85. Scholten DJ, Morgan RE, Davis AT, Albrecht RM. Failure of BCAA supplementation to promote nitrogen retention in injured patients. J Am Coll Nutr 1990;9:101–106.

86. von Meyenfeldt MF, Soeters PB, Vente JP, et al. Effect of branched chain amino acid enrichment of total parenteral nutrition on nitrogen sparing and clinical outcome of sepsis and trauma: a prospective randomized double blind trial. Br J Surg 1990;77:924–929.

87. Schena F, Guerrini F, Tregnaghi P, Kayser B. Branched-chain amino acid supplementation during trekking at high altitude: the effects on loss of body mass, body composition, and muscle power. Eur J Appl Physiol 1992;65:394–398.

88. Bigard AX, Lavier P, Ullmann L, et al. Branched-chain amino acid supplementation during repeated prolonged skiing exercises at altitude. Int J Sports Nutr 1996;6:295–306.

89. Candeloro N, Bertini I, Melchiorri G, De Lorenzo A. Effects of prolonged administration of branched-chain amino acids on body composition and physical fitness. Minerva Endocrinol 1995;20:217–223.

90. Mourier A, Bigard AX, de Kerviler E, et al. Combined effects of caloric restriction and branched-chain amino acid supplementation on body composition and exercise performance in elite wrestlers. Int J Sports Med 1997;18:47–55.

91. Blomstrand E, Newsholme EA. Effect of branched-chain amino acid supplementation on the exercise-induced change in aromatic amino acid concentration in human muscle. Acta Physiol Scand 1992;146:293–298.

92. MacLean DA, Graham TE, Saltin B. Branched-chain amino acids augment ammonia metabolism while attenuating protein breakdown during exercise. Am J Physiol 1994;267:E1010–E1022.

93. Blomstrand E, Andersson S, Hassmen P, et al. Effect of branched-chain amino acid and carbohydrate supplementation on the exercise-induced change in plasma and muscle concentration of amino acids in human subjects. Acta Physiol Scand 1995;153:87–96.

94. Blomstrand E, Ek S, Newsholme EA. Influence of ingesting a solution of branched-chain amino acids on plasma and muscle concentrations of amino acids during prolonged submaximal exercise. Nutrition 1996;12:485–490.

95. Freyssenet D, Berthon P, Denis C, et al. Effect of a 6-week endurance training programme and branched-chain amino acid supplementation on histomorphometric characteristics of aged human muscle. Arch Physiol Biochem 1996;104:157–162.

96. Van Koevering M, and S Nissen. Oxidation of leucine and a-ketoisocaproate to b-hydroxy-b-methylbutyrate in vivo. Am J Physiol 1992;262:E27–E31.

97. Chua BH. Specificity of leucine effect on protein degradation in perfused rat heart. J Mol Cell Card 1994;26:743–751.

98. Torres N, Tovar AR, Harper AE. Leucine affects the metabolism of valine by isolated perfused rat hearts: relation to branched-chain amino acid antagonism. J Nutr 1995;125:1884–1893.

99. McDowell HE, Christie GR, Stenhouse G, Hundal HS. Leucine activates system A amino acid transport in L6 rat skeletal muscle cells. Am J Physiol 1995;269:C1287–C1294.

100. Zawalich WS. Time-dependent potentiation of insulin release induced by alpha-ketoisocaproate and leucine in rats: possible involvement of phosphoinositide hydrolysis. Diabetologia 1988;31:435–442.

101. Pell JM, Caldarone EM, Bergman EN. Leucine and alpha-ketoisocaproate metabolism and interconversions in fed and fasted sheep. Metab Clin Exp 1986;35:1005–1016.

102. Harper AE, Benjamin E. Relationship between intake and rate of oxidation of leucine and alpha-ketoisocaproate in vivo in the rat. J Nutr 1984;114:431–40.

103. Istfan NW, Ling PR, Bistrian BR, Blackburn GL. Systemic exchangeability of enteral leucine: relationship to plasma flux. Am J Physiol 1988; 254: R688–R698.

104. Yu YM, Young VR, Tompkins RG, Burke JF. Comparative evaluation of the quantitative utilization of parenterally and enterally administered leucine and L-[1-13C,15N]leucine within the whole body and the splanchnic region. JPEN 1995;19:209–215.

105. Papet I, Glomot F, Grizard J, Arnal M. Leucine excess under conditions of low or compensated aminoacidemia does not change skeletal muscle and whole-body protein synthesis in suckling lambs during postprandial period. J Nutr 1992;122:2307–2315.

106. Helland SJ, Ewan RC, Trenkle A, Nissen S. In vivo metabolism of leucine and alpha-ketoisocaproate in the pig: influence of dietary glucose or sucrose. J Nutr 1986;116:1902–1909.

107. Oh HY, Fadda GZ, Smogorzewski M, et al. Abnormal leucine-induced insulin secretion in chronic renal failure. Am J Physiol 1994;267:F853–F860.

108. Mitch WE, Walser M, Sapir DG. Nitrogen sparing induced by leucine compared with that induced by its keto analogue, alpha-ketoisocaproate, in fasting obese man. J Clin Invest 1981;67:553–562.

109. Sapir DG, Stewart PM, Walser M, et al. Effects of alpha-ketoisocaproate and of leucine on nitrogen metabolism in postoperative patients. Lancet 1982;1(8332):1010–1014.

110. Mendell JR, Griggs RC, Moxley RT, et al. Clinical investigation in Duchenne muscular dystrophy: IV. Double blind controlled trial of leucine. Muscle Nerve 1984;7:535–541.

111. Millikan WJ Jr, Henderson JM, Galloway JR et al. In vivo measurement of leucine metabolism with stable isotopes in normal subjects and in those with cirrhosis fed conventional and branched-chain amino acid-enriched diets. Surgery 1985;98:405–413.

112. Essen P, Heys SD, Garlick P, Wernerman J. The separate and combined effect of leucine and insulin on muscle free amino acids. Clin Physiol 1994;14(5):513–525.

113. Mero A, Pitkanen H, Oja SS, et al. Leucine supplementation and serum amino acids, testosterone, cortisol and growth hormone in male power athletes during training. J Sports Med Phys Fitness 1997;37:137–145.

114. Mori E, Hasebe M, Kobayashi K. Metabolic effect of short-term total parenteral nutrition highly enriched with leucine or valine in rats recovering from severe trauma. JPEN 1992;16:236–240.

115. Satoh T, Narisawa K, Tazawa Y, et al. Dietary therapy in a girl with propionic acidemia: supplement with leucine resulted in catch up growth. Tohoku J Exp Med 1983;139:411–415.

116. Chevalier P, Aschkenasy A. Hematological and immunological effects of excess dietary leucine in the young rat. Am J Clin Nutr 1977;30:1645–1654.

117. Nishihira T, Takagi T, Mori S. Leucine and manifestation of antitumor activity by valine-depleted amino acid imbalance. Nutrition 1993;9:146–152.

118. Wendel U, Langenbeck U. Intracellular levels and metabolism of leucine and alpha-ketoisocaproate in normal and maple syrup urine disease fibroblasts. Biochem Med 1984;31:294–302.

119. Miller RH, Harper AE. Regulation of valine and alpha-ketoisocaproate metabolism in rat kidney mitochondria. Am J Physiol 1988;255:E475–E481.

120. Mitch WE, Chan W. Alpha-ketoisocaproate stimulates branched-chain amino acid transaminase in kidney and muscle. Am J Physiol 1979;236:E514–E518.

121. Lembert N, Idahl LA. Alpha-ketoisocaproate is not a true substrate for ATP production by pancreatic beta-cell mitochondria. Diabetes 1998;47:339–344.

122. Leclercq-Meyer V, Marchand J, Leclercq R, Malaisse WJ. Calcium deprivation enhances glucagon release in the presence of 2-ketoisocaproate. Endocrinology 1981;108:2093–2097.

123. Welsh M, Hellerstrom C, Andersson A. Respiration and insulin release in mouse pancreatic islets: effects of L-leucine and 2-ketoisocaproate in combination with D-glucose and L-glutamine. Biochem Biophys Acta 1982;721:178–184.

124. Welsh M, Brunstedt J, Hellerstrom C. Effects of D-glucose, L-leucine, and 2-ketoisocaproate on insulin mRNA levels in mouse pancreatic islets. Diabetes 1986;35:228–231.

125. Ashcroft FM, Ashcroft SJ, Harrison DE. Effects of 2-ketoisocaproate on insulin release and single potassium channel activity in dispersed rat pancreatic beta-cells. J Physiol 1987;385:517–529.

126. Branstrom R, Efendic S, Berggren PO, Larsson O. Direct inhibition of the pancreatic beta-cell ATP-regulated potassium channel by alpha-ketoisocaproate. J Biol Chem 1998;273:14113–14118.

127. Best L. Glucose and alpha-ketoisocaproate induce transient inward currents in rat pancreatic beta cells. Diabetologia 1997;40:1–6.

128. Abumrad NN, Wise KL, Williams PE, et al Disposal of alpha-ketoisocaproate: roles of liver, gut, and kidneys. Am J Physiol 1982;243:E123–E131.

129. Harper AE, Benjamin E. Relationship between intake and rate of oxidation of leucine and alpha-ketoisocaproate in vivo in the rat. J Nutr 1984;114:431–440.

130. Kang CW, Walser M. Nutritional efficiency of alpha-ketoisocaproate relative to leucine, assessed isotopically. Am J Physiol 1985;249:E355–E3559.

131. Kang CW, Tungsanga K, Walser M. Effect of the level of dietary protein on the utilization of alpha-ketoisocaproate for protein synthesis. Am J Clin Nutr 1986;43:504–509.

132. Imura K, Shiota T, Swain LM, Walser M. Utilization for protein synthesis of 2-ketoisocaproate relative to utilization of leucine, as estimated from exhalation of labeled CO2. Clin Sci 1988;75:301–307.

133. Munoz S, Walser M. Effect of experimental liver disease on the utilization for protein synthesis of orally administered alpha-ketoisocaproate. Hepatology 1986;6:472–476.

134. Pell JM, Caldarone EM, Bergman EN. Leucine and alpha-ketoisocaproate metabolism and interconversions in fed and fasted sheep. Metab Clin Exper 1986;35:1005–1016.

135. Shiota T, Yagi M, Walser M. Utilization for protein synthesis in individual rat organs of extracellular 2-ketoisocaproate relative to utilization of extracellular leucine. Metab Clin Exper 1989;38:612–618.

136. Yagi M, Matthews DE, Walser M. Nitrogen sparing by 2-ketoisocaproate in parenterally fed rats. Am J Physiol 1990;259:E633–E638.

137. Flakoll PJ, VandeHaar MJ, Kuhlman G, Nissen S. Influence of alpha-ketoisocaproate on lamb growth, feed conversion, and carcass composition. J Anim Sci 1991;69:1461–1467.

138. Mitch WE, Walser M, Sapir DG. Nitrogen sparing induced by leucine compared with that induced by its keto analogue, alpha-ketoisocaproate, in fasting obese man. J Clin Invest 1981;67:553–562.

139. Dalton RN, Chantler C. Metabolism of orally administered branched-chain alpha-keto acids. Kidney Int Suppl 1983;15:511–515.

140. Sapir DG, Stewart PM, Walser M, et al. Effects of alpha-ketoisocaproate and of leucine on nitrogen metabolism in postoperative patients. Lancet 1983;1(8332):1010–1014.

141. Sandstedt S, Jorfeldt L, Larsson J. Randomized, controlled study evaluating effects of branched chain amino acids and alpha-ketoisocaproate on protein metabolism after surgery. Br J Surg 1992;79:217–220.

142. Kuhlman G, Roth JA, Flakoll PJ, et al. Effects of dietary leucine, alpha-ketoisocaproate and isovalerate on antibody production and lymphocyte blastogenesis in growing lambs. J Nutr 1988;118:1564–1569.

143. Kuhlman G, Roth J, Nissen S. Effects of alpha-ketoisocaproate on adrenocorticotropin-induced suppression of lymphocyte function in sheep. Am J Vet Res 1991;52:388–392.

144. McKenna MC, Sonnewald U, Huang X, et al. Alpha-ketoisocaproate alters the production of both lactate and aspartate from [U-13C]glutamate in astrocytes: a 13C NMR study. J Neurochem 1998;70:1001–1008.

145. Dibner JJ, Ivey FJ. Hepatic protein and amino-acid metabolism in poultry. Poultry Sci 1990;69:1188–1194.

146. Van Koevering M, Nissen S. Oxidation of leucine and a-ketoisocaproate to b-hydroxy-b-methylbutyrate in vivo. Am J Physiol 1992;262:E27–E31.

147. Burke ER. Nutritional ergogenic aids. In: Berning, JR, Steen SN, eds. Nutrition for Sport and Exercise. 2nd ed. Gaithersburg, MD: Aspen Publishers, 1998:119–142.

148. Kreider R. Dietary supplements and the promotion of muscle growth with resistance exercise. Sports Med 1999;27:97–110.

149. Passwater RA, Fuller J Jr. Building Muscle Mass, Performance and Health with HMB. New Canaan, CT: Keats Publishing, 1997.

150. Dibner JJ. Utilization of supplemental methionine sources by primary cultures of chick hepatocytes. J Nutr 1983;113:2116–2123.

151. Dibner JJ, Knight CD. Conversion of 2-hydroxy-4-(methylthio)butanoic acid to L-methionine in the chick: a stereospecific pathway. J Nutr 1984;114:1716–1723.

152. Knight CD, Atwell CA, Wuelling CW, et al. The relative effectiveness of 2-hydroxy-4-(methylthio) butanoic acid and DL-methionine in young swine. J Anim Sci 1998;76:781–787.

153. Saunderson CL. Comparative metabolism of L-methionine, DL-methionine and DL-2-hydroxy 4-methylthiobutanoic acid by broiler chicks. Br J Nutr 1985;54:621–633.

154. Damron BL, Flunker LK. 2-Hydroxy-4 (methylthio) butanoic acid as a drinking water supplement for broiler chicks. Poultry Sci 1992;71:1695–1699.

155. Van Koevering MT, Dolezal HG, Gill DR, et al. Effects of beta-hydroxy-beta-methyl butyrate on performance and carcass quality of feedlot steers. J Anim Sci 1994;72:1927–1935.

156. Nissen S, Faidley TD, Zimmerman DR, et al. Colostral milk fat percentage and pig performance are enhanced by feeding the leucine metabolite beta-hydroxy-beta-methyl butyrate to sows. J Anim Sci 1994;72:2331–2337.

157. Nissen S, Fuller JC Jr, Sell J, et al. The effect of beta-hydroxy-beta-methylbutyrate on growth, mortality, and carcass qualities of broiler chickens. Poultry Sci 1994;73:137–155.

158. Papet I, Ostaszewski P, Glomot F, et al. The effect of a high dose of 3-hydroxy-3-methylbutyrate on protein metabolism in growing lambs. Br J Nutr 1997;77:885–896.

159. Nissen S, Sharp R, Ray M, et al. Effect of leucine metabolite beta-hydroxy-beta-methylbutyrate on muscle metabolism during resistance-exercise training. J Appl Physiol 1996;81:2095–2104.

160. Smith G. Whey protein. World Rev Nutr Diet 1976;24:88–116.

161. Smithers GW, Ballard FJ, Copeland AD et al. New opportunities from the isolation and utilization of whey proteins. J Dairy Sci 1996;79:1454–1459.

162. O'Sullivan AC Delaney RAM. Whey products—established and new. Food Progress 1972;5:1.

163. Morr CV, Swenson PE, Richter RL. Functional characteristics of whey protein concentrates. J Food Sci 1973;38:324.

164. Kar T, Misra AK. Effect of fortification of concentrated whey on growth of Kluyveromyces sp. Rev Argent Microbiol 1998;30:163–169.

165. Petschow BW, Talbott RD. Growth promotion of Bifidobacterium species by whey and casein fractions from human and bovine milk. J Clin Microbiol 1990;28:287–292.

166. Lammers BP, Heinrichs AJ, Aydin A. The Effect of whey protein concentrate or dried skim milk in milk replacer on calf performance and blood metabolites. J Dairy Sci 1998;81:1940–1945.

167. Mee J, O'Farrell K, Reitsma P, Mehra R. Effect of a whey protein concentrate used as a colostrum substitute on calf immunity, weight gain, and health. J Dairy Sci 1996;79:886–894.

168. Seymour WM, Nocek JE, Siciliano-Jones J. Effects of a colostrum substitute and of dietary Brewer's yeast on the health and performance of dairy calves. J Dairy Sci 1995;78:412–420.

169. Mochizuki H, Trocki O, Dominioni L, Alexander JW. Effect of a diet rich in branched chain amino acids on severely burned guinea pigs. J Trauma 1986;26:1077–1085.

170. Poullain M-G, Cezard J-P, Marche C, et al. Dietary whey proteins and their peptides or amino acids: effects on the jejunal mucosa of starved rats. Am J Clin Nutr 1989;49:71–76.

171. Poullain M-G, Cezard J-P, Roger L, Mendy F. Effect of whey proteins, their oligopeptide hydrolysates and free amino acid mixtures on growth and nitrogen balance in fed and starved rats. JPEN 1989;13:382–386.

172. Garlick PJ, McNurlan MA, Ballmer PE. Influence of dietary protein intake on whole-body protein turnover in humans. Diabetes Care 1991;14:1189–1198.

173. Boirie Y, Gachon P, Corney S, et al. Acute postprandial changes in leucine metabolism as assessed with an intrinsically labeled milk protein. Am J Physiol 1996;34:E1083–E1091.

174. Motil KJ, Matthews, DE, Bier DM, et al. Whole-body leucine and lysine metabolism: response to dietary protein intake in young men. Am J Physiol 1981;240:E712–E721.

175. Tessari P, Pehling G, Nissen SL, et al. Regulation of whole body leucine metabolism with insulin during mixed meal absorption in normal and diabetic humans. Diabetes 1988;37:512–519.

176. Boirie Y, Dangin M, Gachon P, et al. Slow and fast dietary proteins differently modulate postprandial protein accretion. Proc Natl Acad Sci USA 1997;94:14930–14935.

177. Bounous G, Baruchel S, Falutz J, Gold P. Whey proteins as a food supplement in HIV-seropositive individuals. Clin Invest Med 1993;16:204–209.

178. Kennedy R, Konok G, Bounous G, et al. The use of a whey protein concentrate in the treatment of patients with metastatic carcinoma: a phase I-II clinical study. Anticancer Res 1995;5:2643–2650.

179. Canciani M, Mastella G. Absorption of a new semielemental diet in infants with cystic fibrosis. J Pediatr Gastroenterol Nutr 1985;4: 735–740.

180. Charlton CP; Buchanan E; Holden CE, et al. intensive enteral feeding in advanced cirrhosis: reversal of malnutrition without precipitation of hepatic encephalopathy. Arch Dis Child 1992;67: 603–607.

181. Swaisgood HE, Catignani GL. Digestibility of modified milk proteins: nutritional implications. J Dairy Sci 1985;68:2782–2790.

182. Silk DB, Clark ML, Marrs TC, et al. Jejunal absorption of an amino acid mixture simulating casein and an enzymic hydrolysate of casein prepared for oral administration to normal adults. Br J Nutr 1975;33:95–100.

183. Jenkin HM, Yang TK, LE Anderson. The effect of partially hydrolyzed casein on the growth of human skin diploid cells. Proc Soc Exp Biol Med 1979;160:59–62.

184. Reecy JM, Williams JE, Kerley MS, et al. The effect of postruminal amino acid flow on muscle cell proliferation and protein turnover. J Anim Sci 1996;74:2158–2169.

185. James KAC, Treloar BP. Incorporation of [14C]leucine into protein of perfused liver of rats fed diets containing casein or lactalbumin. J Nutr 1981;1797–1804.

186. Nam TJ, Noguchi T, Funabiki R, et al. Correlation between the urinary excretion of acid-soluble peptides, fractional synthesis rate of whole body proteins, and plasma immunoreactive insulin-like growth factor-1/somatomedin C concentration in the rat. Br J Nutr 1990;63:515–520.

187. Binoux M, Lassarre C, Hardouin N. Somatomedin production by rat liver in organ culture: III. Studies on the release of insulin-like growth factor and its carrier protein measured by radioligand assays. Acta Endocrinol 1982;99:422–430.

188. Reeves RD, Dickinson L, Lee J, et al. Effects of dietary composition on somatomedin activity in growing rats. J Nutr 1979;109: 613–620.

189. Miura Y, Kato H, Noguchi T. Effect of dietary proteins on insulin-like growth factor-1 (IGF-1) messenger ribonucleic acid content in rat liver. Br J Nutr 1992;67:257–265.

190. Gluckman PD, Barry TN. Relationships between plasma concentrations of placental lactogen, insulin-like growth factors, metabolites and lamb size in late gestation ewes subject to nutritional supplementation and in their lambs at birth. Dom Anim Endocrinol 1988;5:209–217.

191. Ragland-Gray KK, Amos HE, McCann MA, et al. Nitrogen metabolism and hormonal responses of steers fed wheat silage and infused with amino acids or casein. J Anim Sci 1997;75(11):3038–3045.

192. Takenaka A, Takahashi S, Noguchi T. Effect of protein nutrition on insulin-like growth factor-I (IGF-I) receptor in various tissues of rats. J Nutr Sci Vit 1996;42:347–357.

193. Kimura T, Murakawa Y, Ohno M, et al. Gastrointestinal absorption of recombinant human insulin-like growth factor-I in rats. J Pharm Exp Therap 1997;283:611–618.

194. Xian CJ, Shoubridge CA, Read LC. Degradation of IGF-I in the adult rat gastrointestinal tract is limited by a specific antiserum or the dietary protein casein. J Endocrinol 1995;146:215–225.

195. Daniel H, Vohwinkel M, Rehner G. Effect of casein and b-casomorphins on gastrointestinal motility in rats. J Nutr 1990;120: 252–257.

196. Moloney AP, Beermann DH, Gerrard D, et al. Temporal change in skeletal muscle IGF-I mRNA abundance and nitrogen metabolism responses to abomasal casein infusion in steers. J Anim Sci 1998; 76:1380–1388.

197. Silk DB, Marrs TC, Addison JM, et al. Absorption of amino acids from an amino acid mixture simulating casein and a tryptic hydrolysate of casein in man. Clin Sci Mol Med 1973;45:715–719.

198. Ljungqvist BG. Plasma amino acid response to single test meals in humans: I. A background review. Res Exp Med (Berl) 1978;174:1–12.

199. Hubbard RW, Sanchez A. Dietary protein control of serum cholesterol by insulin and glucagon. Monogr Atheroscler 1990;16:139–147.

200. Mahe S, Roos N, Benamouzig R, et al. Gastrojejunal kinetics and the digestion of [15N]B-lactoglobulin and casein in humans: the influence of the nature and quantity of the protein. Am J Clin Nutr 1996;63:546–552.

201. Boirie Y, Dangin M, Gachon P, et al. Slow and fast dietary proteins differently modulate postprandial protein accretion. Proc Natl Acad Sci USA 1997;94:14930–14935.

202. Collin-Vidal C, Cayol M, Obled C, et al. Leucine kinetics are different during feeding with whole protein or oligopeptides. Am J Physiol 1994;30:E907–E914.

203. Fok TF, So LY, Lee NN. Late metabolic acidosis and poor weight gain in moderately pre-term babies fed with a casein-predominant formula: a continuing need for caution. Ann Trop Paediatr 1989;9: 243–247.

204. Sampson HA, Bernhisel-Broadbent J, Yang E, Scanlon SM. Safety of casein hydrolysate formula in children with cow milk allergy. J Pediatr 1991;118:520–525.

205. Saylor JD, Bahna SL. Anaphylaxis to casein hydrolysate formula. J Pediatr 1991;118:71–74.

206. Hermus RJ, West CE, van Weerden EJ. Failure of dietary-casein-induced acidosis to explain the hypercholesterolemia of casein-fed rabbits. J Nutr 1983;113:618–629.

207. Scholz KE, Beynen AC, West CE. Regression of casein and cholesterol-induced hypercholesterolaemia in rabbits. Z Ernahrungswiss 1983;22:85–96.

208. Terpstra AH, Van Tintelen G, West CE. The effect of semipurified diets containing different proportions of either casein or soybean protein on the concentration of cholesterol in whole serum, serum lipoproteins and liver in male and female rats. Atherosclerosis 1982;42:85–95.

209. Van der Meer R, De Vries HT, Van Tintelen G. The phosphorylation state of casein and the species-dependency of its hypercholesterolaemic effect. Br J Nutr 1988;59:467–473.

210. Corpet DE, Chatelin-Pirot V. Cooked casein promotes colon cancer in rats, may be because of mucosal abrasion. Cancer Lett 1997;114: 89–90.

211. Corpet DE, Stamp D, Medline A, et al. Promotion of colonic microadenoma growth in mice and rats fed cooked sugar or cooked casein and fat. Cancer Res 1990;50:6955–6958.

212. Zhang XM, Stamp D, Minkin S, et al. Promotion of aberrant crypt foci and cancer in rat colon by thermolyzed protein. J Natl Cancer Inst 1992;84:1026–1030.

213. Anastasia JV, Braun BL, Smith KT. General and histopathological results of a two-year study of rats fed semi-purified diets containing casein and soya protein. Food Chem Toxicol 1990;28:147–156.

214. Nilausen K, Meinertz H. Lipoprotein (a) and dietary proteins: casein lowers lipoprotein (a) concentrations as compared to soy protein. Am J Clin Nutr 1999;69:419–425.

215. Kitts DD. Bioactive substances in food. Can J Physiol Pharmaol 1994;72:424–434.

216. Grosvenor CE, Picciano MF, Baumracker CR. Hormones and growth factors in milk. Endo Rev 1993;14:710–728.

217. Belford DA, Rogers ML, Regester GO, et al. Milk-derived growth factors as serum supplements for the growth of fibroblast and epithelial cells. In Vitro Cell Dev Biol Anim 1995;31:752–760.

218. Petschow BW, Talbott RD. Growth promotion of Bifidobacterium species by whey and casein fractions from human and bovine milk. J Clin Micro 1990;28:287–292.

219. Petschow BW, Talbott RD. Response of bifidobacterium species to growth promoters in human and cow milk. Pediatr Res 1991; 29:208–213.

220. Talhouk RS, Neiswander RL, Schanbacher FL. Developmental regulation and partial characterization of growth factors in the bovine mammary gland. J Reprod Fert 1996;106:221–230.

221. Gale SM, Read LC, George-Nascimento C, et al. Is dietary epidermal growth factor absorbed by premature human infants? Biol Neo 1989;55:104–110.

222. Iacopetta BJ, Grieu F, Horisberger M, Sunahara GI. Epidermal growth factor in human and bovine milk. Acta Paedia 1992;81: 287–291.

223. Belford DA, Rogers ML, Francis GL, et al. Platelet-derived growth factor, insulin-like growth factors, fibroblast growth factors, and transforming growth factor beta do not account for the cell growth activity present in bovine milk. J Endocrinol 1997;154:45–55.

224. Cox DA, Burk RR. Isolation and characterisation of milk growth factor, a transforming-growth-factor-beta 2-related polypeptide, from bovine milk. Eur J Biochem 1991;197:353–358.

225. Rogers ML, Goddard C, Regester GO, et al. Transforming growth factor beta in bovine milk: concentration, stability and molecular mass forms. J Endocrinol 1996;151:77–86.

226. Pakkanen R. Determination of transforming growth factor-beta 2 (TGF-beta 2) in bovine colostrum samples. J Immunol 1998;19: 23–37.

227. Strydom DJ, Bond MD, Vallee BL. An angiogenic protein from bovine serum and milk–purification and primary structure of angiogenin-2. Euro J Bioch 1997;247:535–544.

228. Hashizume S, Kuroda K, Murakami H. Identification of lactoferrin as an essential growth factor for human lymphocytic cell lines in serum-free medium. Biochem Biophys Acta 1983;763:377–382.

229. Kohno Y, Shiraki K, Mura T, Ikawa S. Iron-saturated lactoferrin as a co-mitogenic substance for neonatal rat hepatocytes in primary culture. Acta Paediatr 1993;82:650–655.

230. Shinoda I, Takase M, Fukuwatari Y, Shimamura S. Lactoferrin promotes nerve growth factor synthesis/secretion in mouse fibroblast L-M cells. Adv Exp Med Biol 1994;357:279–285.

231. Rao RK, Baker RD, Baker SS. Bovine milk inhibits proteolytic degradation of epidermal growth factor in human gastric and duodenal lumen. Peptides 1998;19:495–504.

232. Klagsbrun M, Neumann J. The serum-free growth of Balb/c 3T3 cells in medium supplemented with bovine colostrum. J Supra Struct 1979;11:349–359.

233. Kishikawa Y, Watanabe T, Watanabe T, Kubo S. Purification and characterization of cell growth factor in bovine colostrum. J Vet Med Sci 1996;58:47–53.

234. Shing YW, Klagsbrun M. Human and bovine milk contain different sets of growth factors. Endocrinology 1984;115:273–282.

235. Ginjala V, Pakkanen R. Determination of transforming growth factor-beta 1 (TGF-beta 1) and insulin-like growth factor (IGF-1) in bovine colostrum samples. J Immunol 1998;19:195–207.

236. Eppard PJ, Bauman DE, Bitman J, et al. Effect of dose of bovine growth hormone on milk composition: alpha-lactalbumin, fatty acids, and mineral elements. J Dairy Sci 1985;68:3047–3054.

237. Prosser CG, Fleet IR, Corps AN. Increased secretion of insulin-like growth factor I into milk of cows treated with recombinantly derived bovine growth hormone. J Dairy Res 1989;56:17–26.

238. Epstein SS. Unlabeled milk from cows treated with biosynthetic growth hormones: a case of regulatory abdication. Int J Health Serv 1996;26:173–185.

239. Campbell PG, Baumrucker CR. Insulin-like growth factor-I and its association with binding proteins in bovine milk. J Endocrinol 1989;120:21–29.

240. Collier RJ, Miller MA, Hildebrandt JR, et al. Factors affecting insulin-like growth factor-I concentration in bovine milk. J Dairy Sci 1991;74:2905–2911.

241. D'Angio RG. Is there a role for albumin administration in nutrition support? Ann Pharmacother 1994;28:478–482.

242. Mero A, Miikkulainen H, Riski J, et al. Effects of bovine colostrum supplementation on serum IGF-I, IgG, hormone, and saliva IgA during training. J App Phys 1997;83:1144–1151.

243. Wolk A, Mantzoros CS, Andersson SO et al. Insulin-like growth factor I and prostate cancer risk: a population-based, case-control study. J Natl Cancer Inst 1998;90(12):911–915.

244. Chan JM, Stampfer MJ, Giovannucci E et al. Plasma insulin-like growth factor I and prostate cancer risk: a prospective study. Science 1998;279(5350):563–566.

245. DeMichele SJ, Karlstad MD, Babayan VK, et al. Enhanced skeletal muscle and liver protein synthesis with structured lipid in enterally fed burned rats. Metabolism 1988;37:787–795.

246. DeMichele SJ, Karlstad MD, Bistrian BR, et al. Enteral nutrition with structured lipid: effect on protein metabolism in thermal injury. Am J Clin Nutr 1989;50:1295–1302.

247. Maiz A, Yamazaki K, Sobrado J, et al. Protein metabolism during total parenteral nutrition (TPN) in injured rats using medium-chain triglycerides. Metabolism 1984;33:901–909.

248. Mok KT, Maiz A, Yamakazi K, et al. Structured medium-chain and long-chain triglyceride emulsions are superior to physical mixtures in sparing body protein in the burned rat. Metabolism 1984; 33:910–915.

249. Teo TC, DeMichele SJ, Selleck KM, et al. Administration of structured lipid composed of MCT and fish oil reduces net protein catabolism in enterally fed burned rats. Ann Surg 1989;210: 100–107.

250. Yamazaki K, Maiz A, Sobrado J, et al. Hypocaloric lipid emulsions and amino acid metabolism in injured rats. JPEN 1984;8:361–366.

251. Gollaher CJ, Swenson ES, Mascioli EA, et al. Dietary fat level as determinant of protein-sparing actions of structured triglycerides. Nutrition 1992;8:348–353.

252. Stein TP, Yoshida S, Schluter MD, et al. Comparison of intravenous nutrients on gut mucosal proteins synthesis. JPEN 1994;18:447–452.

253. Selleck KJ, Wan JM-F, Gollaher CJ, et al. Effect of low and high amounts of structured lipid containing fish oil on protein metabolism in enterally fed burned rats. Am J Clin Nutr 1994;60:216–222.

254. Sandstrom R, Hyltander A, Korner U, Lundholm K. Structured triglycerides were well tolerated and induced increased whole body fat oxidation compared with long-chain triglycerides in postoperative patients. JPEN 1995;19:381–386.

255. Bach AC, Babayan VK. Medium chain triglycerides: an update. Am J Clin Nutr 1982;36:950–962.

256. Jandecek RJ, Whiteside JA, Holcombe HN, et al. The rapid hydrolysis and efficient absorption of triglycerides with octanoic acid in the 1 and 3 positions and long-chain fatty acid in the 2 position. Am J Clin Nutr 1987;45:940–945.

257. Needleman P, Raz M, Minkes MS, et al. Triene prostaglandins: prostaglandin and thromboxane biosynthesis and unique biologic properties. Proc Natl Acad Sci USA 1979;76:944–948.

258. Baracos V, Rodemann HP, Dinarello CA, et al. Stimulation of muscle protein degradation and prostaglandin E2 release by leukocytic pyrogen (interleukin-1). N Engl J Med 1983;308:553–558.

259. Swails WS, Kenler AS, Driscoll DF, et al. Effect of a fish oil structured lipid-based diet on prostaglandin release from mononuclear cells in cancer patients after surgery. JPEN 1997;21:266–274.

260. Endres S, Ghorbani R, Kelley VE, et al. The effect of dietary supplementation with n-3 polyunsaturated fatty acids on the synthesis of interleukin-1 and tumor necrosis factor by mononuclear cells. N Engl J Med 1989;320:265–271.

261. Berkenbosch F, van Oers J, del Ray A, et al. Corticotropin-releasing factor-producing neurons in the rat activated by interleukin-1. Science 1987;238:524–526.

262. Bernton EW, Beach JE, Holaday JW, Smallridge RC, Fein HG. Release of multiple hormones by a direct action of interleukin-1 on pituitary cells. Science 1987;238:519–521.

263. Curti BD; Urba WJ; Longo DL et al. Endocrine effects of IL-1 alpha and beta administered in a phase I trial to patients with advanced cancer. J Immunother Emphasis Tumor Immunol 1996;19:142–148.

264. Nordenstrom J, Thorne A, Olivecrona T. Metabolic effects of infusion of a structured-triglyceride emulsion in healthy subjects. Nutrition 1995;11:269–274.

265. Sandstrom R, Hyltander A, Korner U, Lundholm K. Structured triglycerides to postoperative patients: a safety and tolerance study. JPEN 1993;17:153–157.

266. Kenler AS, Swails WS, Driscoll DF, et al. Early enteral feeding in postsurgical cancer patients: fish oil structured lipid-based polymeric formula versus a standard polymeric formula. Ann Surg 1996;223:316–333.

267. Hamada K, Matsumoto K, Okamura K, et al. Effect of amino acids and glucose on exercise-induced gut and skeletal muscle proteolysis in dogs. Metab Clin Exp 1999;48:161–166.

268. Biolo G, Tipton KD, Klein S, Wolfe RR. An abundant supply of amino acids enhances the metabolic effect of exercise on muscle protein. Am J Physiol 1997;273:E122–E129.

269. Volpi E, Ferrando AA, Yeckel CW, et al. Exogenous amino acids stimulate net muscle protein synthesis in the elderly. J Clin Invest 1998;101:2000–2007.

270. Hammarqvist F, Wernerman J, von der Decken A, Vinnars E. Alanyl-glutamine counteracts the depletion of free glutamine and

the postoperative decline in protein synthesis in skeletal muscle. Ann Surg 1990;212:637–644.

271. Naka S, Saito H, Hashiguchi Y, et al. Alanyl-glutamine-supplemented total parenteral nutrition improves survival and protein metabolism in rat protracted bacterial peritonitis model. JPEN 1996;20:417–423.

272. Scrimshaw NS, Wayler AH, Murray E, et al. Nitrogen balance response in young men given one of two isolated soy proteins or milk proteins. J Nutr 1983;113:2492–2497.

273. Wayler AH, Queiroz E, Scrimshaw NS, et al. Nitrogen balance studies in young men to assess the protein quality of an isolated soy protein in relation to meat proteins. J Nutr 1983;113:2485–2491.

274. Young VR, Wayler A, Garza C, et al. A long term metabolic balance study in young men to assess the nutritional quality of an isolated soy protein and beef proteins. Am J Clin Nutr 1984;39:8–15.

275. Gausseres N, Catala I, Mahe S, et al. Whole-body protein turnover in humans fed a soy protein-rich vegetable diet. Eur J Clin Nutr 1997;51:308–311.

276. Deutz NE, Bruins MJ, Soeters PB. Infusion of soy and casein protein meals affects interorgan amino acid metabolism and urea kinetics differently in pigs. J Nutr 1998;128:2435–2445.

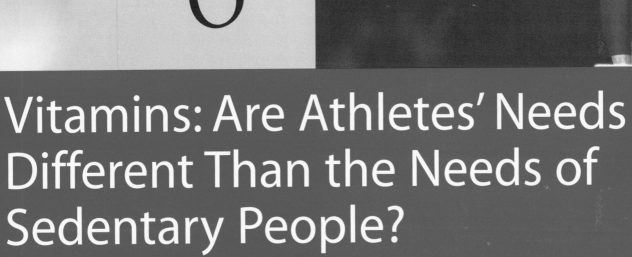

CHAPTER 6

Vitamins: Are Athletes' Needs Different Than the Needs of Sedentary People?

Douglas Kalman

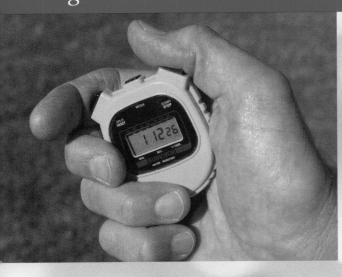

Research Review

Vitamin E—An Anticatabolic Agent?

In a study performed at the German Sport University in Cologne, scientists examined 32 rats that had one of their hindlegs immobilized for 8 days, similar to the way a fractured bone is cast. The other leg was free to move. One group received six intraperitoneal injections of vitamin E in the form of alpha-tocopherol acetate at a dose of 60 mg/kg twice a week. The injections started 2 weeks before the immobilization period. After the treatment period, the animals were sacrificed and their muscles examined.

Levels of oxidative stress were less in the vitamin E group. This supports the role of vitamin E as a potent antioxidant. Muscle fiber measurements of the soleus muscle revealed a 35% decrease in muscle fiber cross-sectional area in the immobilized muscles of animals that did not receive vitamin E. However, the vitamin E–treated group showed only a 12% loss of muscle fiber cross-sectional area.

This study clearly shows that vitamin E plays a role in modulating skeletal muscle mass. In this case, the muscle studied was the predominantly slow-twitch (>90%) soleus muscle. Most muscles in the human body are 50% fast and slow. Would this muscle-protective effect of vitamin E be similar in those muscles that have a greater percentage of fast fibers? Certainly, one should be cautious of over-extrapolating from rodent data to the human condition.

Nevertheless, this study has interesting implications for human athletes (particularly strength-power athletes) who often succumb to injury and have to rest a body part or the entire body for prolonged periods. How much vitamin E should you consume? Right now, scientists do not know the optimal dose for athletes, but many individuals who do not experience any ill effects take doses as high as 200–400 IU per day regularly. Further, you need these doses to attain some degree of cardiovascular disease protection.

Appell HJ, Duarte JA, Soares JM. Supplementation with vitamin E may attenuate skeletal muscle immobilization atrophy. Intern J Sports Med 1997;18:157–160.

Introduction

Whether vitamin needs differ among athletic and sedentary individuals has been an intense area of debate. Coaches, athletes, and parents often search for ways to produce bigger, faster, and stronger athletes. In ancient Greece, this was accomplished by using paidotribes or gymnaste (trainers) and later by the advice of Celcus (24 AD).[1,2]

Celcus has written eight books, which are beautifully detailed in matters of nutrition and exercise. Today, this brings sports nutritionists, trainers, physicians, and exercise physiologists to examine which dietary interventions might produce better performances without impairing health. Some may argue that the different nutritional needs of athletes, although debatable, promote health. From a nutritional standpoint, the basis of health starts with obtaining adequate macronutrient and micronutrient intake. This nutrition is first from food sources, fortified foods second, and then if needed or warranted, from dietary supplements. In essence, the bottom line is whether athletes need a higher intake of any or all of the known vitamins and whether this translates into an improvement in performance or post-exercise recovery.

This chapter will focus on vitamins. Vitamins, initially called *vital amines*, are organic molecules needed in minute quantities. No common molecular structure exists among vitamins. Vitamin intake is often ignored until a deficiency symptom(s) presents itself. Thirteen different vitamins have been characterized and they are divided into two

WATER-SOLUBLE VITAMINS

The water-soluble vitamins are found in bodily fluids; however, they are not stored to any appreciable degree. They act largely as coenzymes that are involved in a host of metabolic reactions (e.g., Krebs cycle, electron transport chain, amino acid metabolism, nucleic acid metabolism, etc.). The water-soluble vitamins are thiamine (B1), riboflavin (B2), pyridoxine (B6), niacin, pantothenic acid, folic acid, biotin, cobalamins, and ascorbic acid (vitamin C).

distinct classes: fat- and water-soluble vitamins. The fat-soluble vitamins are stored within the body's adipose tissue; thus, deficiency symptoms do not occur readily. Water-soluble vitamins, most of which act as coenzymes, are not stored to any great extent. Thus, athletes must be cognizant of consuming a varied diet that provides these vitamins or resort to dietary supplementation.

Thiamin

Thiamin is also known as vitamin B1 or thiamine. Thiamin functions as a component of the coenzyme thiamin pyrophosphate (TPP).[3] At the cellular level, thiamin is important for energy transformation reactions, synthesis of pentoses and NADPH (a coenzyme form of niacin, another B vitamin). Perhaps the most important reaction that thiamin is involved with is the decarboxylation of both pyruvate and α-ketoglutarate. Decarboxylation of pyruvate and α-ketoglutarate is important in producing energy and driving the Krebs cycle forward as well as for the production of fatty acids, cholesterol, and other important compounds. Thiamin is one of the essential cofactors for the production of acetyl-CoA and ultimately the production of adenosine triphosphate (ATP) or energy. Thiamin is a major component of the pyruvate dehydrogenase complex (drives pyruvate into the Krebs cycle as acetyl-CoA). Decarboxylation reactions are also important in amino acid metabolism. Thiamin serves as a cofactor for the production of the keto acid analogues of leucine, isoleucine, and valine. In fact, failure to produce the keto acid analogues of the branched-chain amino acids is known as maple syrup urine disease (MSUD, an inborn error of metabolism).

The synthesis of pentoses is important when considering the hexomonophosphate shunt. This is a pathway where sugars of various carbon lengths are interconverted and NADPH is produced. Pentoses are also used in the production of nucleic acids, whereas NADPH is needed for the synthesis of fatty acids. Furthermore, thiamin is needed for membrane and nerve conduction; however, it is not clear how thiamin functions in regard to nerve conduction.

Sources—Thiamin is widely distributed in foods. Good sources of thiamin are whole grain products, enriched wheat, lean pork, yeast, liver, and nuts. Naturally occurring anti-thiamin factors are present in raw fish but are negated by cooking fish. Thus, these factors are thermolabile. Other foods that contain anti-thiamin factors are tannic and caffeic acids; these are thermostabile and found in coffee, tea, betel nuts, blueberries, black currants, brussel sprouts, and red cabbage. Thiamin destruction can be prevented or reduced if the offending agent is eaten with a food containing vitamin C or citric acid (FIG. 6-1).

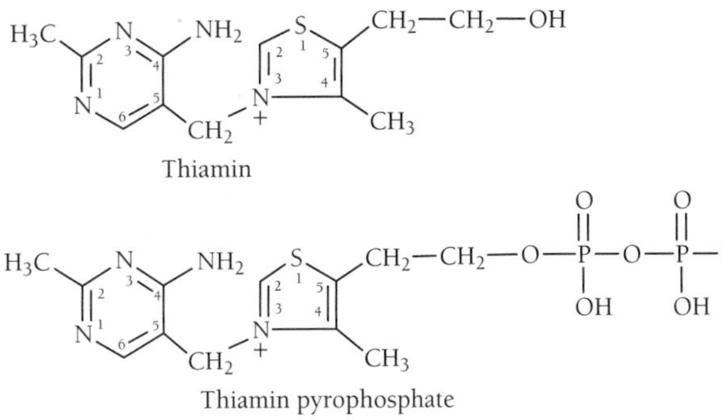

Figure 6-1. The structure of thiamin.

Governmental Recommended Intake—0.5 mg/1000 calories or no less than 1 mg per day.[3] Dietary supplements often contain more than this amount.

Deficiency symptoms—Deficiency is rare. It can occur with long-term extremely low intake or high alcohol intake. The first symptom of deficiency is loss of appetite, progressing to cardiac hypertrophy or dysrhythmia, and neurologic symptoms due to alcoholism (Wernicke's encephalopathy/Wernicke-Korsakoff syndrome). Beriberi (dry, wet, or acute) is a common deficiency identified in older adults.

Human Studies

To date, studies indicate that athletes' intake of thiamin appears to be adequate.[4] However, evidence for an ergogenic effect of thiamin is equivocal. Knippel et al.[5] found that supplementation of 900 mg/day for 3 days enabled trained cyclists to achieve lower blood lactate and heart rate levels during intense exercise. This increase in the lactate threshold was significant. The mechanism(s) for this improvement can be understood because thiamin is one of the cofactors serving as part of the pyruvate dehydrogenase complex (PDHC). PDHC drives the forward reaction of pyruvate to acetyl CoA to produce energy through the Krebs cycle. Theoretically, if less pyruvate is needed for the acetyl CoA product, more may be available for the glucose-alanine cycle and thus less lactate is produced during intense exercise. Studies conducted with pyruvate alone illustrate a possible buffering capacity. However, the current study mentioned above has yet to be replicated.

One could surmise that the need for thiamin might be increased in athletes due to their greater demand for carbohydrates or energy during prolonged endurance events. Because research with pyruvate and dihydroxyacetone (DHA) has shown the benefit for enhancing endurance exercise, future research should examine if a synergy or potentiation of ergogenics can occur by adding thiamin to exogenous pyruvate during intense exercise.

Safety and Toxicity

Toxicity has rarely been seen (with doses as high as 500 times the recommended daily intake).

Is the RDA an Outmoded Term?

Julie J. Bartlett and Ann Grandjean, EdD

In 1941, the Recommended Dietary Allowances, RDAs for short, were created by the Food and Nutrition Board of the National Academy of Sciences. At that time, the primary goal was to prevent diseases caused by nutrient deficiencies. The RDA is the level that is sufficient to meet the nutrient requirements of nearly all (~98%) individuals of a specific age and sex. The foundation for the RDAs is the Estimated Average Requirements, or EAR. The EAR is the level sufficient to meet the requirements of 50% of the individuals of a specific age and sex.

As if that wasn't confusing enough, now we need to learn the AI, the UL, and the DRIs, which are abbreviations for Adequate Intake, Tolerable Upper Intake Level, and Dietary Reference Intakes. Of this pot of alphabet soup, the DRIs are the new way to look at human nutrient requirements. Instead of being concerned primarily about preventing deficiency disease, the DRIs are also aimed at reducing the risk of diet-related chronic conditions such as heart disease, diabetes, hypertension, and osteoporosis. Think of the DRI as an *umbrella* term used to include the EAR, RDA, AI, and UL. The DRIs will include all four values for some nutrients. Why only for *some*? Because the upper limits for some nutrients may not be known. Or, the RDA may not be known. But when there is adequate science, all four values will be determined.

Currently, the Food and Nutrition Board plan to develop DRI reports on seven groups of nutrients. They include the following:

- Calcium, phosphorus, magnesium, vitamin D, and fluoride

- Thiamin, riboflavin, niacin, vitamin B6, folate, vitamin B12, pantothenic acid, biotin, and choline

- Antioxidants such as vitamins C and E, beta-carotene, and selenium

- Macronutrients such as protein, fat, and carbohydrate

- Trace elements such as iron and zinc

- Electrolytes and water

- Other food components such as dietary fiber and phytochemicals

Two reports have been released so far, the group of nutrients related to bone health (calcium, phosphorus, etc.) and the group of B vitamins. For more information on DRIs, go to http://www4.nas.edu/IOM/IOMHome.nsf/Pages/Food+and+Nutrition+Board. To order copies of the reports, call the National Academy Press at 800-624-6242.

So, by now you're asking, "how does this affect me?" "Which number do I use?" Most of us need a standard by which we can evaluate an individual's diet and the RDA is still the one! At least in most cases. For assessment purposes, the EAR, IA, and UL are of limited use without clinical, biochemical, and anthropometric data. So, for those of you working in hospitals or other medical settings, you may find them of value. For those of you working with healthy athletes, fitness clients, or anytime you're evaluating a diet, use the RDA. Nutrients for which an RDA has not been established, use the AI. However, if you have a client that uses a variety of dietary supplements, you may want to check his or her total intake against the UL.

The Nutrition Facts label found on most foods and dietary supplements are values that are still based on Daily Values, which are based on the old RDAs. You just thought you were confused.

One thing in which there is no confusion is the potential *bone health* crisis facing the United States. As shown in the accompanying table, the recommended intake for calcium has been increased significantly for adults. Although to a lesser degree, it has also increased for children and teens. The new calcium levels are important because bones that are calcium rich are less susceptible to fractures.

Dietary Reference Intakes: Selected Recommended Levels for Individual Intakes

Nutrient	Old RDA or ESADDI[a] (25–50 yrs)		New RDA or AI[b] (31–50 yrs)	
	Male	Female	Male	Female
Calcium (mg)	800	800	1000[e]	1000[e]
Phosphorus (mg)	800	800	700	700
Magnesium (mg)	350	280	420	320
Vitamin D (μg)[c]	5	5	5[d]	5[d]
Fluoride (μg)	1.5–4.0[e]	1.5–4.0[e]	4[d]	3[d]
Thiamin (mg)	1.5	1.1	1.2	1.1
Riboflavin (mg)	1.7	1.3	1.3	1.1
Niacin (mg)	19	15	16	14
Vitamin B6 (mg)	2.0	1.6	1.3	1.3
Folate (μg)	200	180	400	400
Vitamin B12 (μg)	2.0	2.0	2.4	2.4
Pantothenic acid (mg)	4–7[e]	4–7[e]	5[d]	5[d]
Biotin (μg)	30–100[e]	30–100[e]	30[d]	30[d]
Choline (μg)	Not determined	Not determined	550[d]	425[d]

[a]RDAs and Estimated Safe and Adequate Daily Dietary Intakes (ESADDIs) published by the Food and Nutrition Board in 1989.
[b]RDA and Adequate Intake (AI) values from the 1997 and 1998 DRI reports.
[c]Vitamin D as cholecalciferol = 400 IU of vitamin D.
[d]AI value.
[e]ESADDI value.

Riboflavin

Riboflavin (vitamin B2) is found in the body as flavin dinucleotide and flavin mononucleotide (FAD and FMN, respectively). Both FAD and FMN play an important role in oxidative enzyme systems, remaining bound to the enzymes during oxidative-reduction reactions. Flavins can act as oxidative agents because they have an ability to accept a pair of hydrogen atoms.

Riboflavin has a broad range of redox potentials and plays a role in intermediary metabolism. Flavoproteins are involved within the electron transport chain in the production of energy. In addition, flavin serves as a coenzyme for fatty acid synthesis, sphingosine synthesis, purine metabolism (via xanthine oxidase) in the liver, vitamin B6 metabolism, synthesis of folate (in its active form of N5-methyl tetrahydrofolate), choline metabolism, dopamine production, and the reduction of glutathione. Because the flavins are integral in numerous energy-producing pathways, they are important for overall energy production (**FIG. 6-2**).

Sources—Dairy products are the richest source of riboflavin. Eggs, meat, and enriched grains also provide riboflavin.

Governmental Recommended Intake—The recommended intake is 0.6 mg/1000 calories or a minimum intake of 1.2 mg/day.[6]

Deficiency symptoms—Deficiency of this vitamin rarely occurs by itself. Clinical symptoms of deficiency include lesions on the outside of the lips (cheilosis) and at the corner of the mouth (angular stomatitis), inflammation of the tongue (glossitis), and other related symptoms. Excretion of riboflavin is enhanced with diabetes, trauma, stress, and the use of oral contraceptive agents.

Human Studies

No conclusive studies have been conducted to date for evaluating possible performance-enhancing effects in healthy athletes. Those who are beginners to exercise have been found to have a reduced or subnormal riboflavin status as measured by erythrocyte glutathione reductase activity (EGRAC). This has also been found in obese healthy subjects.[7,8] It is known that in high ambient temperatures (heated environments) an increase in the rate of riboflavin excretion occurs; therefore, athletes who engage in outdoor sports in warm climates may have increased riboflavin needs. There is also a notion that low riboflavin status may result in hyperexcitability in the muscle, yet no studies have examined the effects of riboflavin on muscle activation.

Safety and Toxicity

No reports on the safety and toxicity of riboflavin have been reported to date.

Niacin

Niacin is actually the name of two compounds, nicotinic acid, and niacinamide. Niacin serves as a precursor to the pyridine nucleotides, which function in energy metabolism. Specifically, the pyridines serve as proton and electron carriers. Niacin also functions as a coenzyme in many oxidative reactions as well as a hydrogen donor for the pentose phosphate pathways. Nicotinic acid is also part of the glucose tolerance factor (along with chromium and glutathione).

Note that over 200 enzymes, which are predominately dehydrogenases, require various forms of niacin for action. These forms, nicotinic acid and niacinamide, are involved with oxidative-reduction reactions, the transfer of electrons to form intermediates within the electron transport chain, and ultimately aid in the production of adenosine triphosphate (ATP). Niacin is involved with glycolysis, β-oxidation of fatty acids, and oxidation of alcohol. In addition, niacin is involved in fatty acid synthesis, cholesterol and steroid hormone synthesis, oxidation of glutamine, indirect reduction of glutathione via glutathione reductase, reduction of vitamin C, the metabolism of folate, protein synthesis, cellular growth and differentiation, and the formation of endogenous tryptophan. Therefore, niacin is an integral part of protein, fat, and carbohydrate metabolism (**FIG. 6-3**).

Sources—The best sources of niacin include tuna, halibut, beef, chicken, and other meats.

Governmental Recommended Intake—Recommended intake for niacin is complicated by the fact that some niacin is derived by the metabolism of the amino acid tryptophan. Niacin requirements are also influenced by protein, energy, pyridoxine (B6), and riboflavin (B2) intake.[9] However, the generally accepted RDI for niacin is 19 mg/day for males and 15 mg/day for females.

Deficiency symptoms—Classic deficiency results in a condition known as pellagra. The signs of pellagra, or

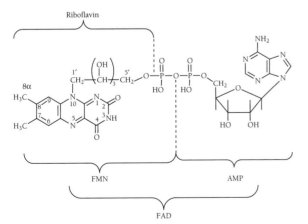

Figure 6-2. The structure of riboflavin.

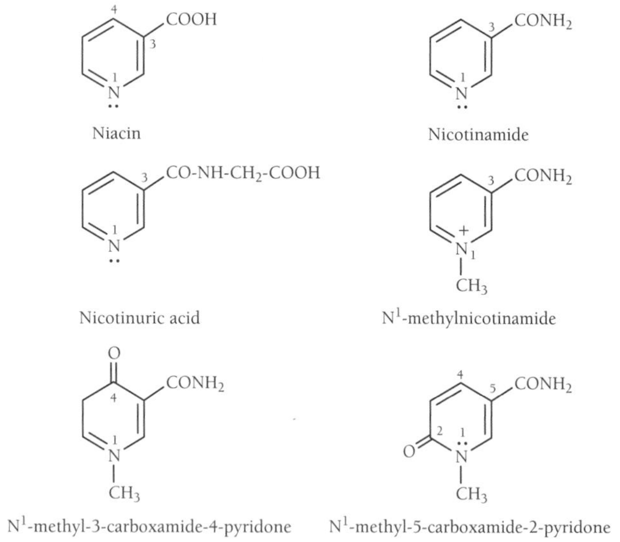

Figure 6-3. The structure of niacin.

advancing deficiency, are dermatitis, dementia, diarrhea, and death. Niacin deficiency can be induced by the anti-tuberculosis medication isoniazid. Malabsorptive conditions can also precipitate a niacin deficiency. In addition, people with stress, trauma, or prolonged fever may have increased niacin needs.[9]

Human Studies

To date, no clear-cut ergogenic benefit has been shown with niacin supplementation. Several studies have indicated that both intravenous and orally ingested niacin can affect free fatty acid (FFA) and muscle glycogen levels during exercise.[10] Some studies demonstrate a lowering of FFA with an increase in the respiratory exchange ratio (RER), indicating relatively greater oxidation of carbohydrates instead of fatty acids. This may not be ideal for prolonged endurance events (e.g., marathon) but it may be of benefit in shorter, more intense aerobic sports (e.g., 1500 meter) that rely predominantly on glycolysis.

Safety and Toxicity

Often, megadoses of nicotinic acid (3 g/day) are used in the treatment of primary hypercholesterolemia. High doses of nicotinic acid can cause abnormal liver function, hyperuricemia, dermatological problems (itching), hyperglycemia, heartburn, nausea, and possibly vomiting. Athletes, particularly bodybuilders, use niacin (nicotinic acid, not niacinamide) to produce vasodilation. Nicotinic acid will cause a release of histamine, which eventually will cause flushing of the skin and improved (temporarily) vascularity. Increasing one's vascularity is thought to be advantageous in bodybuilding competitions.

Pyridoxine

Pyridoxine is also known as vitamin B6. In fact, B6 exists as several vitamers (any one of several compounds that have specific vitamin activity), known as pyridoxal phosphate (PLP), pyridoxamine phosphate (PMP), and pyridoxine phosphate (PNP). These are interchangeable and comparable in their activity. The coenzyme form of B6 is involved with many enzymes. The primary involvement of these enzymes is in protein metabolism. Examples of the interactions with which B6 is involved are transamination, decarboxylation, trans and desulfhydration, cleavage, racemization, and synthesis reactions.[11]

Vitamin B6 is also involved with glycogen and steroid metabolism. Furthermore, it can influence carnitine, histamine, taurine, and dopamine in various metabolic reactions that are mainly neuromodulatory in nature (FIG. 6-4).

Sources—Vitamin B6 and its various vitamers are found in plants, bananas, beans, walnuts, red meat, fish, and chicken. The bioavailability of each vitamer of B6 depends on the processing of that particular food.

Governmental Recommended Intake—The need for vitamin B6 is highly dependent on the level of dietary protein intake. The assumption is that the average male consumes approximately 126 g/day of protein, which translates into needs of 2.0 mg/day of B6. Women tend to take in less protein than men with the upper limit estimated at 100 g/day; the RDI for women is 1.6 mg/day. An intake of 0.02 mg of B6 per gram of protein is sufficient to meet the needs of adults under normal conditions. As the level of dietary protein intake rises, the need for greater B6 intake is generated.

Deficiency symptoms—Deficiency of this vitamin is rare. Groups at risk for B6 deficiency are breast-fed infants, the elderly, people who consume large amounts of alcohol, patients on dialysis, and patients on drug therapy with isoniazid (used for tuberculosis), penicillamine (an antibiotic), corticosteroids (anti-inflammatory), and anticonvulsants (used to treat seizures). For athletes, most of the aforementioned risk factors are not applicable, but warrant the need for awareness. Symptoms of deficiency are sleepiness, fatigue, cheilosis, glossitis, stomatitis, abnormal electrocardiograms, seizures, convulsions, and microcytic anemia.[12] In addition, B6 deficiency will alter calcium and magnesium metabolism and impair niacin synthesis from tryptophan.[13,14]

Human Studies

To date, vitamin B6 supplementation has not been shown to enhance athletic performance. Two studies published in *Medicine in Science, Sports, and Exercise* showed that combining a high-carbohydrate diet with B6 supplementation (8–10 g/day) yields an increase in the use of glycogen stores and a decrease in resting and exercise levels of

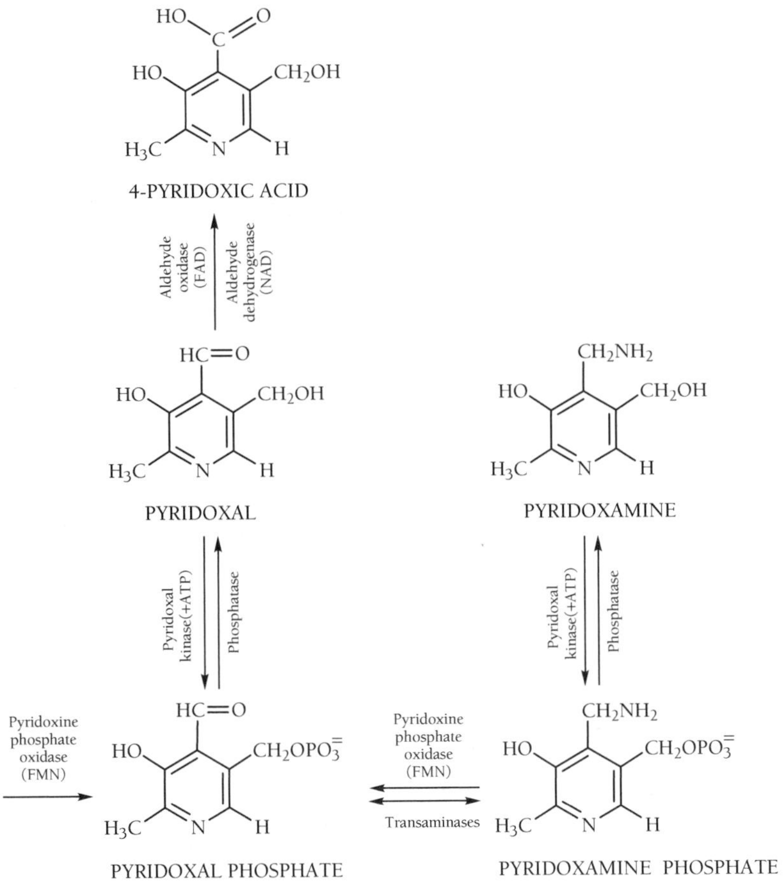

Figure 6-4. The structure of pyridoxine.

FFA.[15,16] This may have implications in athletes who compete in events that use the lactic acid or glycolytic energy systems (e.g., 800-meter run). Other research has indicated a growth hormone potentiating factor by B6 supplementation; this may be beneficial for improving body composition.[17] In a more recent study, researchers found that vitamin B6 (20 mg/day) can alter plasma free fatty acid and amino acid concentrations during exhaustive endurance exercise without affecting endurance.[18] Future research should elucidate the role of B6 supplementation on anaerobic metabolism and exercise performance during high-intensity exercise.

Safety and Toxicity

Toxicity or side effects of megadosing on B6 are seen when ingesting greater than 2 g daily. Recall that the RDI is 2.0 mg/day for males and 1.6 mg/day for females. Two grams is 2000 times the recommended dose! Side effects that are commonly seen with overzealous intake of B6 include unsteady gait, numbness of the hands and feet, impaired tendon reflexes, paresthesia, possible degeneration of the dorsal root ganglia in the spinal cord, loss of myelination, and possible degeneration of sensory fibers in the periphery.[14,19]

Vitamin B12 (Cobalamins)

Functions—Three main enzymatic reactions requiring vitamin B12 have been noted to occur in humans. The first reaction requires methylcobalamin as a coenzyme in the conversion of homocysteine into methionine. This reaction occurs in the cytosol of the cell. The reaction is intrinsic to the production of tetrahydrofolate (THF). The production of THF is irreversible and requires vitamin B12; therefore, a B12 deficiency can trap folate in its methyl form (also known as the folate-methyl trap), which in turn affects purine and thymidylate synthesis.

A second set of reactions requiring B12 are those catalyzed by mutases. These reactions occur within the mitochondria. These include the production of succinyl CoA, a Krebs cycle intermediate. Mutase enzymes are also intrinsic in the oxidation of fatty acids. A defect in mutase activity results in impaired muscle activity and an accumulation of methylmalonyl CoA and methylmalonic acid. The branched-chain amino acid leucine is also catalyzed by a mutase enzyme. Specifically, leucine undergoes isomerization, requiring adenosylcobalamin (FIG. 6-5).

Sources—The only dietary sources of vitamin B12 are animal products. Plants and legumes are not good sources

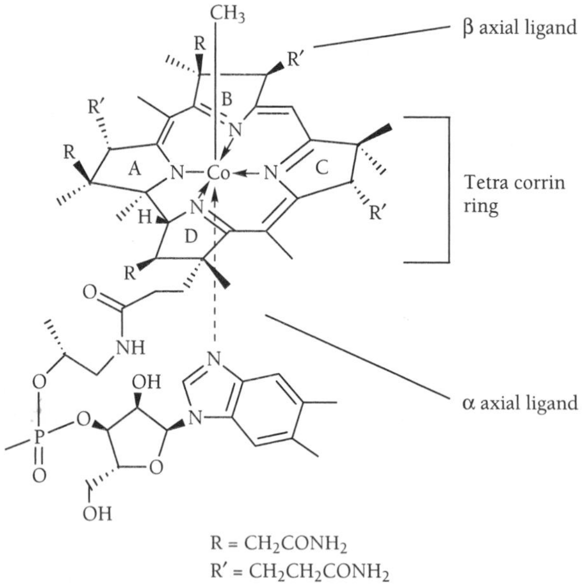

R = CH$_2$CONH$_2$
R' = CH$_2$CH$_2$CONH$_2$

Figure 6-5. The structure of vitamin B12.

of vitamin B12, but may contain small quantities of B12 due to contamination with microorganisms during harvesting. Cobalamins are found in meat, meat products, poultry, fish, clams, oysters, and eggs. The bioavailability of the cobalamins depends on which form they are found in.

Governmental Recommended Intake—Two micrograms daily is the recommended daily intake for vitamin B12. Doses of vitamin C that are greater than 500 mg and taken within 1 hour of eating a meal may impair B12 absorption.[20]

Deficiency symptoms—More than 95% of the B12 deficiencies diagnosed are related to inadequate absorption rather than inadequate dietary intake. Vitamin B12 deficiency occurs in stages of which changes within the cells and blood are primary. Vitamin B12 deficiency later results in megaloblastic anemia (this can also be caused by folate deficiency; therefore, it is best to treat with a combination of B12 and folate). Signs of progressive B12 deficiency include neuropathy, characterized by demyelination of nerves, and hyperhomocystinemia. The populations at greatest risk for a B12 deficiency do not include athletes, but rather the elderly, alcoholics, gastrectomy patients, and strict vegetarians (vegans).

Human Studies

In the late 1980s a popular dietary supplement known as Dibencozide (a coenzyme of vitamin B12) was purported to have *steroid-like properties*. This was anecdotal and was never confirmed by research. Bodybuilders have also been known to use the injectable cyanocobalamin as a stimulant for appetite and muscle gain. This was due to the misunderstood role that B12 has in red blood cell and protein synthesis. To date, there has not been a reputable study illustrating an ergogenic effect of vitamin B12 or any of its cobalamin forms.

Safety and Toxicity

Not one case has been reported on toxicity from excess intake of vitamin B12.

Pantothenic Acid

Functions—Pantothenic acid is a vitamin whose primary function is as a component of coenzymeA (CoA). In fact, CoA is synthesized from pantothenic acid (pantothenate). This reaction requires pantothenic acid, cysteine, and adenosine triphosphate (ATP). This vitamin and coenzyme is essential for the production of energy from carbohydrate, fat, and protein. One should think of pantothenic acid and CoA as one and the same. CoA is needed for many reactions including the formation of thio esters, activation of acids (acetic, malonic, propionic, etc.), and the production of heme (along with vitamin B6 and glycine).

Within energy metabolism, acetyl CoA holds major prominence. Acetyl CoA is formed via condensation along with oxaloacetate to introduce acetate for oxidation in the Krebs cycle. Also, acetyl CoA via a condensation reaction with carbon dioxide forms malonyl CoA, the first step in fatty acid synthesis. Other reactions for which pantothenic acid is important include the formation of β-hydroxy-β-methylglutaryl CoA (HMG-CoA), cholesterol, phospholipids, sphingomyelin, and ketones. Furthermore, pantothenic acid is also used in the production and modification of proteins via an acetylation process (FIG. 6-6).[21]

Sources—Pantothenic acid is widely distributed in many foods, making a deficiency highly unlikely. Meats, liver, egg yolks, legumes, whole grain cereals, and vegetables are all good sources of this vitamin. An interesting dietary supplement or a delicacy to some, royal jelly is another good source of pantothenate.

Governmental Recommended Intake—The government does not recommend a specific amount, but it is generally regarded as safe and adequate to ingest 4–7 mg/day.

Deficiency symptoms—Reports of deficiency are noted in the literature. Symptoms such as altered sensations (hot/cold) in the lower legs and feet (known as *burning feet syndrome*), as well as vomiting, fatigue, and weakness are common in pantothenic acid deficiency. Conditions that are conducive to promoting this vitamin deficiency include alcoholism, diabetes, irritable bowel syndrome, and other gastrointestinal disorders.

Human Studies

Because pantothenic acid is intrinsic in the formation of acetyl CoA (CoA), one might think that athletes might get a performance benefit from supplementing with this vitamin. For instance, supplementing with pantothenate during times of stress (e.g., surgery) enhances recovery time by increasing cellular multiplication.[22] Enhancing

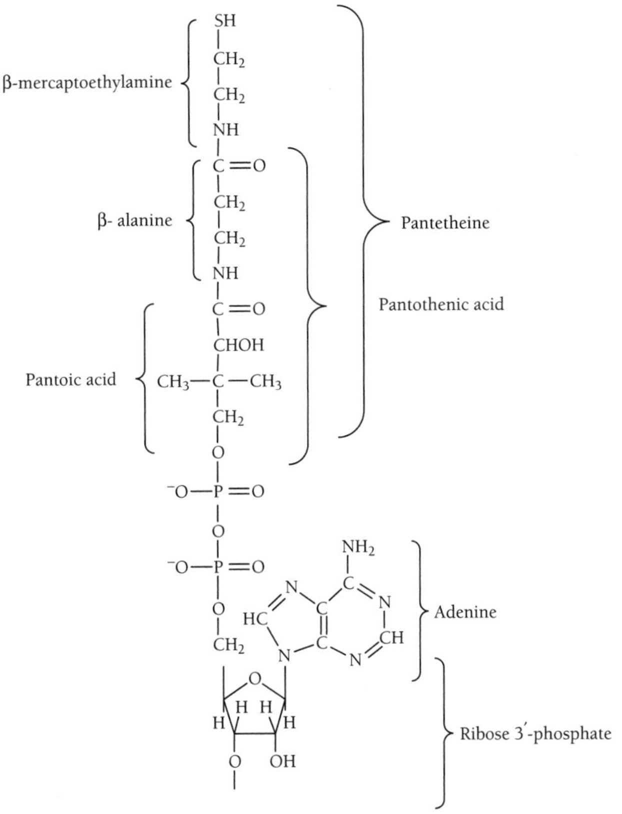

Figure 6-6. The structure of pantothenic acid.

cellular replication may be beneficial postexercise, a period characterized by increased muscle protein synthesis. Would exercise provide a similar metabolic challenge as surgery?

In one study with cyclists, decreased blood lactate and oxygen consumption was found after 2 weeks of supplementation (2 g/day). This suggests that pantothenate supplementation may hold benefit for exercise that is limited by the production of lactate; thus, it might enhance exercise recovery.[23] Future studies should focus on the effect of CoA on anaerobic metabolism.

Safety and Toxicity

There are no reports of toxicity in the literature.

Biotin

Biotin is also known as vitamin H, biocytin, or biotinyllysine. It functions primarily as a coenzyme in protein, fat, and carbohydrate metabolism. To be active within a cell, biotin must react within a magnesium framework requiring ATP to form biotinyl 5′-adenylate. Biotinyl 5′-adenylate is also known as activated biotin. One of the predominant enzymes requiring biotin is carboxylase. Examples of biotin-dependent enzymes include acetyl CoA carboxylase, pyruvate carboxylase, propionyl CoA carboxylase, and β-methylcrotonyl CoA carboxylase. These enzymes are needed for energy production (carbohydrate, protein, and fatty acid metabolism) as well as the catabolism of certain proteins (FIG. 6-7).

Sources—Biotin is widely distributed in foods. The best sources include liver, soybeans, egg yolk, cereal, legumes, and nuts. Biotin is also synthesized by bacteria within

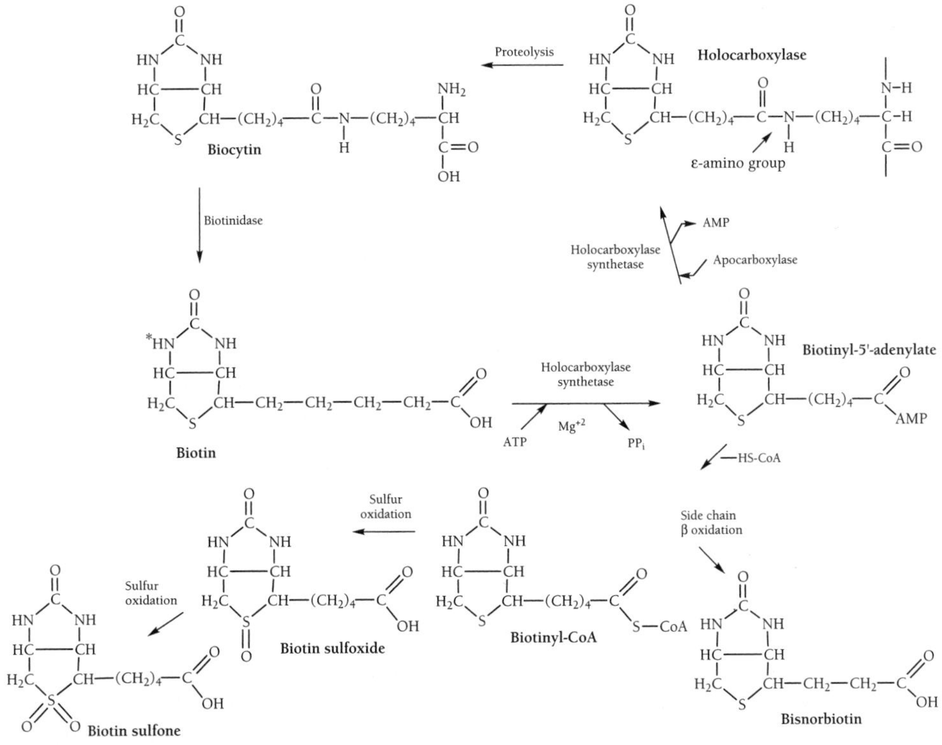

Figure 6-7. The structure of biotin.

the colon. Avidin, a protein found in raw egg whites, can bind to biotin (found in the yolk) and prevent biotin absorption. Besides *Escherichia coli,* this is sufficient reason to refrain from raw whole egg consumption.

Governmental Recommended Intake—In general, the RDI of biotin is 30 to 100 µg/day. The colon does not synthesize enough biotin to meet one's daily needs.[24]

Deficiency symptoms—Biotin deficiency is characterized by symptoms that may include depression, hallucinations, muscle pain, localized paresthesia, anorexia, nausea, alopecia, and scaly dermatitis. Impaired biotin ingestion can cause deficiency. Impaired biotin absorption may be caused by the ingestion of raw eggs, various gastrointestinal disorders, or the use of anticonvulsant medications. Alcoholism also can lead to biotin deficiency.

Human Studies

No exercise training/biotin supplementation studies have been done to date on this nutrient as a single compound.

Safety and Toxicity

No cases have been documented on biotin toxicity.

Folic Acid

Folate and folacin are generic terms for compounds that have a similar structure to folic acid. This group of like compounds are known as pteroylglutamate or pteroylmonoglutamate.

Folic acid and its metabolites (the most common in the body is tetrahydrofolate [THF]) play a major role in amino acid metabolism, specifically the interconversion or synthesis of serine from glycine, methionine reduction from homocysteine, and histidine to formiminoglutamate (FIGLU).

Additionally, folate is essential for cellular division, and purine and pyrimidine synthesis. Particularly, cells that have short life spans, such as enterocytes (cells that line the enteral tract) depend on having an adequate level of folate.

The body is in a dynamic state of being. Every nutrient has its own function and an interaction of some capacity with another nutrient. Folate is no different. Folate is protected from oxidative damage by ascorbic acid (vitamin C), high folate intakes may interfere with zinc absorption (in lab rats), and there is a synergistic relationship between folate and vitamin B12 (FIG. 6-8).[25]

Sources—Folate is available in vegetables, such as mushrooms, turnip greens, spinach, broccoli, brussel sprouts, and asparagus. It is also found in lima beans and organ meats (e.g., liver). Please note that the bioavailability of folate is higher in raw foods rather than cooked. Folate is heat labile and up to 95% of the folate in a food

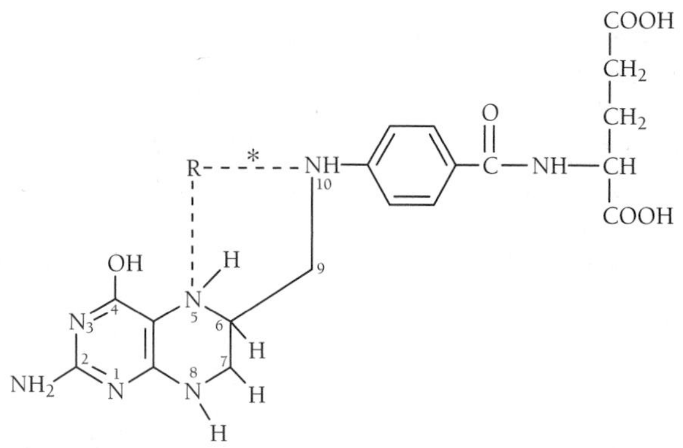

*Broken lines indicate the N^3 and/or N^{10} site of attachment of various 1-carbon units for which THFA acts as a carrier.

5,6,7,8-Tetrahydrofolic Acid (THFA)(FH$_4$)(R=—H)

Figure 6-8. The structure of folic acid.

can be lost in the cooking process. In 1999 the US Government mandated that certain foods (grains) be supplemented with folate.

Governmental Recommended Intake—The current recommended daily intake is 400 µg. This level is both safe and with good reason. Daily intake of 400 µg of folate by women in their childbearing years has been shown to decrease the risks of neural tube defects for the unborn. Furthermore, research has shown that an intake of 800 µg may help decrease the risk of cardiovascular disease associated with high levels of circulating homocysteine.

Deficiency symptoms—Folate deficiency has several aspects. Folate deficiency may be caused by the high intake of conjugase inhibitors. Conjugase inhibitors are naturally occurring enzymes found in foods containing soy. The various types of folate deficiency are characterized by low-plasma folate levels and hypersegmentation of polymorphonuclear leukocytes. It takes about 4 months of a deficiency for this symptom to appear.[26] After 5 months of a folate deficiency, megaloblastic anemia may occur. This type of anemia is common in the United States, but it can also be caused by a vitamin B12 deficiency.

Folate deficiency could play a role in the development of certain types of cancer. Recall that folate is essential for purine and pyrimidine metabolism, and therefore for DNA/RNA actions.[26] Furthermore, certain conditions are associated with folate deficiency including alcoholism, inflammatory bowel syndromes, oral contraceptive use, achlorhydria as well as a few medications.

Human Studies

Studies conducted on folate-deficient nonanemic runners show that folate supplementation produces improvements in folate levels but has no effect on exercise performance.[27] Folate, along with vitamins B12 and B6, can help reduce hyperhomocystinemia, a risk factor for heart disease. In this sense it can be considered an ergogenic aid.

Safety and Toxicity

There are virtually no reports of folate toxicity. However, the use of over 15 mg daily can be toxic in some individuals. The toxic symptoms manifest themselves as insomnia, malaise, irritability, diminished zinc status, and gastrointestinal problems.[28]

Vitamin C

Vitamin C is a unique vitamin in that some species (e.g., primates, dogs, bats, guinea pigs, and some types of birds) can synthesize ascorbic acid and therefore do not need it in their diet.

Vitamin C has a complex role in the body. Historically, vitamin C is known primarily as the cure for scurvy.[29] Additionally, normal development of cartilage, bone, and dentine depends on an adequate level of vitamin C in the diet. The membrane linings of capillaries and endothelial cells as well as scar tissue formation (for healing) require sufficient levels of Vitamin C.

Ascorbic acid has both antioxidant and pro-oxidant activity, which is not unusual for vitamins and minerals to have. As an antioxidant, ascorbic acid (ascorbate) may react with a variety of free radicals and set the reduction potential in cells.[30] The ability of ascorbate to be regenerated through reductase enzymes is important; two such products of this reaction are glutathione and niacin (NADH and NADPH).[29]

Conversely, vitamin C acts as a pro-oxidant by reducing transition metals (copper and iron). A transition metal is one that can operate in more than one state. For example, iron can be Fe^2 or Fe^3 (ferric or ferrous), products that are produced by a reduction reaction. Ferrous and cuprous can cause cell damage through the production of reactive oxygen species (i.e., free radicals). There is a correlation between circulating iron levels in the body and heart disease. In fact, some researchers speculate that high vitamin C intake can cause iron (ferrous) to oxidize LDL, thus leading to an increased risk for heart disease.

Vitamin C is also needed for the synthesis of collagen, carnitine, various neurotransmitters (e.g., norepinephrine and epinephrine), proteoglycans, and bile acids. Furthermore, vitamin C plays an important role in tyrosine synthesis and catabolism, cholesterol degradation, and immune system function.

Vitamin C is also important for the absorption of non-heme iron (iron from sources other than red meat). Vitamin C has been shown to increase the absorption and excretion of heavy metals, such as lead, by forming a chelate.[31] It is also thought that vitamin C is needed to keep folate in its reduced state (tetrahydrofolate, dihydrofolate).

Clearly, vitamin C plays an important role in many processes and interacts with a broad spectrum of other substances within the body; thus, a deficiency might impair overall health and physical performance (FIG. 6-9).

Sources—Dietary sources include papaya, oranges, orange juice, cantaloupe, cauliflower, broccoli, brussel sprouts, green peppers, grapefruit, grapefruit juice, kale, strawberries, and lemons.

Governmental Recommended Intake—Currently, the Recommended Daily Intake is 60 mg/day for nonsmokers and 100 mg/day for smokers. Many exercise scientists and sports nutritionists believe that this is an insufficient amount. Currently, there is a debate within the Institute of Medicine (the group that decides the RDI) about increasing the daily recommended intake to 200 mg/day. Recently, five prominent vitamin researchers supported the idea of increasing the RDI of vitamin C.[32] The standard for determination of adequate vitamin C consumption is a circulating pool of 1500 mg.

Deficiency symptoms—A consistent intake of less than 10 mg/day of vitamin C can lead to scurvy. The likelihood of that occurring in North America is low. Symptoms of scurvy include bleeding gums, small skin discoloration (due to petechiae), sublingual hemorrhages, bruising,

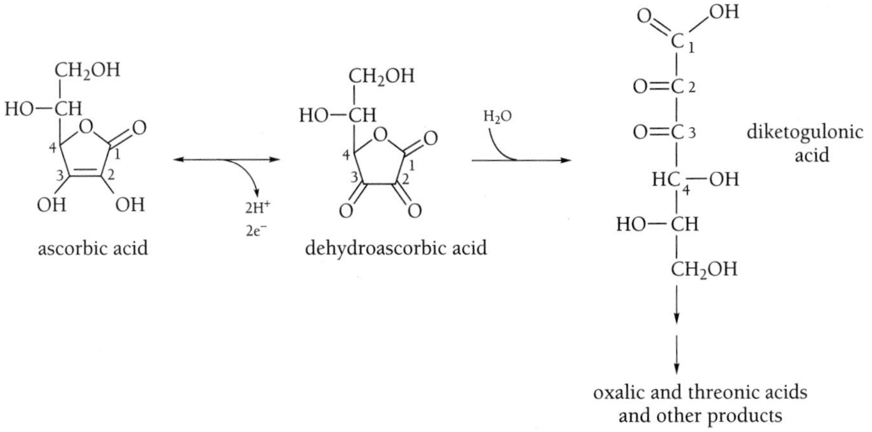

Figure 6-9. The structure of vitamin C.

impaired wound healing, joint pain, decaying or loose teeth, and hyperkeratosis of the hair follicles. As previously indicated, the incidence of scurvy in North America is low; however, suboptimal plasma levels are found in the elderly, people with poor diets, alcoholics, drug addicts, diabetics, and in some types of cancer.[33,34]

Safety and Toxicity

Vitamin C absorption is dose dependent. For the most part, vitamin C is nontoxic. However, with several large doses throughout the day, one increases the relative risk of toxicity.[35] Potential side effects of high-dose vitamin C intake include diarrhea and in some instances, kidney stones. However, it should be clear that this risk has been greatly overstated.

Vitamin C is metabolized into oxalate, and calcium oxalate is a common constituent of kidney stones; however, this does not demonstrate causality. Various studies have demonstrated that with doses of 10 g/day of vitamin C, the amount of oxalate excreted is less than 50 mg. This is the normal amount excreted daily.

Doses of 4 g/day will produce an increase in the amount of uric acid that is released in the urine. This increases the acid content of the urine, which could result in urate crystals being formed. This could conceivably result in urate kidney stones. Again, this association is weak.

There are other reasons to be cautious of high-dose vitamin C intake. One reason is that people who are unable to regulate iron absorption (vitamin C increases the absorption of iron from non-heme sources) can end up with an exacerbation of diseases, such as hemochromatosis, thalassemia, and sideroblastic anemia.[35] Another possible side effect with a high-dose intake of vitamin C is when it is excreted in the urine and feces it can cause false-negatives for fecal occult tests as well as invalidating urinary glucose tests. When ingesting high doses of vitamin C, a rebound of scurvy can occur upon rapid cessation of intake.

Vitamin C and the Strength-Power Athlete

Robert E. Keith, PhD

Although little research has been conducted on the ascorbic acid (vitamin C) needs of strength-power athletes (SPAs), what we know about the functions of ascorbic acid indicate that SPAs should probably be consuming ascorbic acid at levels above the Recommended Dietary Allowance (RDA). Research clearly shows that deficiency, or even marginal ascorbic acid status, can adversely affect physical performance. For example, muscle weakness is a common symptom of vitamin C deficiency.

Vitamin C has several functions that would be important to the performance of SPAs. For example, vitamin C is needed for the integrity and strength of tendons and ligaments. Ascorbic acid also is needed for the synthesis of adrenaline, which is needed to produce the excitatory state before and during performance. Adequate intake of the vitamin causes a lower release of the hormone, cortisol, in response to physical stress. Cortisol is a catabolic hormone that causes the body to break down skeletal muscle. Thus, lower secretion of this hormone may result in better performance. In general, any physical stress could cause an increased need for vitamin C. Finally, ascorbic acid is a powerful water-soluble antioxidant. Research has established that physical training, including weightlifting, causes an increased production of oxidative damage markers. Vitamin C, in its antioxidant capacity, would function to reduce the level of these damage products.

Studies do seem to indicate that strenuous physical activity increases the need for vitamin C. Animal and human studies show reduced tissue levels of ascorbic acid with exercise. Reduced urinary excretion of the vitamin following exercise has also been reported. Several studies show better heat adaptation with improved vitamin C status. One study, using junior elite weightlifters, did report a reduced serum cortisol concentration in the lifters following a training session when the lifters had been consuming a vitamin C supplement versus when they consumed a placebo.

The Recommended Dietary Allowance for vitamin C is 60 mg/day. However, recent studies in nonathletes suggest that an optimal vitamin C intake is more likely to be around 200 mg/day. Because physical training, such as weightlifting, places stress on the body, optimal vitamin C needs in SPAs may be 200 mg or higher. Vitamin C and exercise studies generally indicate that intakes of various athletes should be in the 200–500 mg/day range. Minimal evidence shows that intake of ascorbic acid above 1000 mg daily is beneficial to a person in general or to athletes specifically.

Although vitamin C supplements are inexpensive to purchase and easy to take, many athletes can easily consume 200 mg/day or more in their normal diets. Studies with bodybuilders and football players show normal vitamin C intake to be 180–300 mg/day. A single 8-ounce glass of orange juice will provide approximately 100–120 mg of vitamin C. If the athlete consumes a proper selection of high vitamin C fruits and vegetables, then meeting the 200–500 mg/day intake level should not be a problem. Although ascorbic acid is a nontoxic vitamin, doses above 1 g/day may cause irritation and discomfort to the gastrointestinal system. Again, obtaining the vitamin from proper dietary selection is the best way to proceed.

Keith, RE. Ascorbic Acid, in Sports Nutrition: Vitamins and Trace elements, In Wolinsky I, Driskell JA, eds. Boca Raton: CRC Press, 1997:29–46.

Marsit JL, Conly MS, Stone MH, et al. Effects of ascorbic acid on serum cortisol and the testosterone:cortisol ratio in junior elite weightlifters. J Strength Cond Res. 1998;12:179–184.

Human Studies

Vitamin C as an antioxidant may offer some protection against free radical damage induced by the exercise itself. In a study with cyclists, Dutch researchers gave 500 mg of vitamin C to 20 subjects for 15 weeks. Compared with the placebo, those receiving vitamin C showed a protective effect on respiratory function. In a second study, researchers indicated that vitamin C supplementation enhances recovery, but not exercise performance itself.[36] Studies by Maxwell et al. and Kanter et al. evaluated box-stepping and treadmill running while supplementing with vitamins C, E, and betacarotene. These investigators found an increase in circulating antioxidants, but no improvement in exercise performance.[37,38] In a Finnish research study examining the effects of ascorbic acid (2 g/day) and carbohydrate supplementation in distance runners (greater than 10 km/day), supplementation offered no apparent benefit. The authors concluded that "Vitamin C and carbohydrate do not prevent exercise-induced increase in oxidative stress, but vitamin C, being a potent aqueous antioxidant, seems to decrease the levels of diene conjugation after exercise." They further state that the significance of lowering diene conjugation postexercise deserves further research.[39]

The performance-enhancing role of vitamin C is inconclusive. Some studies show a detriment to muscular strength and $VO_{2\,max}$ with high doses (2 g/day), though a benefit was observed with 500 mg/day.[40]

FAT-SOLUBLE VITAMINS

Fat-soluble vitamins are stored in the body's adipose tissue (fatty tissues). For instance, the liver stores vitamins A and D in appreciable amounts. These vitamins are distributed throughout the body's lipid stores whereas vitamin K is stored in smaller amounts within the liver. Usually, one is warned about the dangers of consuming too much of the fat-soluble vitamins (precisely because they are stored). However, it is clear that one cannot treat all fat-soluble vitamins the same.

Vitamin E

Vitamin E is actually eight different vitamins (i.e., tocols and the tocotrienols). There are four components in each class, therefore equaling eight total vitamers. The biological activity is not equivalent for each vitamer. The hierarchy of activity is as follows α-tocopherol (where the natural L isomer is more active than the synthetic DL form), β-tocopherol, α-tocotrienol, γ-tocopherol, δ-tocopherol, β-tocotrienol, γ-tocotrienol, and δ-tocotrienol.

The principal function of vitamin E is to maintain the integrity and stability of cell membranes.[41] Vitamin E protects cell membranes from destruction via its ability to prevent oxidation of unsaturated fatty acids of the phospholipid bilayer of the cell membrane (i.e., antioxidant). Tissues that are highly susceptible to oxidation include the lungs, brain, and erythrocytes.

The following free radicals can interact with vitamin E: superoxide, peroxide, hydroxide, free hydroxy, perhydroxy, lipid peroxyl radical(s), and many other products or intermediate metabolites of any reduction reaction. Vitamin E, as a free radical scavenger, can be oxidized and therefore needs to be regenerated. The regeneration process requires vitamin C, reduced glutathione, and NADPH.[41] Vitamin E is just one of many cellular defense allies. Some of the other defense systems that interact with vitamin E require minerals or trace minerals for activation. These include iron, selenium, zinc, copper, and manganese.

Vitamin E appears to offer protection against the oxidation of low-density lipoprotein (LDL). Oxidized LDL is partially responsible for atherosclerosis and the relative atherogenicity of reduced macrophage motility in the arterial intima, increased monocyte accumulation in endothelial cells, and cytoxicity of these endothelial cells.[42,43] Vitamin E also demonstrates a protective effect regarding blood sugar regulation in type II diabetics, development of cataracts, and against liver damage caused by iron overload. Further, there is intriguing evidence that it may slow the progression of Alzheimer's disease (FIG. 6-10).[44]

Sources—Vitamin E is distributed in foods but in minute quantities. Plant foods and the oil from these plants are the primary sources of vitamin E. Vitamin E is also found in nuts, seeds, margarine, and vegetable shortening. Restrictive diets limit the nutrient intake of many vitamins, minerals, and phytochemicals. Reduced-calorie diets are problematic regarding adequate vitamin E consumption.

Governmental Recommended Intake—The recommended daily intake is 8 mg α-tocopherol equivalents for adult females and 10 mg for adult males. Labels on vitamins and foods do not express the amount of vitamin E in the product as "mg α-tocopherol equivalents, but the more user-friendly 30 international units (IU); 30 IU equals 100% of the RDI. People who are on low-fat or restrictive diets may need to supplement their diet with vitamin E due to the lack of plant oil and nut consumption.

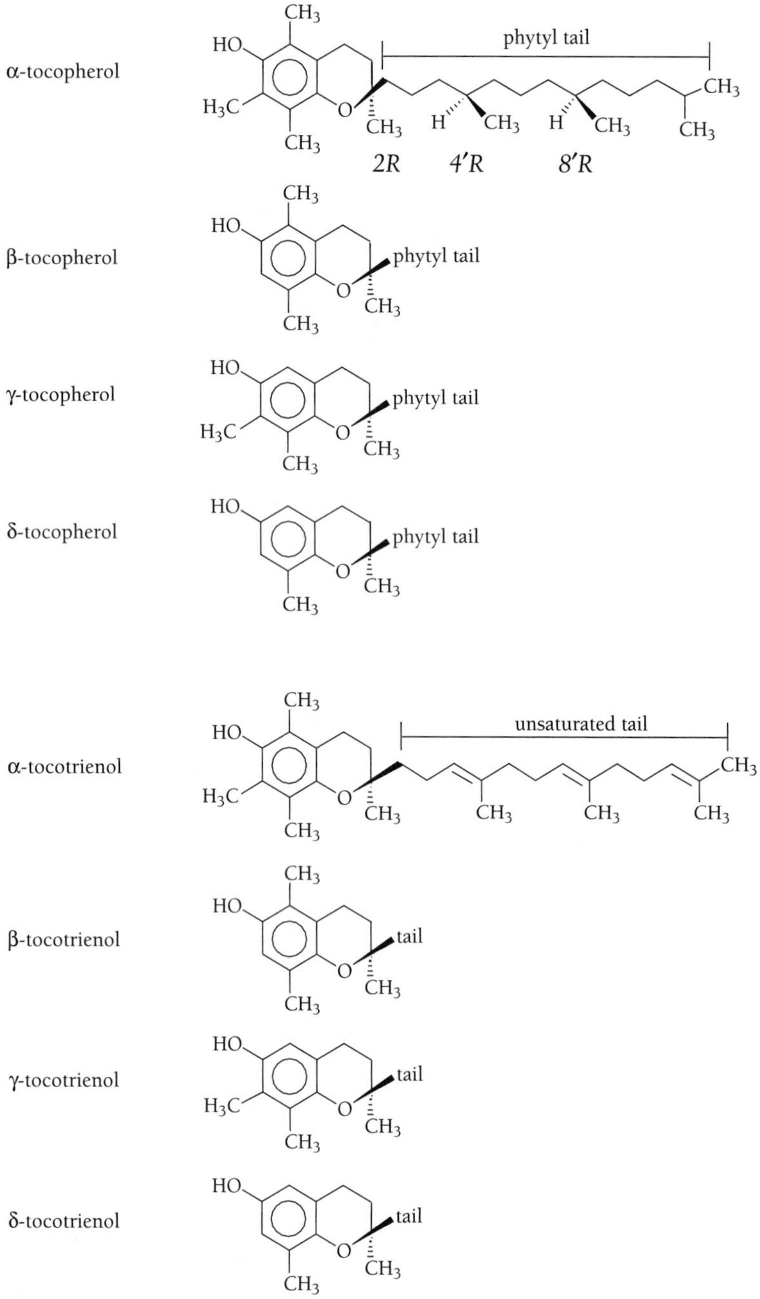

Figure 6-10. The structure of vitamin E.

The Many Faces of Vitamin E

Kristin J. Reimers, MS, RD

Read the label on a vitamin E supplement and chances are it will say *alpha-tocopherol*. Most consumers don't know that alpha-tocopherol is not the only form of vitamin E. In fact, eight different compounds make up the vitamin E family. Those compounds are four tocopherols and four tocotrienols. The four types of each are alpha, beta, gamma, and delta. Early research on vitamin E deficiency found that alpha-tocopherol per se treated vitamin E deficiency, so it was heralded as the *important* form and the other forms were largely ignored. Recent evidence has shown that all types of tocopherols and tocotrienols have specific roles in the body and should not be ignored. In fact, overconsumption of alpha-tocopherol may reduce plasma levels of gamma tocopherol. Furthermore, only gamma-tocopherol was effective in ridding the body of two toxins, whereas alpha-tocopherol was not.

To add to the confusion, alpha-tocopherol is available in supplements in two forms. The natural form is d-alpha and the synthetic form is dl-alpha. It appears that the natural form is more bioavailable than the synthetic form. In its natural form, the vitamin is oil, but it can be dried. So it's hard to tell whether the supplement is gel capsule or a pressed powder tablet. The only way to know if the alpha-tocopherol is natural or synthetic is to look for *d* for natural or *dl* for synthetic.

How Much?

The RDA for vitamin E is 12 IU for women and 15 IU for men. This level is adequate to prevent deficiency, but is a far cry from the levels shown to be protective in studies. Doses in clinical trials range from 100 to 1200 IU alpha-tocopherol per day. Supplements commonly provide 100–400 IU vitamin E. About 12 million Americans take vitamin E, with 400 IU per day as the most common dose.

Reports of adverse effects of vitamin E are rare. One study suggested an increased risk of hemorrhagic stroke, but this has not been replicated. A study on older men did not show any negative side effects of up to 800 IU vitamin E per day for 4 months. The NOAEL (No Observed Adverse Effect Level) for vitamin E has been set at 1200 IU.

Diet versus Supplement

Considering the fact that vitamin E occurs in plant oils in eight different forms and that it is difficult at the current time to find supplements that mimic nature, the argument for obtaining vitamin E from food is strong. Food sources of vitamin E are primarily plant oils like corn, soy, canola, and so forth. Wheat germ is also a source of vitamin E, as are nuts. Although it is easy for those on diets including these foods to consume the levels of vitamin E to avoid deficiency, getting the levels used in research is another matter. To consume even 100 IU would require more than 2 cups of wheat germ or 5 cups of peanuts. Few would argue that supplementing the diet with vitamin E is the only practical way to consume protective amounts.

Although many perceive vitamin E supplementation to be a no-brainer, some still advise caution. The American Heart Association, in its official statement, does not recommend vitamin E supplementation on a population-wide basis because of the lack of data on safety and efficacy. Instead, they encourage the consumption of a balanced diet with plenty of fruits, vegetables, and whole grains.

However, the crux of the matter is that it is impractical to suggest that one can obtain the protective levels of vitamin E from dietary sources, unless one has a penchant for mountains of mayonnaise and margarine. And so for those who are not willing to wait until the last piece of data is in, based on what we know now, supplementation with vitamin E poses benefit and little, if any, risk. Eating a wide variety of foods to get as much of the different forms of vitamin E has merit. But to achieve the levels shown to be protective in research, additional supplementation with natural forms of alpha-tocopherol or ideally with supplements that provide the mix of natural tocopherols and tocotrienols makes sense.

Adams AK, Wermuth EO, McBride PE. Antioxidant vitamins and the prevention of coronary heart disease. Am Fam Physician 1999;60(3):895–904.

Deficiency symptoms—Deficiency is rare. However, you may see deficiency symptoms in low birthweight infants, patients who have lipid disorders, and malabsorptive syndromes. Symptoms include retinal degeneration, hemolytic anemia, muscle weakness, degenerative neurologic problems, cerebellar ataxia, incoordination of extremities, and others.[45]

Human Studies

Dietary vitamin E by itself does not appear to have any ergogenic effects. However, there is exciting clinical evidence that demonstrates the utility of vitamin E supplementation.

In a study conducted at the National Cancer Institute, a daily dose of 50 mg of vitamin E cut the risk of symptomatic illness (prostate cancer) by 32% and reduced the death rate from malignancy by 41%.[46,47] The risk of prostate cancer can be reduced by diets rich in lycopene (an antioxidant), vitamin E, and low-fat foods. In addition to the benefits imparted by vitamin E for the prostate, this vitamin has a demonstrable benefit for the heart. Vitamin E decreases the susceptibility of low-density lipoprotein (LDL) to oxidation by free radicals (unpaired electrons). This action of vitamin E may prevent atherosclerosis. In fact, one large landmark study found that men who ingested 100 IU daily for 2 years enjoyed a 40% risk reduction of heart disease.[43] As previously stated, vitamin E supplementation should be heeded because of its coronary benefits.[47,48]

In an evaluation of vitamin and mineral status in athletes' blood, Fogelholm[49] found little difference between athletes and nonathletes. However, those who do not read this text in depth may take this out of context. Upon further reading, Fogelholm states that there was no correlation between micronutrient status and changes in athletic performance.[49]

One should be mindful that correlating improvements in performance with blood values of particular micronutrients presents only a narrow aspect of an athlete's physiology. Several factors can affect blood levels of a vitamin or mineral without an effect on performance.

In 1995 the Department of Physical Education at Wilfrid Laurier University in Ontario, Canada conducted a study evaluating vitamin E status and response to exercise training. These researchers found that certain indices of tissue peroxidation may be reduced following dietary supplementation of vitamin E. Though the performance benefits of vitamin E supplementation are debatable, supplementation in athletes does not appear to be harmful.[50]

In a review paper by Roy Shepard, MD he states "an increased intake of antioxidants may protect the active person against an augmented production of reactive species associated with an increased tissue metabolism and minor muscle injuries."[51] Mitchell Kanter, PhD raises many good points regarding vitamins in a more recent paper.[52] Although vitamin E supplementation might not have a direct performance-enhancing effect, it does have favorable effects on markers of lipid peroxidation following exercise. In fact, athletes who follow a high-carbohydrate diet typically exhibit suboptimal vitamin E intake and therefore may not recover in the same manner as an athlete who obtains adequate vitamin E. He also raises the following question. Because older athletes benefit from antioxidant supplementation, would their younger counterparts also obtain the similar benefit?[52]

A research group out of Tufts and Harvard University recently demonstrated that vitamin E supplementation can lead to improvement in certain clinically relevant indices of cell-mediated immunity in healthy elderly persons (>64 yrs). In a dose-escalating manner, researchers gave 60 mg, 200 mg, 800 mg, or placebo to 88 healthy older adults for 235 days. Those receiving the 200-mg dose of vitamin E experienced a 65% improvement in their delayed-type hypersensitivity. Delayed-type hypersensitivity skin test is a good marker for overall immune system status as well as a marker for nutrition. These subjects also had significant increases in antibody response to tetanus and hepatitis B vaccines. From an economic viewpoint, one could conclude that supplementation with 200 mg of vitamin E for 1 year time costs much less than three physician visits or 1 day in a hospital; therefore, it is a cost-effective preventive strategy for the elderly.[53]

Although little research has been done on vitamin E supplementation in an athletic population, it is plausible that this vitamin could be tremendously beneficial. Scientists from Pennsylvania State University examined 12 weight-trained males who were divided into two groups. The supplement group received 1200 IU vitamin E daily while the placebo group received a dummy pill. The study lasted 2 weeks. One of the variables they tested included markers of free radical damage (i.e., variables associated with muscle membrane disruption). After 2 weeks of heavy-resistance training and supplementation, researchers found that the group taking vitamin E had a significantly smaller increase in creatine kinase activity at 6 and 24 hours after weightlifting compared with the placebo group. Thus, vitamin E supplementation may decrease muscle membrane disruption. In turn, this may lead to a quicker recovery between heavy-resistance training bouts.[54]

Safety and Toxicity

This is one of the least toxic vitamins. However, in doses above 800 mg of α-tocopherol equivalents, one may experience diarrhea, flatulence, nausea, muscle weakness, and fatigue.[55] Renowned cardiologist, Mitchell Baruchin, MD, FACC of Pavonia Medical Group, Jersey City, NJ states "doses of vitamin E of 1000 IU or greater may act as a weak blood thinner; thus, it is important for a health care practitioner to fully question patients or clients on supplements and medicines that they may take." Nonetheless, vitamin E has so many benefits that it would be wise for all athletes to supplement.

Vitamin D

This vitamin has an interesting history. In the early 20th century scientists deemed any substance which possessed an anti-rickets property as a "vitamin D." This included exposure to the sun. Many scientists placed emphasis on the dietary components that could treat rickets rather than the vitamin derived from the sun.

Many different forms of vitamin D are in the body. The active form is $1,25\text{-}(OH)_2\,D_3$, otherwise known as calcitriol. This vitamin is unique in that it is the only one considered to act as a steroid hormone. Calcitriol is a hormone that is released by the kidney and taken up by other organs in the body. Calcitriol acts on the heart, brain, stomach, intestine, bone, and within the kidney itself. Calcitriol is transported in the blood by a binding protein made in the liver, an α-2 globulin known as vitamin D–binding protein (DBP).

Calcitriol plays a role in the homeostasis of blood calcium concentrations through its interactions with parathyroid hormone (PTH). When there is low blood calcium, stimulation of parathyroid hormone from the parathyroid gland occurs. Consequently, PTH will stimulate 1-hydroxylase in the kidney so that the vitamin D precursor $25\text{-}OH\,D_3$ is converted into active calcitriol. Calcitriol will then act on its target tissues to spur blood calcium and phosphorus concentrations to rise.[56] The site where the interaction of calcitriol acts to cause the stepwise release and increase of calcium and phosphorus levels is the intestine. Calcitriol will interact with receptors within the enterocyte where it is carried to the nucleus interacting with the specific genes that encode for the proteins that are involved with calcium transport.[57] Ultimately, calcium is extracted from the intestinal cell and transported to the bloodstream, where it helps to raise serum calcium concentrations. To keep a balance between calcium and phosphorus in the body, calcitriol will affect the activity of alkaline phosphatase so that a greater hydrolyzation of phosphate-ester bonds occur, allowing for greater phosphorus absorption.

Regarding the effect of calcitriol on the bone, it is thought that calcitriol directs the mobilization of calcium and phosphorus from the bone to the bloodstream. In turn, osteoclastic activity is increased, causing bone reabsorption. Calcitriol also functions within bone metabolism in the synthesis of osteocalcin, a protein found in bone. Osteocalcin is associated with new bone formation. In addition, calcitriol appears to initiate differentiation of stem cells to osteoclasts, which aid in bone resorption and the release of calcium into the bloodstream.[58]

Regarding interaction with other nutrients, it is apparent that the primary interactions of calcitriol are with calcium and phosphorus. However, calcitriol is also involved with vitamin K and iron. In addition, calcitriol also interacts with iron in such a way that if an iron deficiency exists, decreased absorption of vitamin D may occur.

Sources—Vitamin D is found in abundance in meats, eggs, liver, butter, and fatty fish. Milk and margarine also contain vitamin D, but these are fortified with the vitamin. Vitamin D is also formed in the body by exposure to sunlight. The mechanism of action of vitamin D synthesis from exposure to sunlight will not be discussed in this chapter (FIG. 6-11).

Governmental Recommended Intake—The requirement for this vitamin is age dependent. Infants over the age of 6 months need 400 IU daily. The recommended daily intake decreases with the cessation of growth. Adults (>24 yrs) need 200 IU daily. People who do not get much sun exposure as well as the elderly are at risk for vitamin D deficiency.

Deficiency symptoms—Deficiency or suboptimal nutritional status of vitamin D is not uncommon. In infants and children, deficiency results in rickets. Rickets is the failure of the bone to properly mineralize. This is physically apparent by bow-shaped legs, knock-knees once the infant can walk, abnormal curvature of the spine, and deformed thoracic and pelvic regions.

In adults, the deficiency results in impaired calcium status. Evidence shows that phosphorus metabolism may be impaired as well.[59] Calcium interacts with PTH in such a way that if deficient it can affect mineral metabolism. Elevated PTH in the presence of vitamin D deficiency can ultimately lead to a normal bone matrix turnover with poor mineralization. This situation can manifest itself as bone pain and osteomalacia.

Impaired vitamin D absorption may occur with tropical sprue, Crohn's disease, as well as parathyroid, liver, and kidney disease. Certain medications (anticonvulsants) and aging may also affect vitamin D status.

Human Studies

There are no known ergogenic effects of supplemental vitamin D in the athletic population. Nevertheless, those who may benefit from vitamin D supplementation include women who take calcium supplements and the elderly.

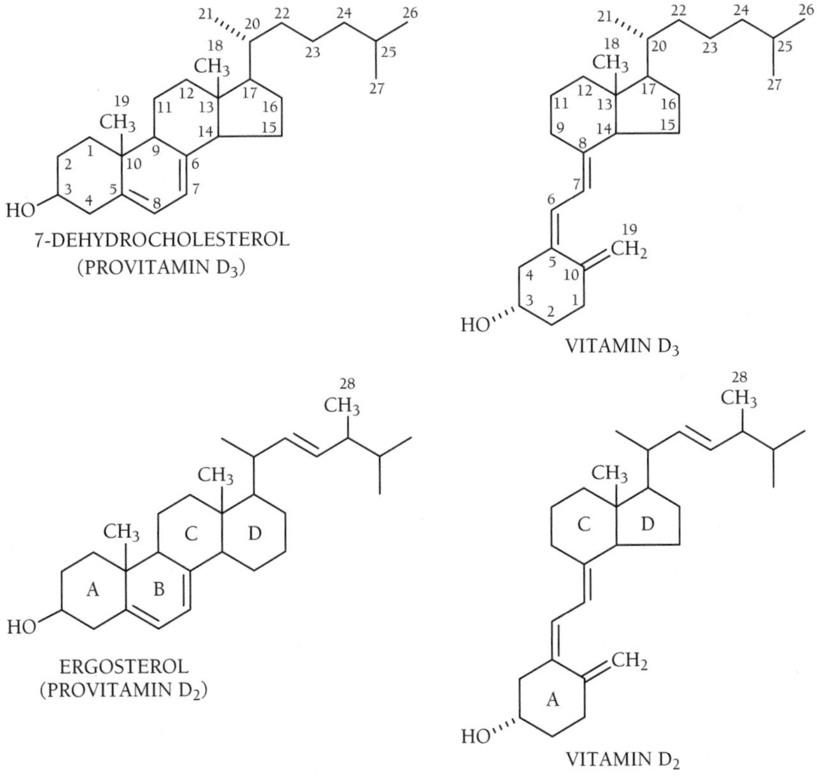

Figure 6-11. The structure of vitamin D.

Safety and Toxicity

The risk of toxicity is relative to the cause. That is, excessive sunlight exposure will not lead to vitamin D toxicity per se, but it may cause skin cancer. Excessive ingestion of dietary or supplemental sources of vitamin D may be harmful.

The symptoms caused by the excessive intake of vitamin D in infants are anorexia, nausea, renal insufficiency, and failure to thrive (the inability to grow or mature as an infant or child). In adults, this situation results in hypercalcemia and possible calcification of soft tissues.[60]

Vitamin K

Vitamin K is made up of many compounds each that contain a 2-methyl-1, 4-napthoquinone ring. These compounds come from many sources but have the same function(s) within the body.[61]

Specifically, vitamin K is necessary for the post-translational carboxylation of specific glutamic acid residues to form γ-carboxyglutamate for normal coagulation of blood. Clotting factors II, VII, IX, and X need vitamin K. These factors are of utmost importance for the production of thrombin. Thrombin is needed for blood clotting (fibrinogen ⇒ soluble fibrin).

Vitamin K interacts with the other fat-soluble vitamins. Both vitamin A and E are antagonistic to vitamin K. Vitamin E is thought to block the regeneration of vitamin K from its reduced state. Because vitamin K and D interact with calcium and have a similar site of action in the kidney, it is thought that an interrelationship exists; however, this interrelationship has not been proven as of yet.[62]

Sources—Vitamin K can be synthesized in the gastrointestinal tract by bacteria. Dietary sources include spinach, broccoli, kale, brussel sprouts, cabbage, and various lettuces. Generally, dark green leafy vegetables are good sources of vitamin K (FIG. 6-12).

Governmental Recommended Intake—The RDI for vitamin K in adult males is 80 μg/day and in females is 65 μg/day. An intake of 1 μg/kg (2.2 pounds) of body weight is a good rule

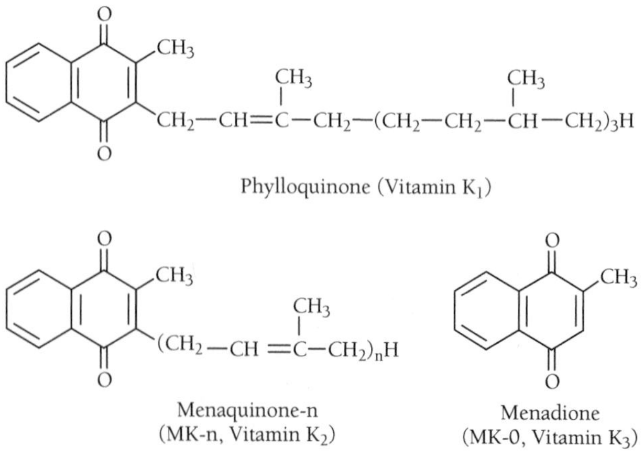

for maintaining optimal clotting time in adults. For children, the recommendation is 0.15 μg/kg body weight per day.[63]

Deficiency symptoms—A deficiency of this vitamin is unlikely. Those who are at greatest risk for a deficiency are newborn infants and individuals with renal insufficiency and those who are treated with long-term antibiotics. Cases have also been documented of people who are on long-term parenteral nutrition developing vitamin K deficiency. Disorders with fat absorption or biliary fistulas, obstructive jaundice, steatorrhea, chronic diarrhea, intestinal bypass surgery, pancreatitis, and liver disease can also cause a vitamin K deficiency.

Human Studies

Vitamin K has never been shown to have any ergogenic effects.

Safety and Toxicity

Two different forms of vitamin K are natural and synthetic. The natural vitamin K has never been associated with toxicity while the synthetic form (menadione) in high doses may cause hemolytic anemia, hyperbilirubinemia, and jaundice.[64]

Vitamin A

Vitamin A or preformed vitamin A is commonly referred to as retinol and retinal. Preformed vitamin A is also known as beta-carotene, as well as the other carotenoids that can be converted in the body to retinol. Vitamin A is absolutely essential for vision as well as cellular differentiation, growth, reproduction, bone development, and the immune system.

Beta-carotene and the other carotenoids function as antioxidants, which possess the ability to quench free radicals. The carotenoids help prevent cellular damage caused by singlet oxygen. Beta-carotene also has the ability to react with peroxyl radicals; thus, it is involved with lipid peroxidation. Similar to vitamin E, the carotenoids may help prevent the oxidation of LDL. This should lead to a decreased risk of arteriosclerosis.

Vitamin A interacts with the other fat-soluble vitamins. Vitamin E is needed for the cleavage of beta-carotene into retinol. Retinol is needed for the vision cycle to occur, as well as other previously mentioned functions. Inadequate protein intake also interferes with the activity of beta-carotene in the body.

Vitamin A also interacts with zinc. If zinc is deficient in the body, growth retardation may occur. In addition, retinol production will be altered. Iron metabolism or storage of iron (as ferritin) may be affected by vitamin A status.

Sources—The primary sources of vitamin A in the diet are beef, liver, sweet potato, carrots, spinach, butternut squash, dandelion greens, and other red, orange, and yellow vegetables (FIG. 6-13).

Phylloquinone (Vitamin K$_1$)

Menaquinone-n
(MK-n, Vitamin K$_2$)

Menadione
(MK-0, Vitamin K$_3$)

Figure 6-12. The structure of vitamin K.

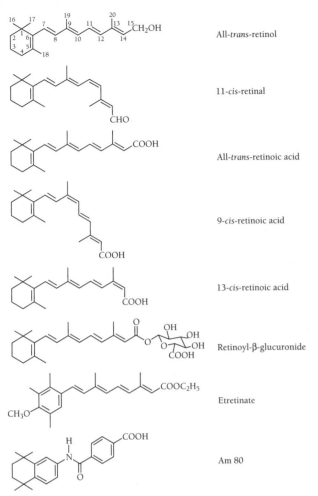

All-*trans*-retinol

11-*cis*-retinal

All-*trans*-retinoic acid

9-*cis*-retinoic acid

13-*cis*-retinoic acid

Retinoyl-β-glucuronide

Etretinate

Am 80

Figure 6-13. The structures of vitamin A.

Governmental Recommended Intake—The RDI of vitamin A (all forms, including retinol, retinal, retinoic acid, and the pro-vitamin carotenoids) is 1000 μg retinol equivalents (RE) for males and 800 μg RE for females.[65]

Deficiency symptoms—Vitamin A deficiency is not common in developed countries. If deficiency occurs in a child less than 5 years old, mortality is increased. Signs of deficiency include anorexia, growth retardation, increased infection rates, and obstruction and enlargement of hair follicles. The most commonly known vitamin A deficiency is night blindness (i.e., xerophthalmia).

Those with malabsorptive disorders, pancreatic, liver, or gallbladder disease, or those who are afflicted with chronic nephritis, acute protein deficiency, intestinal parasites, or acute infections are at increased risk for developing a vitamin A deficiency.[65]

Human Studies

The United States Olympic Committee has a position stand on antioxidants. The recommendations include an upper level for antioxidant supplementation. Although the belief is to get vitamins and minerals from food first, the USOC recommendation for beta-carotene is 3000 to 20,000 μg/day.[66]

Beta-carotene used with other antioxidants have shown an improved antioxidant status and amelioration of markers of oxidative stress induced by exercise.[67] In an elegant review by Kritchevsky,[68] he states that there are several epidemiologic studies that show an inverse association between heart disease and beta-carotene consumption. That is, the more beta-carotene that you consume, the lower your risk of heart disease. On the other hand, randomized clinical trials have not supported such a beneficial effect. The dissimilarities between clinical trials and epidemiologic evidence may be that other carotenoids (that are found in the same foods as beta-carotene) may be more important in reducing the risk of heart disease. This would support the role of eating foods that are rich in carotenoids as opposed to singular supplementation of beta-carotene.

Use of Vitamins by Medical Professionals

It is interesting to see what many medical professionals do regarding vitamin supplementation. Though it may not be common for physicians to *prescribe* vitamins per se, it is certainly clear that a significant number of physicians probably supplement their diets with vitamins. In a study by Frank et al., they examined the supplementation pattern of 4501 female physicians from a nationwide, random sample. They found that over one third of this population regularly consumed a multivitamin/mineral complex (see FIG.). The percentage of female physicians who consumed a multiantioxidant or vitamins A, C, or E was approximately 10–20%. More interesting was the fact that those who supplemented regularly also ate more fruits and vegetables and consumed less fat. Thus, it would seem that at least within this population, the consumption of supplements often goes hand-in-hand with other healthful habits.

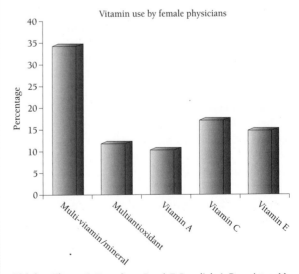

Sidebar Figure 1. Data from Frank E, Bendich A, Denniston M. Use of vitamin-mineral supplements by female physicians in the United States. Am J Clin Nutr 2000;72:969–975.

Although it does not appear that beta-carotene or vitamin A have any ergogenic effect, the health-promoting effects of beta-carotene cannot be ignored. More research is needed on the effects of beta-carotene as a single nutrient in an active or exercising population.

Safety and Toxicity

The best known cause of vitamin A toxicity is Acutane(R). Acutane(R) is also known as 13-cis retinoic acid and is used in the treatment of acne. If used by a pregnant female, teratogenesis (i.e., birth defects) can occur. A chronic intake of high levels of vitamin A can result in anorexia, dry, itchy, flaky skin, alopecia, headaches, bone and muscle pain, and conjunctivitis. Vitamin A toxicity usually slowly disappears when the offending cause is removed.

Beta-carotene toxicity manifests itself as a yellow discoloration of the skin, especially in the palms of the hands and soles of the feet. This too is reversed by the cessation of beta-carotene intake.

SUMMARY

The need for vitamin supplementation in athletes and nonathletes has been the subject of intense debate. Although vitamins do not provide energy or contribute significantly to body mass, they provide functions that are critical for normal energy metabolism. There is little evidence that singular supplementation of vitamins directly improves exercise performance. With that caveat, the question that arises is whether the RDA or RDI is sufficient for aerobic and strength-power athletes. Should we assume that a 25-year-old, 90-kg, 20% body fat, sedentary male whose primary activity is surfing the web has the same dietary needs as a 25-year-old, 90-kg, 5% fat, athletic male who competes in the 100-meter dash at the elite level?

Furthermore, there is ample evidence that the antioxidant properties of vitamins E, C, and A (beta-carotene) have protective functions. These vitamins can ameliorate the free radical damage that results from oxidative stress. Simply as an insurance policy against cancer and heart disease, supplementation of these vitamins may be warranted.

AUTHOR'S RECOMMENDATION

Today, given the freedom to choose and the desire most people have to improve their bodies, performance, and life, it makes perfect sense for them to supplement their diets with a multivitamin. As a practicing sports nutritionist who has had the pleasure of working with athletes from Little League–age children to Olympic athletes, there is one thing that cannot be denied. Few individuals eat perfectly everyday of their life. To put this another way, ask yourself a question, have you eaten at least five fruits and vegetables today? Have you had 20 to 35 grams of dietary fiber today? Have you consumed adequate and wholesome carbohydrates today (not processed grains)? Most of us would not answer yes to all of these questions. Or sadly, many of us would answer no to all of these questions. Because diet is responsible for ~35% of all cancers, and 7 out of the top 10 causes of death in America are diet related, there is a definite need to take an "insurance" pill. That insurance pill is a quality multivitamin with minerals.

The above is not taking into consideration whether vitamin supplementation can aid in exercise performance. Certainly, there is evidence to suggest that certain vitamins can benefit postexercise recovery. Though you will not necessarily run faster or jump higher from vitamin supplementation per se, it would be smart for all athletes to take a quality multivitamin as an insurance policy against poor eating and for the health benefits derived from consuming certain vitamins (e.g., vitamin E's antiatherogenic properties). As far as singular supplementation of vitamins, here is a synopsis.

Thiamin (B1)—If carbohydrate intake is sufficient, there is no compelling evidence to support singular supplementation with this vitamin at this time.

Riboflavin (B2)—If the athlete is restricting his or her caloric intake, supplementing with riboflavin may offer the benefit of maintaining optimal blood values. Otherwise, there is not enough evidence yet to warrant dietary supplementation of this nutrient alone.

Niacin—The question of niacin supplementation for athletes is complicated. For example, niacin helps to bring out or enhance vascularity, which is important for bodybuilders. However, it also causes flushing, itching, and possible liver damage. Furthermore, niacin is considered by some cardiologists to be a first- or second-line aid for lowering cholesterol, triglycerides, and elevating high-density lipoprotein levels. Although controlling high cholesterol may not be a primary concern to an athlete, it might be to an athlete who uses anabolic-androgenic steroids (AAS); AAS are known to negatively impact lipid profiles. Therefore, before using this nutrient as a singular dietary supplement, it may be wise to consult your physician.

Pyridoxine (B6)—This is a vitamin that holds promise in doses less than 100 mg/day for ergogenic effect. It would, however, be best to consume vitamin B6 as part of a multivitamin.

Cobalamin (B12)—At this time, there does not appear to be sufficient evidence to supplement with this vitamin alone. However, anecdotal reports from the strength-training world suggest that parenteral B12 (intramuscular injections) increases appetite.

Pantothenic Acid—The evidence concerning an ergogenic effect of pantothenic acid is sparse. However, it may be worth a *self-experiment* if you are an athlete who trains in, at, or near your lactate threshold.

Biotin—This vitamin has exciting possibilities. Biotin supplementation may aid in the treatment of fatigue. We do know that exercise-induced fatigue is different than chronic fatigue; however, high-dose biotin holds the possibility as an adjunctive treatment.

Folate—Although not an ergogenic property, folate is best used as a single-nutrient supplement (400 μg) by females who are in their childbearing years. Most multivitamin preparations already contain this vitamin. Supplementation does not appear to offer any pure ergogenic effect.

Vitamin C—Several studies show no performance benefit with vitamin C supplementation, but a potential benefit in postexercise recovery. Thus, the utility of vitamin C may be related to its antioxidant capabilities. Lester Packer, PhD of the University of California at Berkeley eloquently stated that "there is little evidence that antioxidant supplementation can improve performance, but a large body of work suggests that bolstering antioxidant defenses may ameliorate exercise-induced damage." Thus, long-term supplementation in the range of 250–1000 mg daily may be warranted by athletes.

Vitamin E—There is overwhelming positive evidence concerning vitamin E supplementation. Because of its potent anticarcinogenic and antiatherogenic effects, vitamin E should be a part of the daily supplementation schedule of athletes. Doses in the range of 400 to 1000 IU are commonly consumed by athletes.

Vitamin D—As a rule of thumb, individual supplementation of this vitamin is not recommended. Vitamin D that is found within multivitamins is usually acceptable.

Vitamin K—Vitamin K is usually found in adequate amounts in a multivitamin. Vitamin K should not be supplemented on an individual basis, unless suggested by a physician.

Vitamin A—It appears to be safer to use the non-meat sources of vitamin A (namely the carotenoids, of which beta-carotene is the primary carotenoid) than pure vitamin A. Research with beta-carotene in both the healthy and ill populations has yielded conflicting results. One study suggested that if you smoke or are exposed to asbestos and take beta-carotene, you would increase your chances of developing lung cancer. There are no conclusive studies with beta-carotene in athletes; therefore, the recommendation is that this pro-vitamin is best obtained through the diet first (e.g., fruits and vegetables). Because most multivitamin supplements contain at least 5000 μg per serving, and there have been no clinical evaluations of beta-carotene within athletic populations, athletes who chose to supplement should obtain beta-carotene from a multivitamin.

FUTURE RESEARCH

Regarding B-complex vitamins, the preponderance of data show that additional supplementation beyond the body's needs does not confer an ergogenic benefit. Nonetheless, it would seem plausible that active individuals would have a greater need for vitamins than their sedentary counterparts. Though there are no studies that have closely examined such a question, common sense would dictate that indeed a difference should exist. Certainly, this could be met with a multivitamin supplement.

Research into the benefits of multivitamin supplementation should focus on chronic consumption (i.e., years) rather than the traditional model of 8–12 week exercise plus dietary intervention. Such short-term studies produce a vague snapshot of what is truly going on within the human body. Regarding vitamins C and E (and perhaps beta-carotene), the evidence is strong enough to support supplementation above the RDA. However, as with the B-complex vitamins, research should focus on the long-term effects of these vitamins, particularly as it applies to musculoskeletal, cardiovascular, and immune system health.

REFERENCES

1. Robinson RS. Sources for the history of Greek athletics. Chicago: Ares Publishers, 1955:118.
2. Celcus D, DeMedicina, Volumes I, II, English translation by Spencer, WG. Cambridge: Harvard University Press, 1935, 1938.
3. Groff JL, Gropper SS, Hunt SM. Advanced Nutrition and Human Metabolism. 2nd Ed. St. Paul: West Publishing, 1995:237–243.
4. Wolinsky I. Nutrition in Exercise and Sport. 3rd Ed. Boca Raton: CRC Press, 1998:181.
5. Knippel M, Mauri L, Bellushi R, Bana G. The action of thiamin on the production of lactic acid in cyclists. Med Sports 1986; 39(1):11.
6. Groff JL, Gropper SS, Hunt SM. Advanced Nutrition and Human Metabolism. 2nd Ed. St. Paul: West Publishing, 1995:243–247.
7. Soares MJ, Satyanarayana K, Bamji MS, et al. The effect of exercise on the riboflavin status of adult men. Br J Nutr 1993; 63: 541–551.
8. Winters LR, Yoon JS, Kalwarf HJ, et al. Riboflavin requirements and exercise adaptation in older women. Am J Clin Nutr 1992;56: 526–532.
9. Groff JL, Gropper SS, Hunt SM. Advanced Nutrition and Human Metabolism. 2nd Ed. St. Paul: West Publishing, 1995:247–252.
10. Wolinsky I. Nutrition in Exercise and Sport. 3rd Ed. Boca Raton: CRC Press, 1998:184–185.
11. Groff JL, Gropper SS, Hunt SM. Advanced Nutrition and Human Metabolism. 2nd Ed. St. Paul: West Publishing, 1995:277–283.
12. Coombs GF. The Vitamins. San Diego: Academic Press, 1992: 311–328.
13. Turland JR, Betschart AA, Liebman M, Kretsch MJ. Vitamin B6 depletion followed by repletion with animal or plant source diets and calcium and magnesium metabolism in young women. Am J Clin Nutr 1992;56:905–910.
14. Leklem JE. Vitamin B6. In: Machlin LJ, ed. Handbook of Vitamins. 2nd ed. New York: Dekker, 1991:341–392.
15. deVos AM, Leklem JE, Campbell DE. Carbohydrate loading, vitamin B6 supplementation and fuel metabolism during exercise in man. Med Sci Sports Exerc 1982;14:137.
16. Manore M, Leklem JE. Effect of carbohydrate and vitamin B6 on fuel substrates during exercise in women. Med Sci Sports Exerc 1988; 20:233–241.
17. Moretti C, Fabbri A, Gnessi L, Bonifacio V. Pyridoxine suppresses the rise in prolactin and increases the rise in growth hormone induced by exercise. N Engl J Med 1982;307(7):444–445.
18. Virk RS, Dunton, NJ, Young JC, Leklem JE. Effect of vitamin B-6 supplementation on fuels, catecholamines, and amino acids during exercise in men. Med Sci Sports Exerc 1999;31(3):400–408.
19. Groff JL, Gropper SS, Hunt SM. Advanced Nutrition and Human Metabolism. 2nd Ed. St. Paul: West Publishing, 1995:276–283.
20. Herbert V. Vitamin B12. In: Brown ML, ed. Present Knowledge in Nutrition. 6th ed. Washington, DC: The Nutrition Foundation, 1990:170–178.
21. Groff JL, Gropper SS, Hunt SM. Advanced Nutrition and Human Metabolism. 2nd Ed. St. Paul: West Publishing, 1995:252–256.
22. Aprahamian M, Dentiger A, Stock-Damge C, et al. Effects of supplemental pantothenic acid on wound healing: Experimental study in rabbit. Am J Clin Nutr 1985;41:578–589.
23. Litoff D, Scherzer H, Harrison J. Effects of pantothenic acid supplementation on human exercise. Med Sci Sports Exerc 1985; 17:287.
24. Bonjour JP. Biotin. In: Machlin LJ, ed. Handbook of Vitamins. 2nd ed. New York: Dekker 1991:393–427.
25. Groff JL, Gropper SS, Hunt SM. Advanced Nutrition and Human Metabolism. 2nd ed. St. Paul: West Publishing, 1995:262–270.
26. Hine RJ. Folic acid: contemporary clinical perspective. Persp Appl Nutr 1993;1:3–14.
27. Matter M, Stittfall R, Graves J, et al. The effect of iron and folate therapy on maximal exercise performance in female marathon runners with iron and folate deficiency. Clin Sci 1987;72:415.
28. Krumdieck CL. Folic acid. In: Brown ML, ed. Present Knowledge in Nutrition. 6th ed. Washington, DC: The Nutrition Foundation, 1990:179–188.
29. Basu TK, Schorah CJ. Vitamin C in Health and Disease. Westport, CT: AVI, 1982.
30. Passmore R. How vitamin C deficiency injures the body. Nutr Today 1997;12:6–11,27–31.
31. Moser U, Bendich A. Vitamin C. In: Machlin LJ, ed. Handbook of Vitamins. 2nd ed. New York: Dekker, 1991:195–232.
32. Levine M, Conry-Cantilena C, Wang Y, et al. Evidence for a recommended daily allowance for vitamin C from pharmacokinetics. Proc Natl Acad Sci 1996;93:3704–3709.
33. Levine M. New concepts in the biology and biochemistry of ascorbic acid. N Engl J Med 1986;314:892–902.
34. Vera JC, Rivas CI, Zhang RH, Golde DW. Colony-stimulating factors for increased transport of vitamin C in human host defense cells. Blood 1998;91(7):2536–2546.
35. Groff JL. Gropper SS, Hunt SM. Advanced Nutrition and Human Metabolism. 2nd Ed. St. Paul: West Publishing, 1995:235.
36. Arbor Clinical Nutrition Update—*http://arborcom./frame/63032/u1.htm*
37. Maxwell SRJ, Jakeman P, Thomson H, et al. Changes in plasma antioxidant status during eccentric exercise and the effect of vitamin supplementation. Free Radic Res Commun 1993;19:191–201.
38. Kanter MM, Nolte LA, Holloszy JO. Effects of an antioxidant vitamin mixture on lipid peroxidation at rest and post-exercise. J Appl Physiol 1993;74:965–969.
39. Vasankari T, Kujala U, Sarna S, Ahotupa M. Effects of ascorbic acid and carbohydrate ingestion on exercise induced oxidative stress. J Sports Med Phys Fitness 1998;38(4):281–285.
40. Bramich K, McNaughton L. The effects of two levels of ascorbic acid on muscular endurance, muscular strength and on VO2 max. Int Clin Nutr Rev 1987:7:5.
41. Diplock AT. Vitamin E. In: Diplock AT, ed. Fat-Soluble Vitamins. Lancaster, PA: Technomic, 1984:154–224.
42. Stampfer MJ, Hennekens CH, Mansone JE, et al. Vitamin E consumption and the risk of coronary disease in women. N Engl J Med 1993;328:1444–1449.
43. Rimm EB, Stampfer MJ, Ascherio A, et al. Vitamin E consumption and the risk of coronary disease in men. N Engl J Med 1993;328: 1450–1456.
44. Groff JL, Gropper SS, Hunt SM. Advanced Nutrition and Human Metabolism. 2nd ed. St. Paul: West Publishing, 1995:308–310.
45. Diplock AT. Vitamin E. In: Diplock AT, ed. Fat-Soluble Vitamins. Lancaster, PA: Technomic, 1984:154–224.
46. Albanes D, Heinonen OP. J Natl Can Inst 1998;90:440–446.
47. McKinney M. Vitamin E may prevent prostate cancer. Medical Tribune 1998;39(8)1,5.
48. Lieberman S. The Real Vitamin and Mineral Book. 2nd ed. Garden City, NJ: Avery Publishing, 1997:76–83.
49. Fogelholm M. Indicators of vitamin and mineral status in athletes' blood: a review. Int J Sports Nutr 1995;5(4):267–284.
50. Tiidus PM, Houston ME. Vitamin E status and response to exercise training. Sports Med 1995;20(1):12–23.
51. Shepard RJ, Shek PN. Heavy exercise, nutrition and immune function: is there a connection? Int J Sports Med 1995;16(8): 491–497.
52. Kanter M. Free radicals, exercise and antioxidant supplementation. Proc Nutr Soc 1998;57(1):9–13.
53. Meydani SN, Meydani M, Blumberg J. Vitamin E supplementation and in vivo immune response in healthy elderly. JAMA 1997;277: 1380–1386.
54. McBride JM, Kraemer WJ, McBride TT, Sebastianelli W. Effect of resistance exercise on free radical production. Med Sci Sports Exerc 1998;30(1):67–72.
55. Combs GF. The Vitamins. New York: Academy Press, 1992:179–203.
56. Groff JL, Gropper SS, Hunt SM. Advanced Nutrition and Human Metabolism. 2nd ed. St. Paul: West Publishing, 1995:299–306.
57. Haussler MR. Vitamin D receptors: nature and function. Ann Rev Nutr 1986;6:527–562.
58. Holick MF. Vitamin D. In: Shils ME, Olson JA, Shike M, eds. Modern Nutrition in Health and Disease. 8th ed. Philadelphia: Lea and Febiger, 1994:308–325.
59. Groff JL, Gropper SS, Hunt SM. Advanced Nutrition and Human Metabolism. 2nd ed. St. Paul: West Publishing, 1995:304–306.
60. Council on Scientific Affairs, American Medical Association. Vitamin preparations as dietary supplements and as therapeutic agents. JAMA 1987;257:1929–1936.
61. Suttie JW. Vitamin K. In: Diplock AT, ed. Fat-Soluble Vitamins. Lancaster, PA: Technomic, 1985:235–311.
62. Price PA. Role of vitamin-K dependent proteins in bone metabolism. Ann Rev Nutr 1988;8:565–583.

63. National Research Council. Recommended dietary allowances. 10th ed. Washington DC: National Academy Press, 1989: 107–114.

64. Combs GF. The Vitamins. New York: Academy Press, 1992: 205–222.

65. National Research Council. Recommended dietary allowances. 10th ed. Washington DC: National Academy Press, 1989:78–92.

66. Evans W. The protective role of anti-oxidants on exercise induced oxidative stress. Task Force on Guidelines for Dietary Supplementation, USOC, 1993.

67. Bucci L. In: Wolinsky I, ed. Nutrition in exercise and sport. 3rd ed. Boca Raton: CRC Press, 1998:329–330.

68. Kritchevsky SB. Beta-carotene, carotenoids and the prevention of coronary heart disease J Nutr 1999;129(1):5–8.

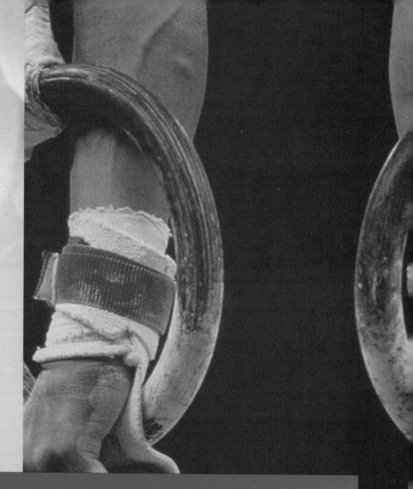

Androgens and GH Releasers

Jose Antonio, Joseph Chromiak, and Chris Street

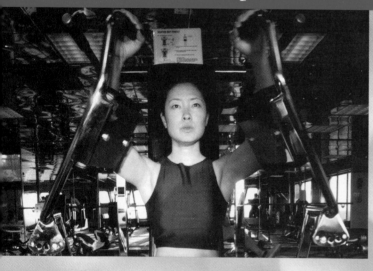

Research Review

Testosterone Enanthate Improves Body Composition and Strength with No Change in Mood or Behavior

The 1985 edition of Goodman and Gilman's *The Pharmacological Basis of Therapeutics* states that "the use of these agents (i.e., androgens) does not cause an increase in muscle bulk, strength, or athletic performance—even when phenomenally large doses are used. The commonly observed increase in body weight (seen secondary to steroid use) is due to the retention of salt and water." This conclusion is based on a review of 25 published papers. Noted scientist Jean Wilson, MD, states in his extensive review of androgens that "After more than 30 years of use, it is still not clear whether androgens do, in fact, enhance athletic performance."[1]

What was so interesting about the aforementioned views on androgen use by athletes was the prevailing notion (among physicians and scientists) that androgens had no ergogenic effect. That notion changed drastically in light of the landmark study by Shalender Bhasin.[2] In this study, 43 normal men were randomly assigned to one of four groups:

1. Placebo–no exercise

2. Placebo–exercise

3. Testosterone–no exercise

4. Testosterone–exercise

Testosterone enanthate (TE) or placebo was given intramuscularly once weekly (600 mg) for 10 weeks. Exercise consisted of traditional weightlifting exercises 3 times per week. Among those in the nonexercise group, TE treatment increased triceps brachii and quadriceps femoris muscle area more than the placebo; furthermore, bench press and squatting exercise strength improved significantly more in the testosterone-treated group. Those assigned TE plus exercise had the greatest improvements in fat-free mass and strength. No change in mood or behavior was seen in any of the men given TE. And perhaps more importantly, there were no significant changes in plasma triglycerides, HDL- or LDL-cholesterol.

Although this study was considered landmark in the field of androgen physiology, for the vast majority of athletes, it was nothing less than a confirmation of what they had already known for the past 40–50 years. An intriguing aspect of Bhasin's study was the fact that skeletal muscle hypertrophy can be induced without an exercise stimulus. This went against the prevailing notion that androgen administration was useful for building muscle mass only when you also engaged in heavy resistance training. Furthermore, the lack of behavioral or mood changes flies in the face of the commonly held idea that androgen use could lead to aggressive behavior, often termed *roid rage* by the uninformed. Though a relationship between testosterone levels and aggressive behavior can often be found in various animal species, it is unclear that such a phenomenon occurs consistently in humans. Perhaps those individuals who are already predisposed to aggressive behavior might become more aggressive under the influence of androgens. Alternatively, we would posit the notion that because androgens contribute to gains in skeletal muscle mass, these individuals (who are now larger) are more apt to act aggressively towards other men (or women) knowing full well they will not be challenged simply due to their greater body size.

A distinct dichotomy exists in how the media, scientists, and physicians view androgen use. Clearly, this study showed a beneficial effect on body composition and muscular strength. However, it is unclear why the media in particular have chosen to ignore the fact that 10 weeks of high-dose TE administration had no harmful side effects. No changes in behavior or plasma lipids were seen. Aren't the two most commonly stated claims of *risk* associated with androgen use *roid rage* and *increased risk of heart disease*?

Furthermore, the hypocrisy of the medical establishment in prescribing estrogen replacement therapy for women while ignoring the potential health benefits of androgen administration in older men is absurd. Only when this topic is devoid of the usual political correctness will health and medical professionals realize that androgen administration might offer enormous benefits.

Bhasin S, Storer TW, Berman N, et al. The effect of supraphysiological doses of testosterone on muscle size and strength in normal men. N Engl J Med 1996;335:1–7.

Prohormones

In 1994, the Dietary Supplement Health and Education Act was signed into law. This act classified substances derived from natural sources as food supplements and made many products otherwise classified as prescription drugs available over-the-counter (OTC) at health food and nutrition stores. In what could only be interpreted as a government mix-up, DHEA and other hormones (e.g., androstenedione, norandrostenedione, pregnenolone) remained legal and available as food supplements. Despite the Anabolic Steroid Control Act of 1990, which requires any substance related to testosterone that possesses anabolic properties to be scheduled as an anabolic steroid, the Drug Enforcement Agency (DEA) has no plans to schedule these supplements as controlled substances. The following sections will go into detail on the OTC androgens and attempt to shed light on a topic that has received a great deal of media attention primarily because of Mark McGuire's highly publicized use of androstenedione.

Androgens (i.e., anabolic steroids) have been used extensively as an ergogenic aid for athletes, particularly strength-power athletes. Recently, certain OTC androgen preparations (e.g., androstenedione) have been sold and marketed based on the assumption that because they serve as immediate precursors to testosterone they too should exert anabolic effects assuming they readily convert to testosterone. Thus, the closer a hormone's precursor is to the end product (i.e., testosterone), the greater the conversion of that precursor to the end product. For instance, the following compounds should convert more readily to testosterone based on their proximity to testosterone in the metabolic pathway for its formation (from greatest conversion to least): androstenedione > DHEA > 17-OH-pregnenolone > pregnenolone > cholesterol. Obviously, this is a simplistic model inasmuch as consuming a large amount of cholesterol is not a recommended method of

inducing plasma testosterone increases. But it is clear that androstenedione can convert to testosterone. Whether this conversion has a physiologically significant effect on the hypertrophic process of skeletal muscles is not known. The scientific study of androstenedione and other prohormones is still in its infancy (FIG. 7-1).

Thus, the focus of this section will not be on the illicit hormones per se (i.e., anabolic steroids) but rather on the legal, over-the-counter prohormones currently sold. It is clear that the self-administration of androgens (i.e., illicit

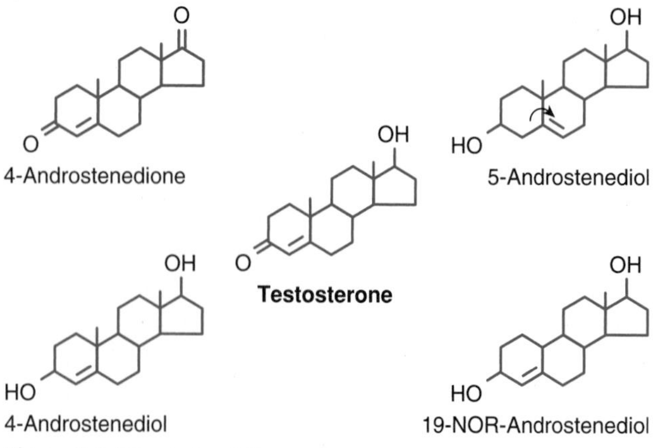

Figure 7-1. What's the difference?

Older Men and Androstenedione

In a recent study from the *Journal of Clinical Endocrinology and Metabolism*, 30– to 56-year-old men consumed 100 mg of androstenedione three times daily for 28 days. They found no change in total testosterone, or prostate-specific antigen levels; however, there were elevated serum concentrations of androstenedione (300%), free testosterone (45%), dihydrotestosterone (83%), and estradiol (68%). Serum HDL-cholesterol decreased by 10%. There was no change in mood states, health, or libido in these men. The significance of these changes is unclear. Would the drop in HDL concentration increase cardiovascular disease risk? Would the increase in free testosterone translate into an eventual gain in skeletal muscle protein? Or does a dramatic rise in serum androstenedione itself have any long-term physiological effects? A similar investigation by Broeder et al. examined the effect of 200 mg/day of androstenediol or androstenedione on 35– to 65-year-old men over a 12-week treatment period. In conjunction with resistance training, they found a significant increase in estrone and estradiol in both groups (no change in the placebo group). Interestingly, total testosterone increased in the androstenedione group (+16%) after 1 month of use but by the end of 12 weeks, it had returned to baseline levels. Furthermore, luteinizing hormone levels decreased (androstenedione group) by 18–33%, thus indicating a suppression of hypothalamic-pituitary function. More importantly, (from an athlete's point of view) there were no differences in exercise performance or body composition between the androstenedione, -diol, or placebo groups. Thus, the preponderance of evidence suggests that supplementation with these prohormones (at the doses suggested) is ineffective for increasing lean body mass and decreasing fat mass. The long-term health implications are not entirely clear.

Broeder CE, Quindry J, Brittingham K, et al. The Andro project. Arch Intern Med 2000;160:3093–3104.
Brown GA, Vukovich MD, Martini ER, et al. Endocrine responses to chronic androstenedione intake in 30–56-year-old men. J Clin Endocrinol Metab 2000;85:4074–4080.

anabolic-androgenic steroids) exerts potent ergogenic effects (see the Research Review). To dispute that would border on folly. For more extensive information on androgens, there are several excellent reviews that we suggest to our readers.[1-4]

Androstenedione and Androstenediol

The initial studies done on prohormones (i.e., over-the-counter androgens or testosterone precursors) examined the acute hormonal response to their ingestion (FIG 7-2).

Androstenedione became famous through professional baseball's single-season home run king, Mark McGuire. His admission that he consumed *andro,* as it's commonly referred to by the lay press, set off a firestorm of scrutiny. At the time, no studies were available to assess the effectiveness of this particular prohormone. However, there have been several published reports (abstracts and full-length papers) which have examined plasma hormone levels (acute and chronic responses), body composition, and exercise performance changes after prohormone supplementation.

Earnest et al.[5] examined the acute effects of androstenedione and -diol administration on eight young men (24 yrs). Using a double-blind, placebo-controlled, crossover design, eight men ingested a placebo, androstenedione (200 mg), and androstenediol (200 mg). Blood was sampled at 30, 60, 90, and 120 minutes. They found that the mean area under the curve for total testosterone was greater in the androstenedione group versus the placebo; however, there was no difference between the androstenedione and -diol groups. A similar pattern was seen in the free testosterone data. However, "the appearance and apparent conversion to total and free testosterone over 90 min was stronger in the [androstenedione] treatment (r = 0.91, P < 0.045) than the [androstenediol] treatment (r = 0.69, NS)" according to Earnest et al.[5]

In a study at the International Conference on Weight Lifting and Strength Training in Finland,[6] Dr. Tim Ziegenfuss of Eastern Michigan University examined temporal changes in plasma testosterone following the ingestion of two different over-the-counter androgen preparations. Using a double-blind, placebo-controlled, crossover design, seven healthy male subjects (mean age ~28 yrs, weight ~78 kg) ingested each of the following in a randomized order: 1) placebo;

2) 100 mg of Androstene™ (4-androstene-3,17-dione or 4-androstenedione); 3) 100 mg of Androdiol™ (4-androstene-3-beta, 17-beta-diol or 4-androstenediol).

Androstene (4-androstenedione) had no significant effect on total or free testosterone concentrations. On the other hand, Androdiol (4-androstenediol) produced significant increases in total and free testosterone. At 60 and 90 minutes post-ingestion, total testosterone increased 40% and 48%. At 60 and 90 minutes post-ingestion—free testosterone increased 29% and 43%. They found no changes in heart rate, blood pressure, or rate-pressure product during the testing period.

The effects of an androgen administered as a sublingual/buccal agent were also examined by Ziegenfuss et al.[7] Eight men were administered a placebo and 150 mg of various androgens (Androstat6) in a counterbalanced fashion. The 150 mg of androgens were comprised of the following: 125 mg of 4-androstene-3, 17-diol—and 5 mg each of 4-androstene-3,17-dione, 5-androstene-3,17-dione, 5-androstene-3,17-diol, 19-nor-4-androstene-3,17-dione, and 19-nor-5-androstene-3,17-diol.

Fasting venous blood samples were collected at 0, 10, 20, 40, 60, 90, 120, and 180 minutes post-ingestion. An increase in total testosterone values peaked at 40 minutes (98% increase); however, by 180 minutes values returned to baseline. Furthermore, this acute dose of sublingual androgens had no effect on isometric strength, vertical jump, or a 30-second bicycle sprint.

Ziegenfuss[8] examined the effects of a much higher dose of the same sublingual androgen preparation. Fourteen recreationally active, eugonadal men (~24 yrs) were given a placebo or 450 mg of the sublingual androgen preparation (divided into three 150-mg doses) for 4 weeks. Various performance and blood chemistry parameters were measured. The androgen-supplemented group had significant increases in body mass (1.8 kg, 2.3%), fat-free mass (0.8 kg, 1.1%), vertical jump (5.1 cm, 9.3%), total body water (5.4 L, 10.5%), and extracellular fluid volume (2.3 L, 11.8%). No changes occurred in the placebo group for any of these measures.

There were no changes in basal hormone concentrations (i.e., testosterone, estradiol, LH) for either group. This would suggest that despite the anabolic properties of this androgen preparation, there was no negative feedback effect on the hypothalamic-pituitary-gonadal axis. Furthermore, there was no change in either group for serum cholesterol, triglycerides, LDL-C, and organ function (i.e., blood urea nitrogen, creatinine, aspartate aminotransferase, alanine aminotransferase, lactate dehydrogenase, and creatine kinase). Oddly, however, HDL-C concentrations increased in both the placebo and androgen-supplemented group.

In a series of case studies using the same sublingual androgen preparation, six male Caucasian bodybuilders (age range = 21–25 yrs; weight range = 82.05–105.45 kg; body mass index range = 24.5–30.7) were monitored for

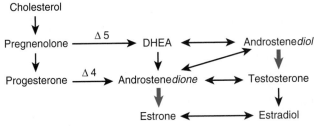

Figure 7-2. Simplified androgen pathways.

6–10 weeks in which they self-administered 150 mg of the steroid daily.[9] Physical performance (1-RM bench press, right knee extensor peak torque) and body composition (dual x-ray absorptiometry analysis and skinfolds) were assessed pre- and post-treatment. There was little change in body weight (−0.52 kg), body mass index (−0.15), lean body mass (−0.22 kg), fat mass (+0.28 kg), and percentage fat (+0.4%). The mean change in 1-RM bench press strength and peak torque was +7.95 kg and +4.9 kg-m, respectively. Thus, in this small population of well-trained male bodybuilders, supplementation with 150 mg/day of this steroid for up to 2 months has no effect on body composition and only a slight effect on muscular power and strength. In a case study performed on a highly trained bodybuilder (28 yrs, 92.3 kg, 5–7% fat via DEXA and skinfolds, >10 years resistance-training experience), androstenedione supplementation at a dose ranging from 200–400 mg per day over an 11-week period resulted in a rise in percentage body fat and a loss of lean body mass (FIG. 7-3).[12] However, there were no changes in liver function or blood lipids.

Perhaps the most publicized study in the ephemeral history of prohormone research was the *JAMA* study by King and associates.[10] This study will be reviewed in detail because of the tremendous publicity generated by it. Some have viewed this experiment as *proof* that androstenedione was a harmful and useless ergogenic aid.

In this investigation, they took 30 untrained, normotestosterogenic men (19–29 yrs) who were not taking any dietary supplements including hormones. Twenty subjects performed 8 weeks of whole-body resistance training. During weeks 1, 2, 4, 5, 7, and 8 men (randomly assigned) consumed either androstenedione (300 mg/day) or placebo. Also, the effect of a single dose of 100 mg of androstenedione was assessed in 10 men.

In essence, they found that short-term administration of androstenedione had no effect on acute hormone concentrations (i.e., free and total testosterone). However,

serum estradiol concentrations were higher after 2, 5, and 8 weeks compared with baseline values in the androstenedione group. Also, serum estrone was higher at weeks 2 and 5 in the androstenedione group but by week 8, there were no differences in serum estrone between groups. Body composition, muscle fiber cross-sectional area, and exercise performance (i.e., knee extension strength) improved similarly in both groups. The increase in lean body mass and drop in fat mass were similar between groups. Regarding serum chemistry, there were no changes in LDL-C, VLDL-C, triglycerides, liver function enzymes, or iron and red blood cell status. However, there was a significant 12% decrease in HDL-C after 2 weeks and this remained depressed at weeks 5 and 8.

On the surface, it seems that androstenedione is useless for improving body composition and exercise performance; further, its effects on HDL-C concentrations may have cardiovascular health implications. However, there are a few salient points that are worth mentioning concerning this study.

First, the subjects in this study were untrained and fat (mean percentage fat = 21.3 and 23.5%, for placebo and androstenedione groups, respectively). Untrained subjects will likely improve their body composition and exercise performance from training alone. This might mask any possible ergogenic effect of the supplement. Also, the body fat levels of these subjects might explain in part why they had unusually high estrogen concentrations (normal range = 40–120 pmol/L (Clinical Laboratory Tests, 2nd edition, Springhouse Corporation, 1995). Serum estradiol concentrations of these subjects were >200 pmol/L. There is an enhanced conversion of androstenedione to estrogens in obese males.[11] Also, it is not known why the androstenedione-supplemented group had higher plasma testosterone concentrations at baseline and at the end of the study than the placebo group. From these data, it is clear that androstenedione does not cause a depression of plasma testosterone and does not have a negative effect on the hypothalamic-pituitary-gonadal axis (i.e., no change in LH or FSH concentrations).

Regarding body composition data, it is true that there were no statistically significant differences between groups (both improved); however, it is worth noting that the androstenedione-supplemented group had an average fat mass loss of 2.2 kg, whereas the placebo group lost an average of 0.8 kg.

With the limited data available, there are a few points that can be made. First, oral and sublingual androstenedione and -diol ingestion can produce a transient increase in plasma testosterone concentrations. Whether this increase translates into a meaningful change in body composition is debatable. Data from Ziegenfuss[7,8] suggest that high doses of a sublingual androgen preparation can improve body composition within 4 weeks while much lower doses have no effect on bodybuilders.[9] On the other hand, King et al.[10] show no effect of androstenedione in

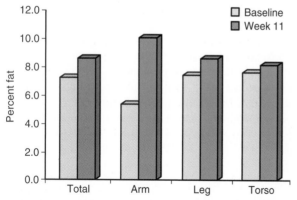

Figure 7-3. Body fat changes in bodybuilder after two cycles of andro. (Data from Antonio J, Sanders M. Effects of self-administered androstenedione on a young male bodybuilder: a single-subject study. Curr Ther Res 1999;60:486–492.)

DHEA: A Prohormone That May Have Health Benefits

Chris Street, MS, CSCS

DHEA was banned from over-the-counter sales in 1985 by the FDA. Because of the Dietary Supplement Health and Education Act, DHEA was reclassified as a food supplement. This androgen precursor was first identified in 1934 and is produced naturally by the zona reticularis cells of the adrenal glands. The exact function of DHEA in the human body is not fully known, but scientists do know that it is a metabolic precursor to testosterone. DHEA may also increase levels of IGF-1 and may have a stimulatory effect on neurotransmitter receptors.

Three biologically active forms of DHEA are found circulating in plasma (DHEA, DHEA-S, and DHEA). Like other sex steroids, DHEA circulates in blood bound to a protein (albumin) and is easily converted to other androgens and estrogen. DHEA and DHEA sulfate (DHEA-S) are converted peripherally to androstenedione, testosterone, and dihydrotestosterone. It can also be aromatized to estrogens via the enzyme P450 aromatase. Factors that influence these conversions are not well understood, but both aerobic and resistance exercise may play a role in the formation of various androgens or a decrease thereof.

The research on DHEA has mostly tested older subjects, not young athletes. For some individuals, supplementing with DHEA might restore feelings of *youthfulness*. A gap in the literature comes when we look at DHEA's effects in younger males, especially bodybuilders. To date, two studies looking at DHEA in those producing normal amounts of the hormone have been conducted. Welle et al. used 1600 mg of DHEA for 4 weeks in a double-blind, placebo-controlled crossover study in men (average age, 26 yrs). With supplementation, serum levels of DHEA increased, but there was no significant effect on body weight, body mass, resting metabolic rate, proteolysis, total energy expenditure, or cholesterol.

In a study by Nestler et al., 10 young men were divided into a placebo versus DHEA-supplemented (1600 mg/day) group for 28-day treatment duration. There was no effect on serum total testosterone, free testosterone, SHBG, estradiol, or estrone concentrations. However, there was a slight decrease in body fat and a decrease in serum low-density lipoprotein cholesterol in the DHEA-supplemented men. Tissue sensitivity to insulin remained unchanged. This study and the one discussed previously illustrate that DHEA research is still in its infancy. Previous data from animal research by Han et al. showed that DHEA might be a potent *anti-obesity* agent. However, at best DHEA produces only modest changes in body composition in humans. Thus, DHEA's applications in medicine could be far-reaching, but it is not clear whether DHEA is useful as an ergogenic aid.

Han DH, Hansen PA, Chen MM, Holloszy JO. DHEA treatment reduces fat accumulation and protects against insulin resistance in male rats. J Gerontol A Biol Sci Med Sci 1998;53(1):B19–24.

Nestler JE, Barlascini CO, Clore JN, Black WG. Dehydroepiandrosterone reduces serum low-density lipoprotein levels and body fat but does not alter insulin sensitivity in normal men. J Clin Endocrinol Metab 1988;66(1):57–61.

Welle S, et al. Failure of dehydroepiandrosterone to influence energy and protein metabolism in humans. J Clin Endocrinol Metab 1990;71:1259–1264.

Androstenedione: Creative Marketing?

Conrad Earnest, PhD

On August 16, 1999, the *Wall Street Journal* published a report on General Nutrition Center (GNC) decision to carry androstenedione as a nutritional supplement. Oddly enough, this occurred hot on the heels of a paper in *Journal of the American Medical Association (JAMA)* by King et al. showing it to have no effect on body composition or exercise performance. The gist of the article went on to recount GNC's tale of *scientific justification* to carry a product that they felt to be both beneficial and free of risk. GNC *solidified* its position with references. What truly raised my curiosity was the citing of my research (from the *Journal of Parenteral and Enteral Nutrition*) to justify the product's effectiveness and safety. Why should I be curious? Perhaps it had something to do with the fact that my research never examined safety or efficacy issues.

However, I did feel honored for a couple of reasons. First, as a scientist, it is nice to have your name and research associated with product development. More importantly, however, I had now been elevated to a status in sports nutrition that is only rivaled by several countries. In a unique combination owing to (a) the findings of my research and (b) the poor interpretation by GNC of my data, I was now achieving fame due to guilt by association. Yes, my name was now being championed in a marketing campaign that was up there with the ever-popular buzzwords for muscle enhancement—Russia, East Germany, and Bulgaria. For, as everybody knows (but never really tells), if you don't have a product that works, you can always rely on these terms to promote your product due to the *communist-guarded mystique* associated with these former communist countries.

To say the least, the last few years in the natural products industry have been interesting. Still piggybacking the industry high brought on by creatine sales, more companies are continually scrambling to find the next blockbuster product. What makes creatine so great is that regardless of how much criticism you throw at it, science keeps giving it right back in terms of validating its safety and benefits.

Despite the myriad of prohormones that have captured the interest of the health supplement industry, the one thing that many of the prohormones do not have is adequate scientific evidence. Sure, we have an interesting study from 1962 in four women and intriguing in vitro findings. But we still have no evidence to support prohormones as being beneficial. In review, all prohormones either directly form testosterone or emulate testosterone by differing only modestly in molecular structure. So, why shouldn't they be used? These are issues challenging both scientists and practitioners alike. After all, as everybody knows, more testosterone means more muscle—right?

Because androstenedione lies in such close proximity to testosterone in the body (one step away), it has become a popular nutritional supplement marketed for muscle growth. From a formation standpoint, the closer a hormone's precursor lies within a pathway to the end product, the more pronounced the conversion to the end result should be. In essence, DHEA should produce greater quantities of testosterone than that of its upstream precursors, such as pregnenolone. Likewise, androstenedione should produce greater quantities of testosterone than DHEA because it lies one step away from testosterone, whereas DHEA is two steps away. In test tubes this appears to be the case. In an elegant series of studies using testicular incubations, the conversion to testosterone was more readily apparent from DHEA than any of its precursors and androstenedione was converted more readily than DHEA.

Whether this occurs in the body is not well determined and currently has produced conflicting results regarding its ability to increase testosterone concentrations. Formerly, the best available reports were testimonials gathered from former East German Republic Olympic athletes and one scientific paper examining the supplementation of androstenedione in women (see Mahesh and Greenblatt). In the former example, Olympic teams first reported the use of androstenedione during the 1970s. In an effort to justify sales promotions, many companies quoted East German patent claims stating that 50 mg of androstenedione increased plasma testosterone concentrations from 140% to 183%. Better yet, 100 mg of androstenedione increased the concentrations from 211% to 337%. A funny thing though, no evidence for this claim is readily available in the scientific literature. Well, here's an information tidbit for you: Just because it appears on a patent doesn't mean it has been scientifically validated. In truth, one can obtain a patent on novel theory alone. No *real* data are actually needed.

Recently, however, investigators at the University of Texas (Arlington) performed a double-blind, crossover, pilot study and found that androstenedione supplementation produced a slightly higher level of total testosterone (18–23%) after the ingestion of 200 mg of androstenedione. Although statistically *significant*, these results are not even close to patent claims and it is likely that these findings have no practical significance. In fact, a good weight training session alone will raise testosterone by over 30%. As more evidence has become available, contrasting reports show that androstenedione has no real effect at raising testosterone, increases estrogen concentrations, has no effect on muscle mass or strength, and even decreases net protein synthesis.

How this will affect future sales is currently a matter of debate. For now, based on the studies in hand, the industry has a hard time justifying the product. Fortunately, this does not fall under the ever-popular scapegoat of an FDA conspiracy. Instead, it is brought about and fully borne from the evidence derived through scientific inquiry showing the product to be ineffective. Hopefully, the industry will not ride out the storm while promoting all the other prohormones that have not accumulated any science because the reports will be coming out soon. Some have already begun as the 19-norandrostenedione/diol products are now attracting scientific scrutiny.

Many of these prohormones do not even contain what is claimed on the label. If you are still tempted to ask yourself why the FDA is so determined to regulate our industry, perhaps you should ask yourself why we are so determined to extend such an open invitation to do so. It comes down to this: either we regulate ourselves by doing the science or we have a government agency do it for us. It is just a matter of time.

Cowan DA, Kicman AT. Doping in sport: misuse, analytical tests, and legal aspects [editorial]. Clin Chem 1997;43:1110–1113.

Colker CM, Kalman DS, Antonio J. Pharmacokinetics of orally ingested 19-nor-4-androsten-3,17-diol and 19-nor-4-androsten-3,17-dione in healthy resistance-trained adult males. FASEB 1999;13:A1043.

Earnest CP, Olson MA, Beckham SG, et al. Oral 4-androstene-3,17-dione and 4-androstene-3,17-diol supplementation in young males. J Paren Ent Nutr 1999;23:S62.

King DS, Sharp RL, Vukovich MD, et al. Effect of oral androstenedione on serum testosterone and adaptations to resistance training in young men: a randomized controlled trial [see comments]. JAMA 1999;281:2020–2028.

Lee EK, Starcevic S, Catlin DH. Effects of dietary supplements, 19-norandrostenedione, androstenediol and androstenedione on the profile of urine steroids. J Invest Med 1999;47:62A.

Mahesh VB, Greenblatt RB. The in vivo conversion of dehydroepiandrosterone and androstenedione to testosterone in humans. Acta Endocrinol 1962;41:400–406.

Rasmussen BB, Volpi E, Gore DC, Wolfe RR. Androstenedione does not stimulate muscle protein synthesis. FASEB J 1999;13:LB46.

Rogol AD, Yesalis CE. Anabolic-androgenic steroids and athletes: what are the issues? J Clin Endocrinol Metab 1992;74(3):465–469.

Street C, Antonio J, Cudlipp D. Androgen use by athletes: a reevaluation of the health risks. Can J Appl Physiol 1996;21(6):421–440.

Yanaihara T, Troen P. Studies of the human testis. I. Biosynthetic pathways for androgen formation in human testicular tissue in vitro. J Clin Endocrinol Metab 1972;34:783–792.

Yanaihara T, Troen P. Studies of the human testis. II. A study of androstenediol and its monosulfate in human testes in vitro. J Clin Endocrinol Metab 1972;34,793–800.

Yanaihara T, Troen P, Troen BR, Troen ML. Studies of the human testis. 3. Effect of estrogen on testosterone formation in human testis in vitro. J Clin Endocrinol Metab 1972;34:968–973.

Yesalis CE. Medical, legal, and societal implications of androstenedione use [editorial; comment]. JAMA 1999;281:2043–2044.

Current Controversy: Andro

Timothy Ziegenfuss, PhD

Despite a dearth of information on their effects, supplementation with *andro*-compounds has become widespread. Unlike synthetic anabolic-androgenic steroids, these precursor androgens are produced endogenously by adrenal, gonadal, and peripheral steroidogenic pathways as part of the normal sexual and reproductive hormonal milieu. It has been suggested that peripheral enzymatic conversion of these *prohormones* to testosterone (via ingestion of androstenedione/diol) or nor-testosterone (via ingestion of 19-nor-androstenedione/diol) might lead to anabolic and/or ergogenic effects. Beyond the narrow scope of performance enhancement, it has also been alleged that supplementation with prohormones might be useful in correcting the gradual decline in testosterone and DHEA concentrations that accompany the aging process. None of these claims have been proven or adequately examined to date.

The biosynthesis of testosterone from the -dione and -diol prohormones is controlled by the ubiquitous enzymes 17- and 3-beta-hydroxysteroid dehydrogenase, respectively. Because these enzymes exist as a family of multiple isozymes, each with a specific oxidative/reductive activity, substrate specificity, and cell-specific expression, prohormone ingestion might, either directly or indirectly, affect the formation of a number of sex steroids other than testosterone (e.g., DHEA, estrone, estradiol, etc.). Initial research in men using single and repeated 100-mg oral doses of androstenedione reported no effect on testosterone concentrations or rates of muscle protein synthesis. Subsequent studies have indicated that oral doses of 200–300 mg are capable of increasing serum testosterone modestly, i.e., up to 34% when mean-area-under-the-curve values are compared. A relatively consistent finding in most studies thus far,

however, has been increases in serum estrone and estradiol. These aforementioned results are not surprising given the known (poor) bioavailability of orally administered androgens and the high aromatase activity of hepatic tissue. Collectively, recent data from our research group and others examining the acute and chronic effects of oral, sublingual, and transbuccal prohormone administration in men suggest that 1) any increase in serum testosterone concentrations from acute, oral androstenedione administration are overshadowed by larger increases in circulating estrogen(s); 2) daily ingestion of androstenedione during intense resistance training does not lead to greater gains in strength or hypertrophy, at least at dosages between 100–300 mg/day; and 3) short-term sublingual and transbuccal administration of androstenediol, on the other hand, may significantly elevate serum testosterone without effects on estradiol concentrations or lipid, renal, and hepatic profiles.

Given the popularity of prohormones and the wide array of clinical effects that androgens may have on health (e.g., alterations in blood lipids, cardiovascular disease risk, bone density, immunocompetence, libido, visceral adiposity, insulin sensitivity, etc.) more research in this area is needed. Admittedly, this will be a complex task because of the numerous interrelated factors that are known to influence individual responses to androgen administration, most notably the genetic polymorphisms of the androgen receptor and potential hormonal interconversions at the paracrine level. Nevertheless, appropriately controlled human trials involving large sample sizes, dose response, duration of use issues, and documentation of side effects must be conducted before the risk-to-benefit ratio of prohormone use can be accurately determined.

untrained males. A case study in a highly trained bodybuilder showed that androstenedione supplementation increased fat mass and decreased lean body mass.[12] Inasmuch as bodybuilders and athletes in general are the primary consumers of these products, one might question the relevance of studies performed on untrained individuals. Nonetheless, the data on *andro* are far from promising. As far as potential health concerns, there is little evidence that prohormone consumption has permanent harmful effects. However, further studies using trained subjects, higher doses, and longer treatment durations are needed to fully assess the effects of these compounds.

GH Enhancers

Various substances, including amino acids, increase circulating growth hormone (GH) concentrations and are referred to as growth hormone secretagogues. Many athletes use specific amino acids to stimulate GH secretion, believing that this practice will promote greater gains in muscle mass and strength. Exercise, including strength-training exercise, also induces an increase in serum GH concentrations. Amino acids may be used before a workout in an attempt to further accentuate the exercise-induced GH release. This section will examine amino acids and other substances that might be used by athletes to stimulate GH release. Because the literature is fairly extensive and there are likely to be significant differences in the regulation of GH release between animals and man, only scientific papers dealing with GH release in humans are included here.

The use of protein or specific amino acids to induce GH release apparently originated with the use of arginine infusion[13] or orally administered protein[14] as tests for GH secretion. Intravenous infusion of 30 g of arginine increases serum GH concentrations[15,16] by suppressing endogenous somatostatin secretion.[15] Intravenous administration of 12 g of ornithine per square meter of body surface area increases serum GH levels.[17] Infusion of 30 g of methionine also induces a consistent and relatively large increase in GH levels, while infusion of leucine or valine promote rather small (~10%) increases in GH levels.[18] The most commonly studied amino acids, and possibly the most widely used, for their effects on GH release are arginine, lysine, and ornithine.

Effect of Amino Acid Ingestion on GH Release

Ingestion of 1.5 g of L-arginine and L-lysine by young adults (age, 22.4 ± 0.8 yrs; mean ± SE) increased GH concentrations 2.7-fold at 60 minutes post-consumption, although GH levels were not elevated 30 minutes or 90 minutes after ingestion.[19] Ingestion of 1.2 g of arginine and 1.2 g of lysine by males, 15 to 20 years of age, resulted in a significant increase in GH concentrations after 30 minutes.[20] Plasma GH concentration was increased nearly eightfold 90 minutes post-ingestion. The combination of 1.2 g each of arginine and lysine was more potent at stimulating GH release than either amino acid alone. Either 1.2 or 2.4 g of arginine or 1.2 mg of lysine did not increase plasma GH concentrations.

These studies clearly demonstrate that arginine and lysine can induce increases in circulating GH concentrations when ingested orally. The GH response appears to be reduced in exercise-trained individuals. Consumption of 2.4 g of arginine and lysine, or 1.85 g of ornithine and tyrosine did not induce a statistically significant increase in serum GH concentrations in young male bodybuilders (age, 22.6 ± 1.0 yrs; mean ± SE) over a 3-hour period, even though GH concentrations increased in five of the seven subjects.[21] Subjects were tested in the morning following an overnight 8-hour fast. There was a large inter-subject variability in GH concentrations between the subjects. For example, 3 hours after ingestion of arginine and lysine there was a 26-fold difference in GH concentrations between the subjects with the lowest and highest GH concentrations. This may be explained in part by the pulsatile release pattern of GH. These results are consistent

with observations that trained individuals have a lower GH response to various stimuli compared to untrained individuals.

Not all amino acids appear to be effective GH releasing agents. Ingestion of 10 g of aspartic acid, glutamic acid, or cysteine did not alter serum GH concentrations.[22] Interestingly, ingestion of a mixture of branched-chain amino acids (BCAAs) immediately before 1 hour of running resulted in lower GH levels post-exercise.[23] High serum BCAA levels may reduce synthesis of serotonin, a stimulator of GH release, in the brain.

Various factors appear to modify the GH response to amino acids and protein, including training status, sex, diet, and age. Larger amounts of amino acids may be necessary to elicit GH release in exercise-trained adults. Consumption of 170 mg of ornithine per kilogram of body weight significantly increased serum GH in male and female bodybuilders.[24]

Nine male (mean age, 28.1 yrs) and three female (mean age, 34.3 yrs) bodybuilders ingested 40, 100, and 170 mg/kg ornithine after an overnight fast on three separate occasions. These dosages are approximately 3, 7, and 12 g for a 70-kg reference man. Ninety minutes after ingestion of the 170-mg/kg dose, serum GH concentration was increased from 2.2 ng/mL at baseline to 9.2 ng/mL. Growth hormone levels were not altered significantly by the 40- or 100-mg/kg doses. However, at the highest dose all subjects experienced mild to severe stomach cramping and diarrhea.

Females show more consistent and greater overall increases in GH concentrations than men in response to arginine infusion.[25] Intravenous administration of 183 mg/kg of arginine significantly increased plasma GH concentrations in females, age 17 to 35 years, after 60 minutes, but not in males.[25] A dosage of 367 mg/kg, infused over a 30-minute period, was necessary for elevating GH levels in males of similar age. At dosages of 76 mg/kg and 550 mg/kg, the increase in GH concentration was substantially greater in females compared with males.

Furthermore, females showed less variability in the GH response to arginine. Ninety-seven percent of females infused with 367 mg/kg or 550 mg/kg had increases in plasma GH concentrations of 5.0 μg/mL or greater but only 56% of males had increases of 5.0 μg/mL or greater. These results are consistent with the reported increased GH release in all women, but only 20% of men, who consumed Bovril.[14] Bovril contains 7.8 g of protein, including 438 mg of arginine and 412 mg of lysine, and has been used as a test for GH secretion. The elevation in plasma GH levels in response to arginine infusion was more than doubled in males pretreated with stilbestrol, an estrogen receptor agonist.[13] This suggests that estrogen enhances GH release, possibly by antagonizing peripheral GH action.

The magnitude of the GH response to various stimuli, including some amino acids, may be accentuated in young subjects. Arginine infusion stimulated GH secretion in

100% of subjects aged 14 to 19 years, but in subjects 20 to 29 years of age, arginine infusion stimulated GH release in approximately 50% of the subjects.[26] Ingestion of 1.5 g of arginine and 1.5 g of lysine increased GH release in approximately 50% of subjects aged 20–25 years.[19] Administration of 3 g of arginine and lysine for 14 days did not significantly affect GH levels in elderly subjects (age: x = 69 yrs).[27] However, a relationship between serum GH and serum arginine was noted, suggesting that the impaired response to arginine/lysine in the elderly is due in part to decreased gastrointestinal absorption.[27]

A diet high in protein has been reported to result in significantly greater basal GH levels compared with a normal, balanced diet.[28] Ingestion of approximately 18 g of arginine per day for 7 days increased the sleep-related GH spike.[29] The acute GH response to amino acid ingestion may be influenced by the amount of dietary protein or amino acid supplementation. Lambert et al.[21] and Fogelholm et al.[30] found no statistically significant effect of amino acid ingestion on GH release in male weightlifters who consumed 1.58 g/kg/day and 2.2 g/kg/day of protein, respectively. This suggests that the use of specific amino acids to induce GH release may not be effective in strength-trained individuals consuming high-protein diets. Whether amino acids are ingested following an overnight fast or at some other time of day is likely to affect the GH response. If one were to consume a low-carbohydrate diet, the low blood glucose concentration could accentuate the effects of pharmacological or physiological stimulation of GH secretion.[31,32] However, the benefits of eating small to moderate amounts of calories on a regular schedule are likely to outweigh any benefits from attempting to accentuate an amino acid or exercise-induced GH response by fasting.

Exercise-Induced Alterations in Circulating GH Concentration

Exercise of sufficient intensity and/or duration can induce GH release. The first report of exercise as a physiological stimulus to GH secretion was in 1963.[33] The exercise-induced rise in GH is related to exercise intensity[16] and duration.[34] In men aged 21 to 24 years, 20 minutes of exercise on a cycle ergometer at 900 kpm/min induced a dramatic increase in serum GH concentration, which peaked 5 to 15 minutes after cessation of the exercise. The GH response during and after cycling at 600 kpm/min was much lower than cycling at 900 kpm/min, and exercise at 300 kpm/min did not induce a significant change in GH levels.

Serum GH concentrations increase in response to moderate- and high-intensity resistance exercise. The increase appears to be regulated by the characteristics of the resistance-training protocol, including exercise duration, number of sets and repetitions, rest periods between sets, and type of exercises performed.[35–38] The intensity of the resistance-training workout is positively related to the amplitude of GH release. Performing vertical leg lifts at 85% of 1-repetition maximum (1-RM) increased circulating GH concentration, but the same exercise done at 28% of 1-RM had no effect on GH levels.[38] Because high-intensity exercise is a potent stimulus for GH release, the ingestion of specific amino acids before exercise may not further elevate GH levels. For example, cycling at approximately 75–90% of maximal oxygen uptake for 20 minutes resulted in increases in GH concentrations comparable to insulin-induced hypoglycemia and greater than that induced by infusion of 30 g of arginine.[16] Other factors such as sex[35] and training status affect the exercise-induced increase in GH. The exercise-induced rise in GH levels is greater in untrained individuals than in trained cyclists.[39]

The physiological purpose of the exercise-induced increase in GH is unclear. GH acts both as an anabolic hormone (via insulin-like growth factor-1) to increase protein synthesis, and as a metabolic hormone to reduce carbohydrate metabolism to maintain blood glucose levels. GH stimulates amino acid movement from the small intestines into the blood,[40] and from the blood into skeletal muscle. The GH response to exercise may help promote an optimal nutritional environment for protein synthesis and muscle growth, or simply to maintain circulating blood glucose levels.

Exercise and Amino Acids

When subjects experienced with weight-training exercises performed a workout lasting approximately 45 minutes, GH levels were dramatically elevated during the workout and remained higher for approximately 70 minutes post-exercise.[19] Subjects performed 3 sets to voluntary exhaustion at 70% of their 1-RM for seven different exercises. Although GH concentrations were increased 2.7-fold 60 minutes after consumption of 1.5 g of arginine plus 1.5 g of ornithine, ingestion of arginine and lysine before the workout did not result in greater increases in GH concentrations than exercise alone.[19] Blood GH concentration was elevated in four male throwers 2 hours after a weight-training circuit, which was performed following an overnight fast.[41] Consumption of an amino acid combination of 1.8 g of L-arginine, 1.2 g of L-ornithine, 0.48 g of L-methionine, and 0.12 g of L-phenylalanine did not alter GH concentration during the workout compared with exercise alone. A protein supplement ingested immediately before exercise and 2 hours after resistance-training exercise had no effect on post-exercise changes in GH concentrations.[42] Exercise is a potent stimulus for GH release and amino acids may not further augment GH release during or after exercise.

Administration of 20 g of arginine and glutamate to highly trained cyclists (VO$_{2\text{ max}}$: 69–80 mL/kg/min) approximately 2 hours before cycling at 75–83% of maximal aerobic power for 60 minutes greatly reduced the rise in plasma GH concentration.[43] In the placebo condition, GH levels peaked after 30 minutes of exercise before beginning to decline, but were still significantly elevated 30 minutes post-exercise. Ingestion of arginine and glutamate significantly decreased the exercise-induced rise in GH. The blunted GH response to arginine-glutamate may be due to the highly trained status of the cyclists, or more likely that glutamate reduces the GH stimulatory effect of exercise.

The effects of consumption of 6 g of amino acids daily for 4 days on GH release was examined in highly trained weightlifters (age: x = 25 y).[30] One gram each of arginine, lysine, and ornithine were consumed at 1 PM and again at 9 PM daily. Subjects also performed a 90-minute weight-training session with resistances of 70–80% of maximal load beginning at 1 PM. The pattern and magnitude of GH secretion over a 24-hour period was not different between placebo and amino acid–supplemented conditions. Subjects in this study consumed high-protein diets of 2.2 g/kg/day (19% of total energy intake). This might mask or blunt a possible effect of amino acids on GH secretion.[23]

Amino acid supplementation did not affect GH concentrations before or after 7 days of high-volume weightlifting in elite junior weightlifters.[44] Although this study is sometimes cited as showing that amino acids do not alter GH release, the purpose of this study was not to examine the effects of amino acids as growth hormone releasing agents. Furthermore, the total amount of arginine, ornithine, and lysine ingested was only 2082 mg daily. An amino acid supplement of 2.368 g was consumed before each of three daily meals and included 694 mg of arginine, ornithine, and lysine. Also, 2.1 g of branched-chain amino acids and 50 mg of glutamine were consumed before each workout. Consumption of branched-chain amino acids or glutamine may reduce the GH response to exercise.

It has been suggested that failure to find an enhancement of the acute GH response to exercise when arginine and lysine were ingested immediately before exercise may be related to a reduction in gastrointestinal tract blood flow. During exercise, blood flow is directed away from the gastrointestinal tract toward active muscles. Thus, absorption of arginine and lysine could be attenuated. A relationship between blood amino acid and GH levels has been reported in the elderly.[27] However, infusion of 30 g of arginine, 20 minutes after the completion of 20 minutes of brisk walking, was not effective in increasing the GH response to exercise.[25] Arginine infusion was used to bypass absorption issues. Larger doses taken orally of arginine and lysine could be given in conjunction with exercise to

enhance the acute GH response to exercise. However, large doses may exceed bowel tolerance and cause intestinal disturbances.[45]

The anabolic effects of GH are mediated by insulin-like growth factor-1 (IGF-1); therefore, the timing of amino acid ingestion to elevate GH and IGF-1 levels is uncertain. Increases in somatomedin A, an earlier designation for IGF, were not detected when blood was sampled from 30 minutes to 2 hours after administration of 1.2 g each of arginine and lysine. However, somatomedin-A levels were elevated threefold at the 8-hour time point.[20] Additional studies are needed to assess both the GH and IGF-1 response to amino acids and exercise.

Effects of Arginine and Ornithine Supplementation on Body Composition

No evidence based on properly conducted, rigorous scientific study suggests that the use of amino acid supplements in conjunction with strength-training increases muscle growth or lean body mass to a greater extent than strength training alone. Two studies that reported greater increases in body mass and reduction in percent body fat,[46] and gains in total body strength, lean body mass, and reduced urinary hydroxyproline excretion[47] as a result of arginine and ornithine supplementation were seriously flawed. In these studies, untrained adult males (mean ages, 38.3 and 37.2 yrs, respectively) trained 3 days per week for 5 weeks. Body composition was assessed using skinfolds and body girths, but not hydrostatic weighing. Subjects in the experimental groups ingested 500 mg each of arginine and ornithine twice daily. In the first study,[46] the statistical procedure used in data analysis was reported as an analysis of variance (ANOVA) using a 2 × 3 factorial design. However, data in the paper were given as absolute change for body mass, percent body fat, and body girths. It appears that each of the dependent variables measured was used within the same ANOVA, thus the "3" in the 2 × 3 statistical analysis. This is clearly an inappropriate statistical analysis. Furthermore, t-tests of the data shown in the paper show no difference for body mass, percent body fat, and the sum of body girth measurements between placebo and amino acid–supplemented groups. In the second study,[47] only the data collected after 5 weeks of training were used in the analysis. The authors reported using a two-way ANOVA with group (amino acid or placebo) and the dependent variables (strength, lean body mass, hydroxyproline excretion) used in the analysis. Again, this is an incorrect statistical procedure. Although it was suggested that the effects of amino acid supplementation could have been due to the effects of arginine and ornithine on GH, the conclusion is not supported by the data.[46,47] Again, there are no properly designed studies demonstrating greater gains in strength or lean body mass in individuals using specific amino acids as GH secretagogues in conjunction with strength training.

Peptide and Nonpeptide GH Secretagogues

The development of orally active peptide and nonpeptide compounds that stimulate the secretion of endogenous GH is a reasonable alternative to GH treatment, because of cost and the requirement for parenteral administration of GH.[48] GH is released episodically in vivo; therefore, it is hypothesized that GH-releasing factors that mimic or amplify the pulsatile release of GH could be more effective than a single injection of GH.[49] There are no reports of athletes obtaining and using these orally active GH secretagogues, but it is common for athletes to obtain any compounds that they believe will enhance muscle mass, strength, and performance. Availability of these GH secretagogues would greatly increase the complexities of drug testing, because they are small molecules that stimulate GH release after intravenous, subcutaneous, oral, and intranasal administration.[50]

Although their exact mechanism(s) of action has not been elucidated, both peptide and nonpeptide GH secretagogues bind to a specific receptor that is distinct from the GH-releasing hormone (GHRH) receptor on both the pituitary and hypothalamus.[50–52] It is thought that they act by inhibiting somatostatin and/or possibly by a GHRH-mediated mechanism.[52] The effects of GH secretagogues are synergistic with GHRH.[50] Although there is some desensitization to these GH secretagogues, IGF-1 concentrations remain elevated during long-term, intermittent oral administration.[50,53]

Growth hormone-releasing peptides (GHRPs) are a series of hepta- (GHRP-1) and hexapeptides (GHRP-2, GHRP-6, hexarelin) that have a dose-dependent effect on GH secretion in man after intravenous, subcutaneous, intranasal, and oral administration.[51] GH-releasing peptide-6 (GHRP-6), a synthetic hexapeptide first identified in the early 1980s,[54] has been shown to be a potent, relatively selective, GH secretagogue in humans.[55–57] The GH release induced by intravenous administration of 1 μg/kg iv hexarelin is greater than that elicited by 1 g/kg GHRH, and larger doses of hexarelin induce greater increases in GH.[58] Intranasal administration of 60 μg/kg hexarelin 3 times daily for up to 8 months to prepubertal short children, aged 4 to 11.6 yrs, increased IGF-1 levels 36%, linear growth velocity 56%, and reduced skinfold thickness.[59] However, treatment of adults with 1.5 μg/kg of hexarelin by subcutaneous injection twice daily for 16 weeks did not alter total body fat or lean body mass.[60]

Absorption of the GH-releasing peptides rarely exceeds 1% of the administered dose[61]; therefore, nonpeptide oral GH secretagogues that have reasonable oral absorption and high potency were developed. These nonpeptide GH secretagogues, including L-692,429, L-692,585, and MK-677 were discovered using GHRP-6 as a template.[51] MK-677, is a nonpeptide spiropiperidine that was developed by Merck Research Laboratories (Rahway, New Jersey), and is one of the more commonly known nonpeptide GH secretagogues. MK-677 synergizes with GHRH through a receptor and signal transduction pathway that is distinct from that of GHRH and is antagonistic to somatostatin.[49] MK-677 increases circulating GH and IGF-1 concentrations in calorie-restricted subjects,[48] obese young and middle-aged adults,[43] and in GH-deficient men.[62] MK-677 administration for a 7-day period reversed the negative nitrogen balance induced by caloric restriction in healthy young subjects.[48] In obese males, treatment with MK-677 for 8 weeks increased fat-free mass by 3 kg, but did not alter total and visceral fat.[53] The increased fat-free mass did not appear to be due to an increase in body water based on estimations of total body water.

MK-677 was being developed for possible treatment of GH deficiency in children and the frail elderly, as well as reduction of tissue wasting caused by trauma or disease. MK-677 may be advantageous to GH since it results in a more physiological GH release pattern that might be associated with smaller effects on blood glucose and fluid retention. Although MK-677 showed some promise, further evaluation has been suspended. Merck did not provide any reason for suspension of testing. Additional GH secretagogues may be developed. For example, L-692, 429 is a substituted benzolactam, which stimulates pulsatile GH secretion and increases circulating GH concentrations when infused in healthy older adults.[62,63]

There are no reports of athletes obtaining and using these newer GH secretagogues. Although they can increase circulating GH and IGF-1 levels, there are no published studies regarding their effects on individuals undergoing rigorous athletic training.

Other GH-Releasing Agents

Additional substances, such as clonidine,[64,65] L-dopa,[16] and methylphenidate[66,67] have been shown to induce GH release. Oral administration of clonidine for 6 months to short children without GH deficiency did not alter growth velocity.[68] Although L-dopa induces an increase in GH concentration and has been used as a provocative test of GH release,[69] it is often associated with nausea and vomiting.[16] Apparently, some athletes have used L-dopa to stimulate GH release.[70] Studies examining its effectiveness in athletes have not been done. These compounds are not recommended for use by athletes attempting to increase GH release.

Current Controversy: Drug Testing in Sport

Michael H. Stone, PhD, CSCS

One of the characteristics of competitive sport that distinguishes it from other forms of physical activity is the importance of winning. Indeed, in many countries 2nd place is referred to as the *first loser*. In this context an athlete purposefully chooses to strive for performance excellence. It is likely that a large part of the emphasis on winning and excellence of performance stems from an intrinsic motivating factor (i.e., some people simply hate to lose). Other extrinsic factors can also play a major role. For example, sports fans prefer and even expect their teams to be winners regardless of the competitive level. Some countries, both past and present, have used sport as a political tool often to the detriment of sport (e.g., Soviet Union's boycott of the 1984 Summer Olympics in Los Angeles). Because of these factors even *amateur* sport with its myriad of governing bodies has become a big business with high stakes for those involved. Thus, because of both intrinsic and extrinsic factors it is incumbent upon the athlete to be a winner.

Despite the efforts of most sports organizations and the medical community anabolic steroids remain on the sports/recreation landscape. The potential danger of high-dose/long-term usage has been well documented but the relatively modest and generally reversible negative side effects of short-term/low-dose use make the ergogenic effects attractive to thousands of users. Recent research points out beneficial effects for some medical conditions. Further research is indicated to define the benefits and risks of usage. While they remain illegal and unethical, the sports and medical community have a responsibility to provide the most honest and accurate information on anabolic steroids. We cannot eradicate use but we must strive to eliminate abuse.
–Norman D. Wathen, MS, ATC, CSCS, NSCA-CPT, 1999-2000 President of the National Strength and Conditioning Association

et al., 1996). This is not to suggest that ergogenic aids cannot cause harm, but rather to place them in a more appropriate context. Certainly, one could posit that certain ergogenic aids such as androgens might offer some protection against injury due to their anabolic properties. Indeed, the misinformation concerning androgens has been so persuasive, pervasive, and prevalent that one would expect high rates of mortality associated with their use. However, there are no data that support this notion. The fear of harmful effects as a result of androgen use, along with the fear of being found positive on a drug test has often precluded their beneficial use for medical reasons (Beiner et al., 1999). Perhaps a reevaluation of the relationship between health and competitive athletics is necessary and reasonable.

Other issues that are somewhat disturbing regard the attitudes held by International and National Governing Bodies (NGBs) towards the use of ergogenic aids. For instance, the idea that one can earn a medal in an event such as weightlifting without the use of androgens (or other illicit substances) has been put forth by the NGBs. This, despite the fact that athletes believe that taking illicit ergogenic aids actually *levels the playing field* rather than provides an undue advantage. Consider men's weightlifting as an example. Within weightlifting circles, it has been suspected for some time that weightlifters in certain countries, particularly in Eastern Europe, regularly use small doses of androgens in conjunction with intense training. Canada, Great Britain, Finland, Sweden, Norway, and the USA have about 7000 weightlifters, yet they do not win medals in the World Championships or the Olympics. Eastern European countries have traditionally been dominant in weightlifting. It is unlikely that Eastern Europeans are genetically superior. Nor is it likely that Eastern Europeans have discovered a vastly superior training program that has been kept secret for 20 years. What is interesting, however, is that Canada, Great Britain, Finland, Sweden, Norway, and the USA all have had strict doping control

business with high stakes for those involved. Thus, because of both intrinsic and extrinsic factors it is incumbent upon the athlete to be a winner.

Hypocrisy Regarding Drug Testing?

The International Olympic Committee's policy on doping has been instituted partly to protect the athlete's health; however, high-level athletic competition is often an inherently unhealthy endeavor. If health is a factor then why are certain sports with high injury rates or the potential for serious injury allowed at all? For example, many linemen playing American football weigh over 135 kg. These higher body weights are necessary to be successful at this sport; however, gaining large amounts of weight is unhealthy. Boxing is universally considered to be a dangerous sport, but is part of the Olympic program. Interestingly, there are no studies currently available which compare the harmful effects of sports with ergogenic aids. On the other hand, there is information that suggests that the harmful effects of ergogenic aids, particularly androgens have been exaggerated (Street

procedures in place for 20 years. Weightlifting's finances (mostly derived through NGBs) as with other sports are usually directly related to how well they perform and to how many medals they produce in major events (i.e., World Championships and Olympics). Thus, governing bodies expect medals to be won knowing that it is extremely unlikely that their athletes can compete on an equal basis. This problem is not isolated to weightlifting.

There is still a great deal of argument over what constitutes an ergogenic aid both among sport scientists and sport administrators. However, there are extremes. Some sports officials have argued that almost anything that is not directly shown to be a *naturally* occurring nutrient should be banned. This would include vitamins and artificially packaged or refined substances including sports drinks. At the other extreme are those who would allow the use of any method of potentially increasing performance. Although the latter stance is clear-cut, the former is not, as it requires definitions of what constitutes an ergogenic aid. Although most sporting authorities and sport scientists are not at either extreme they will tend to choose one side over the other. Thus, defining ergogenic aids is not a simple proposition.

For instance, androstenedione, DHEA, and a few related compounds can be legally sold without a physician's prescription in the United States and several other countries. Whether they work as ergogenic aids is subject to debate (King et al., 1999). The IOC and its related governing bodies ban these compounds as they are related to androgens (which are ergogenic). Baseball, the NHL, and a few other governing bodies for professional sports do not ban them. In 1998, Randy Barnes, the world record holder in the shot-put, incurred a lifetime ban for taking androstenedione; Mark McGuire, who admitted taking androstenedione, broke a long-standing home run record. According to the mainstream media, Randy Barnes was deemed a disgraced cheater whereas Mark McGuire was a hero, even though they used the *same* substance.

The IOC's policy on doping basically states that the use of an "expedient substance or method" to gain a performance advantage is against the rules. The use of birth control pills to control the menstrual period during training and competition is not banned, yet clearly places women in an unnatural state. The argument in support of this practice is that the hormones supplied by the birth control pills basically represent replacement therapy (Reis et al., 1999). Increased training volume or intensity has been shown to decrease the testosterone concentrations in males and has been associated with symptoms of overtraining and overstress (Hakkinen et al., 1987; Stone et al., 1991). However, the use of exogenous testosterone in males, even as replacement therapy, is banned. One could interpret this information to indicate that ergogenic hormone therapy is acceptable for women but not for men.

False Positives

In any discussion of ergogenic aids and doping one must consider the tests and the testing procedures themselves. Science is based on probabilities, not absolutes. There is always a degree of error in the tests and testing procedures. Consider the following. Because there is always a degree of error, this means that there will always be false positives and false negatives. However, the IOC and its subsidiaries have released little or no data on its testing procedures dealing with athletes. Most of the published data on testing, particularly with anabolic steroids, have been carried out with small numbers of untrained nonathletes. Thus, the exact degree of error is unknown. For the sake of argument, assume that the chance of a false positive is 0.0015% (Denhennin and Scholler, 1990). This seems quite small; however, if 10,000 athletes were to be tested in a year, one might expect as many as 15 false-positive tests. In reality this means that, potentially, 15 athletes will be wrongly accused of violating the rules governing their sport. Furthermore, as of 1996 the degree of agreement among six IOC laboratories was not acceptable (Catlin et al., 1996). Thus, the degree of error is not consistent between laboratories and the chance of a false positive may be greater in some laboratories. This clearly may exacerbate the problem.

Certain drugs such as cocaine are not found naturally occurring (as far as we know) in humans. Thus, detection of these substances is relatively easy. Many hormones, when used as ergogenic aids, are quite difficult to detect (e.g., growth hormone). Also, certain androgens have been recently shown to occur naturally (i.e., nandrolone); thus, cutoff limits for drug testing must be established.

Several problems arise from the testing of androgens. First consider testosterone (T). Because T is produced in relatively large amounts naturally, simply finding an amount that is somewhat over the average limits cannot be considered positive. Currently the test for the use of exogenous testosterone is the testosterone:epitestosterone ratio. In normal untrained adult humans the ratio of production is approximately 1:1. This ratio may be disturbed slightly by alcohol ingestion (especially in women), aging (Starks et al., 1996; Karila et al., 1996), physical activity, sexual activity, etc. The established ratio for testing positive is 6:1. The use of this ratio in drug testing is greatly complicated because there is evidence that at least 1 in 2000 (0.0005%) men are deficient in the enzyme(s) necessary for the production of epitestosterone (Eichner, 1997); this would suggest that their

T:E ratio will be higher than 6:1. The likelihood of finding athletes with high T:E ratios is illustrated by the Swedish anti-doping program. As reported in 1996, 28 out of 8946 samples (0.3%) produced T:E ratios higher than 6; however, only one of these 28 samples was conclusively considered to be the result of exogenous testosterone use (Garle et al., 1996). This study not only points out the difficulty of determining whether exogenous testosterone was used, but also suggests that the actual incidence of naturally occurring high T:E ratios may be as high as 0.3% in athletes. Detection of exogenous testosterone use can be further complicated if the athlete simultaneously uses exogenous epitestosterone (Denhennin and Peres, 1996). Because it is difficult to determine the difference between natural and synthetic T using the T:E ratio, alternate or additional methods are being considered such as using a testosterone: luteinizing hormone ratio (Perry et al., 1997). Another alternative is the use of carbon isotope ratios. Differences in the ratio of carbon isotopes are used to construct T synthetically and the ratio found in naturally occurring T. However, the isotope ratio method of determining these differences is not any more accurate than using the T:E ratio at present. Furthermore, the carbon isotope ratio (C12:C13) may be affected by diet (Shakleton et al., 1997).

Recently, the sporting world has been shocked by the number of positive doping tests for nandrolone. Included in these positive tests are several superstars of track and field including Linford Christie and Merlene Ottey. Nandrolone is typically injected in an oil base and is the primary anabolic agent, which has been avoided by athletes subject to drug tests because it is easily detected even months after injection (Kintz et al., 1999). It has only been within the last 2–3 years that nandrolone has been shown conclusively to be a naturally occurring steroid and the IOC has adopted a doping positive cutoff of 2 ng/mL (Kintz et al., 1999; Dehennin et al., 1999). It is interesting that many of the positive tests produced concentrations of only 8–12 ng/mL. This suggests several possibilities. First, the tests are becoming more sensitive (i.e., the IOC position) and the athletes were taking a banned substance. Second, the test doesn't work and is showing false positives (i.e., the position of some athletes, coaches, and scientists). Third, the athletes were taking (legally purchased) over-the-counter food supplements that contained a substance which produces nandrolone or its metabolites unknown to them (i.e., the position of some athletes, coaches, and scientists). The stature and number of athletes being tested positive have raised questions about the validity of the tests, questions that have reached national government levels. To date (August 1999), the IOC has released little information on the testing program, which would allow independent verification of its testing procedures (Sport:

Demands Grow for Drug Test Review, BBC Online News, August 5, 1999; Sport: Call for Fail Safe Drug Tests, BBC Online News, August 4, 1999). Certainly, with the potential problems seen with drug testing (i.e., false positives), it is not difficult to legally challenge the veracity of such tests.

Flawed Process?

In the process of drug testing, two samples of urine are collected and stored. If a positive test occurs for sample A, the NGB and the athlete are notified. The athlete or their representative can observe sample B being tested. If both samples are positive, the test results are subsequently made public. The athlete has a right to arbitration (i.e., a *trial*). In many sports there are two trials. First is the trial within the athletes' governing body and then there can be a trial within the international body. This system then places the athlete and their NGB in adversarial roles. For example, in track and field the International Athletics Federation (IAAF) is the international governing body. First the athlete must go through arbitration within their NGB (UK Athletics or USA Track and Field, for example). The results of this trial are then forwarded to the IAAF. Rarely, if ever, does the IAAF accept an NGB arbitration verdict that the athlete was innocent of doping (e.g., Dennis Mitchell and Dougie Walker). The stated position of the IAAF is that the athlete is guilty until proven innocent and that it does not matter how the substance got there (Athlete guilty until proven innocent/Doug Gillon, August 20, 1999, The Electronic Herald). Thus, the second trial begins with the IAAF. Rarely, if ever, do the athletes prove themselves not guilty to the IAAF (e.g., Dennis Mitchell and Dougie Walker). A number of reasons can be given for a false positive including individual differences in metabolism, taking a legal supplement that contains a banned (or the building blocks) substance, and sabotage (e.g., Tonya Harding). None of these reasons are sufficient in the eyes of the IOC/IAAF.

What is unfortunate is that after the myriad of legal maneuvers, the athlete's reputation can be damaged and a considerable amount of time, money, and effort are spent. The athlete (e.g., Diane Modahl) might win the lawsuit and then the NGB loses a great deal of money; however, the IAAF and IOC have so far been protected. Even when a national court finds in favor of an athlete (e.g., Butch Reynolds) the IOC/IAAF, etc. may not meet their obligations openly or fairly.

Summary

Although many other issues could be discussed, there are clearly problems with doping tests. Pointing out these problems is not a blanket indictment of doping control but rather an attempt to identify deficiencies.

There is little doubt that ergogenic aids will continue to be used, as will banned substances until adequate testing methods can be devised. Perhaps the vast majority of athletes would not use banned substances if they believed that the playing field was level. Certainly, the current testing methods do not work well. Consider the following:

1. The IOC testing procedures should be reviewed by independent agencies. The IOC should release data on athletic testing (especially for nandrolone) to independent agencies for evaluation and validation.

2. Until adequate tests can be devised for testosterone, it should be removed from the banned list.

3. An independent agency should take over doping control that will remove suspicion from the athletic governing bodies and eliminate the current adversarial role of the national and international governing bodies.

Beiner JM, Jokl P, Cholewicki J, Panjabi MM. The effect of anabolic steroids and corticosteroids on healing of muscle contusion injury. Am J Sports Med 1999;27(1):2–9.

Catlin DH , Cowan DA, de la Torre R, et al. Urinary testosterone (T) to epitestosterone (E) ratios by GC/MS. Initial comparison of uncorrected T\E in six international laboratories. J Mass Spectros 1996;31(4):397–402.

Dehennin L, Peres G. Plasma and urinary markers of oral testosterone misuse by healthy men in presence of masking epitestosterone administration. Int J Sports Med 1996;17(5):315–319.

Dehennin L, Scholler R. Detection of self-administration of testosterone as an anabolic by determination of the ratio of urinary testosterone to urinary epitestosterone in adolescents. Pathol Biol 1990;38(9):920–922.

Dehennin L, Bonnaire Y, Plou P. Urinary excretion of 19-norandrosterone of endogenous origin in man: quantitative analysis by gas chromatography-mass spectrometry. J Chromatog Biomed Appl 1999;72:301–307.

Eichner ER. Ergogenic aids: what athletes are using—and why. Phys Sports Med 1997;25(4):70–77.

Garle MR, Ocka E, Palonek I. Bjorkhem. Increased urinary testosterone:epitestosterone ratios found in Swedish athletes in connection with a national control program: evaluation of 28 cases. J Chromatog Biol Biomed Appl 1996;687(1):55–59.

Hakkinen K, Pakarinen A, Alen M, et al. Relationships between training volume, physical performance capacity, and serum hormone concentrations during prolonged training in elite weightlifters. Int J Sports Med 1987;1:61–65.

Karila T, Kosumen V, Leinomen A, et al. High doses of alcohol increase urinary testosterone-to-epitestosterone ratio in females. J Chromatog Biol Biomed Appl 1996;687(1):109–116.

King DS, Sharp RL, Vukovich MD, et al. Effect of oral androstenedione on serum testosterone and adaptations to resistance training in young men. JAMA 1999;28(21):2020–2028.

Kintz P, Crimele V, Ludes B. Norandrostenolone and noretiocholanolone: metabolite markers. Acta Clin Belg (Suppl) 1999;1:68–73.

Levine BD, Stray-Gundersen J. Living high–training low: effect of moderate altitude acclimatization with low-altitude training on performance. J Appl Physiol 1997;83(1):102–112.

Perry PJ, MacIndoe JH, Yates WR, et al. Detection of anabolic steroid administration: ratio of urinary testosterone:epitestosterone vs the ratio of urinary testosterone to luteinizing hormone. Clin Chem 1997 May;43(5):731–735.

Reis E., Frick U, Scimidtbleicher D. Frequency variation of strength training sessions triggered by the phases of the menstrual cycle. Int J Sports Med 1995;16(8):545–550.

Shakleton CH, Phillips A, Cahng T, Li Y. Confirming testosterone administration by isotope ratio mass spectrometric analysis of urinary androstenediols. Steroids 1997;62(4):379–387.

Starka L, Hill M, Lapcik O, Hampl R. Epitestosterone as an endogenous antiandrogen in men. Vnitr Lek 1996;43(9):620–623.

Stone MH, Keith R, Kearney JT, et al. Overtraining: a review of the signs and symptoms of overtraining. J Appl Sports Sci 1991;5(1):35–50.

Street C, Antonio J, Cudlipp D. Androgen use by athletes: a reevaluation of the health risks. Can J Appl Physiol 1996;21(6):421–440.

SUMMARY

Data on prohormones are at best sparse. We do know that transient elevations in serum testosterone can be achieved with oral or sublingual androstenedione and -diol consumption. It is not known if transient elevations in serum testosterone confer a long-term anabolic effect. Furthermore, there are currently no human data on norandrostenedione and norandrostenediol. So, in this case, one can *rely* only on anecdotal reports. Low doses of sublingual androgens (primarily 4-androstenediol) do not seem to have an effect on body composition in trained bodybuilders. However, preliminary evidence suggests that higher daily doses (~450 mg) may be effective in augmenting lean body mass. The evidence for androstenedione having an ergogenic effect is nonexistent. Within the limitations of the King et al.[10] study, it is apparent that androstenedione is ineffective. Furthermore, the

case study of the well-trained bodybuilder gaining fat mass and losing lean body mass after two 4-week cycles of androstenedione does not bode well for this supplement.

The practice of consuming specific amino acids, particularly arginine, lysine, and ornithine to increase GH levels during or after exercise does not appear to be effective. Although consumption of specific amino acids at high doses can increase GH concentrations,[24] this response is affected by training status, sex, and diet. Furthermore, exercise is a potent stimulant for GH release, and amino acids have not been shown to augment the exercise-induced increase.[19,41] Also, the significance of the exercise-induced elevation in GH levels is not clear, and studies need to examine the effect of exercise and amino acid supplementation on IGF-1 levels. Finally, there is no evidence that supplementation with arginine, ornithine, or lysine is effective in altering body composition. The primary side effects of consuming large quantities of amino acids are stomach cramping and diarrhea.

The peptide and nonpeptide GH secretagogues can increase circulating GH and IGF-1 levels,[48,53,62] even with long-term administration. Even though these GH secretagogues have been shown to improve body composition in some studies,[53,59] there are no studies examining their effectiveness in recreational or highly trained athletes. The side effects of these compounds can include impaired glucose tolerance and other side effects associated with GH use. These agents enhance the normal pulsatile secretion of GH; therefore, they

are likely to have lesser side effects than a single daily bolus injection of GH.

Additional compounds can increase GH levels, but the long-term effects on GH release and body composition have not been studied. Because of the nausea and vomiting associated with L-dopa it is unlikely to be used routinely for physique enhancement.

Finally, the administration of GH to individuals undergoing strength training has not been shown to result in greater gains in strength or mass than strength training alone.[71,72] The use of amino acids and other GH secretagogues to promote greater gains in muscle mass and strength and to alter body composition is not recommended.

AUTHORS' RECOMMENDATIONS

The use of prohormones as a means of increasing skeletal muscle mass is largely untested. With the limited data that exist, relatively high doses of 4-androstenediol are ostensibly effective in improving lean body mass in young males. However, androstenedione is ineffective as an ergogenic aid and would not be recommended. Whether norandrostenedione and -diol are equally effective (or ineffective) awaits further research. It is not known if an ergogenic effect of prohormone supplementation would be more easily achieved in older men, hypogonadal men, or women. One would suspect that individuals who have low plasma testosterone concentrations might benefit from prohormone supplementation.

The consumption of single amino acids for improving body composition and exercise performance (vis-a-vis elevations in plasma GH) is not supported by the literature. On the other hand, there are single amino acids that might confer an ergogenic effect based on their anticatabolic properties (i.e., branched-chain amino acids, glutamine, etc.) (see Chapter 5). Inasmuch as exercise and sleep are potent stimulators of GH release, consuming high-dose amino acids as a strategy to increase GH levels and therefore improve body composition would seem expensive and fruitless. Certainly, there are easier ways to improve body composition.

FUTURE RESEARCH

Because the primary consumers of prohormones and GH enhancers are young male athletes, it would seem sensible that future research uses trained men as their study population. Although untrained subjects are readily available for scientific study, the relevance of data derived from these individuals is highly questionable. The following variables need to be elucidated regarding these supplements.

1. Is there a dose-related response? That is, would androstenedione, a largely ineffectual supplement at doses less than 500 mg, promote gains in lean body mass if used at high doses (>500 mg daily)?

2. Is there a population-specific response? Would older men or hypogonadal men respond favorably to prohormone supplementation (see Sidebar "Older Men and Androstenedione")? Women?

3. What is the minimal and optimal treatment duration for the prohormones?

4. Does prolonged use of prohormones affect the hypothalamic-pituitary-gonadal axis?

5. Is there a differential response with the various prohormones regarding body composition, blood chemistry, etc?

REFERENCES

1. Wilson JD. Androgen abuse by athletes. Endo Rev 1988;9(2): 181–199.
2. Bhasin S, Storer TW, Berman N, et al. The effect of supraphysiological doses of testosterone on muscle size and strength in normal men. N Engl J Med 1996;335(1):1–7.
3. Street C, Antonio J, Cudlipp D. Androgen use by athletes: a reevaluation of the health risks. Can J Appl Physiol 1996;21(6):421–440.
4. Rogol AD, Yesalis CE. Anabolic-androgenic steroids and athletes: what are the issues? J Clin Endocrinol Metabol 1992;74(3):465–469.
5. Earnest CP, Olson MA, Broeder CE, et al. Oral 4-androstene-3,17-dione and 4-androstene-3,17-diol supplementation in young males. Eur J Appl Physiol 2000;81:229–232.
6. Ziegenfuss TN, Lambert CP, Lowery LM. Oral administration of testosterone precursors elevates plasma androgens in men. Abstract presented at the International Conference on Weight Lifting and Strength Training. Finland, 1998.
7. Ziegenfuss TN, Kerrigan DJ, Ehrman JK, Lowery LM. Physiological responses to a novel testosterone precursor. Abstract presented at the International Conference on the Physiology and Pyschology of Sport. Anchorage, Alaska, 1999.
8. Ziegenfuss TN, Kerrigan DJ. Safety and efficacy of prohormone administration in men. J Exerc Physiol 1999.
9. Antonio J, Uelmen J, Ehler L, et al. Case reports: Sublingual androgen use in six male bodybuilders, 2000.
10. King DS, Sharp RI, Vukovich MD, et al. Effect of oral androstenedione on serum testosterone and adaptations to resistance training in young men. JAMA 1998;281:2020–2028.
11. Kley HK, Desalaers T, Peerenboom H, Kruskemper HL. Enhanced conversion of androstenedione to estrogens in obese males. J Clin Endocrinol Metab 1980;51:1128–1132.
12. Antonio J, Sanders M. Effects of self-administered androstenedione on a young male bodybuilder: a single-subject study. Curr Ther Res 1999; 60:486–492.
13. Merimee TJ, Lillicrap DA, Rabinowitz D. Effect of arginine on serum-levels of human growth-hormone. Lancet 1965;2:668–670.
14. Jackson D, Grant DB, Clayton BE. A simple oral test of growth-hormone secretion in children. Lancet 1968;373–375.
15. Alba-Roth J, Muller OA, Schopohl J, Werder K. Arginine stimulates growth hormone secretion by suppressing endogenous somatostatin secretion. J Clin Endocrinol Metab 1988;67:1186–1189.
16. Sutton J, Lazarus L. Growth hormone in exercise: comparison of physiological and pharmacological stimuli. J Appl Physiol 1976;41: 523–527.
17. Evain-Brion D, Donnadie M, Roger M, Job JC. Simultaneous study of somatotrophic and corticotrophic pituitary secretions during ornithine infusion test. Clin Endocrinol 1982;17:119–122.
18. Knopf RF, Conn, JW, Fajans SS, et al. Plasma growth hormone response to intravenous administration of amino acids. J Clin Endocrinol 1965;25:140–144.
19. Suminski RR, Robertson RJ, Goss FL, et al. Acute effects of amino acid ingestion and resistance exercise on plasma growth hormone concentration in young men. Int J Sports Nutr 1997;7:48–60.
20. Isidori A, Lo Monaco A, Cappa, M. A study of growth hormone release in man after oral administration of amino acids. Curr Med Res Opin 1981;7:475–481.
21. Lambert MI, Hefer JA, Millar RP, Macfarlane PW. Failure of commercial oral amino acid supplements to increase serum growth hormone concentrations in male bodybuilders. Int J Sports Nutr 1993;3:298– 305.
22. Carlson HE, Miglietta JT, Roginsky MS, Stegnik LD. Stimulation of pituitary hormone secretion by neurotransmitter amino acids in humans. Metabolism 1989;38:1179–1182.
23. Carli G, Bonifazi M, Lodi L, et al. Changes in the exercise-induced hormone response to branched chain amino acid administration. Eur J Appl Physiol Occup Physiol 1992;64:272–277.
24. Bucci L, Hickson Jr JF, Pivarnik JM, et al. Ornithine ingestion and growth hormone release in bodybuilders. Nutr Res 1990;10:239–245.
25. Merimee TJ, Rabinowitz D, Fineberg SE. Arginine-initiated release of human growth hormone. N Eng J Med 1969;280:1434–1438.
26. Tanaka KS, Inoue J, Shiraki T, et al. Age-related decreases in plasma growth hormone: response to growth hormone-releasing hormone, arginine, and L-dopa in obesity. Metabolism 1991;40:1257–1262.
27. Corpas E, Blackman MR, Roberson R, et al. Oral arginine-lysine does not increase growth hormone or insulin-like growth factor-I in old men. J Gerontol 1993;48:M128–M133.
28. Sellini M, Fierro A, Marchesi L, et al. Behavior of basal values and circadian rhythm of ACTH, cortisol, PRL, and GH in a high-protein diet. Boll Soc Ital Biol Sper 1981;57:963–969.
29. Besset A, Bonardet A, Rondouin G, et al. Increase in sleep related GH and Prl secretion after chronic arginine aspartate administration in man. Acta Endocrinol (Copenh) 1982 Jan;99(1):18–23.
30. Fogelholm GM, Naveri HK, Kiilavuori KTK, Harkonen MHA. Low-dose amino acid supplementation: no effects on serum human growth hormone and insulin in male weightlifters. Int J Sports Nutr 1993;3:290–297.
31. Galbo H, Christensen NJ, Mikines KJ, et al. The effect of fasting on the hormonal response to graded exercise. J Clin Endocrinol Metab 1981;52:1106–1112.
32. Quirion A, Brisson G, De Carufel D, et al. Influence of exercise and dietary modifications on plasma human growth hormone, insulin and FFA. J Sports Med Phys Fitness 1988;28:352–353.
33. Hunter WM, Fonseka CC, Passmore R. Growth hormone: important role in muscular exercise in adults. Science 1963;150:1051–1053.
34. Sutton JR, Lazarus L. Effect of adrenergic blocking agents on growth hormone responses to physical exercise. Hormone Metab Res 1974; 6:428–429.
35. Kraemer WJ, Gordon SE, Fleck,SJ, et al. Endogenous anabolic hormonal and growth factor responses to heavy resistance exercise in males and females. Int J Sports Med 1991;12:228–235.
36. Kraemer RR, Kilgore JL, Kraemer GR, Castracane VD. Growth hormone, IGF-1, and testosterone response to resistive exercise. Med Sci Sports Exerc 1992;24:1346–1352.
37. Kraemer WJ, Marchtelli LJ, Gordon SE, et al. Hormonal and growth factor responses to heavy resistance exercise protocols. J Appl Physiol 1990;69:1442–1450.
38. Vanhelder WP, Radomski MW, Goode RC. Growth hormone responses during intermittent weight lifting exercise in men. Eur J Appl Physiol 1984;53:31–34.
39. Bloom SR, Johnson RH, Park DM, et al. Differences in the metabolic and hormonal response to exercise between racing cyclists and untrained individuals. J Physiol 1978;258:1–18.
40. Inoue Y, Copeland EM, Souba WW. Growth hormone enhances amino acid uptake by the human small intestine. Ann Surg 1994;219: 715–722.
41. Fricker PA, Beasly SK, Copeland, IW. Physiological growth hormone response of throwers to amino acids, eating, and exercise. Austr J Med Sport 1988;20:21–23.
42. Chandler RM, Byrne HK, Patterson JG, Ivy, JL. Dietary supplements affect the anabolic hormones after weight-training exercise. J Appl Physiol 1994;76:839–845.
43. Eto B, Gisele LM, Porquet D, Peres G. Glutamate-arginine salts and hormonal response to exercise. Arch Physiol Biochem 1995;103: 160–164.
44. Fry AC, Kraemer WJ, Stone MH, et al. Endocrine and performance responses to high volume training and amino acid supplementation in elite junior weightlifters. Int J Sports Nutr 1993;3:306–322.
45. Bucci L, Hickson Jr JF, Wolinsky I, Pivarnik JM. Ornithine supplementation and insulin release in bodybuilders. Int J Sports Nutr 1992;2:287–291.
46. Elam RP. Morphological changes in adult males from resistance exercise and amino acid supplementation. J Sports Med Phys Fitness 1988;28:35–39.
47. Elam RP, Hardin DH, Sutton RAL, Hagen L. Effect of arginine and ornithine on strength, lean body mass and urinary hydroxyproline in adult males. J Sports Med Phys Fitness 1989;29:52–56.
48. Murphy MG, Plunkett LM, Gertz BJ. MK-677, and orally active growth hormone secretagogue, reverses diet-induced catabolism. J Clin Endocrinol Metab 1998;83:320–325.
49. Smith RG, Pong SS, Hickey G, et al. Modulation of pulsatile GH release through a novel receptor in hypothalamus and pituitary gland. Recent Prog Horm Res 1996;51:261–285.
50. Ghigo E, Arvat E, Camanni F. Orally active growth hormone secretagogues: state of the art and clinical perspectives. Ann Med 1998;30: 159–168.
51. Camanni F, Ghigo E, Arvat E. Growth hormone-releasing peptides and their analogs. Frontiers Neuroendocrinol 1998;19:47–72.

52. Ghigo E, Arvat E, Muccioli G, Camanni F. Growth hormone-releasing peptides. Eur J Endocrinol 1997;136:445–460.

53. Svensson J, Lonn L, Jansson J-O, et al. Two-month treatment of obese subjects with the oral growth hormone (GH) secretagogue MK-677 increases GH secretion, fat-free mass, and energy expenditure. J Clin Endocrinol 1998;83:362–369.

54. Bowers C, Momany F, Chag D, et al. Structure-activity relationships of a synthetic pentapeptide that specifically releases GH in vitro. Endocrinology 1980;106:663–667.

55. Bowers CY, Reynolds GA, Durham D, et al. Growth hormone (GH)-releasing peptide stimulates GH release in normal men and acts synergistically with GH-releasing hormone. J Clin Endocrinol Metab 1990;70:975–982.

56. Bowers CY, Alster DK, Frentz JM. The growth hormone-releasing activity of a synthetic hexapeptide in normal men and short statured children after oral administration. J Clin Endocrinol Metab 1992;74:292–298.

57. Ilson BE, Jorkasky DK, Curnow RT, Stote RM. Effect of a new synthetic hexapeptide to selectively stimulate growth hormone release in healthy human subjects. J Clin Endocrinol Metab 1989;69:212–214.

58. Ghigo E, Arvat E, Gianotti L, et al. Growth hormone-releasing activity of Hexarelin, a new synthetic hexapeptide, after intravenous, subcutaneous, intranasal and oral administration in man. J Clin Endocrinol Metab 1994;78:693–698.

59. Laron Z, Frenkel J, Deghenghi R, et al. Intranasal administration of the GHRP hexarelin accelerates growth in short children. Clin Endocrinol 1995;43:631–635.

60. Rahim A, O'Neill PA, Shalet SM. Growth hormone status during long-term hexarelin therapy. J Clin Endocrinol Metab 1998;83:1644–1649.

61. Deghendhi R. The development of 'impervious peptides' as growth hormone secretagogues. Acta Paediatr Suppl 1997;423:85–87.

62. Chapman IM, Pescovitz OH, Murphy G, et al. Oral administration of growth hormone (GH) releasing peptide-mimetic MK-677 stimulates the GH/insulin-like growth factor-I axis in selected GH-deficient adults. J Clin Endocrinol Metab 1997;82:3455–3463.

63. Aloi JA, Gertz BJ, Hartman ML, et al. Neuroendocrine responses to a novel growth hormone secretagogue, L-692,492, in healthy older subjects. J Clin Endocrinol Metab 1994;79:943–949.

64. Cassanueva FF, Villanueva L, Cabranes JA, et al. Cholinergic mediation of growth hormone secretion elicited by arginine, clonidine, and physical exercise in man. J Clin Endocrinol Metab 1984;59:526–530.

65. Hunt GE, O'Sullivan BT, Johnson GF, Smythe GA. Growth hormone and cortisol secretion after oral clonidine in healthy adults. Psychoneuroendocrinology 1986;11:317–325.

66. Brown WA, Williams BW. Methylphenidate increases serum growth hormone concentration. J Clin Endocrinol Metab 1976;43:937–939.

67. Joyce PR, Donald RA, Nicholls MG, et al. Endocrine and behavioral responses to methylphenidate in normal subjects. Biol Psychiatry 1986;21:1015–1023.

68. Allen DB. Effects of nightly clonidine administration on growth velocity in short children without growth hormone deficiency: a double-blind, placebo controlled study. J Pediatr 1993;122:32–36.

69. Boyd AE, Lebovitz HE, Pfeiffer JB. Stimulation of human-growth-hormone by L-DOPA. N Engl J Med 1970;283:1425–1429.

70. Di Pasquale M. Amino acids and proteins for the athlete. Boca Raton, FL: CRC Press, 1997:103.

71. Crist DM, Peake GT, Egan PA, Waters, DL. Body composition response to exogenous GH during training in highly conditioned adults. J Appl Physiol 1988;65:579–584.

72. Yarasheski KE, Campbell JA, Smith K, et al. Effect of growth hormone and resistance exercise on muscle growth in young men. Am J Physiol 1992;262:E261–E267.

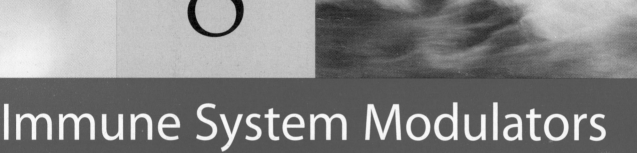

CHAPTER

8

Immune System Modulators

Marian Kohut

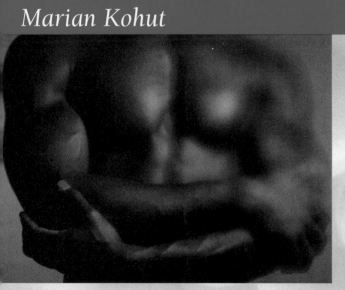

Research Review

Whey Protein Increases Longevity in Old Mice

The effects of a whey-rich diet (20 g/100 g diet) compared with that of Purina mouse chow or a casein-rich diet (20 g/100 g diet) were examined for 6.3 months in old male mice. Heart and liver tissue glutathione content were significantly higher in the whey-fed versus the casein diet–fed and Purina-fed mice in mice 17–20 months of age. Mice fed the whey protein diet at the onset of senescence or old age (84 weeks) exhibited increased longevity as compared to mice fed Purina mouse chow. The average survival time of mice fed the casein diet is almost identical to that of Purina-fed controls. Body weight curves were similar in all three dietary groups. Therefore, a whey protein diet appears to enhance the liver and heart glutathione concentration in aging mice and to increase longevity in older mice.

Certainly, the evidence in mice is intriguing; however, studies need to be repeated in elderly humans to see if similar effects are seen. At this point, it is not known if whey protein consumption affects human longevity. One could speculate that the increased glutathione levels seen in these mice played a role in their increased longevity. Glutathione is the cell's main antioxidant and is found in almost all mammalian cells. The liver has a tremendous amount of glutathione, which makes it to detoxify your body of various drugs, toxins, and other pollutants. Glutathione, a compound produced from three amino acids—cysteine, glutamic acid, and glycine—is a fairly large molecule that is not well absorbed from the GI tract. Thus, oral supplementation of glutathione is largely ineffective.

Bounous G, Gervais F, Amer V, et al. The influence of dietary whey protein on tissue glutathione and the diseases of aging. Clin Invest Med 1989;12:343–349.

Introduction

Many individuals seek to use nutritional supplements in an attempt to *boost immunity* in the hope that a particular supplement will prevent or reduce susceptibility to infection. Years of research have established that nutritional deficiencies are associated with compromised immune function and in some instances, increased susceptibility to infection. However, it has been much more difficult to demonstrate that a particular supplement enhances immune function AND reduces the susceptibility to or severity of infection in healthy well-nourished individuals. Many published studies report an enhancement of various immune responses in association with nutritional supplements; however, it has been much more difficult to demonstrate that these alterations of immune response have clinical relevance in terms of disease outcome. This is an important point to keep in mind when reviewing the literature regarding nutrition and immunity. Sometimes, an enhancement of immune function is observed in association with a particular supplement *in vitro* or in an animal model, but fails to produce the same results in humans. Another assumption that is often made relates to the clinical significance of studies in humans. It is often assumed that an enhancement of a particular immune response observed in association with the consumption of a nutritional supplement will directly result in increased resistance to infection. More often than not, an effect is found with respect to the immune parameter being measured, but no effect is found in relation to disease incidence or severity. The reader may question why this apparent inconsistency is observed. One

possibility is that most studies examine only one or two particular immune responses or changes in cell numbers, yet the immune system is a vast and complex network of cells, organs, and molecules that work together to defend the body against foreign invaders (viruses, bacteria, parasites, etc.). The response of one cell may not reflect this complex interaction and therefore an assumption made regarding the entire immune system based on the response of one cell may be inaccurate. At this time, the complex interactions between cells and molecules of the immune system and how they respond to hormones and/or other biochemical signals are not completely understood. Therefore, we often rely on clinical trials to determine whether an observed change in one immune parameter is associated with improved resistance to infection.

The Immune System

A brief review of the immune system may provide some information that could be helpful in analyzing the literature on nutrition and immunity. The immune system has the ability to recognize millions of foreign invaders. When the immune system encounters a foreign invader, an immune response is initiated, and anything that triggers an immune response is referred to as an *antigen*. The immune system has many different ways of preventing invaders from getting into the body (skin, mucous membranes) and if the microbe passes through these barriers, different methods may be used to destroy or eliminate an antigen.

The immune system is often divided into *nonspecific* defenses and *specific* immune responses. Nonspecific defenses which include phagocytic cells (granulocytes, monocytes, macrophages), natural killer cells, and a group of chemicals referred to as complement, are ready to attack and destroy any foreign invader. In other words, specific antigen markers on the foreign invader are not necessary to trigger the response of these cells and chemicals. They will attempt to destroy any bacteria or virus that tries to invade the body. The macrophage may digest these invaders and then display the foreign antigens in such a way as to involve the specific immune system.

In contrast, the specific immune system requires the recognition of specific antigen markers on the invader before an immune response can be initiated. The specific immune system can recognize and respond to millions of different antigens. B cells and T cells, both lymphocytes, are cells of the specific immune system. B cells secrete antibodies that circulate in body fluids and can attach to and destroy antigens. Each B cell is genetically programmed to secrete one specific antibody and this response occurs when the B cell encounters a specific antigen. After the antigen is encountered, if the B cell receives appropriate signals from other immune cells it will proliferate, producing plasma cells which secrete large amounts of the identical antibody that the original B cell was programmed to secrete. T cells have several functions. Some T cells (helper T cells) act to help other cells of the immune system by producing chemicals known as cytokines. Other T cells (cytotoxic T cells) can attack and eliminate virus-infected cells or cancer cells. The nonspecific and specific immune systems often work together to eliminate an invader. Communication between the nonspecific and specific immune systems may involve the release of chemicals called cytokines. Each cell of the immune system can release an array of cytokines, which have different functions such as recruiting other cells to the site of infection or helping other cells become active to assist in destroying an invader. Although we understand some of the functions and interactions between cells of the immune system, additional research will provide more information as to how all of these cells and chemicals work together to destroy pathogens.

The immune system is not an isolated system, but rather a bi-directional communication exists between the neuroendocrine system and the immune system. Therefore, the immune system responds not only to foreign invaders, but the immune system can also be modulated by neuropeptides and hormones and vice versa, resulting in a complex network. With this in mind, it may be easier to understand why one might observe an enhancement in one of the functions of a particular immune cell in association with the consumption of a nutritional supplement, yet no effect on resistance to infection. The response of one cell is just a small piece of a large and complicated puzzle and certainly one should be cautious in assuming that a change in a single parameter will completely alter the way the body responds to infectious agents.

It may also be beneficial to briefly review the typical immune measures used in many studies to assess immune

response. This brief discussion will be confined to those measures most often used in studies with human subjects. In general, blood is collected from human subjects and the cells are used in a number of assays. Typically, the measures of immune function in humans are limited to those that can be assayed in the blood. For ethical reasons, other immune tissues such as spleen or lymph nodes cannot be collected from humans. This is one limitation to studying human subjects (i.e., responses in blood immune cells may not reflect responses in other immune tissues).

Lymphocytes may be isolated from blood and often these cells are then stimulated with compounds called mitogens. Mitogens cause the cells to proliferate and release cytokines, similar to the proliferation that is observed when these cells encounter an invader such as a virus or bacteria. However, one important difference is that the markers recognized by a lymphocyte in the mitogen-induced proliferation and cytokine release are not the same as the markers used by the lymphocyte in response to a specific antigen (virus, bacteria, etc.). Therefore, the use of an antigen-specific measure is probably more physiologically relevant than mitogen-induced immune stimulation. It has also been shown that stress-induced alterations in mitogen-induced immune response differ from the antigen-induced response.[1] This is important to keep in mind, considering that many studies of exercise and immune function use mitogen-induced proliferation to assess lymphocyte function. This measure of immune function in association with exercise, which can be considered a stress, may therefore be completely different from antigen-specific immune response (most likely a better predictor of how the body actually responds to virus or bacteria). Mitogens stimulate the production of different cytokines. Often, different mitogens are used to assess cytokine production. However, the same precautions with respect to mitogen-induced or antigen-specific cytokine production need to be considered. Antibody levels in serum or saliva can also be measured. Again, the production of specific antibodies (e.g., in response to tetanus vaccine) may be used to predict antigen-specific response.

Another type of assay often used is the assessment of natural killer (NK) cell cytoxicity. NK cells can destroy virus-infected or tumor cells in a nonspecific manner. In this assay, NK cells are usually incubated with radiolabeled tumor cells for some period of time, and the degree of tumor cell killing (cytotoxicity) is measured. This assay is used often with respect to exercise immunology. One important aspect to keep in mind is that the number of circulating NK cells changes with exercise. Consequently, if one observes a change in cytoxicity, it is important to determine whether this is due to more NK cells in the assay or whether each cell has a greater killing capacity.

Monocytes or granulocytes including neutrophils may phagocytize (digest and destroy) foreign particles. Often potent chemicals are released in this process and many assays of neutrophil function will either assess phagocytosis and/or produce the reactive chemicals. Monocytes and granulocytes derived from human blood may also release different cytokines upon appropriate stimulation.

In summary, although there are numerous other immune functions that can be assessed, we have described the ones that are most often encountered with studies involving human subjects. Ideally, a study will incorporate several measures of immune function and also determine whether these changes have any clinical relevance in terms of disease outcome. The incidence of infection, such as cold or flu, is often used as an outcome measure, which may be diagnosed by a physician or simply reported by the subjects. Some studies may also examine the actual number of days of illness or number and severity of symptoms. Several of both clinical and immune measures can be used in these studies to provide information regarding the potential effect of nutritional supplements. The most convincing evidence with respect to an immunomodulatory effect of a supplement should include not only measures of immune function and alterations in susceptibility to or severity of disease, but also evidence that without the immunomodulatory effect, there is no change in clinical outcome. These types of studies are difficult, time consuming, and expensive and as a result, few of these studies have been done.

Dietary Supplementation and the Immune System

Unfortunately, there are few data regarding the role of many of the nutritional supplements reviewed in this chapter and how they might alter the immune system in association with exercise. The small amount of data that exists on this topic has usually been generated from studies of endurance activities. Therefore, for each supplement, studies regarding the potential immunomodulatory effect of the supplement are reviewed first. If there are any data available on how exercise might alter the effect of the supplement on immune response, these data are presented. The reader will find that there is a lack of data regarding strength-types of activities, immune function, and nutritional supplementation. Suggestions for future research are provided; unfortunately, recommendations regarding the role of these supplements in terms of enhanced immunity in the strength or power athlete cannot be made at this time due to the lack of data.

Arginine

Arginine is classified as a nonessential amino acid and therefore can be synthesized in the body in amounts adequate for the average, healthy adult. Interest in arginine as a supplement for athletes who are involved in sprint or power sports may be related to its involvement in the synthesis of creatine. The results from several studies also suggest that arginine may have some effects on immune function. These effects may be independent of or related to nitric oxide (NO) synthesis. Arginine functions as a precursor in the formation of NO. NO has several different functions in the body and one of these functions is to act as an important immune effector molecule. NO is formed from arginine and oxygen by nitric oxide synthase (NOS). There are several types of NOS, but the one that is important with respect to immune function is inducible NOS (iNOS). Microorganisms or cytokines produced by the immune system induce the formation of iNOS, which eventually results in the synthesis of NO. NO acts as a cytotoxic molecule and in that capacity can destroy tumor cells, invading microorganisms, and viral-infected cells.

Immune Effects

Although arginine is a precursor in the synthesis of NO, we are not aware of any studies to date that have demonstrated an increased production of NO, in either individuals or animals consuming additional arginine in the diet. Recall that the NO produced by immune cells is dependent on iNOS. The gene product iNOS is triggered by an encounter with microorganisms, or induced by cytokines. Typically, cytokines are released in response to immune activation, such as exposure to an infectious agent. Therefore, because NO production is dependent on immune activation, in the healthy state, it may be less likely to find an effect of arginine supplementation on NO production. In states of illness, injury, or patients undergoing surgery, some studies have demonstrated that arginine supplementation does enhance certain aspects of immune response. Surgical patients or breast cancer patients as well as injured animals demonstrate enhanced lymphocyte response to stimulation with mitogens.[2–5] Other studies have found no effect on lymphocyte proliferation.[6] Arginine supplementation may also have an antitumor effect in animal models, perhaps related to enhanced macrophage or NK cell cytotoxicity. However, arginine has also been shown to promote tumor growth and therefore the effect of arginine supplementation on tumor growth may be dependent on the type of tumor.[7–9]

Fewer studies have been performed to evaluate the effect of arginine supplementation in healthy individuals. However, the findings from several studies show that approximately 30 g of arginine HCl or arginine aspartate supplementation for 1 to 2 weeks increases lymphocyte proliferation and wound healing in both young[10,11] and elderly humans.[12] We are unaware of any studies of healthy individuals that have demonstrated an enhanced resistance to infection in association with dietary arginine supplementation. One study did examine arginine plus zinc supplementation in the elderly as a potential method of increasing antibody response to influenza vaccination in the elderly. This study found no benefit of supplementation on antibody response.[13] Arginine supplementation could have harmful effects. Excessive doses of arginine supplementation *in vitro* may inhibit or suppress immune response[14] and an appropriate *in vivo* dose has not been determined. It is important to be aware that arginine supplementation may potentially be harmful for some types of patients, in particular those suffering from sepsis. This possibility is an important area of study and it has been suggested that the effects of arginine supplementation on NO production in septic burn patients be carefully evaluated.[15]

The findings demonstrating an enhancement of immune function with arginine supplementation must be interpreted with caution. The mechanism(s) by which arginine may alter immunity are unknown. The level of other nutrients has not always been well controlled in these studies and therefore the immune effects that were observed may be related to a lack of certain nutrients or adequate nitrogen in the control diets. It has also been suggested that arginine, by itself, does not alter immunity, but in combination with other nutrients may have an effect on immune response.[5,16] Another possibility to consider is that the immunomodulatory effects of arginine are indirect and may result from the altered hormonal pattern following arginine intake. Catecholamines, corticosteroids, growth hormone, insulin, and prolactin release may be altered by arginine and each of these neuroendocrine factors has been shown independently to alter immunity. Therefore, the effects of arginine could be related to changes in the concentrations of these hormones and to our knowledge this possibility has not yet been investigated.

In conclusion, arginine supplementation may show some promise as to its potential enhancement of immune response particularly in those patients suffering from certain types of illness or injury. In healthy individuals, dietary supplementation with arginine requires further research before any clear conclusions can be made with respect to enhanced immunity. The role of supplemental arginine and the potential effects it may have in athletes remain to be established.

Vitamin A, C, E (Antioxidants)

Vitamin C, vitamin E (tocopherols), and some precursors to vitamin A (the carotenoids) exhibit antioxidant activity. Each of these vitamins has independently been shown to alter immunity. The antioxidant function of these vitamins is of interest to some athletes primarily because exercise increases the production of reactive oxygen species (ROS) which have been associated with muscular fatigue and muscular damage. In addition, neutrophils and macrophages produce ROS. The ROS produced by the immune system may have a role in modulating postexercise muscle damage.

The other reason that vitamins A, C, and E may be of interest to athletes relates to their potential immunostimulatory properties. The antioxidant properties of the vitamins may differ from the immunomodulatory effects and therefore will be discussed separately.

Reactive oxygen species (ROS) are produced during strenuous exercise, result in oxidative stress, and are associated with a depletion of antioxidants, muscle damage, and fatigue. High concentrations of antioxidants may protect against the damaging effects of ROS. An assumption has been made that a high intake of vitamins A, C, E, or beta-carotene may protect against the exercise-induced oxidative stress and several studies have examined this possibility. Vitamin E (alpha-tocopherol) is considered the most important scavenger of ROS at the level of membranes and is probably the most well studied with respect to exercise.

Several studies have established that exercise training is associated with a decrease in the accumulation of the products used to assess oxidative stress or an enhancement of antioxidant enzymes.[17–19] The findings from some studies suggest that vitamin E supplementation may protect against the oxidative damage induced by exercise.[20] However, the results from both human and animal studies show that vitamin E supplementation does not improve performance[21–25] and may not attenuate muscular damage following a marathon.[26]

An understanding of interactions between the immune system, ROS production, and muscle damage may provide some insight regarding antioxidants and exercise-induced muscle damage. Although these interactions are not completely understood at this time, it appears that the production of ROS by cells of the immune system may be an important part of the postexercise muscle repair process. Neutrophils and macrophages appear to infiltrate sites of postexercise muscle damage[27] and both of these cell types produce ROS. The release of ROS can enhance the release of cytokines[28,29] and cytokines can induce the production of ROS.[30,31] The release of both cytokines and ROS are important in removing damaged muscle tissue and may assist in the repair process.[27] The findings from a recent study suggest that the generation of ROS postexercise may be beneficial in the repair process. In this study, normal mice demonstrated greater oxidative stress postexercise than mice with inhibited neutrophil function; however, 4 days later normal mice showed evidence of less muscle damage.[32,33] Based on this evidence and findings from other studies mentioned previously, it should be noted that the production of free radicals or ROS during exercise may be an important part of the muscle tissue repair process and the consumption of high levels of antioxidants may not necessarily be beneficial.

Some researchers have examined life span and whether it can be extended by increased antioxidant intake. The evidence from two recent studies suggests that supplementing diets with high levels of antioxidants does not increase maximum life span[34] and exercised rodents fed a diet containing additional antioxidants did NOT have a greater life span than exercised rodents on a normal diet.[35] It appears that although exercise may be associated with a greater production of ROS, this does not result in a shortened life span and the consumption of additional antioxidants confers no additional increase in longevity.

Taken together, the findings from the studies above suggest that additional antioxidants do not improve performance, do not appear to improve muscle tissue repair postexercise, and are not beneficial in terms of increasing life span in exercised rodents. Although the interactions between the immune system and ROS produced during exercise need further research, at this time it does not appear that additional antioxidants will enhance immune responses such as postexercise muscle tissue repair. (For further information on antioxidants, see Chapter 12).

Vitamin A

Several approaches have been taken in an attempt to determine whether Vitamin A supplementation enhances immune response and resistance or recovery from infection. In some investigations, researchers have attempted to correlate plasma concentrations of beta-carotene or retinol with immune response or susceptibility to infection. One limitation of this approach is related to the fact that plasma concentrations may have depressed plasma retinol levels as a result of disease. Therefore, it is not possible to establish whether low plasma retinol levels resulted in suppressed immune response or if plasma retinol levels decreased in response to disease or infection. Another approach used is to supplement the diet with retinol precursors and examine immune response at a later time point. This approach may be useful in examining the particular aspects of immunity that may be altered by supplementation, but additional studies are necessary to determine whether these effects have clinical significance in terms of disease outcome. Vitamin A has been fairly well studied in terms of its immunomodulatory effects, and we will review the evidence from randomized controlled trials as well as potential mechanisms of action.

Vitamin A supplementation may afford some protection from infection in malnourished individuals, but the potential benefits of supplementation in normal wellnourished individuals remain to be established. There is evidence from several studies that suggests that vitamin A deficiency is associated with depressed immune function[36–39] and an impaired response to influenza infection.[40] Supplementation of vitamin A is associated with a reduction of mortality and morbidity among certain populations.[41] It appears that populations suffering from malnutrition may benefit from adequate or additional vitamin A supplementation. However, it is less clear if normal, healthy, well-nourished individuals will benefit from additional supplementation with respect to enhanced immunity. The results from several studies involving beta-carotene supplementation in the diet of healthy individuals suggest

that certain aspects of innate immunity, such as NK cytotoxicity and monocyte production of the cytokine TNFα, are enhanced.[42–44] It appears that lymphocyte subsets or the lymphocyte response to mitogens are not altered.[45,46] In addition, one study of healthy older individuals found that vitamin A supplementation was associated with a reduction in the number of T lymphocytes.[47] Whether these observed changes of immune function in response to supplementation actually result in reduced susceptibility to infection in healthy individuals is not well established. The results from one study demonstrated no association between vitamin A supplementation and incidence of bacterial infection.[48] We are not aware of any long-term, randomized clinical trials that have evaluated the incidence of viral infection in response to supplementation with vitamin A alone. However, several studies have examined the possibility that supplementation with several multivitamins and or trace elements such as zinc, may alter susceptibility to infection. In general, the findings from these studies show no protection from infection in association with vitamin intake, but a slight decrease in the incidence of infection in those individuals consuming supplemental trace elements such as zinc and selenium.[49–51] At this time, the potential benefits of vitamin A supplementation for healthy well-nourished individuals regarding susceptibility to infection remain to be established.

A high beta-carotene intake has also been associated with a reduced risk of cancer. Earlier epidemiological studies suggested a high natural (fruits and vegetables) intake of beta-carotene was associated with reduced risk of cancer. However, more recent studies have not observed any benefit of beta-carotene intake on incidence of cancer[52,53] and two studies actually observed an increased incidence of lung cancer in those participants consuming beta-carotene supplements.[54,55] The presence of other carotenoids in fruits and vegetables has been suggested to be the protective factor in regards to cancer incidence in the early epidemiological studies.[56] Based on the findings from these recent studies, dietary supplementation with high doses of synthetic beta-carotene may be contraindicated for smokers. As a reminder, it has been known for some time that a high intake of vitamin A results in adverse effects (neurologic, dermatologic, musculoskeletal, gastrointestinal, birth defects) and the results from the most recent studies suggest a potential risk of high doses of synthetic beta-carotene in certain populations. At this time it is probably safest to follow the National Cancer Institute recommendations that suggest five or more servings of fruits and vegetables per day.

Immune Effects and Exercise

We are currently aware of only one study that has examined whether vitamin A supplementation is associated with a reduced incidence of infection in athletes. Several studies have shown that the risk of upper respiratory infection is increased following competition in marathons or ultramarathons.[57–59] However, vitamin A supplementation before marathon competition did not reduce the incidence of infection in the post-race period.[60] Therefore, to our knowledge, vitamin A supplementation has not been associated with enhanced resistance to infection in healthy athletes.

Vitamin C

Although vitamin C has long been touted as a preventive measure against the common cold, the available evidence from several large-scale randomized controlled trials does not support this claim. Several studies conducted awhile ago have shown that vitamin C supplementation can enhance certain aspects of immune response such as lymphocyte proliferative response, neutrophil function, and hypersensitivity response,[61–63] although not all parameters of immunity are enhanced.[61] It has been suggested that vitamin C and vitamin E supplementation together may have a greater effect on immune responsiveness than vitamin C alone,[64] but further research on this topic is warranted. Although supplementation of vitamin C has been shown to enhance certain aspects of immune function, this does not appear to result in a reduced incidence of the common cold in humans[65] or a reduced incidence of influenza in an animal model.[66] However, a recent review of placebo-controlled trials suggests that vitamin C may decrease the duration or severity of the common cold in certain populations such as children.[67] Also, some recent evidence suggests that populations undergoing heavy physical stress (running a marathon) may benefit from vitamin C supplementation.[59,68,69]

Immune Effects and Exercise

The results from a few studies suggest that vitamin C supplementation may be beneficial in reducing the incidence or severity of upper respiratory infection following strenuous, prolonged exercise. Several epidemiological studies have indicated that the risk of developing an upper respiratory infection (URI) is increased in the week or two following a session of prolonged exercise such as running a marathon.[57–59] However, runners who consumed a 600-mg supplement of vitamin C for 21 days before competing in an ultramarathon race reported fewer symptoms and a shorter duration of URI than the runners who consumed placebo.[59] There was no difference in the incidence of symptoms of URI before the race, suggesting that perhaps the benefits of vitamin C supplementation are more pronounced during periods of heavy physical stress. The same group of investigators examined whether different antioxidant preparations may provide additional benefits in regards to reduced URI in the postcompetition period. In this study runners received one of the following supplements for 21 days before competition: 500 mg vitamin C; 500 mg vitamin C and 400 IU vitamin E; 300 mg vitamin C, 300 IU vitamin E, and 18 mg beta-carotene; or

placebo. The results from this study again showed that vitamin C had a protective effect in terms of reduced incidence of URI symptoms, but the addition of vitamin E or beta-carotene did not confer any additional benefits.[70] Others have reported that vitamin C consumption in the range of 600 mg—1 g per day was associated with a decrease in symptoms of the common cold compared with subjects consuming placebo.[68] However, others have reported that prophylactic administration of vitamin C (2 g/day) for an 8-week period in marine recruits was not associated with decreased incidence or duration of colds, although the vitamin C group rated their colds as being less severe.[71] At this time, the results from several studies suggest that vitamin C supplementation may reduce the incidence and/or severity of URI during times of heavy physical stress. None of these studies explored changes in immune function that could potentially be associated with reduced incidence or severity of infection. One recent study examined the effects of vitamin C supplementation for 8 days on a range of immune responses before performing a 2.5-hour run at a high intensity. No change was observed in NK cell cytotoxicity, lymphocyte proliferative response to mitogens, granulocyte phagocytosis, or production of the cytokine IL-6.[72] These findings may not appear to be consistent with the previous studies that observed an effect of supplementation on the incidence of infection. However, a longer period of supplementation could have been necessary (21 days, rather than 8 days). The study of immune measures did not assess antigen-specific immune responses and that the antigen-specific immune response could be altered by vitamin C supplementation, resulting in fewer infections. It is also important to note that a change or lack of change in immune parameters measured does not necessarily relate to disease outcome. Other factors may mediate disease outcome. For example, the findings from some recent studies suggest that dietary oxidative stress from vitamin deficiency changes the genome of a virus, resulting in increased virulence.[73] Vitamin C concentration in plasma has been shown to decline following long-term endurance exercise and this short-term decrease could be associated with increased susceptibility to infection.[74] Although the findings from the vitamin C supplementation studies in those individuals undergoing heavy physical exertion are promising, further research is needed to confirm these findings and to explore potential mechanisms mediating the change in susceptibility to infection. Also, to our knowledge the role of vitamin C supplementation in preventing infection in athletes participating in heavy resistance training or bodybuilding has not been studied.

Vitamin E

Vitamin E deficiency is associated with impaired immune responsiveness and increased severity of infection.[75] Vitamin E deficiency has resulted in impaired bactericidal activity of phagocytes, reduced lymphocyte response to mitogens, decreased production of the cytokine IL-2, altered T cell differentiation in the thymus, and increased myocardial injury during viral infection.[76–78] Supplementation with vitamin E during viral or bacterial infection (influenza, murine AIDS, herpes simplex virus, *Staphylococcus aureus*, parainfluenza, *Clostridium perfringens*) has been shown to decrease mortality rate or severity of infection in several different animal models.[79–84] However, not all studies have found an improved resistance to infection from vitamin E supplementation[85] and we are not aware of any human studies that have tested this theory by infecting human subjects and then assessing disease incidence and/or severity.

It is less clear whether intake of vitamin E above the RDA enhances resistance to infection in healthy individuals. The most promising results have come from studies involving elderly human subjects. In several randomized controlled trials, various doses of vitamin E were administered to elderly individuals for different periods of time and immune responses were measured. Two studies that administered supplements (100–800 mg/day) for at least 6 months found an enhancement of several immune parameters including dihydrotestosterone (DTH) response, mitogen-induced IL-2 production, and increased antibody titer to hepatitis B and tetanus vaccine.[86,87] One of these studies found optimal results in those subjects receiving 200 mg/day of vitamin E, but higher levels of vitamin E (800 mg/day) were not associated with an additional improvement of immune response.[86] The results from one study failed to find an enhancement of immune response in elderly subjects consuming 100 mg/day.[88] However, in this study, subjects received the supplement for only 3 months and perhaps a longer period of supplementation is necessary to observe an effect. The results from two additional studies found enhancement of several immune parameters (LPS-induced production of IL-1, TNFα, mitogen-induced lymphocyte proliferation, neutrophil phagocytosis) when vitamin C (1 g/day) and vitamin E (200–400 mg/day) were administered to healthy young and elderly adults.[64,89] The mechanisms by which vitamin E supplementation may alter immune response remain to be established. Currently, it is thought that one potential mechanism may involve the production of prostaglandin E$_2$ (PGE$_2$). PGE$_2$, produced by macrophages, is known to suppress some lymphocyte responses. Some recent evidence suggests that aged animals fed additional vitamin E have a reduction of macrophage PGE$_2$ production.[90] The immune response may be enhanced through the reduction of PGE$_2$. Further research on potential mechanisms will provide important information with respect to an understanding of vitamin E–associated immunomodulation. The findings from these studies show promise with respect to vitamin E supplementation and enhanced immune function, particularly in the elderly. However, we are not aware of any randomized clinical trials that have shown a decreased incidence of infection in

association with vitamin E supplementation alone (without other vitamins or trace nutrients). The findings from one of the studies described above suggested a trend (p = 0.098, not statistically significant) towards reduced incidence of infectious disease in the elderly.[86]

The results from animal studies suggest that in some instances, the incidence of disease is reduced with vitamin E supplementation. A reduced incidence of infection, however, was observed in chickens consuming diets supplemented with vitamin E.[83] One study involving calves did not find a reduction in disease incidence in those animals fed additional vitamin E.[91] Thus, the results from animal studies are similar to the human studies in that a beneficial effect of vitamin E supplementation has been found, although the finding is not consistent. At this time, the results regarding vitamin E supplementation and immunity in the elderly human population are promising. However, additional large-scale randomized controlled trials are necessary before it is possible to determine whether vitamin E supplementation results in reduced susceptibility to infection.

Immune Effects and Exercise

Although vitamin E has been studied in relation to exercise, most studies have focused on the potential antioxidant effects of vitamin E supplementation, which was discussed above. Others have examined various physiological changes regarding vitamin E supplementation and exercise and found no change in neuroendocrine profile[92] but a slight reduction in the incidence of gastrointestinal complications in those marathon runners consuming vitamin E for 2 weeks before the race.[93] The only study we are aware of that examined immunity and vitamin E supplementation with exercise found that vitamin E and C supplementation before competing in an ultramarathon reduced the incidence of URI symptoms in the post-race period.[70] However, it was thought that this effect was related to vitamin C rather than vitamin E because the post-race reduction in symptoms of URI was not lower with vitamin E + C than vitamin C alone. To our knowledge, we are not aware of any studies that have explored potential associations between vitamin E supplementation alone and immune response in regards to exercise. Perhaps this area of research may show some promise in the elderly.

Zinc

Zinc is an essential nutrient that has an important role in the growth and development of many cells, tissues, and the immune system. Zinc is considered a cofactor for over 300 metalloenzymes and one of the symptoms of zinc deficiency is an increased frequency of bacterial and viral infections. The effects of zinc and immune function have been well studied. The cellular and molecular effects of zinc on immunity are beyond the scope of this review and the reader is referred to several recent reviews for additional information.[23,94–96]

Zinc deficiency may impair nonspecific and specific immune responses. Nonspecific defenses that may be impaired by zinc include NK cytotoxicity, macrophage phagocytosis, neutrophil oxidative burst, and chemotaxis. Other observations include thymic atrophy, decreased DTH, reduction in peripheral T-cell count, decrease in T helper cell and T cytotoxic cell functions, and reduced antibody production.[95] It is apparent that zinc deficiency affects multiple aspects of host immunity and therefore it is not surprising that an increased frequency of infection is observed in deficient individuals. Zinc supplementation of deficient individuals has been shown to reduce the incidence and severity of infection, especially in children.[97–99]

Although it is clear that malnourished individuals suffer impaired immunity due in part to zinc deficiency, the question of relevance to normal well-nourished healthy individuals is whether zinc supplementation can enhance immunity. Several studies in the elderly have shown that zinc supplementation is associated with an increased number of T cells, improved delayed dermal hypersensitivity, DTH response, and antibody production to tetanus vaccine.[100–102] The elderly may suffer from mild zinc deficiency and therefore may benefit from supplementation.

Recently, there has been an interest in the potential role of zinc supplementation in reducing the duration of symptoms associated with the common cold. Some studies have demonstrated that zinc gluconate lozenges administered within 24 hours of the onset of symptoms of the common cold reduced the duration of cold symptoms.[103,104] However, this is not a consistent finding[105,106] and a recent meta-analysis that reviewed a number of clinical trials concluded that solid evidence for the effectiveness of zinc lozenges in reducing the duration of common colds is lacking.[107]

Immune Effects and Exercise

Many athletes may be tempted to try zinc supplementation while experiencing symptoms of the common cold in the hope that the duration of cold symptoms will be reduced. Short-term supplementation is probably not harmful; however, high-dose zinc supplementation is associated with immunosuppression.[108] It is not known if zinc supplementation can reduce the incidence of infection in healthy well-nourished individuals. Some evidence supports the concept that zinc supplementation may be considered potentially beneficial during episodes of the common cold, in terms of decreased symptoms or duration. However, there is no evidence that zinc can reduce the incidence of the common cold among healthy individuals.

One potential area of consideration for some athletes regarding zinc is the finding that some athletes, particularly endurance athletes, may suffer from mild zinc deficiency.[109–111] This population may be similar to elderly individuals regarding mild zinc deficiency and therefore may benefit from supplementation. However, to our knowledge this possibility has not been tested. Also, keep in mind that the elderly experience an age-associated decline in immune responsiveness and therefore zinc supplementation of younger individuals may not show similar benefits.

One study did compare the postexercise immune response in those individuals who consumed zinc and placebo. The subjects consuming zinc did not experience an exercise-induced increase in neutrophil production of ROS.[112] It is possible that this change may alter exercise-induced tissue damage. It is not clear at this time how the change in neutrophil function may relate to susceptibility to infection or disease outcome. Again, further research is certainly warranted considering that some athletes may experience mild zinc deficiency and adequate zinc intake is essential for optimal immune response and resistance to infection.

Whey Protein

Bovine milk whey protein consists of various amino acids, and the amount of each amino acid differs from the concentrations found in other proteins such as soy. The components of whey protein contain α-lactalbumin, β-lactoglobulin, bovine serum albumin, immunoglobulins, lactoferrin, and lactoperoxidase. In animal models, diets consisting of whey protein rather than other types of protein have been shown to modulate immune function; however, it is not known if the immune effects are related to the differing concentration of amino acids or the potential immunomodulatory properties of lactoferrin or lactoperoxidase.

Immune Effects

Several studies using animal models have shown that diets consisting of whey protein rather than soy or casein protein enhance certain aspects of immune response. Several studies have indicated that a diet containing 20% whey protein enhanced humoral (antibody) immune response in mice.[113–115] Neutrophil function and cell-mediated immune responses are also enhanced by whey protein,[115,116] although others have failed to find an enhancement of cell-mediated immunity.[113] In addition, a diet containing 20% whey protein decreased tumor incidence and size of a chemically induced carcinoma in mice.[117] As mentioned previously, it is not known which component(s) of whey protein may enhance immune function. One recent study showed that two of the components, lactoperoxidase and lactoferrin, impaired mitogen-induced

Whey Protein: Immune Enhancer?

Gustavo Bounous, MD, FRCS

In the early 1980s, it was discovered that normal mice that were fed a whey protein concentrate (WPC) as 20% of a formula diet exhibited a marked increase in antibody production in response to a T-cell–dependent antigen. The immunosustaining effect of this WPC, unrelated to its nutritional efficiency, was confirmed by the protective effect of this dietary treatment against pneumococcal infection. The cysteine content of WPC was found to play a crucial role in the bioactivity of the diet.

Optimization of the immune response in animals that were fed WPC is attributed to a greater production of glutathione (GSH) in the lymphocytes, through dietary provision of supplementary doses of the GSH precursor, cysteine.

In fact, it has been demonstrated that the ability of lymphocytes to offset oxidative damage during their oxygen-requiring clonal expansion, and following that expansion in the production of antibodies, is measured by determining the capacity of these cells to regenerate intracellular stores of GSH. Therefore, this would allow them to respond more fully to the antigenic stimulus.

More evidence for the involvement of GSH in the modulation of immune function comes from human studies related to HIV infection. Staal et al. showed that HIV-infected individuals have lower GSH concentrations in their blood lymphocytes. Moreover, a recent study indicates that the more GSH that patients carry in their CD4 helper T-cells, the cells targeted primarily by the HIV virus, the longer these patients are likely to survive. Conditions that facilitate cellular GSH replenishment or maintenance are thus expected to optimize the activity of the immune system.

A slightly modified version of WPC used in our experimental studies (Immunocal[R]) was given to adult HIV-positive patients and in children with AIDS. The GSH content of blood mononuclear cells was below normal values in all patients at the onset of the study. Over a 3–6 month period, GSH levels increased and in some cases reached normal values with a concomitant increase in body weight, CD4 cells, decrease in viral load, and overall clinical improvement.

Bounous G, Batist G, Gold P. Immunoenhancing property of dietary whey protein in mice: role of glutathione. Clin Invest Med 1989;12:154–161.

Bounous G, Letourneau L, Kongshavn PAL. Influence of dietary protein type on the immune system of mice. J Nutr 1983; 113:1415–1421.

Bounous G, Stevenson MM, Kongshavn PAL. Influence of dietary lactalbumin hydrolysate on the immune system of mice and resistance to Salmonellosis. J Infect Dis 1981;144:281.

Staal FJ, Roederer M, Israelski DM, et al. Intracellular glutathione levels in T cell subsets decrease in HIV-infected individuals. AIDS Res Hum Retroviruses 1992;8:305–311.

lymphocyte proliferation and cytokine production, whereas another component, α-lactalbumin, enhanced cytokine production.[116] It is also possible that the particular combination of amino acids present in whey protein confers enhanced immunity, and it has been suggested that the greater concentration of cysteine in whey protein is associated with improved immunity[118] (see sidebar by Gustavo Bounous, MD). These studies can still be considered preliminary and additional research may clarify the mechanism of immunomodulation.

The findings from the few animal studies are promising regarding potential immunomodulatory effects of whey protein. However, we are not aware of any studies that have shown enhanced immune function in humans with dietary whey protein. Also, note that the animal studies tested diets consisting of whey protein (20% protein) as the sole source of dietary protein. These studies did not assess the potential immunomodulatory role of additional dietary supplementation with whey protein above and beyond the normal protein intake. In addition, we are not aware of any studies that have tested potential clinical outcomes of the potential immunomodulatory properties of whey protein. In other words, does a diet consisting of whey protein increase resistance to infection? At this time, the findings regarding potential immunomodulatory effects of whey protein should be considered preliminary.

Additional studies are needed to determine whether diets consisting of whey protein enhance immunity in humans and decrease susceptibility to or severity of infection. Future studies should also clarify whether the same immunomodulatory effects can be observed by supplementing the normal diet with additional whey protein. The role of whey protein combined with exercise and immunity has also not yet been studied. Finally, the potential mechanisms of immune enhancement associated with whey protein remain to be established.

Dehydroepiandrosterone (DHEA)

Dehydroepiandrosterone (DHEA) is a steroid produced by the adrenal gland. DHEA is often measured in human serum as DHEA-sulfate (DHEAS) and serum levels of DHEAS decline with age. It has therefore been proposed that supplementation with DHEA may benefit the elderly to a greater degree than younger individuals. The physiological function(s) of DHEA remains to be determined. To date, studies have shown that DHEA may have neurological, immunological, cardiovascular, metabolic, and oncologic effects; refer to the review by Svec and Porter.[119]

DHEA may be of interest to strength athletes because DHEA can be considered a precursor to testosterone. However, DHEA may also follow different biochemical pathways and is not necessarily converted to testosterone. Although most of the research on DHEA has been conducted recently, the studies performed in the early 1990s suggested promising immunological effects. The findings from more recent studies in humans question the clinical significance of the proposed immunological benefits. Recent studies using animal models have also examined the immunological effects of DHEA derivatives, including androstenediol and androstenetriol. The preliminary results of these findings suggest that these compounds may enhance immune function to a greater degree than DHEA, although these studies have yet to be conducted in humans.

A number of studies in mice have indicated that DHEA treatment (usually by injection) can increase resistance or improve antibody response to a number of pathogens such as herpesvirus, coxsackievirus, tuberculosis, and *Enterococcus faecalis*.[120,121] The immune response to vaccination is often impaired in the elderly and DHEA supplementation has been proposed as a method of enhancing the response to immunization. Several studies using the mouse model have shown that the immune response (antibody production, antigen-specific activation of T-helper cells) to immunization of influenza virus or hepatitis B is improved in mice receiving DHEA treatment.[122–124] Researchers have also demonstrated that administration of DHEA to mice is associated with a greater production of IL-2, mitogen-induced lymphocyte proliferation, monocyte antitumor function (cytotoxicity) monocyte cytokine, and reactive nitrogen intermediate release, IFN-γ production.[125–128] Interestingly, the studies that examined the effect of DHEA *in vitro* tended to show either no effect of DHEA or a suppression of immune response (decreased lymphocyte proliferation, and decreased IL-2 and IL-3 production).[121,124,129] These contrasting findings, immunoenhancement *in vivo* and immunosuppression *in vitro*, suggest that the effects of DHEA treatment *in vivo* may be indirect. Perhaps DHEA administration alters other neuroendocrine or biochemical factors, ultimately resulting in altered immune response. This hypothesis has not yet been tested to our knowledge. Taken together, the findings from the studies using animal models appear promising with the exception of *in vitro* findings. Not only do these studies demonstrate enhancement of immune response, but also this enhancement is associated with a beneficial clinical outcome in terms of disease resistance and immunological response to infection.

The immunomodulatory role of DHEA supplementation in humans is much less promising than the findings from the mice studies. The findings from earlier studies suggested a benefit of supplementation on some immune parameters; however, more recent findings tend to show no benefit in terms of antigen-specific immunity (response to flu vaccine). Although the human research is not as extensive as animal research, the findings from one study of aged men showed that oral administration of 50 mg/day of DHEA was associated with enhanced T and B cell mitogenic response, increased number of T cells expressing the IL-2 receptor, and increased concentration of IL-2 receptor in serum.[130] DHEA treatment of postmenopausal women with adrenal androgen insufficiency resulted in a decreased number of helper T cells, decreased T cell mitogenic response, but increased NK cell cytotoxicity.[131] Lymphocytes obtained from humans and then cultured with DHEA *in vitro* produced more IL-2.[132]

The results from these earlier studies suggest that DHEA supplementation may be associated with an enhancement of certain immune parameters in specific human populations. Researchers have extended this earlier research by testing the possibility that DHEA administration in elderly humans might enhance immune response to vaccination. Recall that elderly individuals have lower levels of DHEA and the animal experiments showed that DHEA administration improved immune response to immunization. In contrast to the animal experiments, four studies have demonstrated that DHEA administration to the elderly did NOT improve immune response.[133–136] In fact, a decrease in the antibody response to one strain of influenza was found in subjects consuming DHEA.[133] One study also examined immune response to tetanus vaccine and also found that DHEA did not improve vaccine effectiveness.[136] Therefore, at this time, DHEA supplementation does not appear to have clinical benefits in humans regarding the immune response following immunization. We are not aware of any studies in humans that have examined the role of DHEA supplementation in terms of reducing susceptibility to infection. This question has recently been tested in an animal model and the authors concluded that lifelong treatment with oral DHEA does not prevent the age-associated decline of immune function, does not prevent disease, and does not improve survival.[137]

To conclude, early experiments using animal models suggested that DHEA has important benefits in terms of immunoenhancement. However, the most recent studies in humans showed no clinical benefits from DHEA supplementation. Why these differences exist between the animal and the human studies is unknown. Plasma levels of DHEA are much lower in rodents than in humans and the tendency for DHEA to follow a given biochemical pathway in humans may also differ from rodents. It is also unclear how DHEA exerts its effects on immune function. A greater understanding of this process might provide an explanation for the discrepancies between animal and human studies.

Immune Effects and Exercise

We are not aware of any studies that have directly examined DHEA and immunity in the context of exercise.

However, in a related area, DHEA administration or treatment with the related compound, androstenediol, has been shown to decrease the stress-induced susceptibility to viral infection and improve antiviral response in mice.[138] Different stressors, including prolonged, exhaustive exercise are associated with increased susceptibility to infection.[57,58] Stress may result in an increase of the concentration of plasma glucocorticoids and it has been suggested that DHEA may counteract the immunosuppressive effects of glucocorticoids. Lymphocytes obtained from mice treated with DHEA and then cultured with glucocorticoids *in vitro* were more resistant to the immunosuppressive effects of the glucocorticoids than those in mice that did not receive DHEA.[125,139] It is therefore possible that DHEA administration may have some immunological benefit in individuals with high plasma levels of glucocorticoids, such as athletes involved in certain types of competition. However, this hypothesis remains to be tested in humans.

Finally, it is important to note that there are several reports of enhanced immune function and resistance to infection in mice treated with androstenediol and androstenetriol.[120,124,140,141] Androstenediol and androstenetriol may improve immune response to a greater degree than DHEA.[124,140,142] At this time, we are not aware of any human studies that have tested the effects of androstenediol or androstenetriol on immune function, but this area of research might prove promising.

Current Controversy: Does Glutamine Enhance Immune Function?

Prolonged exercise may deplete glutamine, resulting in a glutamine deficiency for cells that rely on glutamine as a fuel (e.g., cells of the immune system, GI tract). Glutamine is an amino acid that serves as a metabolic fuel for lymphocytes, macrophages, and cells lining the intestine. Glutamine is considered a nonessential amino acid, although some evidence suggests that additional glutamine may be beneficial in terms of immune function during periods of severe stress, including critical illness, sepsis, and surgery. Skeletal muscle synthesizes and stores glutamine, and is considered a site of glutamine reserves. The concentration of glutamine in plasma has been suggested to represent a *metabolic link* between skeletal muscle and cells of the immune system. In other words, the function of cells of the immune system may be influenced by the plasma concentration of glutamine, which is dependent on the rate of glutamine synthesis and release by skeletal muscle. Low plasma concentrations of glutamine are found during certain types of catabolic stress such as sepsis, burns, trauma, and surgery. Periods of catabolic stress may be associated with suppression of immune function. The findings from some studies show a decrease in plasma glutamine concentration following prolonged endurance exercise and therefore it has been proposed that prolonged exercise is another type of catabolic stress that may be associated with immunosuppression. Prolonged exercise (marathon running) has been associated with an increased incidence of upper respiratory infection in the week or two following the event. In an attempt to coun-

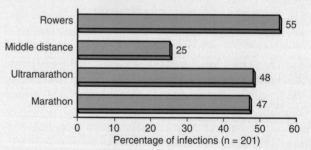

Incidence of infections in athletes 7 days after different types of exercise. (*Data from* Castell LM, Poortmans JR, Newsholme EA. Does glutamine have a role in reducing infections in athletes? Eur J Appl Physiol 1996;73:488–490.)

teract the suggested postexercise immunosuppression, several investigators have administered supplemental glutamine before and/or after exercise. There is some evidence that supports the theory that additional glutamine may enhance resistance to infection, although at

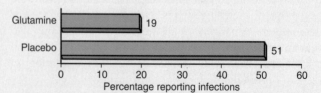

Effect of glutamine vs placebo during 7 days in runners after a marathon or ultramarathon event; compiled from eight different studies. (*Data from* Castell LM, Poortmans JR, Newsholme EA. Does glutamine have a role in reducing infections in athletes? Eur J Appl Physiol 1996;73:488–490.)

this time, there are more studies suggesting that supplemental glutamine does not alter the exercise-associated changes in immune function.

Evidence For/Against the Glutamine Hypothesis?

Although the possibility that glutamine may alter the immune response has received much attention, and has been the topic of at least five review articles, we are aware of only ONE study in healthy humans that has demonstrated a positive effect of glutamine supplementation. In this particular study athletes participating in either a marathon or ultramarathon were given either a placebo or 5 g of glutamine within 2 hours postexercise and the incidence of reported infections (cough, cold, sore throat, flu) was monitored for 7 days after the event (see figures). Approximately 20% of the subjects consuming glutamine reported an infectious episode whereas approximately 50% of the subjects consuming placebo reported an infection during this time ($p < 0.001$). A separate study of swimmers examined plasma glutamine levels during a period of intensified training and found a decrease in glutamine concentration at one time point in overtrained swimmers, but found no association between plasma glutamine and the incidence of upper respiratory infection. One other study in support of the glutamine hypothesis examined the lymphocyte response to 60 minutes of treadmill exercise using a rat model and found that rats consuming a glutamine diet did not exhibit a post-exercise suppression of mitogen-induced lymphocyte proliferation. Evidence against the glutamine hypothesis comes from six other studies which indicated that glutamine supplementation had no effect on the exercise-induced alterations of immunity. The results from three human studies showed that glutamine supplementation before prolonged exercise (marathon, 2 hours exercise at 75% VO_{2max}, repeated bouts of exercise over 2 hours total time at 75% VO_{2max}) prevented the exercise-induced decline in plasma glutamine but did not alter mitogen-induced lymphocyte proliferation, lymphokine-activated killer cell function, percentage of leukocyte subpopulations, NK function, or salivary IgA concentration. The findings from another study showed that glutamine supplementation after a marathon did not alter lymphocyte subpopulations, although in this study glutamine supplementation did not prevent the exercise-induced decrease in plasma glutamine postexercise. Glutamine supplementation *in vitro* of peripheral blood mononuclear cells obtained from HIV patients postexercise did not alter the exercise-induced decline in mitogen-stimulated lymphocyte proliferation. The effect of glutamine supplementation during a 21-day period of intense exercise training (swimming 2 or 4 hours per day) was tested in a rat model. The results from this study showed no benefit of glutamine supplementation on immune response and, in fact, an impairment of NK cytotoxicity was observed in the exercised rats receiving glutamine. At this time, it appears that the weight of the evidence does not support the glutamine hypothesis and the potential reasons for the discrepancies in the findings are discussed below.

One potential reason for the opposing results of the human studies may be related to the outcome measures, and it is possible that the findings from all the studies may be valid. One study found a benefit of glutamine supplementation *in vivo* in terms of reduced incidence of infection, whereas four studies observed no effect on the immune parameters measured. It is possible that the reduced incidence of infection is not related to the specific immune parameters measured. Perhaps glutamine supplementation alters resistance to infection by another mechanism such as a reduction in viral pathogenesis and is not reflected in the immune measures. The immune measures that were evaluated in these studies did not assess antigen-specific immune response and the immune response to viral infection is an antigen-specific response. Therefore, immune function may have changed, but this change is not reflected in the immune measures that were assessed in these studies. Further research is needed to clarify these possibilities. Ideally, the effects of glutamine supplementation on both measures of antigen-specific immune function and susceptibility to infection postexercise would be assessed in the same study.

Potential problems with the statistical design of the human study showing a benefit of glutamine could have also led to inaccurate conclusions. The results from eight separate studies were combined and it is not clear whether the investigators accounted for potential differences between these eight studies. To date, we are not aware of any other published findings that have replicated the results of this study in terms of reduced susceptibility to infection. The findings from the study by Castell et al. are promising with respect to the potential role of glutamine, but should be replicated before a recommendation can be made regarding supplemental glutamine for participants of long endurance exercise.

There are additional issues to address regarding the type of athlete and the potential role of supplemental glutamine. Note that plasma glutamine concentration does not always decrease following exercise. It appears that the decline is found in prolonged endurance exercise, such as running marathons or completing a triathlon. Exercise at a lower intensity (55% VO_{2max}), but for a long period of time, approximately 3 hours or upon reaching fatigue, can also result in reduced plasma glutamine levels. Short-term exercise (less than 2 hours) does not appear to decrease plasma glutamine levels unless the exercise intensity is $\geq 90\%$ VO_{2max}. Overtraining has been suggested to be associated with decreased plasma glutamine concentration. One investigation compared plasma glutamine levels during a 4-week period of intensified training and classified their subjects as either well trained or overtrained. At the 2-week time point, plasma glutamine was lower in the overtrained group, but this difference was not apparent at 4 weeks. In addition, there was no association between plasma glutamine levels and the incidence of upper respiratory infection. It is not clear whether activities such as strength training alter plasma glutamine. Severe eccentric exercise did not alter glutamine levels in one study; however, the results from a separate study demonstrated a decline in plasma glutamine following eccentric exercise, although the decrease was not correlated with markers of skeletal muscle damage. In a cross-sectional comparison of different athletes, power lifters were found to have a lower plasma concentration of plasma glutamine than healthy nonathletes. Interestingly, in the same study, cyclists were found to have the greatest plasma concentration of glutamine, an activity thought to rely on protein as an energy source, due to the prolonged duration and volume of training. In this study, a significant negative correlation between plasma glutamine concentration and dietary protein intake $(g \cdot kg^{-1} \cdot day^{-1})$ was observed. That is, the athletes with the greatest intake of protein had the lowest level of plasma glutamine. The authors proposed that the high protein intake might result in enhanced renal uptake of glutamine, in an attempt to maintain acid-base balance. Regarding the role of supplemental glutamine in strength or power sports, at this time future research is needed to determine whether there is a change in the requirement for glutamine and whether this relates to immune function.

And finally, keep in mind that although glutamine supplementation has been shown to be beneficial in terms of immune response and infection in catabolic patients as recently reviewed by Sacks, it may not be valid to compare endurance exercise with the catabolic state observed in patients suffering from sepsis, critical illness, burns, etc. For example, pro-inflammatory cytokines (IL-1, IL-6, TNFα) are often elevated in catabolic states such as critical illness, sepsis, trauma, etc. These pro-inflammatory cytokines along with glucocorticoids and altered insulin action are involved in skeletal muscle proteolysis, and the potential development of cachexia. Not only are the levels of pro-inflammatory cytokines increased during catabolic states such as

sepsis or trauma, but also a range of immune functions are dysregulated as recently reviewed by Catania and Chaudry. The immune and hormonal changes that occur during these catabolic states may be considered extreme and different from the immunological changes, which accompany prolonged exercise. For example, with the pro-inflammatory cytokines, an increase in plasma IL-6 is typically observed postexercise, but most studies do not report an increase in plasma TNFα or IL-1. Some studies report a slight decrease in cell-mediated immunity postexercise; this decrease is short term and returns to normal within hours, whereas the immunosuppression associated with catabolic states persists. Given the major immunological and physiological differences between the postexercise state and other catabolic states such as sepsis, trauma, burns, etc., it may not be valid to compare the role of glutamine supplementation in these catabolic states to that of healthy individuals in the postexercise state.

Alverdy JA, Aoys E, Weiss-Carrington P, Burke DA. The effect of glutamine-enriched TPN on gut immune cellularity. J Surg Res 1992;52:34–38.

Askanazi J, Carpentier YA, Michelson CB, et al. Muscle and plasma amino acids following surgery. Ann Surg 1980;192:78–85.

Antonio J, Street C. Glutamine: a potentially useful supplement for athletes. Can J Appl Physiol 1999;24:1–14.

Castell LM, Newsholme EA. Glutamine and the effects of exhaustive exercise upon the immune response. Can J Physiol Pharmacol 1998;76:524–532.

Castell LM, Poortmans JR, Leclercq R, et al. Some aspects of the acute phase response after a marathon race, and the effects of glutamine supplementation. Eur J Appl Physiol 1997;75:47–53.

Castell LM, Poortmans JR, Newsholme EA. Does glutamine have a role in reducing infections in athletes? Eur J Appl Physiol 1996;73:488–490.

Catania RA, Chaudry IH. Immunological consequences of trauma and shock. Ann Acad Med Singapore 1999;28:120–132.

Chang HR, Bistrian B. The role of cytokines in the catabolic consequences of infection and injury. JPEN 1998;22:156–166.

Gleeson M, Walsh NP, Blannin AK, et al. The effect of severe eccentric exercise-induced muscle damage on plasma elastase, glutamine and zinc concentrations. Eur J Appl Physiol 1998;77:543–546.

Grizard J, Dardevet D, Balage M et al. Insulin action on skeletal muscle protein metabolism during catabolic states. Reprod Nutr Dev 1999;39:61–74.

Hiscock N, Mackinnon LT. A comparison of plasma glutamine concentration in athletes from different sports. Med Sci Sports Exerc 1998;30:1693–1696.

Hasselgren PO. Glucocorticoids and muscle metabolism. Curr Opin Clin Nutr Metab Care 1999;2:201–205.

Keast D, Arstein D, Harper W, et al. Depression of plasma glutamine concentration after exercise stress and its possible influence on the immune system. Med J Aust 1995;162:15–18.

Krzykowski K, Wolsk Peterson W, Ostrowski K, et al. Effects of glutamine and protein supplementation on exercise-induced decrease in lymphocyte function and salivary IgA [abstract]. Presented at International Society of Exercise and Immunology. Rome, Italy, May, 1999.

Mackinnon L, Hooper S. Plasma glutamine and upper respiratory infection during intensified training in swimmers. Med Sci Sports Exerc 1996;28:285–290.

Miles MP, Naukam RJ, Hackney AC, Clarkson PM. Blood leukocyte and glutamine fluctuations after eccentric exercise. Int J Sports Med 1999;20:322–327.

Moriguchi S, Miwa H, Kishino Y. Glutamine supplementation prevents the decrease of mitogen response after a treadmill exercise in rats. J Nutr Sci Vitaminol 1995;41:115–125.

Nehlsen-Cannarella SL, Fagoaga OR, Nieman DC, et al. Carbohydrate and the cytokine response to 2.5 hours of running. J Appl Physiol 1997;82:1662–1667.

Newsholme EA. Biochemical mechanisms to explain immunosuppression in well-trained and overtrained athletes. Int J Sports Med 1994;S142–S147.

Nieman DC, Johansen LM, Lee JW, Arabtzis K. Infectious episodes in runners before and after the Los Angeles Marathon. J Sports Med Phys Fitness 1990;30:316–328.

Northoff H Berg A. Immunologic mediators as parameters of the reaction to strenuous exercise. Int J Sports Med 1991;12:S9–14.

Parry-Billings M, Budgett R, Koutedakis Y, et al. Plasma amino acid concentration in the overtraining syndrome: possible effects on the immune system. Med Sci Sports Exerc 1992;24:1353–1358.

Parry-Billings M, Evans J, Calder PC, Newsholme EA. Does glutamine contribute to immunosuppression after major burns? Lancet 1990;336:523–525.

Peters EM, Bateman ED. Ultramarathon running and upper respiratory infections. S Afr Med J 1983;64:582–584.

Powell H, Castell LM, Parry Billings M, et al. Growth hormone suppression and glutamine flux associated with cardiac surgery. Clin Physiol 1994;14:569–580.

Robson PJ, Blannin AK, Walsh NP, et al. Effects of exercise intensity, duration and recovery on in vitro neutrophil function in male athletes. Int J Sports Med 1999;20:128–135.

Rohde T, Asp S, MacLean DA, Pedersen BK. Competitive sustained exercise in humans, lymphokine activated killer cell activity, and glutamine—an intervention study. Eur J Appl Physiol 1998;78:448–453.

Rohde T, MacLean DA, Hartkopp A, Pedersen BK. The immune system and serum glutamine during a triathlon. Eur J Appl Physiol 1996;74:428–434.

Rohde T, MacLean DA, Pedersen BK. Effect of glutamine supplementation on changes in the immune system induced by repeated exercise. Med Sci Sports Exerc 1998;30:856–862.

Rohde T, Ullum H, Rasmussen JP, et al. Effects of glutamine on the immune system: influence of muscular exercise and HIV infection. J Appl Physiol 1995;79:146–150.

Rowbottom DG, Keast D, Morton AR. The emerging role of glutamine as an indicator of exercise stress and overtraining. Sports Med 1996;21:80–97.

Sacks GS. Glutamine supplementation in catabolic patients. Ann Pharmacother 1999;33:348–354.

Shewchuck LD, Baracos VE, Field CJ. Dietary L-glutamine does not improve lymphocyte metabolism or function in exercise-trained rats. Med Sci Sports Exerc 1997;4:474–481.

Sprenger H, Jacobs C, Nain M, et al. Enhanced release of cytokines, interleukin-2 receptors, and neopterin after long-distance running. Clin Immunol Immunopathol 1992;63:188–195.

Ullum H, Haahr PM, Diamant M, et al. Bicycle exercise enhances plasma IL-6 but does not change IL-1α, IL-1β, IL-6, or TNFα pre-mRNA in BMNC. J Appl Physiol 1994;77:93–97.

Walsh NP, Blannin AD, Robson PJ, Gleeson M. Glutamine, exercise and immune functions: links and possible mechanisms. Sports Med 1998;26:177–191.

New Trends in Nutritional Supplementation That May Alter Immunity: HMB and Carbohydrates

Recently, investigators have been studying the potential immunomodulatory role of carbohydrate supplementation in endurance performance with interesting results. Carbohydrate supplementation during prolonged exercise (2.5 hours running or a triathalon) attenuated some of the exercise-induced alterations of immune response.[72,143–145] The exercise-induced increase in the number of circulating leukocytes, plasma IL-6 concentration, plasma IL-1 receptor antagonist concentration, NK cell activity, and granulocyte and monocyte phagocytosis were attenuated by carbohydrate supplementation, whereas the exercise-induced decline in neutrophil elastase production was attenuated with carbohydrate supplementation. Others have shown that a high-carbohydrate diet for 48 hours (after glycogen-depleting exercise) also attenuated the exercise-induced increase in circulating leukocyte number and subsets.[146] These and other studies have shown that carbohydrate supplementation alters the neuroendocrine response to exercise—for example,

lower cortisol, epinephrine, and growth hormone, but higher levels of plasma glucose and insulin.[147] Each of these hormones has been shown to alter immune function and therefore it is likely that the effect of carbohydrate supplementation during exercise on immune response is related to the different hormonal milieu. These recent findings are likely to be most applicable to the endurance athlete, assuming that the mechanism of immune modulation is related to changes in the neuroendocrine profile.

The other relatively new supplement that may be consumed by strength and power athletes is β-hydroxy β-methylbutyrate (HMB). One recent study showed that HMB supplementation in subjects initiating a weight-training program may partially attenuate exercise-induced proteolysis, as assessed by urinary markers of muscle breakdown, and was associated with larger gains in muscle.[148] The effects of HMB supplementation in humans with respect to immune function have not been tested to our knowledge. However, the results from a number of animal studies show that HMB can enhance immune function, may attenuate the stress-induced alterations of immunity, and may reduce mortality.[149–151] Exercise is often considered a type of stress and therefore this supplement could alter the immune response in human subjects participating in prolonged or intense exercise; however, this hypothesis remains to be tested.

SUMMARY

Vitamin, mineral, and protein malnutrition are associated with immune dysfunction and illness; however, there is currently not sufficient evidence to conclude that any of the supplements reviewed in this chapter can improve immunity, resist infection, or enhance the muscle repair process in strength/power athletes. Although many vitamins, minerals, and nutritional supplements may modulate immune function, in this chapter, we reviewed the immunomodulatory effects of those supplements most likely to be consumed by strength/power athletes. The supplements reviewed in this chapter are arginine, antioxidants including vitamin A, C, and E, zinc, whey protein, dehydroepiandrosterone (DHEA), glutamine, and β-hydroxy β-methylbutyrate (HMB).

Under conditions of heavy stress, which may include strenuous weight training, evidence from human studies suggests that vitamin C supplementation may reduce the duration and/or severity of cold symptoms. Animal models using conditions of stress have demonstrated that supplementation with DHEA or a related compound, androstenediol, may reduce susceptibility to viral infection and improve antiviral immune response. Vitamin E supplementation may protect against oxidative damage induced by exercise. However, evidence using animal models suggests that generation of reactive oxygen species produced during strenuous exercise may be beneficial in the muscle repair process. In certain populations including the elderly, and injured or ill patients, supplementation with vitamin E, zinc, arginine, and glutamine may enhance immunity, but this effect has not been clearly demonstrated in young, healthy individuals. Findings using laboratory animals indicate a potential immunomodulatory role of HMB, whey protein, and compounds related to DHEA, including androstenediol and androstenetriol. These supplements, to our knowledge, have not been tested in humans for potential immunomodulatory effects and therefore further research using humans is necessary before any conclusions can be made. Future research may identify the supplements that could be beneficial to the strength athletes, in terms of reduced susceptibility to infection, and perhaps as a method of improving the muscle damage/repair process.

AUTHOR'S RECOMMENDATIONS

In general, research regarding nutritional supplementation and immunity in strength or power athletes is currently limited and we cannot make any conclusive recommendation for supplementation at this time. Although there are numerous nutritional supplements, vitamins, and minerals that may modulate immune function, only a few of these have documented clinical benefits, and these benefits have been demonstrated in select populations (elderly, ill, or injured individuals). At this time, we can only speculate that the supplements shown to have some benefit under conditions of heavy stress may hold some promise for strength/power athletes involved in strenuous, intense training. In humans, vitamin C supplementation during periods of heavy physical stress has been shown to reduce the duration of cold symptoms. However, vitamin C supplementation has not been tested in strength/power athletes to our knowledge. Results from animal studies suggest that DHEA and the chemically related steroid, androstenediol, may reduce the stress-induced susceptibility to viral infection. No human studies that we are aware of have attempted to test whether DHEA can attenuate immunosuppressive effects of heavy physical stress. And the remaining supplement that may show promise in conditions of heavy eccentric exercise (downhill running) is vitamin E. Supplementation with vitamin E may attenuate the oxidative damage associated with eccentric exercise. However, more recent studies using animal models indicated that the production of reactive oxygen species is beneficial in terms of removing and/or repairing damaged muscle tissue. Therefore, until further research is performed in humans, recommendations regarding vitamin E cannot be made, and until further research is completed, no firm recommendations can be made for strength or power athletes regarding nutritional supplementation and potential improvement in immunity or muscle repair processes.

FUTURE RESEARCH

Currently, there is minimal information published regarding the potential effects of nutritional supplementation on the immune response in strength/power athletes. Therefore, many avenues of research remain open to investigation. Two important areas of concern for strength athletes are 1) a reduction in incidence and/or severity of illness, especially during periods of competition, and 2) methods of enhancing the muscle repair process.

Athletes may benefit from future research that is focused on studying those supplements that may prevent or shorten illness during periods of intense training. As competition nears, athletes often increase the intensity of training and the incidence of colds often increases. Although there is little evidence to suggest that healthy, well-nourished younger individuals can reduce the incidence of colds by taking nutritional supplements, athletes undergoing physical and mental stress associated with intense training could benefit from nutritional supplementation. Future studies may focus on the supplements that have been shown to reduce the severity of colds in endurance athletes (vitamin C) and the supplements shown to reduce the severity of viral infection in animal models under stress (DHEA and androstenediol). Other vitamins, minerals, or nutritional supplements could also benefit the

strength/power athlete in terms of reduced severity of colds; however, these have not yet been studied. Currently, the list of supplements with the potential to enhance immunity in competing athletes is very long, and it is only through future research that this list will be shortened with more conclusive evidence for or against various nutritional supplements.

Also of interest to strength/power athletes is the role of the immune system in the muscle damage and repair process. Immune cells infiltrate sites of postexercise muscle injury and produce chemical mediators that are important in removing and/or repairing damaged muscle. Future research may concentrate on the role of nutritional supplements (antioxidants) and the production of reactive oxygen species by cells of the immune system. Further information on the function of immune cells at the site of postexercise muscle damage is also necessary. It is important for this process to be clarified before one may determine whether nutritional supplementation can enhance the repair process. Given that the research on the basic mechanisms of the postexercise immune-mediated muscle repair process is ongoing, it may be some time before the potential effects of nutritional supplementation in modifying this process are understood.

REFERENCES

1. Kusnecov AW, Rabin BS. Inescapable footshock exposure differentially alters antigen- and mitogen-stimulated spleen cell proliferation in rats. J Neuroimmunol 1993;44:33–42.
2. Barbul A, Wasserkrug HL, Yoshimura N, et al. High arginine levels in intravenous hyperalimentation abrogate post-traumatic immune suppression. J Surg Res 1984;36:620–624.
3. Barbul A, Fishel RS, Shimazu S, et al. Intravenous hyperalimentation with high arginine levels improves wound healing and immune function. J Surg Res 1985;38:328–334.
4. Daly JM, Reynolds J, Thom A, et al. Immune and metabolic effects of arginine in the surgical patient. Ann Surg 1988;208:512–523.
5. Sigal RK, Shou J, Daly JM. Parenteral arginine infusion in humans: nutrient substrate or pharmacologic agent? J Parenter Enter Nutr 1992;16:423–428.
6. Ronnenberg AG, Gross KL, Hartman WJ, et al. Dietary arginine supplementation does not enhance lymphocyte proliferation or interleukin-2 production in young and aged rats. J Nutr 1991;121:1270–1278.
7. Ma Q, Hoper M, Anderson N, Rowlands BJ. Effect of supplemental L-arginine in a chemical-induced model of colorectal cancer. World J Surg 1996;20:1087–1091.
8. Reynolds JV, Daly JM, Zhang S, et al. Immunomodulatory mechanisms of arginine. Surgery 1988;104:142–151.
9. Reynolds JV, Thom AK, Zhang SM, et al. Arginine, protein malnutrition, and cancer. J Surg Res 1988;45:513–522.
10. Barbul A, Sisto DA, Wasserkrug HL, Efron G. Arginine stimulates lymphocyte immune response in healthy human beings. Surgery 1981;90:244–251
11. Barbul A, Lazarou SA, Efron DT, et al. Arginine enhances wound healing and lymphocyte immune responses in humans. Surgery 1990;108:331–336.
12. Kirk SJ, Hurson M, Regan MC, et al. Arginine stimulates wound healing and immune function in elderly human beings. Surgery 1990;114:155–159.
13. Provinciali M, Montenonvo AD, Di Stefano, et al. Effect of zinc or zinc plus arginine supplementation on antibody titer and lymphocyte

subsets after influenza vaccination in elderly subjects: a randomized controlled trial. Age Ageing 1998;27:715–722.
14. Wiebke EA, Grieshop NA, Sidner RA, et al. Effects of L-arginine supplementation on human lymphocyte proliferation in response to nonspecific and alloantigenic stimulation. J Surg Res 1997;70:89–94.
15. De-Souza DA, Greene LJ. Pharmacological nutrition after burn injury. J Nutr 1998;128:797–803.
16. Anonymous. Does supplemental arginine alter immune function following major surgery? Nutr Rev 1993;51:54–56.
17. Hellsten Y, Apple F, Sjodin B. Effects of sprint cycle training on activities of antioxidant enzymes in human skeletal muscle. J Appl Physiol 1996;81:1484–1487.
18. Ji LL. Exercise and oxidative stress: role of the cellular antioxidant systems. In: Holloszy JO, ed. Exercise and Sport Science Reviews. Baltimore: Williams & Wilkins, 1995:135–166.
19. Sen CK. Oxidants and antioxidants in exercise. J Appl Physiol 1995;79:675–686.
20. Meydani M, Evans W, Handelman G, et al. Protective effect of vitamin E on exercise-induced oxidative damage in young and older adults. Am J Physiol 1993;264:R992–R998.
21. Lawrence JD, Bower RC, Riehl WP, Smith JL. Effects of alpha-tocopherol acetate on the swimming endurance of trained swimmers. Am J Clin Nutr 1975;28:205–208.
22. Rokitzki L, Logemann E, Huber G, et al. Alpha-tocopherol supplementation in racing cyclists during extreme endurance training. Int J Sports Nutr 1994;4:253–264.
23. Shewchuck LD, Baracos VE, Field CJ. Dietary L-glutamine does not improve lymphocyte metabolism or function in exercise-trained rats. Med Sci Sports Exerc 1997;4:474–481.
24. Sumida S, Tanaka K, Kitao H, Nakadomo F. Exercise-induced lipid peroxidation and leakage of enzymes before and after vitamin E supplementation. Int J Biochem 1989;21:835–838.
25. Tiidus PM, Houston ME. Vitamin E status does not affect the response to exercise training and acute exercise in female rats. J Nutr 1993;123:834–840.
26. Kaikkonen J, Kosonen L, Nyyssonen K. et al. Effect of combined coenzyme Q10 and d-α-tocopherol acetate supplementation on

exercise-induced lipid peroxidation and muscular damage: a placebo-controlled double-blind study in marathon runners. Free Rad Res 1998;29:85–92.

27. Evans W, Cannon J. Metabolic effects of exercise-induced muscle damage. In: Holloszy JO, ed. Exercise and Sport Science Reviews. Baltimore: Williams & Wilkins, 1991:99–125.

28. Chaudhri G, Clark IA. Reactive oxygen species facilitate the in vitro and in vivo lipopolysaccharide-induced release of tumor necrosis factor. J Immunol 1989;143:1290–1294.

29. DeForge LE, Fantone JC, Kenney JS. Oxygen radical scavengers selectively inhibit IL-8 production in human whole blood. J Clin Invest 1992;90:2123–2129.

30. Farante A, Nandoskar M, Walz A, et al. Effects of tumor necrosis factor alpha and interleukin-1 alpha and beta on human neutrophil migration, respiratory burst and degranulation. Int Arch Allergy Appl Immmunol 1988;86:82–91.

31. Lamas S, Michel T, Brenner BM, et al. Nitric oxide synthesis in endothelial cells: evidence for a pathway inducible by TNFα. Am J Physiol 1991;261:C634–C641.

32. Duarte J, Carvalho F, Bastos M, et al. Do invading leukocytes contribute to the decrease in glutathion concentration indicating oxidative stress in exercising muscle, or are they important for its recovery? Eur J Appl Physiol 1994;68:45–53.

33. Tiidus PM. Radical species in inflammation and overtraining. Can J Physiol Pharmacol 1998;76:533–538.

34. Meydani M, Lipman RD, Han SN, et al. The effect of long-term dietary supplementation with anti-oxidants. Ann NY Acad Sci 1998;854:352–360.

35. Holloszy JO. Longevity of exercising male rates: effect of an antioxidant supplemented diet. Mech Aging Dev 1998;100:211–219.

36. Coutsoudis A, Kiepiela P, Coovadia HM, Broughton M. Vitamin A supplementation enhances specific IgG antibody levels and total lymphocyte numbers while improving morbidity in measles. Pediatr Infect Dis J 1992;11:101–107.

37. Ross CA, Hammerling UG. Retinoids and the immune system. In: Sporn MB, Roberts AB, Goodman DS, eds. Biology, Chemistry, and Medicine. New York: Raven Press, 1994:521–543.

38. Semba RD, Muhilal A, Scott AL, et al. Depressed immune response to tetanus in children with vitamin A deficiency. J Nutr 1992;122:101–107

39. Semba RD, Graham NM, Caiaffa WT, et al. Increased mortality associated with vitamin A deficiency during human immunodeficiency virus type 1 infection. Arch Intern Med 1993;153:2149–2154.

40. Gangopadhyay NN, Moldoveanu Z, Stephensen CB. Vitamin A deficiency has different effects on immunoglobulin A production and transport during influenza A infection in BALB/c mice. J Nutr 1996;126:2960–2967.

41. Humphrey JH, Agoestina T, Wu L, et al. Impact of neonatal vitamin A supplementation on infant morbidity and mortality. J Pediatr 1996;128:489–496.

42. Hughes DA, Wright AJ, Finglas PM, et al. The effect of beta-carotene supplementation on the immune function of blood monocytes from healthy male nonsmokers. J Lab Clin Med 1997;129:309–317.

43. Sacks GS. Glutamine supplementation in catabolic patients. Ann Pharmacother 1999;33:348–354.

44. Santos MS, Gaziano JM, Leka LS, et al. Beta-carotene-induced enhancement of natural killer cell activity in elderly men: an investigation of the role of cytokines. Am J Clin Nutr 1998;68:164–170.

45. Dauda PA, Kelley DS, Taylor PC, et al. Effect of a low beta-carotene diet on the immune functions of adult women. Am J Clin Nutr 1994;60:969–972.

46. Santos MS, Leka LS, Ribaya-Mercado JD, et al. Short and long-term beta-carotene supplementation do not influence T cell-mediated immunity in healthy elderly persons. Am J Clin Nutr 1997;66:917–924.

47. Fortes C, Forastiere F, Agabiti N, et al. The effect of zinc and vitamin A supplementation on immune response in an older population. J Am Geriatr Soc 1998;46:19–26.

48. Murphy S, West KP, Greenough WB, et al. Impact of vitamin A supplementation on the incidence of infection in elderly nursing-home residents: a randomized controlled trial. Age Ageing 1992;21:453–459.

49. Girodon F, Lombard M, Galan P, et al. Effect of micronutrient supplementation on infection in institutionalized elderly subjects: a controlled trial. Ann Nutr Metab 1997;41:98–107.

50. Girodon F, Galan P, Monget AL, et al. Impact of trace elements and vitamin supplementation on immunity and infections in institutionalized elderly patients: a randomized controlled trial. Arch Intern Med 1999;159:748–754.

51. Johnson MA, Porter KH. Micronutrient supplementation and infection in institutionalized elders. Nutr Rev 1997;55:400–404.

52. Christen WG, Buring JE, Manson JE, Hennekens CH. Beta-carotene supplementation: a good thing, a bad thing, or nothing? Curr Opin Lipidol 1999;10:29–33.

53. Hennekens CH, Buring JE, Manson JE, et al. Lack of effect of long-term supplementation with beta carotene on the incidence of malignant neoplasms and cardiovascular disease. N Engl J Med 1996;334:1145–1149.

54. Omenn GS, Goodman GE, Thornquist MD, et al. Effects of a combination of beta carotene and vitamin A on lung cancer and cardiovascular disease. N Engl J Med 1996;334:1150–1155.

55. The Alpha Tocopherol, Beta Carotene Prevention Study Group. The effect of vitamin E and beta carotene on the incidence of lung cancer and other cancers in male smokers. N Engl J Med 1994;330:1029–1035.

56. Hinds TS, West WL, Knight EM. Carotenoids and retinoids: a review of research, clinical, and public health applications. J Clin Pharmacol 1997;37:551–558.

57. Nieman DC, Johansen LM, Lee JW, Arabtzis K. Infectious episodes in runners before and after the Los Angeles Marathon. J Sports Med Phys Fitness 1990;30:316–328.

58. Peters EM, Bateman ED. Ultramarathon running and upper respiratory infections. S Afr Med J 1983;64:582–584.

59. Peters EM, Goetzsche J, Grobbelaar, B, Noakes TD. Vitamin C supplementation reduces the incidence of post-race symptoms of upper-respiratory-tract infection in ultramarathon runners. Am J Clin Nutr 1993;57:170–174.

60. Peters EM, Cambell A, Pawley L. Vitamin A fails to increase resistance to upper respiratory infection in distance runners. S Afr J Sports Med 1992;7:3–7.

61. Kennes B, Dumont I, Brohee D, et al. Effect of vitamin C supplements on cell-mediated immunity in old people. Gerontology 1983;29:301–310.

62. Patrone F. Effects of ascorbic acid on neutrophil function: studies on normal and chronic granulomatous disease neutrophils. Acta Vitaminol Enzymol 1982;4:163–168.

63. Prinz W. The effect of ascorbic acid supplementation on some parameters of the human immunological defense system. Int J Vit Nutr Res 1977;47:248–257.

64. Jeng KC, Yang CS, Siu WY, et al. Supplementation with vitamins C and E enhances cytokine production by peripheral blood mononuclear cells in healthy adults. Am J Clin Nutr 1996;64:960–965.

65. Hemila H. Vitamin C intake and susceptibility to the common cold. Br J Nutr 1997;77:59–72.

66. Ganguly R, Park J. Immunostimulating agents against influenza virus infection in senescent rats. Allerg Immunol 1988;34:239–247.

67. Hemila H. Vitamin C supplementation and common cold symptoms: factors affecting the magnitude of the benefit. Med Hypotheses 1999;52:171–178.

68. Hemila H. Vitamin C and common cold incidence: a review of studies with subjects under heavy physical stress. Int J Sports Med 1996;17:379–383.

69. Peters, EM. Exercise, immunology and upper respiratory tract infections. Int J Sports Med 1997;18:S69–S77.

70. Peters EM, Goetzsche JM, Joseph LE, Noakes TD. Vitamin C as effective as combinations of anti-oxidants nutrients in reducing symptoms of upper respiratory tract infections in ultramarathon runners. S Afr J Sports Med 1996;4:23–27.

71. Pitt HA, Costrini AM. Vitamin C prophylaxis in marine recruits. JAMA 1979;241:908–911.

72. Nieman DC, Henson DA, Butterworth DE, et al. Vitamin C supplementation does not alter the immune response to 2.5 hours of running. Int J Sports Nutr 1997;3:173–184.

73. Beck MA, Levander OA. Dietary oxidative stress and the potentiation of viral infection. Annu Rev Nutr 1998;18:93–116.

74. Gleeson M, Robertson JD, Maughan RJ. Influence of exercise on ascorbic acid status in man. Clin Sci 1987;73:510–515.

75. Beharka A, Redican S, Leka L, Meydani SN. Vitamin E status and immune function. Methods Enzymol 1997;282:247–263.

76. Beck MA, Kolbeck PC, Rohr LH, et al. Vitamin E deficiency intensifies the myocardial injury of coxsackievirus B3 infection of mice. J Nutr 1994;124:345–358.

77. Moriguchi S, Oonishi K, Kishino Y. Vitamin E is an important factor in T cell differentiation in the thymus of F 344 rat. J Nutr Sci Vitaminol 1993;5:451–463.

78. Wu D, Mura C, Beharka AA, et al. Age-associated increase in PGE2 synthesis and COX activity in murine macrophages is reversed by vitamin E. Am J Physiol 1998;275:C661–C668.

79. Hayek, MG, Taylor SF, Bender BS, et al. Vitamin E supplementation decreases lung virus titers in mice infected with influenza. J Infect Dis 1997;176:273–276.

80. Reffett JK, Spears JW, Brown TT. Effects of dietary vitamin E and selenium on the primary and secondary immune response in lambs challenged with parainfluenza virus. J Anim Sci 1988;66:1520–1528.

81. Smith KL, Harrison JH, Hancock DD. Effect of dietary vitamin E and selenium supplementation on incidence of clinical mastitis and duration of clinical symptoms. J Dairy Sci 1984;67:1293–1300.

82. Tengerdy RP, Meyer DL, Lauerman LH, et al. Vitamin E enhances humoral antibody response to clostridium perfringens type D in sheep. Brit Vet J 1983;139:147–152.

83. Tengerdy RP, Nockels CF. Vitamin E or vitamin A protects chickens against E. coli infection. Poult Sci 1975;54:1292–1296.

84. Wang Y, Huang DS, Wood S, Watson RR. Modulation of immune function and cytokine production by various levels of vitamin E supplementation during murine AIDS. Immunopharmacology 1995;29:225–233.

85. Sell JL, Trampel DW, Griffith RW. Adverse effects of Escherichia coli infection of turkeys were not alleviated by supplemental dietary vitamin E. Poult Sci 1997;76:1682–1687.

86. Meydani SN, Meydani M, Blumberg JB, et al. Vitamin E supplementation and in vivo immune response in healthy elderly subjects: a randomized controlled trial. JAMA 1997;277:1380–1386.

87. Pallast EG, Schouten EG, de Waart FG, et al. Effect of 50 and 100 mg vitamin E supplements on cellular immune function in noninstitutionalized elderly persons. Am J Clin Nutr 1999;69:1273–1281.

88. De Waart FG, Portengen L, Koekes G, et al. Effect of 3 months vitamin E supplementation on indices of the cellular and humoral immune response in elderly subjects. Br J Nutr 1997;78:761–774.

89. De la Fuente M, Ferrandez MD, Burgos MS, et al. Immune function in aged women is improved by ingestion of vitamins C and E. Can J Physiol Pharmacol 1998;76:373–380.

90. Wong CW, Liu AH, Regester GO, et al. Influence of whey and purified whey proteins on neutrophil functions in sheep. J Dairy Res 1997:64:281–289.

91. Pehrson B, Hakkarainen J, Tornquist M, et al. Effect of vitamin E supplementation on weight gain, immune competence, and disease incidence in barley-fed beef cattle. J Dairy Sci 1991;74:1054–1059.

92. Singh A, Papanicolaou DA, Lawrence LL, et al. Neuroendocrine responses to running in women after zinc and vitamin E supplementation. Med Sci Sports Exerc 1999;31:536–542.

93. Buchman AL, Killip D, Ou CN, et al. Short-term vitamin E supplementation before marathon running: a placebo-controlled trial. Nutrition 1999;15:278–283.

94. Prasad AS. Zinc and immunity. Molec Cell Biochem 1998;188:63–69.

95. Wellinghausen N, Kirchner H, Rink L. The immunobiology of zinc. Immunol Today 1997;18:519–521.

96. Wellinghausen N, Rink L. The significance of zinc for leukocyte biology. J Leuk Biol 1998;64:571–578.

97. Sazawal S, Jalla S, Maxumder S, et al. Effect of zinc supplementation on cell-mediated immunity and lymphocyte subsets in pre-school children. Indian Pediatr 1997;34:589–596.

98. Sazawal S, Black RE, Jalla S, et al. Zinc supplementation reduces the incidence of acute lower respiratory infections in infants and preschool children: a double-blind, controlled trial. Pediatrics 1998;102:1–5.

99. Sempertegui F, Estrella B, Correa E, et al. Effects of short-term zinc supplementation on cellular immunity, respiratory symptoms, and growth of malnourished Ecuadorian children. Eur J Clin Nutr 1996;50:42–46.

100. Bogden JD, Oleske JM, Lavenhar MA, et al. Zinc and immunocompetence in elderly people: effects of zinc supplementation for 3 months. Am J Clin Nutr 1988;48:655–663.

101. Bogden JD, Oleske JM, Lavenhar MA, et al. Effects of one year of supplementation with zinc and other micronutrients on cellular immunity in the elderly. J Am Coll Nutr 1990;9:214–225.

102. Duchateau J, Delepesse G, Vrijens R, Collet H. Beneficial effects of oral zinc supplementation on the immune response of old people. Am J Med 1981;70:1001–1004.

103. Al-Nakib W, Higgins PG, Barrow I, et al. Prophylaxis and treatment of rhinovirus colds with zinc gluconate lozenges. J Antimicrob Chemother 1987;20:893–901.

104. Mossad SB, Macknin ML, Medendorp SV, Mason P. Zinc gluconate lozenges for treating the common cold: a randomized, double blind, placebo-controlled study. Ann Intern Med 1996;15:81–88.

105. Farr BM, Conner EM, Betts RF, et al. Two randomized controlled trails of zinc gluconate lozenge therapy of experimentally induced rhinovirus colds. Antibmicrob Agents Chemother 1987;31:1183–1187.

106. Macknin ML, Piedmonte M, Calendine C, et al. Zinc gluconage lozenges for treating the common cold in children: a randomized controlled trial. JAMA 1998;279:1961–1967.

107. Jackson JL, Peterson C, Lesho E. A meta-analysis of zinc salts lozenges and the common cold. Arch Intern Med 1997;157:2373–2376.

108. Chandra RK. Excessive intake of zinc impairs immune responses. JAMA 1984;252:1443–1446.

109. Deuster PA, Day BA, Singh A, et al. Zinc status of highly trained women runners and untrained women. Am J Clin Nutr 1989;49:1295–1301.

110. Dressendorfer RH, Sockolov R. Hypozincemia in runners. Physician Sportsmed 1980;8:97–100.

111. Haralambie G. Serum zinc in athletes in training. Int J Sports Med 1981;2:135–138.

112. Singh A, Failla ML, Deuster P.A. Exercise-induced changes in immune function: effect of zinc supplementation. J Appl Physiol 1994;76:2298–2303.

113. Bounous G, Kongshavn PA. Differential effect of dietary protein type on the B-cell and T-cell immune responses in mice. J Nutr 1985;115:1403–1408.

114. Parker NT, Goodrum KJ. A comparison of casein, lactalbumin, and soy protein effect on the immune response to a T-dependent antigen. Nutrition Res 1990;10:781–792.

115. Wong CW, Watson DL. Immunomodulatory effects of dietary whey protein in mice. J Dairy Res 1995;62:359–368.

116. Wong CW, Seow HF, Husband AJ, et al. Effects of purified bovine whey factors on cellular immune functions in ruminants. Vet Immunol Immunopathol 1997;56:85–96.

117. Papenburg R, Bounous G, Fleiszer D, Gold P. Dietary milk proteins inhibit the development of dimethylhydrazine-induced malignancy. Tumour Biol 1990;11:129–136.

118. Bounous G, Batist G, Gold P. Immunoenhancing property of dietary whey protein in mice: role of glutathione. Clin Invest Med 1989;12:154–161.

119. Svec F, Porter JR. The actions of exogenous dehydroepiandrosterone in experimental animals and humans. Proc Soc Exp Biol Med 1998;218:174–191.

120. Hernandez-Pando R, De La Luz Sterber M, Orozco H, et al. The effects of androstenediol and dehydroepiandrosterone on the course and cytokine profile of tuberculosis in BALB/c mice. Immunology 1998;95:234–241.

121. Loria RM, Padgett DA, Huynh PN. Regulation of the immune response by dehydroepiandrosterone and its metabolites. J Endocrinol 1996;150:S209–S220.

122. Araneo BA, Woods ML, Daynes RA. Reversal of the immunosenescent phenotype by dehydroepiandrosterone: hormone treatment provides an adjuvant effect on the immunization of aged mice with recombinant hepatitis B surface antigen. J Infect Dis 1993;167:830–840.

123. Danenberg HD, Ben-Yehuda A, Zakay-Rones Z, Friedman G. Dehydroepiandrosterone (DHEA) treatment reverses the impaired immune response of old mice to influenza vaccination and protects from influenza infection. Vaccine 1995;13:1445–1448.

124. Padgett DA, Loria RM. In vitro potentiation of lymphocyte activation by dehydroepiandrosterone, androstenediol, and androstenetriol. J Immunol 1994;153:1544–1552.

125. Daynes RA, Dudley DJ, Araneo B. Regulation of murine lymphokine production in vivo II. Dehydroepiandrosterone is a natural enhancer of interleukin 2 synthesis by helper T cells. Eur J Immunol 1990;20:793–802.

126. Inserra P, Zhang Z, Ardestani SK, et al. Modulation of cytokine production by dehydroepiandrosterone (DHEA) plus melatonin supplementation of old mice. Proc Soc Exp Biol Med 1998;218:76–82.

127. McLachlan JA, Serkin CD, Bakouche O. Dehydorepiandrosterone modulation of lipopolysaccharide-stimulated monocyte cytotoxicity. J Immunol 1996;156:328–335.

128. Weindruch R. McFeeters G, Walford RL. Food intake reduction and immunologic alterations in mice fed dehydroepiandrosterone. Exp Gerontol 1984;19:297–304.

129. Pahvlani MA, Harris MD. Effect of dehydroepiandrosterone on mitogen-induced lymphocyte proliferation and cytokine production in young and old F344 rats. Immunol Lett 1995;47:9–14.

130. Khorram O, Vu L, Yen SS. Activation of immune function by dehydroepiandrosterone (DHEA) in age-advanced men. J Gerontol A Biol Sci Med Sci 1997;52:M1–7.

131. Casson PR, Andersen RN, Herrod HG, et al. Oral dehydroepiandrosterone in physiologic dose modulates immune function in postmenopausal women. Am J Obstet Gynecol 1993;169:1536–1539.

132. Suzuki T, Suzuki N, Daynes RA, Engleman EG. Dehydroepiandrosterone enhances IL-2 production and cytotoxic effector function of human T cells. Clin Immunol Immunopathol 1991;61:202–211.

133. Ben-Yehuda A, Denenberg HD, Zakay-Rones Z, et al. The influence of sequential annual vaccination and of DHEA administration on the efficacy of the immune response to influenza vaccine in the elderly. Mech Ageing Dev 1998;102:299–306.

134. Danenberg HD, Ben-Yehuda A, Zakay Rones Z, et al. Dehydroepiandrosterone treatment is not beneficial to the immune response to influenza in elderly subjects. J Clin Endocrinol Metab 1997;82:2911–2914.

135. Degelau J, Guay D, Hallgren H. The effect of DHEAS on influenza vaccination in aging adults. J Am Geriatr Soc 1997;45:747–751.

136. Evans TG, Judd ME, Dowell T, et al. The use of oral dehydroepiandrosterone sulfate as an adjuvant in tetanus and influenza vaccination in the elderly. Vaccine 1996;14:1531–1537.

137. Miller RA, Chrisp C. Lifelong treatment with oral DHEA sulfate does not preserve immune function, prevent disease, or improve survival in genetically heterogeneous mice. J Am Geriatr Soc 1999; 47:960–966.

138. Padgett DA, Sheridan RF. Androstenediol prevents neuroendocrine-mediated suppression of the immune response to an influenza viral infection. J Neuroimmunol 1999;98:121–129.

139. Blauer KL, Poth M, Rogers WM, Bernton EW. Dehydroepiandrosterone antagonizes the suppressive effects of dexamethasone on lymphocyte proliferation. Endocrinology 1991;129:3174–3179.

140. Loria RM, Padgett DA. Androstenediol regulates systemic resistance against lethal infections in mice. Arch Virol 1992;127:103–115.

141. Padgett DA, Loria RM, Sheridan JF. Endocrine regulation of the immune response to influenza virus infection with a metabolite of DHEA-androstenediol. J Neuroimmunol 1997;78:203–211.

142. Padgett DA, Loria RM. Endocrine regulation of murine macrophage function: effects of dehydroepiandrosterone, androstenediol, and androstenetriol. J Neuroimmunol 1998;84:61–68.

143. Nehlsen-Cannarella SL, Fagoaga OR, Nieman DC, et al. Carbohydrate and the cytokine response to 2.5 hours of running. J Appl Physiol 1997;82:1662–1667.

144. Henson DA, Nieman DC, Parker JC, et al. Carbohydrate supplementation and the lymphocyte proliferative response to long endurance running. Int J Sports Med 1998;19:574–580.

145. Henson DA, Nieman DC, Blodgett AD, et al. Influence of exercise mode and carbohydrate on the immune response to prolonged exercise. Int J Sports Nutr 1999;9:213–238.

146. Mitchell JB, Pizza FX, Paquet A, et al. Influence of carbohydrate status on immune responses before and after endurance exercise. J Appl Physiol 1998;84:1917–1925.

147. Nieman DC. Influence of carbohydrate on the immune response to intensive prolonged exercise. Exerc Immunol Rev 1998;4:64–76.

148. Nissen S, Sharp R, Ray M, et al. Effect of leucine metabolite β-hydroxy β-methylbutyrate on muscle metabolism during resistance exercise training. J Appl Physiol 1996;81:2095–2104.

149. Nissen S, Fuller JC, Sell J, et al. The effect of β-hydroxy β-methylbutyrate on growth, mortality, and carcass qualities of broiler chickens. Poult Sci 1994;73:137–155.

150. Peterson AL, Qureshi MA, Ferket PR, Fuller JC. In vitro exposure with β-hydroxy-β-methylbutyrate enhances chicken macrophage function. J Vet Immunol Immunopathol 1999;67–78.

151. Talleyrand V, Dorn A, Frank D, et al. Effect of feeding β-hydroxy β-methylbutyrate on immune function in stressed calves. FASEB J 1994;8:A951.

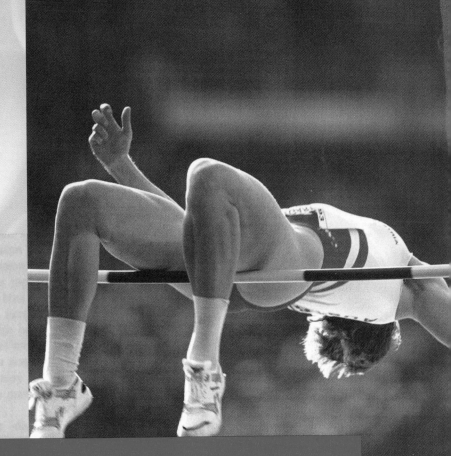

CHAPTER

9

Nutritional Considerations for Preventing Overtraining

Richard B. Kreider and Brian Leutholz

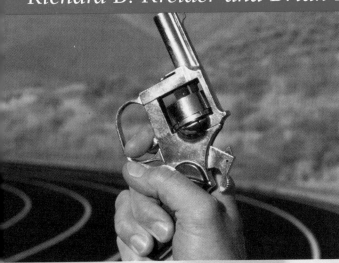

Introduction

To enhance athletic performance, athletes must optimally train. Athletes who do not train enough may not reach their potential. However, athletes who train too often and/or too intensely may experience negative training adaptations leading to short-term (overreaching) or long-term (overtraining) decrements in performance capacity.[1] The reduced exercise capacity may or may not be associated with a myriad of reported physiological, psychological, and/or immunological signs and symptoms of overreaching and overtraining. Once performance is diminished, it may take several weeks or months to fully recover. For this reason, determining the appropriate training volume/intensity necessary to optimize performance without leading to overtraining is one of the foremost challenges for athletes and coaches.[1] Although the specific reason some athletes become overtrained is not well understood, research has determined a number of strategies that athletes and coaches can use in an attempt to reduce the incidence of overtraining among athletes. This chapter describes the physiological and psychological symptoms of overreaching/overtraining as well as nutritional strategies that have been suggested to help decrease the incidence of overreaching/overtraining in sport.

Overtraining In Sport

The phenomenon of overreaching and overtraining is not new to sport. Athletes involved in intense training often experience short-term and/or long-term decrements in performance. In fact, coaches and athletes often plan intensified periods of training in hopes that the training will promote greater training adaptations.[2,3] Unfortunately, while some athletes respond well to the intensified training, others may become overreached and/or overtrained. According to Kreider,[1] overreaching is an accumulation of training and/or nontraining stress resulting in a short-term decrement in performance capacity with or without related physiological and psychological signs and symptoms of overtraining in which restoration of performance capacity may take from several days to several weeks. More severely, overtraining is an accumulation of training and/or nontraining stress resulting in a long-term decrement in performance capacity with or without related physiological and psychological signs and symptoms of overtraining in which restoration of performance capacity may take several weeks or months.

Although the specific etiology of overtraining is unclear, there are basically two types of overtraining described in the literature—sympathetic and parasympathetic.[3,4] See Table 9-1 for a list of some of the characteristics related to these types of overtraining. Sympathetic overtraining is typically associated with anaerobic strength-power training whereas parasympathetic overtraining is usually associated with endurance exercise training. In sympathetic-type overtraining, performance is decreased and response to training stimulus is delayed. Athletes may also exhibit signs/symptoms of increased irritability, disturbed patterns of sleep, weight loss, increased resting heart rate and blood pressure, and/or impaired recovery during training. In parasympathetic-type overtraining, performance capacity is decreased and response to training is also delayed with decreases in heart rate, blood pressure, and suppressed neuromuscular excitability. Other factors that can result in a decrease in performance are fatigue, depression, and altered endocrine function.[1,3,4]

Additionally, a number of physiological, biochemical, immunological, and psychological signs and symptoms of overtraining have been described in the literature (SEE TABLE 9-1). Although some overreached/overtrained athletes experience a decrease in performance without any signs/symptoms of overtraining, most will exhibit some of these overt signs. However, there does not appear to be any consistent pattern of symptoms of overtraining among athletes.[1,2,5,6] Therefore, although some markers have been proposed, there are presently no valid markers of overreaching and overtraining other than reductions in exercise capacity[6] (SEE TABLE 9-1).

Several factors have been suggested to increase the susceptibility of athletes to become overtrained (SEE TABLE 9-2). Care should be taken to plan training carefully so that the athletes are progressing properly from various training phases to avoid sudden increases in training volume and/or intensity.[2,3] Care should also be taken to ensure that there is enough recovery time during training to optimize physiological adaptations. Additionally, one must consider that the athlete not only must endure the physical stress of training but that the psychological stress of competition, school, work, social environment, or personal life may add to the physical stress of training.[6] Coaches and trainers should be aware of these psychological stressors and alter training volume and intensity as necessary.[1,2,5]

It is also clear that during periods of increased physical or psychological stress, athletes often do not eat enough calories to offset energy expenditure.[7] The result is that the athlete maintains a negative energy status that may further compromise training adaptations. Consequently, coaches and trainers should ensure that the athlete is well-fed during periods of intensified training. Finally, it is recommended that coaches and athletes closely monitor signs and symptoms of overtraining during training.[1,2,6] Research has indicated that some psychological signs (e.g., general fatigue, lethargy, disinterest in training, etc.) may often precede physiological symptoms of overreaching/overtraining.[1,2] Therefore, simply monitoring how athletes feel, how they perceive they are responding to training, and performance markers can serve as valuable feedback in understanding how athletes are tolerating training so that training volume/intensity can be altered accordingly.

Table 9-1 The Major Signs/Symptoms of Overtraining

Physiological/Performance

Decreased performance

Inability to meet previously attained performance standards/
criteria

Recovery prolonged

Reduced toleration of loading

Decreased muscular strength

Decreased maximum work capacity

Loss of coordination

Decreased efficiency/decreased amplitude of movement

Reappearance of mistakes already corrected

Reduced capacity of differentiation and correcting technical
faults

Increased difference between lying and standing heart rate

Abnormal T wave pattern in ECG

Heart discomfort on slight exertion

Changes in blood pressure

Changes in heart rate at rest, exercise, and recovery

Increased frequency of respiration

Perfuse respiration

Decreased body fat

Increased oxygen consumption at submaximal workloads

Increased ventilation and heart rate at submaximal workloads

Shift of the lactate curve towards the x-axis

Decreased evening post-workout weight

Elevated basal metabolic rate

Chronic fatigue

Insomnia with and without night sweats

Feels thirsty

Anorexia nervosa

Loss of appetite

Bulimia

Amenorrhea/oligomenorrhea

Headaches

Nausea

Increased aches and pains

Gastrointestinal disturbances

Muscle soreness/tenderness

Tendonostic complaints

Periosteal complaints

Muscle damage

Elevated C-reactive protein

Rhabdomyolysis

Psychological/Information Processing

Feelings of depression

General apathy

Decreased self-esteem/worsening feelings of self

Emotional instability

Difficulty in concentrating at work and training

Sensitive to environmental and emotional stress

Fear of competition

Changes in personality

Decreased ability to narrow concentration

Increased internal and external distractibility

Decreased capacity to deal with large amounts of information

Gives up when the going gets tough

Immunological

Increased susceptibility to and severity of illness/colds/allergies

Flu-like illnesses

Unconfirmed glandular fever

Minor scratches heal slowly

Swelling of the lymph glands

One-day colds

Decreased functional activity of neutrophils

Decreased total lymphocyte counts

Reduced response to mitogens

Increased blood eosinophil count

Decreased proportion of null (non-T, non-B lymphocytes)

Bacterial infection

Reactivation of herpes viral infection

Significant variations in CD4:CD8 lymphocytes

Biochemical

Negative nitrogen balance

Hypothalamic dysfunction

Flat glucose tolerance curves

Depressed muscle glycogen concentration

Decreased bone mineral content

Delayed menarche

Decreased hemoglobin

Decreased serum iron

Decreased serum ferritin

Lowered TIBC

Mineral depletion (Zn, Co, Al, Mn, Se, Cu, etc.)

Increased urea concentrations

Elevated cortisol levels

Elevated ketosteroids in urine

Low free testosterone

Increased serum hormone binding globulin

Decreased ratio of free testosterone to cortisol of more
than 30%

Increased uric acid production

Data from Fry RW, Morton AR, Keast D. Overtraining in athletes: an update. Sports Medicine 1991;12:32–65. Reprinted with permission from Adis Press International.

Table 9-2 Factors Contributing to Overreaching/ Overtraining

- Sharp increases in training volume/intensity
- Training too often, too intensely, & too frequently
- Lack of rest/recovery days during training
- Inadequate diet leading to negative energy states, glycogen depletion, and/or central fatigue
- Training boredom/monotony
- Compulsive behavior toward training
- Excessive competitiveness
- Poor performance
- Ignoring signs/symptoms of overtraining

Data from Kreider RB, Fry AC, O'Toole ML, eds. Overtraining in Sport. Champaign: Human Kinetics, 1998.

Role of Nutrition in Central Fatigue and Immune Function

During prolonged exercise, athletes become fatigued. For many years, exercise scientists believed that fatigue was simply related to peripheral muscle glycogen depletion and perhaps the hypoglycemia which may occur during prolonged exercise.[7–9] However, more recent studies indicated that athletes fatigue even though blood glucose levels were maintained during exercise and a sufficient amount of glycogen was available in the muscle. These findings suggested that fatigue could not simply be explained by peripheral adaptations but that other factors may be involved in the fatigue process during prolonged exercise.[7–9] The following discusses the potential role that central fatigue may play in overtraining, and dietary strategies that may help delay central fatigue.

Central Fatigue Hypothesis

Newsholme, Blomstrand, and colleagues[10–13] initially advanced the theory that fatigue during prolonged exercise may be partly related to exercise-induced alterations in the central nervous system. The theory suggests that as muscle glycogen levels decline during exercise, there is an increased oxidation of fat and the branched-chain amino acids (BCAAs) leucine, isoleucine, and valine as fuel substrates. As a result, free fatty acid (FFA) levels in the blood gradually increase while the availability of BCAAs in the blood decreases. The increase in FFA levels in the blood is accompanied by a release of the amino acid tryptophan from albumin, serving to increase the level of free tryptophan in the blood. The result is that as one exercises, the ratio of free tryptophan to BCAA steadily increases.

Increases in the ratio of free tryptophan to BCAA have been shown to increase the entry of tryptophan into the brain.[10] Increased concentrations of tryptophan in the brain have been reported to promote the formation of the neurotransmitter 5-hydroxytryptamine (serotonin). Increased levels of serotonin in the brain and peripheral tissues have been reported to induce sleep, depress motor neuron excitability, influence autonomic and endocrine function, and suppress appetite in animal and human studies. Consequently, an exercise-induced imbalance in the ratio of free tryptophan to BCAA has been implicated as a possible cause of acute physiological and psychological fatigue (central fatigue). It has also been hypothesized that chronic elevations in serotonin levels, which may occur in athletes who overtrain, may explain some of the reported signs and symptoms of the overtraining described above.[10]

Although the central fatigue theory seems straightforward, there has been debate in the scientific community regarding the validity of the hypothesis.[14–17] Segura and Ventura[17] hypothesized that the increase in the free tryptophan to BCAA ratio may help to decrease the perception of pain, thus improving exercise performance by increasing the pain threshold. However, given the most recent research there is more sound scientific evidence to support the theory that central influences during exercise may play a role in the onset of fatigue under certain conditions. However, because the potential causes of overtraining are multifaceted and have yet to be fully understood, the degree to which central fatigue may contribute to overreaching and/or overtraining remains to be determined.[15,16]

Nutritional Needs of the Immune System

Although moderate exercise has been reported to enhance immunity, intense prolonged exercise has been found to temporarily suppress the immune system.[18,19] For example, research has indicated that following intense exercise, the immune system may be depressed for as long as 6 hours. This *open window* of suppressed immune function may allow the body to be more susceptible to acquiring host infections.[18,19] To support this theory, several studies have reported that following intense exercise like a marathon, athletes have a greater incidence of upper respiratory tract infections (URTIs) for several weeks following the event. Additionally, athletes who overreach and/or overtrain often get URTIs, ear infections, and/or colds.[19] This suggests that athletes who train too often or too intensely may experience a chronically suppressed immune system.

The primary metabolic fuel for the lymphocyte is glutamine.[16,20,21] The availability of glutamine affects lymphocytic function. In this regard, *in vitro* and *in vivo*, evidence suggests that increasing the availability of glutamine enhances immune function while decreasing glutamine levels suppresses immune function.[21] During high-intensity intermittent and prolonged exercise, it has been suggested that glutamine levels decline in the blood.[16] The reason for this is that glutamine, like BCAAs, readily serves as a metabolic substrate during exercise.[20,21] The exercise-induced hypoglutaminia has been reported to last up to 6 hours following high-intensity intermittent exercise.[22] Moreover, some overtrained athletes have been reported to have chronically low glutamine levels.[21] Consequently, one theory of exercise-induced immunosuppression is that decreased glutamine availability following exercise may serve to suppress lymphocytic function, making it more difficult to respond to immune challenges.[16,20,21] Athletes involved in periods of intensified training that often involves training more than once per day may therefore be more susceptible to a hypoglutaminia-induced immunosuppression.

Dietary Strategies that May Help Prevent Overtraining

A number of the physiological and psychological symptoms and signs of overreaching/overtraining have been suggested to be partly due to a chronic energy deficit, an inadequate availability of specific nutrients, or both. This may affect the body's response to intensified training. The following describes some of the general dietary strategies that athletes can use to prevent overtraining.

Energy Intake

The first nutritional strategy to prevent overtraining is to make sure that athletes consume enough calories to offset energy demands or maintain energy balance.[7–9,23] Daily caloric intake for untrained individuals typically ranges between 1900 to 3000 kcals/day (i.e., 25 to 45 kcals/kg/day for a 70-kg person).[7,24,25] Exercise training obviously increases energy expenditure. The longer and more intense an athlete exercises, the greater the energy expenditure. Energy expenditure estimates for athletes have ranged from 3500 kcals/day (50 kcals/kg/day) for individuals training 30 to 60 min/day up to 12,000 kcals/day (i.e., 170 kcals/kg/day) for cyclists competing in the Tour de France (cycling 4 to 6 hrs/day).[7,16,23,26] For most high school and college athletes training 2–2.5 hrs/day, energy expenditure estimates range between 60 to 80 kcal/kg/day.[24] Despite this energy requirement, athletes often do not consume enough calories to offset energy demands.[7,8] This may result in a chronic deficit in energy intake and has been implicated as one potential causative factor to overtraining.[1,7,8]

Athletes particularly susceptible to maintaining negative energy intakes during training include runners, cyclists, swimmers, triathletes, gymnasts, skaters, dancers, wrestlers, and boxers.[7] Additionally, female athletes have been reported to have a high incidence of eating disorders.[7] Consequently, the parent and/or coach should ensure that athletes are well fed and consume enough calories to offset the increased energy demands of training. Although this sounds relatively simple, intense training often suppresses appetite and/or alters hunger patterns.[7] Some athletes do not like to exercise within several hours after eating because of sensations of fullness and/or a predisposition to cause gastrointestinal distress. Further, travel and training schedules may limit food availability and/or the types of food athletes are accustomed to eating. This means that care should be taken to plan meal times in concert with training as well as make sure athletes have sufficient availability of nutrient-dense foods throughout the day for snacking between meals (e.g., drinks, fruit, carbohydrate/protein bars, etc.).[7,9,23]

Macronutrient Intake Guidelines

The second nutritional strategy to prevent overtraining is to ensure that athletes consume the proper amounts of carbohydrate, protein, and fat in their diet. Research has indicated that athletes should ingest between 8 to 10 g/day of carbohydrate during intense periods of training to help maintain carbohydrate stores.[9,23] To do so, athletes are recommended to eat frequently (e.g., 4 to 6 meals per day) and ingest high-calorie carbohydrate foods and/or concentrated carbohydrate drinks. Preferably, the majority of dietary carbohydrate should come from complex carbohydrates with a low to moderate glycemic index (e.g., grains, starches, fruit, maltodextrins, etc.).

There has been considerable debate regarding protein needs of athletes.[16,27,28] Initially, it was recommended that athletes do not need to ingest more than the RDA for protein (i.e., 0.8 to 1.0 g/kg/day for children, adolescents, and adults). However, research over the last decade has indicated that athletes engaged in intense training need to ingest about 1.5–2 times the RDA of protein in their diet (1.5 to 2.0 g/kg/day) to maintain protein balance.[16,27,29,30] If an insufficient amount of protein is obtained from the diet, an athlete will maintain a negative nitrogen balance which can increase protein catabolism and slow recovery. Over time, this may lead to lean muscle wasting and training intolerance.[7,16,29]

Although most athletes ingest this amount of protein in their normal diet, there are some athletes who are susceptible to protein malnutrition (e.g., runners, cyclists, swimmers, triathletes, gymnasts, dancers, skaters, wrestlers, boxers, etc.). Therefore, care should be taken to ensure that these types of athletes consume a sufficient amount of quality protein in their diet to maintain nitrogen balance

supplements during training may be more effective than simply adding carbohydrate to the diet.[37–39]

Glucose/Electrolyte Drinks

It is well known that ingesting GES drinks during prolonged exercise may help spare muscle glycogen and prevent dehydration. However, the use of GES drinks during endurance exercise has also been shown to blunt increases in FFAs and attenuate increases in the ratio of free tryptophan to BCAAs, enhancing endurance capacity.[40] These findings suggest that the use of GES drinks during endurance exercise may be an effective nutritional strategy to delay the onset of fatigue via both peripheral and central mechanisms. Additionally, there is some recent evidence that suggests ingesting GES drinks during exercise may lessen the effects that intense exercise has on the immune system.[41] Theoretically, use of GES drinks during training may help an athlete maintain glycogen and hydration levels, delay peripheral and central fatigue, and/or stay healthier. However, although there is a significant body of evidence to support use of GES drinks during prolonged intermittent and endurance exercise, there is little evidence that use of GES drinks during training will help athletes tolerate training to a greater degree and/or lessen the severity of symptoms of overtraining. Nevertheless, we believe that if an athlete is training more than 1 hour per day, frequent use of GES drinks or gels should be encouraged, particularly when training in hot and humid environments.

Amino Acids

Several amino acids have been theorized to help decrease the incidence of overtraining.[16,32] As stated earlier, BCAA supplementation before and/or during exercise has been suggested to be an effective nutritional strategy to delay the onset of central fatigue. Although there is strong theoretical rationale to support the potential use of BCAAs as an ergogenic aid, research investigating the effects of BCAA supplementation on physiological and psychological responses to exercise and exercise performance is mixed. Several studies indicate that BCAA supplementation before or during exercise increases BCAA levels, minimizes increases in the free tryptophan to BCAA ratio, and may affect physiological and psychological responses to exercise.[11–13,16,42–49] However, other studies have found limited effects[40,41,50,51] and few studies have found that BCAA supplementation actually improves exercise performance capacity.[43,48] Studies that have reported improved physiological and/or psychological responses to exercise typically involve ingesting 4 to 21 g/day BCAA during training and/or 2 to 4 g/hr of BCAA with a 6–8% GES drink before and during prolonged exercise. Additionally, there are several studies that indicate that ingesting carbohydrate with BCAA and/or protein before and/or

following exercise during training helps promote greater training adaptations.[37–39] In our view, the greatest potential application of BCAA supplementation is to help athletes tolerate training to a greater degree rather than a performance enhancement supplement. However, more research is needed to determine the role of BCAA on exercise capacity and markers of overtraining before definitive conclusions can be drawn.

The second amino acid that may help lessen the incidence of overtraining is glutamine.[52] As stated earlier, glutamine serves as the primary fuel for the lymphocyte. Some have suggested that glutamine supplementation may help athletes maintain immune function because exercise has been reported to decrease glutamine availability and immune function.[20,21,32,52] Additionally, glutamine has been reported to regulate cellular hydration status, which has been shown to be an important regulator of protein synthesis.[53–55] Consequently, glutamine supplementation (e.g., 6 to 12 g/day) has become popular among athletes attempting to increase muscle mass and/or maintain a healthy immune system during training.[27] Although there is a strong scientific basis to support a theoretical use of glutamine in athletes, studies on athletes are mixed or lacking. Several studies indicate that BCAA and glutamine supplementation can preserve and/or increase glutamine levels during exercise. Theoretically, a maintenance and/or increase in glutamine levels should help lessen the negative impact of intense exercise on immune function. Studies investigating this hypothesis, however, have not consistently observed improved immune status.[54,56] We are also not aware of any study that has evaluated the effects of glutamine alone on strength and muscle mass alterations during training. Consequently, additional research is necessary to determine whether glutamine supplementation may affect immune function and training adaptations before conclusions can be drawn.

Another compound that may play a role in lessening the incidence of overtraining is creatine. Classified as a methylglycocynamine, creatine supplementation has been shown to increase intramuscular creatine and phosphocreatine stores and improve performance capacity during intermittent high-intensity exercise.[39,40,57] Additionally, creatine supplementation has been reported to allow athletes to maintain greater training volume and promote greater gains in strength and muscle mass.[39,40,57] These findings suggest that creatine supplementation may allow an athlete to tolerate a greater training volume while maintaining positive training adaptations. Although it is unclear whether creatine supplementation may have a direct role in preventing overtraining, creatine supplementation during intensified periods of training may help an athlete tolerate training to a greater degree and thereby lessen the susceptibility to overtraining. More research is needed to investigate this hypothesis.

Can amino acid supplementation help prevent overtraining? Although more research is needed to determine the potential ergogenic value of BCAA, creatine, and glutamine supplementation, it is our view that athletes involved in intense training should ingest a diet high in BCAAs, creatine, and glutamine. This can be accomplished either by selecting high-quality protein sources in the diet (e.g., caseine, whey protein, etc.) and/or by ingesting carbohydrate/protein supplements that contain quality protein, BCAAs, and glutamine.[29,30] It is also our view that given the evidence regarding the ergogenic value and medical safety, creatine supplementation can serve as an effective ergogenic aid for athletes involved in high-intensity training. Whether creatine has a role in lessening the impact of overtraining remains to be determined.

Nutrients that Support the Immune System

In addition to glutamine, there has been interest in determining the role that other nutrients may have on immune function. From these studies, there appear to be several nutrients and/or herbs that may help athletes maintain a healthier immune system during training. The first nutrient reported to enhance immune function is protein.[29,30,32] Studies indicate that immunosuppressed patients are often protein malnourished. Additionally, athletes who maintain a negative energy balance during training may also be susceptible to become protein malnourished.[7] Protein supplementation in protein-malnourished patients has been shown to improve immune status.[32] Consequently, it is important that athletes eat enough quality protein in their diet to maintain a healthy immune system.

The second nutrient that may affect immune responses during training is vitamin C. Vitamin C is involved in the synthesis of epinephrine, iron absorption, and is an antioxidant.[23] There is also evidence that vitamin C may enhance immune function.[58] With regards to athletes, vitamin C supplementation (600 mg/day for 3 weeks) following an ultramarathon race was found to decrease the incidence of URTI by 33% following the event in comparison to athletes given a placebo.[59] These findings have led some to contend that athletes engaged in intensified periods of training should supplement their diet with vitamin C to help decrease the incidence of URTI.

More recently, zinc supplementation (25 to 100 mg/day) during the onset of symptoms of a cold or URTI has been reported to decrease the severity and length of the cold/infection.[60] Athletes have been reported to be commonly zinc deficient. Theoretically, zinc supplementation during intensified periods of training and/or as athletes experience symptoms of a cold may help athletes stay healthier. To support this theory, one study reported that zinc supplementation (25 mg/day) during training minimized exercise-induced changes in immune function.[61] However, more research is needed to test this hypothesis.

The last supplement that may be beneficial for athletes to enhance immune function is echinacea. Echinacea is a popular herb that has been reported to enhance the immune system in a similar manner as an antibiotic. Evidence suggests that echinacea can reduce the incidence, severity, and duration of colds and infections.[62] Theoretically, echinacea supplementation during periods of intensified training and/or as an athlete experiences symptoms of a URTI may help athletes stay healthy during training. However, although there is scientific support for use of echinacea, we are not aware of a study that has evaluated whether echinacea supplementation during training affects the incidence of URTI in athletes.

SUMMARY

Overtraining represents a maladaptation to training stress that results in a long-term decrement in performance. Overtraining is often manifested in athletes with various physiological and/or psychological signs and symptoms. The most prevailing theory is that overtraining is a result of a chronic suppression in hypothalamic function that chronically alters hormonal responses to stress. Although the etiology of overtraining is not well understood, research has indicated that there are several nutritional factors that may play a role in overtraining. The most important nutritional factors appear to be that athletes need to eat enough calories to offset energy expenditure and that their diet provides sufficient amounts of carbohydrate and protein. Moreover, a number of nutritional strategies have been proposed to help delay peripheral and/or central fatigue as well as help athletes tolerate training. Analysis of the literature indicates that under the conditions described, some of these nutritional strategies may help athletes tolerate training and/or maintain a healthy immune system. Theoretically, these strategies may help lessen the incidence of overtraining. However, more research is needed to understand the role of nutrition in potentially preventing overtraining before definitive conclusions can be drawn.

AUTHORS' RECOMMENDATIONS

- Athletes engaged in intense training should ensure that they eat enough calories to offset energy expenditure. For most athletes training 2 to 3 hrs/day, this typically ranges between 60 and 80 kcal/kg/day.

- Since the caloric needs of athletes are often high, athletes should eat 4 to 6 meals per day and ingest carbohydrate/protein snacks between meals to offset energy expenditure.

- For athletes involved in intense training, the diet should consist primarily of carbohydrate (8 to 10 g/kg/day), enough high-quality protein to maintain a positive nitrogen balance (1.5 to 2 g/kg/day), and low to moderate fat intake.

- Ingesting a light carbohydrate/protein snack or supplement (e.g., 50 g of carbohydrate and 5 to 10 g of protein) 30 to 60 minutes before exercise can help reduce catabolism during exercise.

- Athletes should ingest a carbohydrate/protein snack or supplement (e.g., 1.5 g/kg of carbohydrate with 0.5 g/kg of protein) within 30 minutes following exercise and eat a high-carbohydrate meal within 2 hours after exercise to promote glycogen resynthesis and recovery.

- Use of vitamin- and mineral-fortified supplements containing carbohydrate and quality protein can serve as an effective and convenient means of increasing caloric intake as well as increasing the availability of various nutrients (e.g., BCAAs, glutamine, creatine, etc.).

- Ingesting GES drinks during exercise may help delay peripheral and/or central fatigue.

- Ingesting BCAAs with a GES before and during exercise may improve physiological and/or psychological responses to exercise but there appears to be limited ergogenic value.

- Glutamine, protein, vitamin C, zinc, and echinacea have been reported to enhance immune status under certain conditions. Theoretically, supplementation of these nutrients during intense training and/or upon the onset of symptoms of URTI may help maintain a healthy immune system.

- Athletes and coaches should monitor signs and symptoms of overtraining so that training programs can be altered and/or dietary strategies used to prevent overtraining.

REFERENCES

1. Kreider RB, Fry AC, O'Toole ML. Overtraining in Sport. Champaign: Human Kinetics, 1998.
2. Foster C. Monitoring training in athletes with reference to overtraining syndrome. Med Sci Sports Exerc 1998;30(7):1164–1168.
3. Lehmann M, Foster C, Gastmann U, et al. Physiological responses to short- and long-term overtraining in endurance athletes. In: Kreider RB, Fry AC, O'Toole ML, eds. Overtraining in Sport. Champaign: Human Kinetics, 1998:29–46.
4. Keizer H. Neuroendocrine considerations. In: Kreider RB, Fry AC, O'Toole ML, eds. Overtraining in Sport. Champaign: Human Kinetics, 1998:145–168.
5. McKenzie DC. Markers of excessive exercise. Can J Appl Physiol 1999;24(1):66–73.
6. Rowbottom DG, Keast D, Morton AR. Monitoring and prevention of overreaching and overtraining in endurance athletes. In: Kreider RB, Fry AC, O'Toole ML, eds. Overtraining in Sport. Champaign: Human Kinetics, 1998:47–68.
7. Berning JR. Energy intake, diet, and muscle wasting. In: Kreider RB, Fry AC, O'Toole ML, eds. Overtraining in Sport. Champaign: Human Kinetics, 1998:275–288.
8. Snyder AC. Overtraining and glycogen depletion hypothesis. Med Sci Sports Exerc 1998;30(7):1146–1150.
9. Sherman WM, Jacobs, KA, Leenders N. Carbohydrate metabolism during endurance exercise. In: Kreider RB, Fry AC, O'Toole ML, eds. Overtraining in Sport. Champaign: Human Kinetics, 1988:289–308.
10. Newsholme EA, Parry-Billings M, McAndrew M, et al. Biochemical mechanism to explain some characteristics of overtraining. In: Brouns F, ed. Medical Sports Science Advances in Nutrition and Top Sport. Basel, Switzerland: Karger, 1991:79–93.
11. Blomstrand E, Celsing F, Newshome EA. Changes in plasma concentrations of aromatic and branch-chain amino acids during sustained exercise in man and their possible role in fatigue. Acta Physiol Scand 1988;133:115–121.
12. Blomstrand E, Hassmen P, Ekblom B, et al. Administration of branch-chain amino acids during sustained exercise: effects on performance and on plasma concentration of some amino acids. Eur J Appl Physiol 1991;63:83–88.
13. Blomstrand E, Hassmen P, Newsholme E. Effect of branch-chain amino acid supplementation on mental performance. Acta Physiol Scand 1991;143:225–226.
14. Davis JM. Carbohydrates, branched-chain amino acids, and endurance: the central fatigue hypothesis. Int J Sports Nutr 1991;5(suppl);29–38.
15. Gastmann UA, Lehmann MJ. Overtraining and the BCAA hypothesis. Med Sci Sports Exerc 1998;30:1173–1178.
16. Kreider RB. Central fatigue hypothesis and overtraining. In: Kreider RB, Fry AC, O'Toole M, eds. Overtraining in Sport. Champaign: Human Kinetics, 1998:309–331.
17. Segura R, Ventura J. Effect of L-tryptophan supplementation on exercise performance. Int J Sports Med 1988;9:301–305.
18. Nieman DC, Pedersen BK. Exercise and immune function, recent developments. Sports Med 1999;27:72–80.
19. Nieman DC. Effects of athletic endurance training on infection rates and immunity. In: Kreider RB, Fry AC, O'Toole ML, eds. Overtraining in Sport. Champaign: Human Kinetics, 1998:193–218.
20. Newsholme EA, Calder PC. The proposed role of glutamine in some cells of the immune system and speculative consequences for the whole animal. Nutrition 1997;13:728–730.
21. Parry-Billings M, Budgett R, Koutedakis K, et al. Plasma amino acid concentrations in the overtraining syndrome: possible effects on the immune system. Med Sci Sports Exerc 1992;24:1353–1358.
22. Kargotich S, Rowbottom DG, Keast D, et al. Plasma glutamine changes after high intensity exercise in elite male swimmers. [abstract]. Med Sci Sports Exerc 1996;28(Suppl 133).

23. Leutholtz B, Kreider RB. Optimizing nutrition for exercise and sport. In: Temple N, Wilson T, eds. Frontiers in Nutrition. Totowa, NJ: Humana Press. In press.

24. American College of Sports Medicine. Encyclopedia of Sports Sciences and Medicine. New York: Macmillan, 1999:1128–1129.

25. Food and Nutrition Board. National Research Council: Recommended Dietary Allowances, Revised. Washington, DC: National Academy of Sciences, 1989.

26. Kreider RB. Physiological considerations of ultraendurance performance. Int J Sports Nutr 1991;1:3–27.

27. Kreider RB. Dietary supplements and the promotion of muscle growth. Sports Med 1999;27:97–110.

28. Williams MH. Facts and fallacies of purported ergogenic amino acid supplements. Clin Sports Med 1999;18:633–649.

29. Di Pasquale MG. Proteins and amino acids in exercise and sport. In: Driskell JA, Wolinsky I, eds. Energy-Yielding Macronutrients and Energy Metabolism in Sports Nutrition. Boca Raton, FL: CRC Press, 1999:119–162.

30. Bucci LR, Unlu LM. Proteins and amino acid supplements in exercise and sport. In: Driskell JA, Wolinsky I, eds. Energy-Yielding Macronutrients and Energy Metabolism in Sports Nutrition. Boca Raton, FL: CRC Press, 1999:191–212.

31. Miller WC, Koceja DM, Hamilton EJ. A meta-analysis of the past 25 years of weight loss research using diet, exercise or diet plus exercise intervention. Int J Obes Relat Metab Disord 1997;21:941–947.

32. Kreider RB, Miriel V, Bertun E. Amino acid supplementation and exercise performance: proposed ergogenic value. Sports Med 1993; 16:190–209.

33. Carli G, Bonifazi M, Lodi L, et al. Changes in exercise-induced hormone response to branched chain amino acid administration. Eur J Appl Physiol 1992;64:272–277.

34. Zawadzki KM, Yaspelkis BB, Ivy JL. Carbohydrate-protein complex increases the rate of muscle glycogen storage after exercise. J Appl Physiol 1992;72:1854–1859.

35. Kraemer WJ, Volek JS, Bush JA, et al. Hormonal responses to consecutive days of heavy-resistance exercise with or without nutritional supplementation. J Appl Physiol 1998;85:1544–1555.

36. Brouns F, Saris WH, Beckers E, et al. Metabolic changes induced by sustained exhaustive cycling and diet manipulation. Int J Sports Med 1989;10(suppl l);49–62 .

37. Cade JR, Reese RH, Privette RM, et al. Dietary intervention and training in swimmers. Eur J Appl Physiol Occup Physiol 1991;63: 210–215.

38. Kreider RB, Klesges R, Harmon K, et al. Effects of ingesting supplements designed to promote lean tissue accretion on body composition during resistance training. Int J Sports Nutr 1996;6: 234–246.

39. Kreider RB, Klesges RC, Lotz D, et al. Effects of nutritional supplementation during off-season college football training on body composition and strength. J Exerc Physiol Online 1999;2(2):24–39. Available: http://www.css.edu/users/tboone2/asep/aprilr.htm

40. Davis JM, Baily SP, Woods JA, et al. Effects of carbohydrate feedings on plasma free tryptophan and branched-chain amino acids during prolonged cycling. Eur J Appl Physiol 1992;65:513–519.

41. Henson DA, Nieman DC, Blodgett AD, et al. Influence of exercise mode and carbohydrate on the immune response to prolonged exercise. Int J Sports Nutr 1999;9(2):213–228.

42. Kreider RB, Miller GW, Mitchell M, et al. Effects of amino acid supplementation on ultraendurance triathlon performance. In: Proceedings of the World Congress on Sport Nutrition. Barcelona, Spain: Enero, 1992:488–536.

43. Hefler SK, Wildman L, Gaesser GA, et al. Branched-chain amino acid (BCAA) supplementation improves endurance performance in competitive cyclists. Med Sci Sports Exerc 1993;25:24.

44. Kreider RB, Jackson CW. Effects of amino acid supplementation on psychological status during and intercollegiate swim season [abstract]. Med Sci Sports Exerc 1994;26:115.

45. Hassmen P, Blomstrand E, Ekblom B, Newsholme EA. Branched-chain amino acid supplementation during 30-km competitive run: mood and cognitive performance. Nutrition 1994;10(5):405–410.

46. Coombes J, McNaughton L. The effects of branched chain amino acid supplementation on indicators of muscle damage after prolonged strenuous exercise [abstract]. Med Sci Sports Exerc 1995;27:149.

47. Mourier A, Bigard AX, de Kerviler E, et al. Combined effects of caloric restriction and branched-chain amino acid supplementation on body composition and exercise performance in elite wrestlers. Int J Sports Med 1997;18(1):47–55.

48. Mittleman KD, Ricci MR, Bailey SP. Branched-chain amino acids prolong exercise during heat stress in men and women. Med Sci Sports Exerc 1998;30(1):83–91.

49. Calders P, Matthys D, Derave W, Pannier JL. Effect of branched-chain amino acids (BCAA), glucose, and glucose plus BCAA on endurance performance in rats. Med Sci Sports Exerc 1999;31(4):583–587.

50. Struder HK, Hollmann W, Platen P, et al. Influence of paroxetine, branched-chain amino acids and tyrosine on neuroendocrine system responses and fatigue in humans. Horm Metab Res 1998;30(4): 188–194.

51. Davis JM, Welsh RS, De Volve KL, Alderson NA. Effects of branched-chain amino acids and carbohydrate on fatigue during intermittent, high-intensity running. Int J Sports Med 1999;20(5):309–314.

52. Antonio J, Street C. Glutamine: a potentially useful supplement for athletes. Can J Appl Physiol 1999;24:1–14.

53. Low SY, Taylor PM, Rennie MJ. Responses of glutamine transport in cultured rat skeletal muscle to osmotically induced changes in cell volume. J Physiol (London) 1996;492(pt 3):877–885.

54. Varnier M, Leese GP, Thompson, Rennie MJ. Stimulatory effect of glutamine on glycogen accumulation in human skeletal muscle. Am J Physiol 1995;269(2 pt 1):E309–315.

55. Rennie MJ. Glutamine metabolism and transport in skeletal muscle and heart and their clinical relevance. J Nutr 1996;126(4) (Suppl):1142–1149.

56. Rohde T, Asp S, MacLean DA, et al. Competitive sustained exercise in humans, lymphokine activated killer cell activity, and glutamine: an intervention study. Eur J Appl Physiol 1998;78:448–453.

57. Williams MH, Kreider RB, Branch D. Creatine: The Power Supplement. Champaign, IL: Human Kinetics, 1999:252.

58. Hemila, H. Vitamin C and common cold incidence: a review of studies with subjects under heavy physical stress. Int J Sports Med 1996;17:379–383.

59. Peters EM, Goetzsche JM, Grobbelaar B, Noakes TD. Vitamin C supplementation reduces the incidence of postrace symptoms of upper-respiratory-tract infection in ultramarathon runners. Am J Clin Nutr 1993;57:170–174.

60. Prasad AS. Zinc and immunity. Mol Cell Biochem 1998;188(1–2): 63–69.

61. Singh A, Failla ML, Deuster PA. Exercise-induced changes in immune function: effects of zinc supplementation. J Appl Physiol 1994;76:2298–2303.

62. Brinkeborn RM, Shah DV, Degenring FH. Echinaforce and other echinacea fresh plant preparations in the treatment of the common cold: a randomized, placebo controlled, double-blind clinical trial. Phytomedicine 1999;6:1–6.

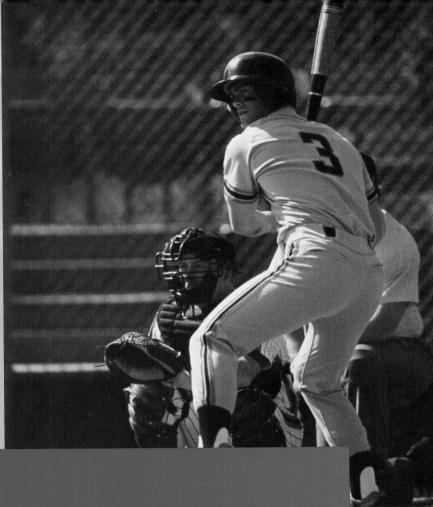

Hydration and Regulation of Cell Size

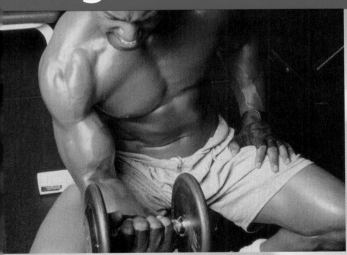

PART I
Hydration

*Jun Ma and
Nancy M. Betts*

Part II
Regulation of Cell Size via
Hydration Status

Thomas Incledon

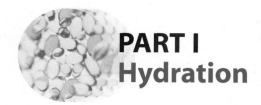

PART I
Hydration

Research Review
Fluid Replacement

The American College of Sports Medicine summarized the current state of the research in their 1996 position stand on exercise and fluid replacement. Typically, humans do not voluntarily consume sufficient water to maintain optimal fluid balance. Superimposing exercise on less than adequate fluid balance, especially in warm environmental conditions, leads to dehydration and performance reductions. Prolonged exercise with profuse sweating and limited fluid replacement can lead to cardiovascular strain and life-threatening heat injury. Following exercise bouts, replacement of fluid losses before the next exercise session is critical to prevent thermal injury and to maximize performance.

Although sweat losses include electrolytes, the concentration of osmotically active ions in sweat is lower than that of the fluid compartments of the body. As the volume of fluid in the blood declines (hypovolemia) and the electrolyte concentration of body fluids rises (hypertonicity), the movement of fluid to the skin for dry heat exchange and evaporative heat exchange (sweating) is impaired. The heat produced by exercising muscle cannot be effectively dissipated when the amount of sweat declines and the body temperature for initiating sweating increases. The resulting increase in body core temperature can lead to serious heat injuries. Dehydration combined with hypovolemia and hyperthermia results in cardiovascular strain and muscle fatigue.

To prevent thermal injury, cardiovascular strain, and performance decrements, water needs to be replaced before, during, and after exercise. This is especially true for endurance exercise in hot climates. While the recommended rate of fluid replacement is the amount that equals sweat losses, this can be difficult to achieve without an individually based, sport-tailored strategy because of limitations in thirst sensations, real or imagined gastrointestinal discomfort, or restrictive rules of the sport. Fluid replacement strategies should focus on the palatability of the drink, timing of ingestion, electrolyte concentration, and carbohydrate composition. In general, fluids that are noncarbonated, cool (15–20°C), and flavored increase palatability. Fluid absorption is enhanced by a high fluid volume in the stomach, which can be achieved with a glucose or sucrose concentration of 4–8%. Usually, a nutritionally balanced diet provides sufficient electrolyte and carbohydrate replacement but when time between exercise bouts is limited, fluids containing sodium and carbohydrate are recommended. Drinking should start early and be repeated every 15–20 minutes throughout exercise. Complete fluid and electrolyte replacement normally occurs within 24 hours after exercise when a balanced, adequate diet is consumed.

In conclusion, for best exercise performance, normal hydration should be maintained before exercise and regained after exercise, and dehydration should be avoided or minimized during exercise. This can be achieved by establishing and implementing individually based and sport-specific fluid replacement strategies following the American College of Sports Medicine guidelines.

American College of Sports Medicine. Position stand on exercise and fluid replacement. Med Sci Sports Exerc 1996;28:i–vii.

Introduction

Water is not typically thought of as a nutritional supplement. This is true even though exercise, especially in hot weather, forces water to become a nutrient requiring supplementation. Surprisingly, the vital role of water relative to physical performance has often been overlooked in the athletic community. It has only been since the 1970s that fluid requirements of athletes began to attract scientific interest. Now, it is becoming clearer that water is the most essential nutrient for maintaining exercise performance. Water accounts for 50–70% of human body weight, with body water existing in a balance between intra- and extracellular compartments. Nearly all the chemical reactions that occur in the body directly involve water or components dissolved within water and these reactions are disrupted by changes in water balance. Small shifts in water concentration from inside the cells to the extracellular spaces can dramatically affect physical performance. This chapter highlights the regulation of water in the body, and water balance in relation to exercise. Of particular importance are the adverse effects of dehydration on physical performance, and optimal fluid replacement before, during, and after exercise. The chapter will cover the basic concepts behind body fluid balance, exercise and body fluid changes, the effects of dehydration and rehydration on physical performance (especially endurance performance), and the prevention of performance reduction through heat acclimation.

Physiological Importance of Body Fluids

Water is an essential nutrient required for life. It is found in varying degrees within every cell and between cells, not only for filling space, but also for maintaining the cell structure. Water is vital for the formation of the macronutrients: carbohydrates, proteins, and lipids. Digestion, absorption, transportation, utilization, and elimination of all the substances we ingest or produce depends on their ability to dissolve in water.[1]

Water serves as a solvent, creating the environment needed for cellular reactions to occur. Perhaps the most important reactions are those involving the electrolytes and ions, which depend on water balance between the cells and in the extracellular compartments. Shifts in electrolyte concentrations inside and outside the cell create the electrical potentials across the cell membrane, which initiate nerve impulses and muscle contractions. During exercise, the movement of skeletal muscle relies upon swift and precise communications with nerves and this communication is dependent on the flow of electric current within each cell.[2] Excitability of cardiac muscle depends on the ionic gradients that exist across the cell membrane.

Blood serves to transport dissolved substances throughout the body. During exercise, the increased need for oxygen by working muscles requires an increased cardiac output to speed blood transport.[3] Hydrostatic pressure is the primary force that propels blood through the arteries, thus controlling cardiac output. Adequate blood volume is one requirement for maintaining hydrostatic pressure and adequate body water is needed to maintain blood volume; thus, the amount of body water has a direct effect on hydrostatic pressure.

Water serves as the principal mechanism for heat removal during body temperature elevations. Of the energy expended during exercise, about 75–80% is converted to heat.[4] This heat can raise the body temperature dramatically and cause serious heat injury. However, the high specific heat of water and water's high heat of vaporization allows substantial heat removal via dry heat exchange and evaporation of sweat. These form the basis

for thermoregulation.[3,5,6] Finally, water functions as a shock absorber and lubricator of various body compartments and joints.

Regulation of Body Fluid Balance

Water is contained in nearly everything we ingest, from fluids to foods with only vegetable and fish oils containing negligible amounts of water. Food contains water in varying amounts ranging from 90% in some fruits and vegetables to 30% or less in such foods as bread and crackers.[7] The ingestion of liquids and foods accounts for most of our daily water input, which averages about 2 liters per day for a nonexercising, sedentary individual. An often-overlooked source of water is that resulting from metabolic oxidation of macronutrients from food and from released liver glycogen and muscle glycogen. Water produced in the metabolism of the three energy-providing nutrients approximates 0.6 g per gram of carbohydrate, 1.07 g per gram of fat, and 0.41 g per gram of protein.[7] This contributes about 250 mL or 1 cup of fluid per day.[1] In addition, over 2 grams of water are bound to each gram of glycogen, and this water is released when glycogen is used as an energy source. Greenleaf[8] reported that oxidation of 500 grams of muscle glycogen could provide 1500 mL of water.

At rest, the kidneys represent the primary avenue of water output. Typically, urine is produced at a rate of 1 mL/min, which can obviously change with alterations in fluid ingestion and/or behavior patterns (exercise, for example). On a daily basis, about 750 mL of water is lost through the skin by insensible perspiration, which accounts for both fluid diffusion through the epidermis and perspiration through sweat glands. Sweat gland activity can become a main avenue of water loss during exercise and will be discussed later. Water excreted in the feces and exhaled through respiration accounts for minor losses.

As can be seen in TABLE 1, daily water input and output are well balanced so that body water can be maintained at a normal level (euhydration). Water balance in the body is accomplished by normal kidney function, which is regulated by several hormones. The kidneys are the most important organs for long-term water and electrolyte balance. First of all, the kidneys adjust the volume of blood filtered through each nephron, the smallest functional unit of the kidney.[9,10] With hyperhydration, filtration rates are increased and excess water is subsequently eliminated, whereas filtration rates decline during hypohydration so as to conserve water. Kidney function in water balance is controlled by several hormones, but primarily by antidiuretic hormone (ADH), also known as vasopressin. ADH is produced and released from the posterior pituitary gland of the brain in response to a decline in blood pressure and an increase in blood solute concentration (osmolarity). Blood pressure depends largely on blood fluid volume, while osmolarity is mainly determined by the concentration of substances, including ions and proteins,

Table 10-1 Average daily water input and output in a nonexercising man

Water input (mL)	Water output (mL)
Fluids—1500	Kidneys—1500
Water in Food—1000	Skin—750
Metabolic Water—250	Lungs—300
	Feces—200
Total input—2750	**Total output—2750**

in the blood per unit of total volume.[3,7,10] The action of ADH is to enhance the reabsorption of water as it is passing through the collecting tubule of the nephron, which results in conserving body water by reducing the water available in (concentrating) the urine.

Aldosterone, a hormone, which directs the kidney to maintain electrolyte (especially sodium) balance, also acts indirectly to influence water balance.[11] A group of specialized cells in the kidney can detect a decrease in urinary sodium, and this stimulates the secretion of renin by the kidneys followed by a chain of reactions occurring in the blood known as the renin-angiotensin system.[11,12] Aldosterone is produced in the cortex of the adrenal gland in response to increased renin activity. Via the action of aldosterone, the retention of sodium occurs in the distal tubule of the nephron. Worth mentioning, as sodium goes, so does water. Therefore, an indirect benefit of the action of aldosterone is that a significant amount of water is reabsorbed in the same process but independently of ADH.

The mechanisms that stimulate and terminate voluntary fluid intake in humans remain unclear. Changes in plasma volume and osmolarity have been proposed to act alone or together to enhance the sensation of thirst and induce drinking.[13] In stress-free conditions, osmotic stimuli may be more important for driving fluid intake than are volume-based stimuli, which continually change with movement. Regardless of the mechanisms, the sensation of thirst appears to be a poor indicator of water needs in humans, given that the thirst threshold occurs at a dehydration level ranging from 0.5–1.2% body weight loss.[14,15] Most experimental land mammals will immediately correct their fluid deficits if water is readily available, whereas humans take much longer.[16] As a result, involuntary dehydration can easily occur in humans and will be aggravated by exercise.[17]

Body Fluid Compartments

Body fluid is usually thought of as existing in separate compartments.[18] The largest proportion of water, approximately 53%, is found inside cells or within the intracellular compartment. The water located outside the cells is termed *extracellular* and accounts for about 32% of total fluid volume. Extracellular fluids are further compartmentalized

into interstitial (fluid located between tissues) and intravascular (the fluid or plasma portion of the blood) spaces. The interstitial fluid volume accounts for approximately 75% of the extracellular fluid volume with the intravascular fluid volume accounting for 25%. The remaining 15% of the total fluid volume is considered insignificant in terms of exercise and fluid balance, as it exists in the transcellular compartment which includes bone joints, eyes, cerebrospinal areas, the gastrointestinal tract, and the connective tissue. The distribution of total body water is much the same in both men and women. Intracellular fluid volume varies depending on the function of the cell.

Due to the semipermeable property of the cell membrane, water molecules can easily pass from one compartment to another. The direction of water movement is mainly determined by hydrostatic and osmotic pressure gradients.[19] The hydrostatic pressure is a function of blood volume, cardiac output, and peripheral resistance, which can all be affected by exercise. The concentrations of solutes, i.e., dissolved electrolytes and protein molecules, exert osmotic pressures in each fluid compartment.

The ionic solutes, or electrolytes, that make up the intra- and extracellular fluids are distinctly different, with sodium (Na^+, 142 meq/L) and chloride (Cl^-, 103 meq/L) being the major extracellular electrolytes, and potassium (K^+, 160 meq/L) and magnesium (Mg^{++}, 35 meq/L) being the major intracellular electrolytes.[11] The marked differences in sodium and potassium concentrations between the extracellular and intracellular compartments are maintained by the ATPase Na-K pump and are crucial for activities such as nerve impulse transmission and muscular contraction. In spite of greatly different individual solute concentrations, the total equilibrium concentration of cations and anions is approximately the same in each compartment. Large protein molecules manufactured by cells for intracellular or extracellular use serve as an additional solute and also exert an oncotic pressure by attracting water.

Hydrostatic and osmotic pressures are regulated closely by the body through hormonal and renal responses in an effort to maintain fluid and electrolyte equilibrium among all the fluid compartments. This equilibrium, however, can be markedly affected by exercise.

Exercise-Induced Changes in Body Fluids

Of all the exercise-induced body fluid changes during exercise, decreases in vascular blood volume during rhythmic or endurance exercise are of greatest concern. Types of exercises that make use of large muscle groups for a period of time (e.g., running, cycling, walking, swimming) have been the most well researched, with varying results.[18–27] During some types of endurance exercise, it appears that the vascular blood volume undergoes a reduction that can be almost completely attributed to a decrease in plasma volume. This is particularly true for cycling done on a cycle ergometer. [21,22] However, results are inconsistent for treadmill running and walking, in which some investigators showed a plasma volume reduction, [23,24] others an increase, [25] and others reported no changes. [26] McMurray [27] conducted an investigation to evaluate the plasma volume response during distance swimming and found similar plasma volume reductions to those observed during cycling at the same intensity.

Plasma volume is maintained by a combination of opposing forces. These forces are termed *Starling forces* [28] and consist of hydrostatic pressure, osmotic pressure in the interstitial space and their opposing pressures, osmotic pressure in the capillaries, and the tissue pressure surrounding the capillaries. Water exchange between the intravascular and interstitial spaces occurs via the capillaries. Hydrostatic and osmotic pressures in the interstitial space forces water to move from the vascular space to the interstitial space at the arterial end of the capillary. Capillary osmotic pressure and pressure from the tissues surrounding the capillaries force water to return to the vascular space at the venous end of the capillary. Compared with the arterial end of the capillary, the venous end has greater surface area and permeability, which allows for greater return of fluids to the vascular space—an action favoring plasma volume conservation.

During exercise, especially aerobic exercise, blood pressure is elevated to supply adequate blood flow to working muscles. This causes an increase in hydrostatic pressure, which drives fluids out of the capillaries and into the interstitial spaces. Because solutes are released as a result of the energy metabolism of contracting muscle, osmotic pressure in the interstitial space rises. Also, capillary surface area is significantly increased to more efficiently nourish the active muscle mass. All of these actions create an environment more favorable to the reduction of vascular fluid from the plasma portion of the blood. This results in decreased blood volume.

However, there are limits to the amount of fluid that can be lost from vascular plasma. During exercise, the plasma solute concentration will increase for several reasons. First, sodium and potassium are released into the plasma from the skeletal muscle as byproducts of increased metabolic activity during exercise. [29] In addition, glucose and lipids released into plasma from glycogen and fat-tissue breakdown add to the solute load. [9] Water lost in sweat creates a shift in the osmotic pressure gradient favoring the movement of fluids from the plasma to the interstitial spaces. But, as fluid moves from the plasma, plasma osmolarity increases and in doing so, the osmotic pressure shifts back toward moving fluids into the plasma.

Protein oncotic pressure may also play a role in stabilizing blood volume during exercise. [26,30] It is speculated that during exercise, proteins move at a faster rate out of the interstitial space into the blood via the lymphatic system than they can move into interstitial via pinocytosis.

The presence of proteins in the intravascular space exerts a higher oncotic pressure, resulting in the movement of water into the blood. Lastly, the skeletal muscle cells surrounding the capillaries impose tissue pressure and structural limits upon the movement of fluids out of the plasma. Greenleaf et al. [31] found that the upper limit of plasma volume loss due to exercise was approximately 20% of the resting plasma volume.

The magnitude of plasma volume loss appears related to the body position before exercise and the time spent in this position, as well as the mode of exercise (e.g., cycle versus running), intensity of exercise (% VO_{2max}) and hydration status. In short-term exercise, plasma volume decreases result in hemoconcentration, which enhances oxygen-carrying capacity per unit of blood. The Starling forces mentioned above, along with the vascular volume and the concentration of osmotically active particles in plasma return to normal within minutes after the cessation of short-term exercise. Plasma volume deficits, however, may continue if the exercise has been lengthy and/or in the heat, combined with moderate-to-severe sweating and dehydration.

Body Fluid Balance

Body fluid balance becomes a primary concern for the exercising subject when an endurance exercise in any form is carried on for long enough, especially in the heat. Respiratory water loss begins to make an impact because of the overall increase in ventilation and energy expenditure accompanying exercise. However, the greatest and potentially most serious body fluid loss during exercise relates to increased sweat production for thermoregulation.

As mentioned before, only 20% of the energy expended during exercise is used for actual mechanical work, while the rest is released in the form of heat. [4] This heat must be dissipated before the body's core temperature (i.e., the temperature of the cranium, thorax, abdomen, pelvis, and deeper muscle masses) is elevated to a dangerous level. Thermoregulation may be seriously impaired if the core temperature exceeds 106°F (41°C). Increased body temperature initiates vasodilation through sympathetic neural control, causing body heat to be transported from the body core to the shell. Under cool and breezy conditions, most of this heat can then be dissipated through convection and radiation, also called *dry heat exchange*. [32] However, this mechanism diminishes in efficiency as exercise intensity, environmental temperature, and/or humidity increase. When vasodilation is no longer a useful means to dissipate body heat, the secretion and evaporation of sweat becomes the foremost avenue of heat removal.

Sweat gland activity is stimulated when the temperature of the blood flowing through the anterior hypothalamus increases. The hypothalamus also receives impulses from temperature receptors in the skin. [33] For heat to dissipate, secreted sweat on the skin must be evaporated into the surrounding air. About 0.58 kcal are lost for each gram of water evaporated; thus, approximately 580 kcal of heat are removed through the evaporation of every liter of sweat.[34]

The sweat rate may be affected by many factors, including physical activity level, environmental conditions (ambient temperature, humidity, air velocity, and radiant load), individual aerobic fitness, heat acclimatization, and clothing (insulation and moisture permeability). Therefore, great inter- and intra-individual differences may exist in body water loss through sweat. Individuals wearing protective clothing commonly have sweating rates of 1 to 2 L/hr while performing light-intensity exercise.[35] Athletes performing high-intensity exercise in the heat can have sweating rates up to 2.5 L/hr.[36]

The immediate source of water for sweat is from the interstitial fluid, even though each sweat gland is served by capillaries. Because the fluid lost through sweat has a lower solute concentration (hypotonic) than interstitial fluid and plasma,[37] osmotically active particles must be left behind in the cutaneous interstitial space. The osmotic gradient from plasma to the cutaneous interstitial space increases, which results in the movement of fluid from the plasma into the interstitial space. This movement of fluid into the interstitial space increases the osmolarity in the plasma, which in turn shifts the osmotic pressure gradient toward movement of water from the intracellular compartment to the blood.

Research examining the relative contribution of the various body compartments to the fluid lost in sweat has accounted for 30–50% as coming from the intracellular compartment.[29,38] The amount varies depending on the hydration status of the subject. The interstitial fluid contributed 40–60% of the lost water, while plasma contributed approximately 10%. The extracellular fluid is the initial source of water loss from sweating when hydration status is normal; however, the contribution from the intracellular fluid increases as hydration levels decrease.

To compensate for this markedly increased water output through sweat, urine production tends to decrease.[3] Also, renal blood flow is reduced during exercise in response to sympathetic nervous system activity, which leads to a reduction in urine formation and to a conservation of fluid during exercise.[39] As a function of increased energy expenditure, water is produced through the metabolic oxidation of macronutrients and released from muscle glycogen.[26] Although in most cases these additions to total body water supply during exercise are not adequate for fluid replacement, their importance should not be totally ignored. Nevertheless, the maintenance of body fluid balance predominantly relies on fluid ingestion. Studies have shown that ad libitum drinking often only replaces 25–35% of the volume lost as sweat.[40,41]

Exercise, especially when accompanied by heat stress, exerts an intense strain on processes for maintaining normal plasma volume and total body fluid balance. Reductions in plasma volume from water lost in sweat are aggravated when fluid replacement is not adequate. Reduced plasma volume and increased plasma osmolarity due to inadequate hydration status have been well documented as producing adverse effects on thermoregulation, cardiovascular responses, and exercise performance.

The Effect of Dehydration on Physical Performance and Health

Greenleaf[42] defines body fluid levels in terms of euhydration, hypohydration, and hyperhydration. Euhydration refers to *normal* total body water, whereas hypohydration and hyperhydration refer to body fluid deficit and excess, respectively. The more common term *dehydration* refers to the dynamic process of body water loss—the transition from euhydration to hypohydration.

Dehydration has been further delineated as voluntary versus involuntary. Involuntary dehydration occurs during training or competition as a result of substantial sweat production and inadequate fluid replacement. It usually occurs during prolonged exercise, particularly in warm environmental conditions. Voluntary dehydration is commonly used by athletes (such as wrestlers and boxers) to reduce weight quickly to compete at a lower weight class. It is induced intentionally in a variety of ways, for example, exercise-induced sweating (exercising in insulated clothing), thermal-induced sweating using a sauna or steam room, diuretic- or laxative-induced water loss, and restricted intake of food and fluids.

Much of the research concerning dehydration and physical performance has focused on involuntary dehydration in relation to aerobic endurance performance, temperature regulation, and cardiovascular dynamics. The research on voluntary dehydration has focused on wrestlers and their relevant physical performance parameters, such as maximal strength, anaerobic power, and capacity.

Anaerobic Performance and Strength

Rapid weight loss, commonly referred to as "weight-cutting," in certain sports (such as wrestling, boxing, judo, lightweight crew, and 150-pound football) has raised considerable concern about the potential for physiological injury. Weight-cutting practices strive to manipulate body water, glycogen content, and lean body mass.[43,44] These practices are all thought to be incompatible with peak performance. However, available research has produced inconsistent findings, with some studies showing that dehydration had little effect on maximal strength[45] and others showing that it reduces maximal strength.[43,46,47] Research findings on the effect of dehydration on anaerobic performance are also inconsistent. Some researchers reported significant decrements in both anaerobic power and capacity due to dehydration,[47–49] while others found no significant effect of dehydration on the two perform-ance parameters.[43,45] The lack of consistency in previous findings may be related to the variations in weight-cutting procedures used. Also, muscle groups tested for anaerobic performance tend to vary from study to study.

Webster and colleagues[47] examined the effects of a *typical* pre-competition weight loss regimen used by intercol-legiate wrestlers on selected physiological parameters, including strength, anaerobic power, anaerobic capacity, lactate threshold, and peak aerobic power. Body composi-tion was assessed 36 hours before weigh-in, and each wrestler was assigned a body weight that was 5% lower than his initial body weight. To reach the assigned body weight during the 12-hour period before weigh-in, the wrestlers participated in a 1.5-hour wrestling practice followed by a 1–2 hour aerobic exercise session which included running, cycling, and rope-jumping. Rapid weight loss in this study produced a small but significant reduction in strength, which was more pronounced for upper-body strength than for leg strength. Anaerobic power was also reduced, which in combination with the strength result suggested a decrease in the wrestler's ability to develop short-term power after a typical weight-cutting regimen. The results also showed significant decreases in anaerobic capacity, peak lactate levels, and aerobic power.

The deleterious effects of weight cutting on wrestling performance reported in Webster et al.'s [47] study could be due to glycogen depletion rather than dehydration, given the fact that the weight loss was primarily induced by aer-obic exercise. However, the procedures used in the study simulated the typical procedures used by wrestlers before actual competition, and the weight reduction was primari-ly a function of body water reduction. The position of the American College of Sports Medicine that *weight-cutting* produces few, if any, positive performance effects and more likely causes performance reductions[50] seems a valid one.

More research is needed to examine the effects of dehy-dration upon strength and anaerobic performance. Besides wrestling, other forms of sports in which a lower weight classification may serve as an advantage and weight-cutting techniques are often practiced should also be examined. It remains to be tested whether inducing dehydration in different ways within the same sport will affect perform-ance differently. For example, Caldwell et al.[51] noted that diuretic-induced dehydration results in a greater decrement in performance than exercise-induced dehydration. This may be due to the concurrent loss of electrolytes caused by diuretics, leading to a much greater loss of plasma fluid vol-ume than is seen with either exercise or thermal-induced dehydration.[52] How dehydration may affect strength and anaerobic performance is still an open question.

Aerobic Performance

Senay and Pivarnik[18] classified exercise into four cate-gories: short-term exercise (<30 min), intermediate-term exercise (from 30 min to 2 hrs), long-term exercise (runs or walks over distances ranging from 42.2 km to 500 km), and maximal exercise (exercise intensity equal to or exceed-ing VO_{2max}). In this classification, short-term exercise and maximal exercise do not produce sufficient sweating to be of concern. Significant sweating produced in intermediate and long-term exercises depends on exercise intensity and environmental conditions. For a given exercise intensity, the relative heat loss due to sweating (evaporative heat loss) as opposed to dry heat exchange will vary depending on the environmental temperature. The hotter the ambient tem-perature, the greater the dependence on sweating. To avoid sweat-loss–induced (involuntary) dehydration, an adequate amount of water must be consumed. However, individuals engaged in prolonged exercise in hot weather often find that drinking enough fluids to avoid dehydration is nearly impossible.

Several reasons exist for why exercising, heat-stressed humans commonly dehydrate from 2–8% of their body weight.[41,53,54] First, thirst may not provide a good index of body water needs. People often do not perceive thirst until a water deficit of about 2% of body weight has occurred. Also, ad libitum drinking usually results only in a replacement of 1/3 to 2/3 of sweat losses.[40,41] Second, gastrointestinal intolerance to fluids, either perceived or actual, may limit fluid consumption. Because maximal gastric emptying rates decrease during high-intensity exer-cise,[55,56] hypohydration,[57,58] and heat strain,[58] there is an upper limit to both gastric emptying and fluid absorption. Lastly, the rules of the game, particularly in team sports, can sometimes discourage fluid replacement during competition, as in soccer in which games are played in 45-minute halves during which fluids are not permitted on the field, and in cricket in which fluids are only allowed every hour at specified breaks.

Numerous studies conducted with endurance runners and cyclists have shown adverse impacts of hypohy-dration on maximal aerobic power and physical work capacity,[43,47,51,59–63] while a few studies have documented decreased tolerance time for exercise, both in terms of heat stress and physiological tolerance.[35,64–66] It was sug-gested that a critical water deficit of 3% body weight loss might need to exist before hypohydration reduces maxi-mal aerobic power in a temperate environment.[47,51,59] In a hot environment, however, hypohydration levels as low as a 2% loss of body weight can result in a large reduc-tion in maximal aerobic power.[61] Physical work capacity decreases have been seen with marginal (1–2% loss of body weight) water deficits, and the more pronounced the water deficit, the greater the reduction in physical work capacity.[51] Hypohydration also tends to increase the inci-dence of exhaustion from heat strain and reduce time to fatigue.[64–66] The reduction could be as substantial as 2 to 3 hours.[64] In the limited research looking at the effects of hydration on performance specific to team sports, it was found that time to complete soccer-specific tests after a match was increased, although hypohydration may not have been the primary contributing factor.[67,68]

Ever since Costill[69] proposed that hypohydration is one of the possible mechanisms underlying the development of fatigue in prolonged endurance exercise, hydration status has received considerable research attention. Clearly, aerobic performance is adversely affected by hypohydration but the mechanism of this effect is less clear. It was recently suggested that the hypohydration seen with exercise in the heat may be associated with hyperthermia due to impaired thermoregulation which in turn results in disturbed cardiovascular dynamics and muscle metabolism.[70,71]

Dehydration and Thermoregulation

The body's temperature rises during exercise due to heat production from increased muscular activity, and a warm environment accentuates this heat stress. Evaporation of sweat and increased skin blood flow through cutaneous dilation are effective mechanisms for heat dissipation, as triggered and controlled by the hypothalamus. But, hypohydration impairs this process and results in substantial, even dangerous, elevations in core temperature. A water deficit of as little as 1% body weight elevates the core temperature during exercise.[72] Both singular and combined effects of plasma hypertonicity (higher in solutes than plasma under conditions of euhydration) and hypovolemia (low volume) have been suggested as mediating the reduced heat loss response when dehydrated.[73]

As described previously, the initial source of water for sweat comes from the interstitial spaces. The water lost in sweat has a lower osmotic concentration than the cutaneous interstitial space, indicating that electrolytes remain in the interstitial space. This increase in electrolytes produces an osmotic pressure gradient favoring movement of water from the blood into the interstitial spaces which, in turn, produces a low plasma volume (hypovolemia). The concentration of solutes in the plasma has been reported to increase from about 283 mOsm/kg when euhydrated to levels approaching 300 mOsm/kg when hypohydrated by exercise-heat strain.[73,74] Sodium, potassium, and chloride are the primary solutes.[52] It is the elevation in plasma solute levels that mobilizes fluid from the intracellular compartment to the extracellular compartments as a partial defense against the plasma losses in hypohydrated subjects.[43,75,76]

Plasma hypertonicity and hypovolemia have been studied in relation to the thermoregulatory responses of sweating-rate threshold (body temperature in which sweating is initiated), sweating sensitivity (change in sweating response per unit change in body temperature), and skin blood flow. Sawka[73] reviewed findings for threshold, sensitivity, and skin blood flow changes when plasma volume and/or tonicity were altered during hypohydration. The sweating rate threshold values were consistently increased with increases in plasma tonicity but sensitivity was not affected. Conversely, as plasma volume declined, sensitivity also declined but sweating threshold was not affected. Sawka[73] thus concluded that hypertonicity appears to cause the initiation of sweating at a higher body temperature while hypovolemia reduces the sweating response to temperature changes. In addition, hypovolemia forces reductions in skin blood flow, thereby greatly reducing the potential for dry heat exchange. Together, hypertonicity and hypovolemia dramatically raise the body's core temperature by reducing both dry heat exchange and evaporative heat loss.

Results from animal studies suggest that alterations in the initiation of sweating due to osmolar changes are probably mediated by the central nervous system and this may be true for humans as well.[77,78] Some researchers, however, have seen indications of secondary effects from hypertonicity and hypovolemia that further reduce sweating rate.[79,80] In terms of hypertonicity, osmotic pressure shifts could serve to pull fluid away from sweat and back into the interstitial space, thus reducing the sweating rate. The cardiopulmonary and arterial blood pressure reductions accompanying hypovolemia and mediated by the hypothalamus produce a cutaneous vasoconstriction for the purpose of conserving blood flow to exercising muscle and the brain (central blood flow) with a resulting reduction in skin blood flow.[71,74] Hyperthermia results from the greatly diminished ability to dissipate body heat either via dry heat exchange or evaporative heat loss. Taken cumulatively, the body's responses to hypohydration in exercise-heat stress appear to be designed to maintain central blood flow in support of exercising muscles and the brain at the expense of thermoregulation.[73] But, regaining thermoregulation is easily achievable by discontinuing exercise and moving out of the heat. The exerciser who continues exercising in the heat while hypohydrated greatly increases his/her risk for life-threatening thermal injury.

In summary, hypohydration reduces the ability to dissipate body heat and increases the rate of heat storage, thus elevating the core temperature during exercise. The magnitude of core temperature elevation can be up to 0.23°C for every percent body weight lost due to water deficit, and the elevation is greater in hot climates rather than temperate ones.[36] Increases in the magnitude of water deficit are concomitantly associated with a graded elevation of core temperature during exercise-heat stress. Montain et al.[81] report that the core temperature elevation is not affected by exercise intensity. Sweat-induced hypertonicity and hypovolemia contribute to reduced body heat dissipation because of reduced sweating rate and reduced skin blood flow responses for a given core temperature. Increasing levels of hypohydration result in a graded increase in the threshold temperature for the onset of sweating and a graded decrease in the sensitivity of the sweating response during exercise. In turn, reductions in sweating rate and skin blood flow are responsible for the increased body temperature associated with dehydration.

Dehydration and Cardiovascular Drift

Alterations in blood volume due to hypohydration exert a strain on the cardiovascular system that is accentuated by exercise in the heat.[81–87] *Cardiovascular drift* is the term used to describe a phenomenon particularly seen in prolonged exercise-heat stress. It is characterized by gradual elevations in heart rate, progressive decreases in stroke volume, and reductions in central venous, pulmonary, and systemic arterial pressures.[82,83] Although cardiovascular drift may occur to some extent under temperate conditions, it is most pronounced under conditions of climatic heat stress, dehydration, and hypovolemia.

Both dehydration and hyperthermia during exercise individually serve to reduce stroke volume and together their effects are additive. It has been reported that with endurance exercise at 70–72% VO_{2max}, either dehydration or hyperthermia will reduce stroke volume by 7–8%[71,85] and, individually, they will increase the heart rate without compromising the maintenance of cardiac output or mean arterial pressure. However, when dehydration is superimposed on hyperthermia during exercise, the stroke volume declines to a level in which cardiac output is negatively influenced. These effects are related to the reductions in skin blood flow, with the resulting increase in the body's core temperature as described in the previous section. As the body's core temperature rises to critical levels, cutaneous vasodilation occurs in an attempt to move the blood to the skin for heat removal. Vasodilation in turn results in a decrease in venous resistance and pressure. As the central venous pressure declines, so does cardiac filling and together these declines serve to reduce stroke volume and increase heart rate. The increase in heart rate is not of sufficient magnitude to compensate for the large reductions in stroke volume from dehydration and hyperthermia combined and, as a result, cardiac output and mean arterial pressure are compromised.[71,84,85] The hypohydration-mediated reduction in cardiac output generally becomes larger as exercise intensity increases, particularly with high levels of fluid loss (5% body weight loss).[81]

In summary, during exercise-induced dehydration in association with hyperthermia, large reductions in stroke volume and cardiac output are seen along with an elevated heart rate and compromised blood pressure. Although cardiovascular drift may occur during exercise in temperate climate conditions, the imposition of heat stress and dehydration greatly increases the risk. Preserving normal hydration and solute levels prevents cardiovascular drift and maintains normal cardiac output.

Other Effects of Dehydration

Dehydration exerts profound effects, either directly or indirectly, on many physiological responses related to exercise performance. Most notably, these responses include muscle endurance, muscle metabolism, and hormonal/renal responses. To date, the alterations in these physiological responses have not been as well documented as those involved in thermoregulation and cardiovascular output.

It has long been known that hypohydration reduces aerobic exercise performance; however, effects on skeletal muscle performance are not clear. One hypothesis, that hypohydration would cause accelerated energy metabolism and accumulation of the metabolites of energy metabolism in skeletal muscle cells,[88,89] was studied by Montain and colleagues.[65] They produced dehydration of 4% body weight by restricting fluids during a 2- to 3-hour moderate-intensity treadmill and cycling bout in a hot room. In comparison to the same exercise performed in the euhydrated state, hypohydration resulted in a 15% decrease in skeletal muscle endurance. Neither muscle strength nor recovery of muscle strength after exhaustive exercise was affected by hypohydration. Levels of the energy metabolites, hydrogen, and inorganic phosphate were measured using a ^{31}P-magnetic resonance spectroscope because they are indicators of muscle pH and ATP, respectively. The accumulation of these products is believed to be responsible for muscle fatigue during high intensity exercise.[88,89] Montain et al.[65] found no changes in hydrogen and inorganic phosphate levels in their study. Their study identified another physiological system, skeletal muscle, that is adversely affected by dehydration but the mechanism of the effect is not known. Several researchers have suggested that the reduced skeletal muscle endurance is a function of the compromised blood flow to skeletal muscle that occurs with hypohydration.[90,91] Gonzalez-Alonso et al.[90] observed a decrease in free fatty acid uptake and an increase in glucose use in the muscles of dehydrated subjects. Others suggest that alterations in muscle calcium and magnesium levels may be responsible for the muscle fatigue seen in hypohydration.[65,89] Clearly, more research is needed.

As discussed previously, body water and electrolyte balance is closely regulated by several hormones in concert with the kidneys. During exercise-heat stress, dehydration-induced alterations in fluid and electrolyte homeostasis lead to hyperosmotic-hypovolemia and to an increase in the circulating concentrations of the main fluid-regulating hormones, antidiuretic hormone (ADH), and the renin-angiotensin-aldosterone system.[92–94] Upon the release of ADH and aldosterone, water and sodium are conserved by reducing their excretion via the kidney which results in a concentrated urine. Surprisingly, Melin et al.[95] observed decreased renal concentrating ability during exercise in dehydration despite elevated plasma ADH. Dehydration appeared to increase the stress hormones, adrenocorticotropic hormone (ACTH) and cortisol,[93] and catecholamine response.[71,95] Previous research identified cortisol as a sensitive index of heat stress heralding the onset of poor tolerance during exercise,[96] while catecholamine responses were shown to influence vessel resistance and water and electrolyte excretion.[71] The combination of these factors were thought to be responsible for the greater water loss in urine during exercise-induced dehydration.

Heat Illnesses

The heat illnesses that can result from exercising in the heat are caused by the physiological factors discussed in this section, namely, hypovolemia, electrolyte imbalance, and hyperthermia. Dehydration can either cause these factors or accentuate them. It is well known that, unchecked, dehydration during exercise in the heat will cause vasoconstriction and reduced sweating, leading to life-threatening hyperthemia.[7,70–87,97,98] Muscle cramping, commonly called heat cramps, appear to be caused by excessive salt losses through profuse sweating.[97,98] Heat syncope, or fainting, describes a condition in which an athlete collapses during or after exercising in the heat, and may occur from the decrease in blood volume (hypovolemia) resulting from dehydration and high sweat losses. Heat stroke is the most dangerous form of heat illness resulting from exercise in hot conditions because it may lead to death. The combination of extreme environmental heat stress, substantial metabolic heat production, diminished evaporative and dry heat exchanges, and impaired hypothalamic heat-regulating ability can raise the body temperature to a life-threatening level (106°F/41°C or greater) and eventually lead to death.[7,97,98]

In summary, dehydration can exert profound influences on exercise performance, and prolonged exercise in hot conditions is more likely to be adversely influenced by hypohydration than short-term anaerobic exercise tasks. The two major systems most affected by dehydration via alterations of plasma volume and/or tonicity are the thermoregulatory system and the cardiovascular system. Dehydration causes or contributes to a) impaired thermoregulatory processes which decrease endurance and increase the risk of hyperthermia; b) lower plasma and blood volumes which lead to decreased cardiac stroke volume, accelerated heart rate, and an overall diminished cardiac output; c) a reduction in skeletal muscle endurance and decreased aerobic performance; d) elevated corticosteroid and catecholamine hormones leading to diminished renal water and sodium conservation; and e) the development of serious heat illnesses.

Fluid Replacement

Due to the adverse effects of dehydration on physical performance and physiological responses, effective fluid replacement is critical for preventing hypohydration during training or competition. The benefits of fluid consumption in the prevention of dehydration and consequent deterioration in physical performance have been

well documented. Several different approaches have been used to research the effects of rehydration upon physical performance, which are comparable to the methods used to study the effects of dehydration.

One approach is related to the sports which primarily rely on anaerobic efforts, in particular wrestling, whereby attempts are made to rehydrate the individual back to euhydration after weigh-in and study the subsequent effects on performance. As noted earlier, it is common for wrestlers to undergo considerable dehydration to compete at a particular weight class. Wrestlers have a limited time, from 30 minutes to 2 hours depending upon the sport, between weigh-in and competition to replenish body fluids, electrolytes, and glycogen. Whether incomplete rehydration affects anaerobic performance remains an open question with a general lack of consistent research findings.[49,99–102] Nonetheless, evidence to date suggests that rehydration during the interval between weigh-in and competition can, at least partly, reestablish water and electrolyte homeostasis, restore body weight, and increase local muscular endurance to levels above those seen in dehydration.[7,50] However, rehydration in such a limited time period may not be sufficient to support performance equivalent to that seen in the euhydrated state. Because of this the American College of Sports Medicine has taken a strong position stand against the use of dehydration and fluid deprivation to "make weight."[50]

With respect to endurance exercise, it is well documented that fluid ingestion attenuates hyperthermia associated with exercise-induced dehydration and cardiovascular drift.[73–87,103–105] Compared with no fluid intake during exercise, fluid ingestion attenuates the rise in core temperature.[86,103,104] Fluid intake also results in a higher stroke volume, cardiac output, and blood volume, and a lower heart rate.[105,106] In addition to the maintenance of thermoregulatory and cardiovascular functions, rehydration also blunts endocrine responses[93,95] and helps to spare muscle glycogen by enhancing free fatty acid use.[90,107] Endurance performance is therefore enhanced by fluid replacement. Fluid ingestion can improve exercise performance during continuous, long-duration, low-to-moderate-intensity exercise,[53,108–110] intermittent exercise of various intensity,[111] and events lasting over 1 hour.[112,113]

Limiting Factors in Fluid Replacement

As stated, there appears to be significant value in the replacement of body fluids for the purpose of limiting dehydration during exercise. The principal aims of fluid ingestion are to prevent shifts in the plasma solute load that would result in low plasma volume.[114] Numerous studies propose that the optimal rate of fluid replacement is the rate that most closely matches sweat loss, since the magnitude of hyperthermia and cardiovascular drift during prolonged exercise is directly related to the magnitude of dehydration.[72,109,114] Shirreffs[115] even suggested that the volume of drink consumed after exercise-induced dehydration should be greater than the volume of sweat lost because obligatory urine losses persist even in the dehydrated state. However, most athletes do not voluntarily replace all the fluid lost during exercise.[53] Historically, water intake during prolonged athletic events was unfashionable and considered a sign of poor fitness.[116,117] Noakes[114] concluded in his review of fluid replacement research that athletes remain *reluctant drinkers,* voluntarily choosing to drink no more than 500–800 mL/hr during exercise. Involuntary dehydration inevitably develops when fluid ingestion is less than sweat losses, which average 1.2 L/hr. The question of how to achieve better fluid replacement is a valid one that has been studied extensively. Primarily, the research focuses on fluid palatability, composition, volume, and timing as factors influencing fluid replacement.

Fluid Palatability

The American College of Sports Medicine has recognized the role of palatability in sports fluids and concludes that "enhancing palatability of an ingested fluid is one way of improving the match between fluid intake and sweat output."[118] Palatability is determined by a number of physical aspects including temperature, taste, mouth feel, and flavor, all of which have been studied for their role in promoting fluid replacement. Adolph[53] concluded that drink temperature of 60°F/15°C is preferred for consumption, particularly when large quantities must be consumed to reduce dehydration. This was confirmed by Boulze et al.[119] who found that maximal intake occurred at a beverage temperature of 15°C. The American College of Sports Medicine recommends beverages at temperatures ranging from 15–20°C during exercise.[118] Contrary to common belief, beverage temperature has little or no effect on gastric emptying or intestinal absorption rates.[120] Nevertheless, cool beverages enhance palatability and encourage fluid ingestion.

Research has shown that flavored and/or sweetened beverages are preferred and consumed more avidly than plain water during and following physical activity.[118,119,121–123] Rolls[123] concluded that the presence of flavor in a fluid is a major determinant of the amount ingested. But, there seems to be a high inter-individual variation in the preference for a specific drink flavor. Rothstein et al.[124] reported that some flavors (i.e., grape, lemon, and orange) were popular for replacing small water deficits, particularly when warm or salted unpalatable water was an alternate choice. While flavoring of the fluid may help augment fluid intake during and following exercise, other aspects of the beverage may reduce drink acceptability and subsequent intake. For example, carbonated beverages were dramatically underconsumed during exercise because carbonation imparted a feeling of fullness in the stomach and caused gastrointestinal distress.[125,126] Passe et al.[127] concluded that carbonated beverages that contain 2.3-vol CO_2 or greater, typical of many soft drinks, can negatively impact drink acceptability and voluntary fluid intake. Therefore, common soft drinks are not an optimal choice for fluid replacement during or following exercise, especially when a large volume needs to be ingested in a short period of time.

As noted, offering palatably flavored beverages facilitates voluntary rehydration and reduces progressive dehydration. In two recent studies conducted with children during exercise,[121,122] it was demonstrated that progressive dehydration can be prevented by consuming flavored beverages with electrolytes and carbohydrate added. A flavored carbohydrate-electrolyte drink elicited the largest total voluntary fluid intake (1157 mL), followed by a flavored drink with no carbohydrate (1112 mL) and plain water (610 mL).[121] These findings indicate a synergistic effect of flavoring and composition in a fluid replacement beverage. But, whether plain water is the best fluid replacement or whether electrolyte- and/or carbohydrate-containing beverages are more beneficial for enhancing exercise performance has been a topic of controversy.

Composition of the Fluid: Electrolyte Content

A brief review of the mechanisms of thirst and the development of involuntary dehydration can help clarify the importance of electrolytes present in a fluid, most critically, the presence of sodium. Thirst, an adequate stimulus for total fluid replacement at rest, appears to be insufficient in humans under physiological and/or psychological stress conditions, resulting in a delay of voluntary fluid intake which can lead to involuntary dehydration.[42] It has been shown that the drinking behavior of dehydrated subjects is regulated by changes in both plasma osmolarity and plasma volume.[114,128,129] Following exercise-induced dehydration, plasma volume reductions produce a volume-dependent thirst signal and the loss of sodium in sweat produces an osmotic-dependent thirst signal. These two signals interact and become the primary initiators of drinking behavior in dehydrated humans and the signals can be modified by the composition of the fluid ingested. Early in the process of dehydration, loss of fluid from the plasma to the interstitial space increases the concentration of plasma solutes; this higher osmolarity favors water movement from the intracellular area into the plasma. This water shift acts to maintain plasma volume and to reduce the volume-dependent drive for fluid replacement. Similarly, the ingestion of plain water in the later stages of dehydration would prematurely inhibit drinking by moving water into the plasma, thus increasing plasma volume and reducing the volume-dependent thirst signal.[128] The rapid drop in serum osmolarity due to plain water ingestion also decreases the plasma levels of antidiuretic hormone and aldosterone, which promotes a higher urine flow resulting in delayed rehydration.[130] In addition,

Nose et al.[128] documented a selective retention of ingested fluid in the vascular space that diminished the volume-dependent thirst drive. These interactions between thirst stimuli may explain why humans are likely to develop involuntary dehydration during exercise.

The addition of sodium to a fluid replacement beverage helps maintain plasma osmolarity while increasing plasma volume. Research findings indicate that compared with fluid devoid of sodium, a higher plasma osmolarity was maintained with fluid replacement drinks containing sodium, the subjects drank significantly more fluid, and they came closer to meeting their fluid needs.[42,121,128–131]

In addition to stimulating thirst via the osmotic-dependent thirst signal, sodium has also been found to maintain body fluid balance among the compartments. Complete total body water replacement is determined by the ability to restore the ions lost from each compartment (sodium from the extracellular compartments and potassium from the intracellular compartments) and is ultimately a function of the proportional distribution of ingested fluid and electrolytes among the body fluid compartments.[42,112,128–132] Restoration of electrolyte deficits is essential to complete restoration of the fluid deficit.

Ingested sodium also aids in fluid and carbohydrate uptake in the gut. The presence of sodium in the lumen is critical for the absorption of many organic and inorganic solutes, such as glucose. Sodium and glucose are transported across the intestinal membrane via glucose-sodium co-transporters, and the resultant shift in osmotic pressure draws water with them.[133] Sodium and potassium supplemented in fluid help replace the electrolytes lost in sweat. Hyponatremia, or low concentration of sodium in the body fluids, can be a serious medical complication. It is most likely to occur when excessive amounts of plain water are ingested following conditions that caused excessive sodium and water losses.[113–116,134] Even though sweat is hypotonic to plasma, prolonged exercise in the heat results in excessive sodium losses through sweat.[73,98,113–116] Although the typical diet should serve to replace sodium losses, consumption of plain water combined with a low sodium intake can be dangerous.

However, It remains unclear whether sodium and potassium should both be supplemented in sports drinks and if so, how much. Electrolyte needs vary considerably on both an individual basis and by sports, which makes it difficult to recommend a standard fluid replacement beverage. The typical amounts of supplemental sodium chloride found in fluid replacement drinks range from 20–50 mmol/L and this range is thought to improve palatability and augment fluid intake.[129,130] It has been shown that inclusion of 25 mmol/L potassium chloride could be as effective as 60 mmol/L sodium chloride in retaining water ingested after exercise-induced dehydration, but there are no additive effects of combining the two.[131] Because sodium offers benefits not provided by potassium, such as conservation of plasma osmolarity, beverage palatability, and intestinal

fluid uptake, sodium is still the electrolyte of primary importance in a fluid replacement drink.

Maughan et al.[135] found that a meal-plus-water treatment was more effective in restoring water and electrolyte balances after moderate levels of exercise-induced dehydration than was electrolyte-containing fluids. The authors concluded that addition of electrolytes to the ingested fluid is not necessary if sufficient plain water is consumed with solid food, which contains an appropriate electrolyte (i.e., sodium and potassium) content. Thus, the supplementation of sodium in a fluid replacement is important in situations in which solid food is not available or when the exerciser has concerns about food consumption causing gastrointestinal discomforts.

The 1996 American College of Sports Medicine position stand stated that "inclusion of sodium (0.5–0.7 g/L of water) in the rehydration solution ingested during exercise lasting longer than 1 hour is recommended since it may be advantageous in enhancing palatability, promoting fluid retention, and possibly preventing hyponatremia in certain individuals who drink excessive quantities of fluid."[118]

Composition of the Fluid: Carbohydrate Content

Carbohydrate concentration is another consideration with respect to the composition of a fluid replacement drink. Dehydration and carbohydrate depletion are recognized as two major causes of fatigue. The ergogenic effect of carbohydrate feeding during exercise is covered elsewhere in this book. Briefly, research consistently shows that carbohydrate ingestion significantly increases physical performance in exercise bouts lasting from less than 1 hour to 4 or more hours.[113,136] The beneficial effects of carbohydrate are additive to that of fluid replacement.

The addition of carbohydrates to a fluid replacement drink can enhance intestinal absorption of water.[113,118] It appears that carbohydrate in solid form, when supplemented with water ingestion, produces a response equivalent to that seen with carbohydrate-containing beverages.[137,138] However, carbohydrates in beverages are commonly preferred by most exercising subjects for obvious practical reasons. A variety of different carbohydrates including glucose, sucrose, and maltodextrins, either alone or in combination, have been added to fluid replacement solutions and have been shown to enhance water absorption in the intestine.[118,138,139] Fructose, however, is the exception to this. Absorption of fructose is slower than an equivalent amount of glucose due to the difference in intestinal brush border carrier mechanisms for the two monosaccharides.[133,138,140] Because of the slower absorption rate, ingesting large amounts of fructose can cause gastrointestinal distress and consequently hamper performance.[118,138] Therefore, beverages containing a high fructose content are not optimal sports drinks.[133,138,140]

The optimum concentration of carbohydrate to be added to drinks will depend on individual circumstances, and most studies demonstrating improved performance with carbohydrate feedings have given subjects 25–60 g of carbohydrate during each hour of exercise.[136–138] These amounts of carbohydrates can be obtained along with large amounts of fluid if the concentration of carbohydrates is kept below 10% (g/100 mL^{-1}).[118,140] The carbohydrate concentration of a solution is an important factor regulating gastric emptying of fluid ingested. Solutions containing up to 8% carbohydrate appear to have little deleterious influence on the rate of gastric emptying, especially when a high gastric volume is maintained with a set drinking schedule.[137,140] But, carbohydrate concentrations >10% will cause a net movement of fluid into the intestinal lumen due to their high osmolarity and this will delay fluid replacement.[118,137] Low carbohydrate concentrations (i.e., <2%), will require too large a volume of fluid if the demands of exercising muscle are also to be met. For these reasons, a concentration of 4–8% of carbohydrate in the fluid is recommended.[118]

Composition of the Fluid: Alcohol and Caffeine Content

The drinks that contain alcohol or caffeine are usually not recommended when fluid replacement is a priority because of the diuretic properties of these substances. Drinks containing alcohol or caffeine are associated with less effective rehydration largely due to greater urine formation and smaller blood volume restoration.[141,142] Caffeine also causes magnesium and calcium losses with urine.[130] Some investigators speculate that the adverse effects of alcohol and caffeine may be dosage dependent.[142,143] However, the maximum dosage of either alcohol or caffeine that will not exert deleterious effects on rehydration and performance is still an open inquiry. For athletes who choose to drink caffeine and/or alcohol-containing beverages due to personal preference, cultural custom, or in the case of caffeine, ergogenic benefits, the best advice is to do so in moderation and to take extra precautions to ensure adequate hydration before and after the event.

Fluid Volume and Drinking Schedule

The rate at which fluid leaves the stomach, gastric emptying, dictates the upper limit for fluid replacement.[144] The volume of fluid in the stomach has been shown to be the most important factor regulating gastric emptying. As reviewed and summarized by Coyle and Montain,[145] the rate of gastric emptying increases progressively as the volume of a given solution ingested is increased. Therefore, to promote gastric emptying, it is advantageous to maintain the largest volume of fluid that can be tolerated by the individual. Maintaining high gastric fluid volume, however, should be practiced with caution considering the common complaints of gastrointestinal discomfort by athletes,

in particular long-distance runners, when a large fluid volume is consumed during exercise.[114] It is unclear whether those complaints are a function of unfamiliarity of exercising with a full stomach or caused by exercise-induced slowing of gastric emptying and/or intestinal absorption. It has yet to be determined if the ability to tolerate high gastric volumes can be improved by chronically ingesting large volumes of fluid before and/or during training. Inter-individual and sports-specific variations in gastric emptying rates and maximum tolerance to gastric volumes should also be taken into account when recommending the optimum volume of fluid ingestion. Once the ingested fluid moves into the intestine, the availability of fluid for circulation depends on intestinal absorption capacity, which is primarily determined by the composition and osmolarity of the fluid.

A drinking schedule should be adopted for maintaining a normal hydration status. First, individuals appear to benefit from fluid ingested before exercise. For example, water ingested 60 minutes before exercise has been shown to enhance thermoregulatory and cardiovascular functions during exercise.[79,118] However, urine volume will markedly increase with pre-exercise fluid intake. It is recommended in the 1996 American College of Sports Medicine position stand[118] that "individuals drink about 500 mL (about 17 ounces) of fluid about 2 h before exercise to promote adequate hydration and allow time for excretion of excess ingested water." The primary purpose of pre-exercise fluid intake is to ensure a euhydration status for the person at the start of the event. A useful side effect of pre-exercise drinking is to prime the stomach for increased emptying rates.[146]

It has been hypothesized that hyperhydration may be beneficial for exercise performance. However, recent research has shown that hyperhydration provides no thermoregulatory or performance advantages over euhydration.[63] Instead, the individual is burdened with extra weight which may impede his/her performance.[12]

As a practical check on hydration status, athletes should pay attention to the color and volume of their urine because well-hydrated individuals normally void a light-colored urine of normal to above-normal volume.[147] A urine that is dark yellow in color, is of small volume, and has a strong odor indicates likely dehydration.[12,147] Of note, athletes who take vitamin supplements may produce a dark-yellow urine from excretion of excess riboflavin; therefore, urine color, volume, and odor must all be considered as indicators of hydration status.

During exercise, fluid replacement should attempt to equal sweat losses to minimize thermal injury and impairment of exercise performance.[118,148] Early and continued drinking throughout exercise is needed because progressive involuntary dehydration during exercise reduces the rate of gastric emptying.[144]

The quantity of fluid ingested after exercise should be greater than the volume of sweat that has been lost to compensate for obligatory urine losses, which persist even when a person is hypohydrated. It is indicated that ingestion of 150% or more of weight loss may be required to achieve normal hydration within 6 hours following exercise,[115] and it is recommended to "drink at least a pint of fluid for every pound of body weight deficit."[135] Well-formulated carbohydrate-electrolyte beverages should be ingested in situations in which a short period of time is given for rehydration before the next session. Otherwise, sufficient plain water plus a nutritiously balanced diet will be most effective in completely replacing any fluid, electrolyte, and carbohydrate losses.[12,135]

In summary, due to the high probability for involuntary dehydration in endurance exercise and the detrimental effects of progressive dehydration on health and performance, it is imperative to implement strategies that ensure adequate hydration before exercise and rehydration both during and after exercise. Strategies that are in line with the guidelines presented by the 1996 American College of Sports Medicine's position on fluid needs[118] are encouraged. Optimum fluids are solutions that maximize palatability, that provide desirable composition of carbohydrates and electrolytes, that promote or maintain hydration, and that enhance or support performance. However, there is no one standard formula recommended for everyone; instead, the interpretation of general recommendations should be individually based and tailored for the sport. Recording and assessing how much fluid is lost while performing different tasks in different environmental conditions may facilitate predicting fluid needs of the individual. The benefits of fluid replacement on exercise performance will be enhanced by heat acclimatization, which can be achieved by repeated exposures to heat or by consistent training in a warm environment.[3] The process of heat acclimatization improves a person's heat tolerance by initiating the sweat response at a lower core temperature and increasing sweat rates and plasma volume.[3] However, the benefits derived from heat acclimatization can be negated by dehydration.

SUMMARY

High rates of metabolic heat production in environments where the capacity for heat loss is limited exert substantial strains on the thermoregulatory and cardiovascular systems. Dehydration, whether due to sweat losses with limited fluid intake during exercise or voluntarily induced fluid deficits before exercise, can significantly decrease the effectiveness of the heat loss mechanisms by elevating the threshold for the onset of sweating and reducing sweat rates. Dehydration and hyperthermia aggravate the circulatory strain experienced during exercise in a warm environment, resulting not only in increased heart rates but also decreased stroke volumes, reduced mean arterial pressure, and compromised cardiac output. In addition, muscular metabolism, hormonal responses, and kidney function may also be affected by dehydration. A harmful reduction in performance, whether in endurance events or in shorter events of higher intensity, will be inevitable if hypohydration is not avoided and/or corrected.

Ensuring adequate hydration before exercise and ingesting fluids during exercise have shown to improve exercise performance. Although the ingestion of plain water has been shown to be effective, the addition of small amounts of carbohydrate can deliver independent and additive benefits in improving exercise capacity. The importance of consuming electrolyte-containing fluids during exercise is open to debate, although electrolyte supplementation has been shown to enhance fluid palatability and enhance the absorption of both water and carbohydrates. The composition of solutes, electrolytes, and/or carbohydrates determines the rate of intestinal absorption of rehydration beverages; however, gastric emptying, the primary limiting factor in rehydration, largely depends upon the volume of fluid ingested. Several factors, including palatability (i.e., flavor and temperature) and sodium content, will influence the volume of fluid that is voluntarily consumed. The optimum volume of fluid ingested during exercise is that which closely matches sweat losses. The combination of a fluid replacement regimen and an acclimatization strategy will help to minimize the negative effects of adverse climatic conditions on exercise performance and reduce the risk of heat illness, but is unlikely to completely restore performance capacity during exercise. For full recovery after exercise, a nutritious diet and sufficient water intake is the most effective means to replace fluid and electrolyte losses and replenish the body's glycogen stores. However, many training and competition situations call for bouts of exercise to be repeated with relatively short recovery times in which eating is impractical and drinking carbohydrate-electrolyte–containing beverages becomes critical. Cool, flavored, and well-formulated beverages at a volume in excess of sweat losses by at least 50% are required for a full recovery.

⊢ AUTHORS' RECOMMENDATIONS ⊣

Upon the review of previous research, the following general guidelines are recommended and should be adapted to each individual and each sport in different environmental conditions.

• Educate coaches, trainers, and athletes about the adverse consequences of dehydration on physical performance and health.

• Encourage sports' governing bodies to assess and revise rules that limit fluid intake.

• Encourage sensible choices of clothing, strapping, and/or protective gear.

• Increase individual athletes' or active peoples' awareness of their typical sweat losses by encouraging regular weighing before and after exercise sessions.

• Begin each competition or training session well hydrated, particularly in hot conditions. This involves consuming a nutritiously balanced diet and adequate water days before the event, pre-exercise drinking, and appropriate heat acclimation. Athletes should start drinking early and at regular intervals during exercise.

• Optimize opportunities to consume fluids during exercise, i.e., by providing individual drinking bottles to athletes and encouraging frequent drinking behavior during exercise. Individual maximum tolerance for fluid intake should be monitored.

• Optimize palatability of fluids to encourage voluntary intake. Cool, flavored/sweetened drinks should be provided.

• Supplement carbohydrates (i.e., glucose and glucose polymers) and electrolytes (e.g., Na^+ and K^+) if necessary.

• Rehydrate after exercise and before the next exercise bout.

• Develop and follow an individual fluid intake plan.

Guidelines for Sports with Different Durations

	Events lasting <1 hr	Events lasting 1–3 hr	Events lasting >3 hr
1. *Events included in each category*	most team sports (i.e., football, basketball, etc.), racket sports, many cycling events, and track events	soccer game, most marathons	triathalon and other forms of ultramarathons
2. *Exercise intensity*	80–130% VO_{2max}	60–90% VO_{2max}	30–70% VO_{2max}
3. *Primary concern*	fluid replacement to reduce risk of a rise in core temperature due to high-intensity exercise in the heat	fluid replacement to closely match sweat loss; carbohydrate provision to increase fluid volume	fluid and carbohydrate provision; Na^+ provision to enhance fluid retention and prevent hyponatremia
4. *Proposed formulation, frequency, and volume*			
pre-exercise (2 hrs prior)	30–50 g CHO in 300–500 mL H_2O	300–500 mL plain water	300–500 mL plain water
during exercise	plain water 500–1000 mL/hr or 150–350 mL every 50–20 min	4–8% CHO; 10–20 mEq NaCl; 500–1000 mL/hr or 150–350 mL every 15–20 min	4–8% CHO; 20–30 mEq NaCl; 500–1000 mL/hr or 150–350 mL every 15–20 min
5. *Fluid requirement during recovery*	nutritiously balanced diet and sufficient water ingestion is most effective in replacing fluid, energy substrates, and electrolytes; otherwise, beverages providing 50 g/hr CHO and 30–40 mEq NaCl are suitable		

FUTURE RESEARCH

This chapter was written based on information available to date. Many issues remain to be addressed in coming investigations. For instance, what role do protein and oncotic pressure play in maintaining plasma volume during exercise; what determines the inter-individual variability of sweating response; how do the contributions of different body fluid compartments to sweat differ; what mechanisms stimulate and terminate voluntary drinking, and more? Studies on the harmful effects of dehydration on physical performance have paid the most attention to endurance exercise, particularly running and cycling. More research is needed on other modes of endurance exercise, various forms of intermittent exercise, and short-duration exercise of high intensity. Decades of scientific research have established the incomparable value of adequate fluid replacement. However, the precise formulation of the most effective beverage that accounts for variability associated with exercising subjects, exercise intensity, and ambient conditions remains elusive. Additional research is necessary to adequately explore the effects of the interaction of carbohydrates, electrolytes, and flavor intensity on drink acceptability and fluid intake. Also, there remains a need for science to be more effectively translated into practice so that the athletic community understands the benefits of remaining well hydrated.

REFERENCES

1. Kleiner SM. Water: an essential but overlooked nutrient. J Am Diet Assoc 1999;99:200–207.
2. Guyton AE, ed. Human Physiology and Mechanisms of Disease. Philadelphia: WB Saunders, 1982.
3. Pivarnik JM. Water and electrolytes during exercise. In: Hickson JF, Jr, Wolinsky I, eds. Nutrition in Exercise and Sport. Florida: CRC Press, 1989.
4. Fox EL, Mathews DK. The Physiological Basis of Physical Education and Athletics. 3rd ed. Philadelphia: WB Saunders, 1981.
5. Wyndham CH. The physiology of exercise under heat stress. Ann Rev Physiol 1973;35:193–220.
6. Senay LC, Jr. Water and electrolytes during physical activity. In: Wolinsky I. Nutrition in Exercise and Sport. 3rd ed. Florida: CRC Press, 1998.
7. Williams MH. Nutritional Aspects of Human Physical and Athletic Performance. 2nd ed. Illinois: Charles C Thomas, 1985:219–271.
8. Greenleaf J. The body's need for fluids. In: Haskell W, Scala J, Whittam J, eds. Nutrition and Athletic Performance. Palo Alto, CA: Bull Publishing, 1982.
9. Guyton AC. Textbook of Medical Physiology. 8th ed. Philadelphia: WB Saunders, 1991:274–275.
10. Vander AJ. Renal Physiology. 2nd ed. New York: McGraw-Hill, 1980.
11. McDowell LR, ed. Minerals in Animal and Human Nutrition. San Diego, CA: Academic Press, 1992.
12. Murray R. Fluid needs of athletes. In: Berning JR, Steen SN, eds. Nutrition for Sport and Exercise. 2nd ed. Maryland: Aspen, 1998:143–153.
13. Oatley K. Simulation and theory of thirst. In: Epstein AN, Kissileff HR, Stellar E, eds. The Neuropsychology of Thirst: New Findings and Advances in Concepts. Washington, DC: Winston, 1973:199–223.
14. Wolf AV. Osmometric analysis of thirst in man and dog. Am J Physiol 1950;161:75–86.
15. Greenleaf J. Drinking and water balance during exercise and heat acclimation. J Appl Physiol 1983;54:414–419.
16. Wolf AV. Thirst: Physiology of the Urge to Drink and Problems of Water Lack. Illinois: Charles C Thomas, 1958.
17. Sagawa S, Miki K, Tajima F, et al. Effect of dehydration on thirst and drinking during immersion in men. J Appl Physiol 1992;72:128–134.
18. Senay LC Jr, Pivarnik JM. Fluid shifts during exercise. Exerc Sport Sci Rev 1985;13:335–388.
19. Guyton AC, Taylor AE, Granger HJ, eds. Circulatory Physiology II. Dynamics and Control of the Body Fluids. Philadelphia: WB Saunders, 1975.
20. Schneeberger EE. Proteins and vesicular transport in capillary endothelium. Fed Proc 1972;42:2419.
21. Senay LC Jr, Rogers G, Jooste P. Changes in blood plasma during progressive treadmill and cycle exercise. J Appl Physiol 1980;49:59–65.
22. Pivarnik JM, Goetting MP, Senay LC Jr. The effects of body position and exercise on plasma volume dynamics. Eur J Appl Physiol 1986;55:450–457.
23. Galbo HJ, Holst J, Christensen NJ. Glucagon and plasma catecholamine responses to graded and prolonged exercise in man. J Appl Physiol 1975;38:70–76.
24. Wilkerson JE, Gutin B, Horvath SM. Exercise-induced changes in blood, red cell, and plasma volumes in man. Med Sci Sports 1977;9:155–158.
25. Sawka MN, Francesconi RP, Pimental NA, Pandolf KB. Hydration and vascular fluid shifts during exercise in the heat. J Appl Physiol 1984;56:91–96.
26. Pivarnik JM, Leeds EM, Wilkerson JE. Effects of endurance exercise on metabolic water production and plasma volume. J Appl Physiol 1984;56:613–618.
27. McMurray RG. Plasma volume changes during submaximal swimming. J Appl Physiol 1983;51:347–356.
28. Starling EH. Physiological factors involved in the causation of dropsy. Lancet 1896;1:1405.
29. Nose H, Mack GW, Shi X, Nadel ER. Shift in body fluid compartments after dehydration in humans. J Appl Physiol 1988;65:318–323.
30. Senay LC, Jr. Movement of water, protein, and crystalloids between vascular and extravascular compartments in heat exposed men during dehydration and following limited relief of dehydration. J Physiol London 1970;210:617–635.
31. Greenleaf JE, Beaumont W, Brock PJ, et al. Plasma volume and electrolyte shifts with heavy exercise in sitting and supine positions. Am J Physiol 1979;206:236.
32. Kerslake D, ed. The Stress of Hot Environments. London: Cambridge University Press, 1972.
33. Greenleaf JE. Hyperthermia and exercise. In: Roertshaw D, ed. Environment Physiology III. Baltimore: University Park Press, 1979:157–208.
34. Brooks GA, Fahey TD, eds. Exercise Physiology: Human Bioenergetics and its Applications. New York: John Wiley & Sons, 1984.
35. Montain SJ, Sawka MN, Cadarette BS, et al. Physiological tolerance to uncompensable heat stress: effects of exercise intensity, protective clothing, and climate. J Appl Physiol 1994;77:216–222.
36. Sawka MN, Latzka WA, Matott RP, Montain SJ. Hydration effects on temperature regulation. Int J Sports Med 1998;19(suppl):108S–110S.
37. Costill DL. Sweating: its composition and effects on body fluids. In: Milvey P, ed. The Marathon: Physiological, Medical, Epidemiological, and Psychological Studies. New York: New York Academy of Sciences, 1977.
38. Costill DL, Cote R, Fink W. Muscle water and electrolytes during varied levels of dehydration in man. J Appl Physiol 1976;40:6–11.
39. Robinson S, Maletich RT, Robinson WS, et al. Output of NaCl by sweat glands and kidneys in relation to dehydration and salt depletion. J Appl Physiol 1956;615:8–12.
30. Senay LC, Kok R. Body fluid response of heat-tolerant and intolerant men to work in a hot wet environment. J Appl Physiol 1976;40:55–59.
41. Hubbard RW, Sandick BL, Matthew WT, et al. Voluntary dehydration and alliesthesia for water. J Appl Physiol 1984;57:868–875.

42. Greenleaf JE. Problem: Thirst, drinking behavior and involuntary dehydration. Med Sci Sports Exerc 1992;24:645–656.
43. Houston ME, Marrin DA, Green HJ, Thomson JA. The effect of rapid weight loss on physiological functions in wrestlers. Phys Sportsmed 1981;9:73–79.
44. Steen SN, McKinney S. Nutritional assessment of college wrestlers. Phys Sportsmed 1986;14:100–116.
45. Serfass RD, Stull GA, Alexander JF. The effects of rapid weight loss and attempted rehydration and endurance of the handgripping muscles in college wrestlers. Res Q 1984;55:46–52.
46. Bosco JS, Greenleaf JE, Terjung RL. Effects of progressive hypohydration on maximal isometric muscular strength. J Sports Med 1968;8:81–86.
47. Webster S, Rutt R, Weltman A. Physiological effects of a weight loss regimen practiced by college wrestlers. Med Sci Sports Exerc 1990; 22:229–234.
48. Torranin C, Smith DP, Byrd RJ. The effects of acute thermal dehydration and rehydration on isometric and isotonic endurance. J Sports Med 1979;19:1–9.
49. Corrigan D. The effects of dehydration and rehydration on anaerobic exercise performance. Med Sci Sports Exerc 1984;112:16–21.
50. Oppliger RA, Case HS, Horswill CA, et al. ACSM position stand on weight loss in wrestlers. Med Sci Sports Exerc 1996;28:ix–xii.
51. Caldwell JE, Ahonen E, Nousiainen U. Differential effects of sauna-, diuretic-, and exercise-induced hypohydration. J Appl Physiol 1984; 57:1018–1024.
52. Kubica R, Nielsen B, Bonnesen A, et al. Relationship between plasma volume reduction and plasma electrolyte changes after prolonged bicycle exercise, passive heating and diuretic dehydration. Acta Physiol Poland 1983;34:569–579.
53. Adolph EF and associates. Physiology of Man in the Desert. New York: Interscience, 1947.
54. Armstrong LE, Hubbard RW, Jones BH, Daniels JT. Preparing Alberto Salazar for the heat of the 1984 Olympic marathon. Phys Sportsmed 1986;14:73–81.
55. Costill DL, Saltin B. Factors limiting gastric emptying during rest and exercise. J Appl Physiol 1974;37:679–683.
56. Neufer PD, Young AJ, Sawka MN. Gastric emptying during walking and running: effects of varied exercise intensity. Eur J Appl Physiol 1989;58:440–445.
57. Rehrer NJ, Beckers EJ, Brouns F, et al. Effects of dehydration on gastric emptying and gastrointestinal distress while running. Med Sci Sports Exerc 1990;22:790–795.
58. Neufer PD, Young AJ, Sawka MN. Gastric emptying during exercise: effects of heat stress and hypohydration. Eur J Appl Physiol 1989;58:433–439.
59. Buskirk ER, Iampietro PF, Bass DE. Work performance after dehydration: effects of physical conditioning and heat acclimation. J Appl Physiol 1958;12:189–194.
60. Saltin B. Aerobic and anaerobic work capacity after dehydration. J Appl Physiol 1964;19:1114–1118.
61. Craig FN, Cummings EF. Dehydration and muscular work. J Appl Physiol 1966;21:670–674.
62. Pinchan G, Gauttam RK, Tomar OS, Bajaj AC. Effect of primary hypohydration on physical work capacity. Int J Biometerol 1988; 32:176–180.
63. Sawka MN, Francesconi RP, Young AJ, Pandolf KB. Influence of hydration level and body fluids on exercise-performance in the heat. JAMA 1984;252:1165–1169.
64. Sawka MN, Young AJ, Latzka WA, et al. Influence of hydration and aerobic fitness on tolerance to exercise-heat strain [abstract]. Med Sci Sports Exerc 1990;21(suppl):118a.
65. Montain SJ, Smith SA, Mattot RP, et al. Hypohydration effects on skeletal muscle performance and metabolism: a ^{31}P-MRS study. J Appl Physiol 1998;84:1889–1894,
66. Cheung SS, McLellan TM. Influence of hydration status and fluid replacement on heat tolerance while wearing NBC protective clothing. Eur J Appl Physiol 1998;77:139–148.
67. Kblom B. Applied physiology of soccer. Sports Med 1986;3:50–60.
68. Rico-Sanz J, Frontera WR, Rivera MA, et al. Effects of hyperhydration on total body water, temperature regulation and performance of elite young soccer players in a warm climate. Int J Sports Med 1996;17:85–91.
69. Costill D. Muscular exhaustion during distance running. Phys Sportsmed 1974;2:36–41.
70. Hargreaves M, Febbraio M. Limits to exercise performance in the heat. Int J Sports Med 1998;19:115S–116S.
71. Gonzalez-Alonso J. Separate and combined influences of dehydration and hyperthermia on cardiovascular responses to exercise. Int J Sports Med 1998;19:111S–114S.
72. Ekblow B, Greenleaf CJ, Greenleaf JE, Hermansen L. Temperature regulation during exercise dehydration in man. Acta Physiol Scand 1970;79:475–583.
73. Sawka MN. Physiological consequences of hydration: exercise performance and thermoregulation. Med Sci Sports Exerc 1992;24: 657–670.
74. Fortney SM, Nadel ER, Wenger CB, Bowe JR. Effect of blood volume on sweating rate and body fluids in exercising humans. J Appl Physiol 1981;51:1594–1600.
75. Gass GC, Camp EM, Watson J, et al. Prolonged exercise in highly trained female endurance runners. Int J Sports Med 1983;4:241–246.
76. Sawka MN, Knowlton RG, Glaser RG. Body temperature, respiration and acid-base equilibrium during prolonged running. Med Sci Sports Exerc 1980;12:370–374.
77. Kozlowski S, Greenleaf JE, Turlejska E, Nazar K. Extracellular hyperosmolality and body temperature during physical exercise in dogs. Am J Physiol 1980;239:R180–R183.
78. Nakashima T, Hori T, Kiyohara T, Shibata M. Effects of local osmolality changes on medial preoptic thermosensitive neurons in hypothalamic slices, in vitro. Therm Physiol 1984;9:133–137.
79. Greenleaf JE, Castle BL. Exercise temperature regulation in man during hypohydration and hyperhydration. J Appl Physiol 1971; 30:847–853.
80. Nielsen B, Hansen G, Jorgensen SD, Nielsen E. Thermoregulation in exercising man during dehydration and hyperhydration with water and saline. Int J Biometeoral 1971;15:195–200.
81. Montain SJ, Sawka MN, Latzka WA, Valeri CR. Thermal and cardiovascular strain from hypohydration: influence of exercise intensity. Int J Sports Med 1998;19:87–91.
82. Ekelund LG. Circulatory and respiratory adaptations during prolonged exercise. Acta Physiol Scand 1967;70(suppl):5S–38S.
83. Rowell LB. Human cardiovascular control. New York: Oxford University Press, 1993:229.
84. Gonzalez-Alonso J, Mora-Rodriguez R, Below PR, Coyle EF. Dehydration reduces cardiac output and increases systemic and cutaneous vascular resistance during exercise. J Appl Physiol 1995;79: 1487–1496.
85. Gonzalez-Alonso J, Mora-Rodriguez R, Below PR, Coyle EF. Dehydration markedly impairs cardiovascular function in hyperthermic endurance athletes during exercise. J Appl Physiol 1997;82:1229–1236.
86. Montain SJ, Coyle EF. Fluid ingestion during exercise increases skin blood flow independent of blood volume. J Appl Physiol 1992; 73:903–910.
87. Coyle EF. Cardiovascular drift during prolonged exercise and the effects of dehydration. Int J Sports Med 1998;19(suppl):121S–124S.
88. Enoka RM, Stuart DG. Neurobiology of muscle fatigue. J Appl Physiol 1992;72:1631–1648.
89. Fitts RH. Cellular mechanisms of muscle fatigue. Physiol Rev 1994; 74:49–94.
90. Gonzalez-Alonso J, Calbet JA, Nielsen B. Metabolic alterations with dehydration-induced reductions in muscle blood flow in exercising humans [abstract]. Eur Coll Sports Sci 1997;2:492–493.
91. Rowell LB. Competition between skin and muscle for blood flow during exercise. In: Nadel ER, ed. Problems With Temperature Regulation During Exercise. New York: Academic Press, 1977:49–76.
92. Brandenberger G, Candas V, Follenius M, et al. Vascular fluid shifts and endocrine responses to exercise in the heat: effect of rehydration. Eur J Appl Physiol 1986;55:123–129.
93. Brandenberger G, Candas V, Follenius M, Kahn JM. The influence of the initial state of hydration on endocrine responses to exercise in the heat. Eur J Appl Physiol 1989;58:674–679.
94. Follenius M, Candas V, Bothorel B, Brandenberger G. Effect of rehydration on atrial natriuretic peptide release during exercise in the heat. J Appl Physiol 1989;66:2516–2521.
95. Melin B, Jimenez C, Savourey G, et al. Effects of hydration state on hormonal and renal responses during moderate exercise in the heat. Eur J Appl Physiol 1997;320–327.

96. Follenius M, Brandenberger G, Oyono S, Candas V. Cortisol as a sensitive index of heat-intolerance. Physiol Behav 1982;29:509–513.

97. Wyndham CH, Strydom NB. The danger of an inadequate water intake during marathon running. S Afr Med J 1969;43:893–896.

98. Noakes TD. Fluid and electrolyte disturbances in heat illness. Int J Sports Med 1998;19(suppl):146S–149S.

99. Herbert WG, Ribisl PM. Effects of dehydration upon physical work capacity of wrestlers under competitive conditions. Res Q 1972;43:416–422.

100. Vaccaro P, Zauner CW, Cade JR. Changes in body weight, hematocrit and plasma protein concentration due to dehydration and rehydration in wrestlers. Med Sci Sports 1975;7:76.

101. Mnatzakanian P, Vaccaro P. Effects of 4 percent dehydration and rehydration on hematological profiles, urinary profiles, and muscular endurance of college wrestlers. Med Sci Sports Exerc 1982;14:117.

102. Chlad P, Paolone A. The effects of pre-match dehydration and rehydration on plasma volume and electrolytes of college wrestlers. Med Sci Sports Exerc 1984;16:171.

103. Candas V, Libert JP, Brandenberger G, et al. Hydration during exercise: effects on thermal and cardiovascular adjustments. Eur J Appl Physiol Occup Physiol 1986;55:113–122.

104. Costill DL, Kammer WF, Fisher A. Fluid ingestion during distance running. Arch Environ Health 1970;21:520–525.

105. Hamilton MT, Gonzalez-Alonso J, Montain SJ, Coyle EF. Fluid replacement and glucose infusion during exercise prevents cardiovascular drift. J Appl Physiol 1991;71:871–877.

106. Melin B, Cure M, Jimenez C, et al. Effect of ingestion pattern on rehydration and exercise performance subsequent to passive dehydration. Eur J Appl Physiol 1994;68:281–284.

107. Hargreaves M, Dillo P, Angus D, Febbraio MA. Effect of fluid ingestion on muscle metabolism during prolonged exercise. J Appl Physiol 1996;80:363–366.

108. Barr SI, Costill DL, Fink WJ. Fluid replacement during prolonged exercise: effects of water, saline, or no fluid. Med Sci Sports Exerc 1991;23:811–817.

109. Montain SJ, Coyle EF. The influence of graded dehydration on hyperthermia and cardiovascular drift during exercise. J Appl Physiol 1992;73:1340–1350.

110. Coyle EF, Hagberg JM, Hurley BF, et al. Carbohydrate feeding during prolonged strenuous exercise can delay fatigue. J Appl Physiol 1983;55:230–235.

111. Murray R, Eddy DE, Murray TW, et al. The effect of fluid and carbohydrate feedings during intermittent cycling exercise. Med Sci Sports Exerc 1987;19:597–604.

112. Below PR, Mora-Rodriguez R, Gonzalez-Alonso J, Coyle EF. Fluid and carbohydrate ingestion independently improve performance during 1 h of intense exercise. Med Sci Sports Exerc 1995;27:200–210.

113. Gisolfi CV, Duchman SM. Guidelines for optimal replacement beverages for different athletic events. Med Sci Sports Exerc 1992;24:679–687.

114. Noakes TD. Fluid replacement during exercise. In: Holloszy JO, ed. Exercise and Sport Sciences Reviews. Baltimore: Williams & Wilkins, 1993:297–330.

115. Shirreffs SM, Taylor AJ, Leiper JB, Maughan RJ. Post-exercise rehydration in man: effects of volume consumed and sodium content of ingested fluids. Med Sci Sports Exerc 1996;28:1260–1271.

116. Noakes TD, Goddwin N, Rayner BL, et al. Water intoxication: a possible complication during endurance exercise. Med Sci Sports Exerc 1985;17:370–375.

117. Noakes TD. Dehydration during exercise: what are the real dangers? Clin J Sport Med 1995;5:123–129.

118. American College of Sports Medicine. Position stand on exercise and fluid replacement. Med Sci Sports Exerc 1996;28:i–vii.

119. Boulze DP, Montastruc P, Cabanac M. Water intake, pleasure and water temperature in humans. Physiol Behav 1983;30:97–102.

120. Lambert CP, Maughan RJ. Accumulation in the blood of a deuterium tracer added to hot and cold beverages. Scand J Med Sci Sports 1992;2:76–78.

121. Wilk B, Bar-Or O. Effect of drink flavor and NaCl on voluntary drinking and hydration in boys exercising in the heat. J Appl Physiol 1996;80:1112–1117.

122. Rivera-Brown AM, Gutierrez R, Gutierrez JC, et al. Drink composition, voluntary drinking, and fluid balance in exercising, trained, heat-acclimatized boys. J Appl Physiol 1999;86:78–84.

123. Rolls BJ. Palatability and fluid intake. In: Marriott BM, Rosemont C, eds. Fluid Replacement and Heat Stress. Washington, DC: National Academy Press, 1991:1–10.

124. Rothstein A, Adolph EF, Wills JH. Voluntary dehydration. In: Adolph EF, ed. Physiology of Man in the Desert. New York: Interscience, 1947:251–270.

125. Lambert GP, Bleiler TL, Chang RT, et al. Effects of carbonated and noncarbonated beverages at specific intervals during treadmill running in the heat. Int J Sports Nutr 1993;3:177–193.

126. Ryan AJ, Navarre CV, Gisolfi CV. Consumption of carbonated and noncarbonated sports drinks during prolonged treadmill exercise in the heat. Int J Sports Nutr 1991;1:225–239.

127. Passe D, Horn M, Murray R. The effects of beverage carbonation on sensory responses and voluntary fluid intake following exercise. Int J Sports Nutr 1997;7:286–297.

128. Nose H, Mack GW, Shi X, Nadel ER. Role of osmolality and plasma volume during rehydration in humans. J Appl Physiol 1988;65:325–331.

129. Mack GW. Recovery after exercise in the heat: factors influencing fluid intake. Int J Sports Med 1998;19(suppl):139S–141S.

130. Maughan RJ, Shirreffs SM. Recovery from prolonged exercise: Restoration of water and electrolyte balance. J Sports Sci 1997;15:297–303.

131. Maughan RJ, Owen JH, Shirreffs SM, Leiper JB. Post-exercise rehydration in man: effects of electrolyte addition to ingested fluids. Eur J Appl Physiol 1994;69:209–213.

132. Cunningham JJ. Is potassium needed in sports drinks for fluid replacement during exercise? Int J Sports Nutr 1997;7:154–159.

133. Leiper JB. Intestinal water absorption: implications for the formulation of rehydration solutions. Int J Sports Med 1998;19(suppl):129S–132S.

134. McArdle WD, Katch FI, Katch V. Exercise thermoregulation, fluid balance, and rehydration. In: Johnson E, ed. Sports & Exercise Nutrition. Baltimore: Williams & Wilkins, 1999:166–291.

135. Maughan RJ, Leiper JB, Shirreffs SM. Restoration of fluid balance after exercise-induced dehydration: effects of food and fluid intake. Eur J Appl Physiol 1996;73:317–325.

136. Coggan A, Coyle EF. Carbohydrate ingestion during prolonged exercise: effects on metabolism and performance. In: Holloszy JO, ed. Exercise and Sports Science Reviews. Baltimore: Williams & Wilkins, 1991:1–40.

137. Coyle EF, Montain SJ. Benefits of fluid replacement with carbohydrate during exercise. Med Sci Sports Exerc 1992;24(suppl):324S–330S.

138. Shirreffs SM. Effects of ingestion of carbohydrate-electrolyte solutions on exercise performance. Int J Sports Med 1998;19(suppl):117S–120S.

139. Shephard RJ, Leatt P. Carbohydrate and fluid needs of the soccer player. Sports Med 1987;4:164–176.

140. Murray R. Rehydration strategies: balancing substrate, fluid, and electrolyte provision. Int J Sports Med 1998;19(suppl):133S–135S.

141. Gonzalez-Alonso J, Heaps CL, Coyle EF. Rehydration after exercise with common beverages and water. Int J Sports Med 1992;13:399–406.

142. Shirreffs SM, Maughan RJ. The effect of alcohol consumption on the restoration of blood and plasma volume following exercise-induced dehydration in man. J Physiol 1996;491:64–65.

143. Brouns F, Kovacs EMR, Senden JMG. The effect of different rehydration drinks on post-exercise electrolyte excretion in trained athletes. Int J Sports Med 1998;19:56–60.

144. Brouns F. Gastric emptying as a regulatory factor in fluid uptake. Int J Sports Med 1998;19(suppl):125S–128S.

145. Coyle EF, Montain SJ. Carbohydrate and fluid ingestion during exercise: are there trade-offs? Med Sci Sports Exerc 1992;24:671–678.

146. Burke LM. Fluid balance during team sports. J Sports Sci 1997;15:287–295.

147. Armstrong LE, Herrera Soto JA, Hacker FT Jr, et al. Urinary indices during dehydration, exercise, and rehydration. Int J Sports Nutr 1998;8:345–355.

148. Maughan RJ. Fluid balance and exercise. Int J Sports Med 1992;13:132S–135S.

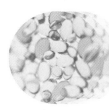

Part II
Regulation of Cell Size via Hydration Status

Research Review

Hyposmolality To Build A Better Body?

Berneis and coworkers examined the effect of acute changes in extracellular osmolality on whole body protein and glucose metabolism in 10 male subjects during conditions of hyperosmolality, hyposmolality, and isosmolality. Simply stated, they altered the hydration state of these subjects by changing the concentration of different osmotic particles in their blood. Hyperosmolality (less water and more particles in the blood) was induced by intravenously infusing a hypertonic solution of NaCl (2–5% weight/volume) and restricting fluid for 17 hours. Hyposmolality (more water and less particles in the blood) was induced by intravenously administering desmopressin (an agent that helps the body to retain water in the vascular compartment), liberal water drinking, and infusion of hypotonic saline (0.4% weight/volume). Isosmolality was induced by allowing the subjects ad libitum oral water intake. The results indicated that during conditions of hyposmolality as induced by this study, leucine release from endogenous proteins (representing protein breakdown) and leucine oxidation (representing a measure of irreversible catabolism) were decreased. In addition, the metabolic clearance rate of glucose (during hyperinsulinemic-euglycemic clamping) increased less during the hyposmolality study than during the isosmolality study. Plasma insulin decreased, while plasma nonesterified fatty acids, glycerol, ketone body concentrations, and lipid oxidation increased during the hyposmolality study. The group concluded that acute alterations of plasma osmolality influence whole body protein, glucose, and lipid metabolism and hyposmolality results in protein sparing associated with increased lipolysis and lipid oxidation and impaired insulin sensitivity. While it has been known for some time that water is important for a variety of health reasons, this is one of the first studies to show that extra water may stimulate protein synthesis. Hopefully, future research will look at whether agents such as glycerol can increase protein synthesis, since it is more readily available and doesn't require an IV infusion to work. Additionally, the longer-term effects of hyposomolality on lean body mass and performance should be investigated.

Berneis K, Ninnis R, Haussinger D, Keller U. Effects of hyper- and hypoosmolality on whole body protein and glucose kinetics in humans. Am J Physiol 1999;276:E188–E195.

Introduction

In 1993 Haussinger, Roth, Lang, and Gerok wrote an article detailing their hypothesis that cellular hydration is an important factor in health and disease.[1] Cell hydration can be influenced within minutes of exposure to amino acids, hormones, and other chemical messengers. This then leads to alterations in cell functions, including protein turnover. An increase in water influx into the cell leads to cell swelling or increased cellular hydration. The increase in cell volume acts as an anabolic signal, which causes an increase in amino acid uptake and protein synthesis. In contrast, an increase in cellular water efflux results in cell shrinkage or decreased cellular hydration. This decrease in cell volume is catabolic and decreases protein synthesis. Ion and substrate transport systems in the plasma membrane are the key factors in determining the cell's hydration state. By acting on various ion channels or influencing concentration gradients for ions, hormones, substrates, and oxidative stress can alter the cellular hydration state within minutes and indirectly affect protein turnover. It is this sequence of events that led Haussinger's group to postulate that a decrease in cellular hydration in liver and skeletal muscle triggers the protein catabolic states that accompany various diseases. More recent evidence indicates that hydration status may have health and potential performance benefits as well. The focus of this section will be to review and possibly apply the effects of altered hydration to skeletal muscle protein synthesis and performance. Because many studies have used liver cells due to their contribution to whole body protein turnover, pertinent references will also be reviewed.

Cell Volume Regulation

A basic understanding of the general principles involved in cell volume regulation is required to appropriately interpret the technical data presented in this chapter (see References 2–6 at the end of this chapter for more detailed reading on cell volume regulation.) In general, the permeability of the cellular membrane to water is high. Water movement across the membrane is influenced by both hydrostatic and effective osmotic gradients. The effective osmotic gradient across the cell membrane is determined by concentration differences across the cell membrane and the reflection coefficient for each solute. By accumulating solutes, cells are able to complete a variety of metabolic functions. The accumulation of solutes, however, results in the formation of an osmotic gradient across the cell membrane, which cells must constantly balance to avoid swelling to the point of lysis. Cells achieve this balance through the active and passive transport of ions and other molecules.

A universal cell is depicted in Figure 10-1 with the primary methods of maintaining cell volume. Three NA^+ ions are actively transported out of the cell in exchange for two K^+ ions transported into the cell. This active transport is accomplished by the Na^+/K^+-ATPase. Since the cell membrane is more permeable to K^+ then Na^+, the chemical gradient for K^+ generates a positive cell membrane potential (the extracellular environment is positive relative to the intracellular environment). Since the internal cellular environment is negative with respect to the extracellular environment, Cl^- ions are driven out of the

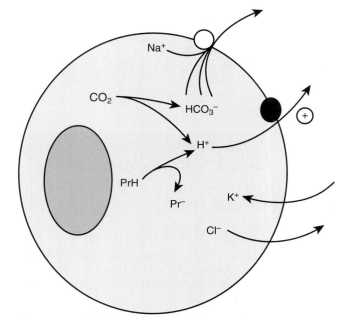

Figure 10-2. Cellular volume maintenance via H^+-ATPase. The extrusion of chloride and $Na(HCO_3^-)$ leads to the intracellular accumulation of K. (*Data from* Lang F. Cell volume regulation. Basel: Karger, 1998.)

cell. The intracellular negatively charged proteins, which have had their H^+ extruded in exchange for NA^+, are neutralized by K^+. While the Na^+/K^+ pump is the primary control for cell volume, other ion pumps can also have a role in cell volume regulation, including the H^+-ATPase, Ca^{++}-ATPase, and exocytosis. (SEE FIGURES 10-1 TO 10-3).

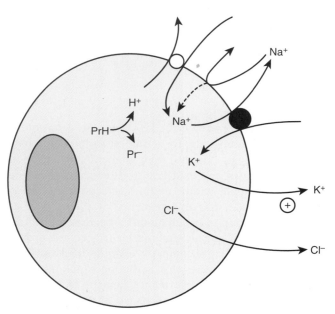

Figure 10-1. Cellular volume maintenance via the sodium–potassium ATPase pump. Sodium (Na^+) exits the cell in exchange for potassium (K^+). K movement through its channels helps drive out chloride. The Na^+–H^+ exchanger helps maintain pH slightly above 7.0. Proteins (Pr^-) help neutralize the positive charge of the intracellular K^+. (*Data from* Lang F. Cell volume regulation. Basel: Karger, 1998.)

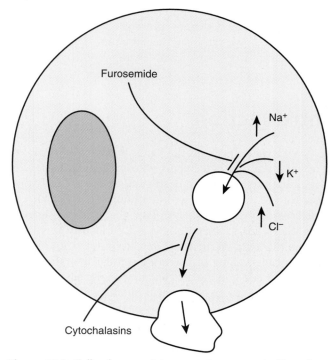

Figure 10-3. Cell volume maintenance via exocytosis. (*Data from* Lang F. Cell volume regulation. Basel: Karger, 1998.)

Regulation of Cell Volume

Cell volume is determined by factors that influence steady-state volume and mechanisms that correct acute perturbations in steady-state volume. Transporters that correct acute changes in cell volume are not usually active at steady-state volume. The current thinking is that cells establish a "set point" or steady-state volume and only activate volume regulatory transporters when cell volume deviates from this set point.[6] Cells suddenly exposed to a hypotonic environment swell. Within minutes, however, they lose most of their volume gain and almost achieve their initial cell volume. This process is called regulatory cell volume decrease. If the same cells are exposed to a hypertonic environment, they initially shrink, only to regain most of their lost volume within minutes. With this basic understanding, it should be noted that extracellular osmolarity is efficiently regulated by the body. Although extracellular osmolarity may be fairly constant, it is the difference between extra- and intracellular osmolarity that determines the cell volume.

In Vitro Studies

Hydration state is thought to be a potential factor that influences cell swelling. To test the effect of hydration state on amino acid uptake, tracer glutamine uptake into primary rat myotubes was studied at external osmolalities of 170, 320, or 430 $mOsm/kg^{-1}$.[7] An inverse relationship between myotube glutamine transport and external osmolality was found after 30 minutes of exposure. During the hyposmotic (170 $mOsm/kg^{-1}$) exposure, cell volume and glutamine transport rapidly increased. Glutamine transport increased transiently during the cell-swelling phase up to approximately 80% at 2 minutes. Glutamine uptake then declined, and after 30 minutes the steady state reflected an elevated baseline. The hyperosmotic (430 $mOsm/kg^{-1}$) exposure rapidly decreased glutamine transport and myotube cell volume by approximately 30% each, for at least 15 minutes. In this study, myotubes exposed to a hyposmotic environment initially swelled and then underwent regulatory cell volume decrease, as mentioned earlier. Despite the changes in cell volume, the myotubes continued to transport glutamine at a higher rate.[7] Glutamine uptake by rat myotubes was consistently greater during conditions of hypoosmolality. The increased glutamine uptake was Na^+ dependent and Li^+ tolerant, with additional characteristics similar to system N^m, an insulin stimulated glutamine transporter in rat skeletal muscle.[8] (It should be noted that the hyposmotic condition used in this study was far below human physiological osmolality levels of 280–320 mOsm/L). The conditions of hypoosomolality and hyperosmolality represent extreme values, with 170 and 500 $mOsm/kg^{-1}$ being the end points of the range, because ". . . beyond these limits, myotubes became dissociated from the culture wells and/or lysed."[7] When 320 $mOsm/kg^{-1}$ was used, there was no change in cell hydration. Additionally, the authors described the cell cultures as "skeletal muscle cells harvested from the thigh muscles of 1-day-old neonatal rats." The extreme conditions of osmolality used, ambiguity in specifically describing the muscle tissues sampled, and the age of the rats, present additional variables to consider when comparing and contrasting these data with future studies on the effects of osmolality.

To determine the mechanisms for cell swelling, Low et al.[9] examined the signaling elements involved in amino acid transport during altered muscle cell volume (using the same study design for cells and osmolalities). Using inhibitors for the various signaling elements involved in cell volume regulation, the group was able to show that system N^m and system A involve phosphatidylinositol 3-kinase (PI_3) but not $p70^{S6}$.[10] System N^m is an Na^+-dependent, insulin-sensitive, glutamine transporter. The signaling pathway to initiate a cell volume response involves PI_3, active G-proteins, and tyrosine kinase(s). Wortmannin (a PI_3 inhibitor), but not rapamycin (an inhibitor of $p70^{S6}$ kinase activation), prevented both the hyposmotic swelling-induced stimulation and the hyperosmotic shrinkage-induced inhibition of Na^+-dependent glutamine uptake in primary cultures of rat skeletal muscle. G-protein inhibitors (cholera, pertussis toxins) abolished the responses of glutamine transport to cell volume changes while G-protein activators (MAS 7, lysophosphatidic acid) sustained the responses. The culture medium from swollen cells had no effect on previously understimulated cells, thus indicating that swelling-induced activation of glutamine transport does not involve the release of autocrine factors. This finding is supported by in vitro work from other labs demonstrating that IGF-1 modulates cardiac myocyte proliferation, but not cellular hypertrophy,[11] and that the anabolic actions of IGF-1 on skeletal muscle burn injury are not mediated by increased cell volume.[12] System A is an Na^+-dependent, insulin-sensitive, methylaminoisobutyric acid (MeAIB) transporter. The system A amino acid transport exhibited the opposite responses to cell volume change compared with those of system Nm, and they were also blocked by wortmannin. Active PI_3 may be required to enable muscle cells to exhibit rapid, volume-induced changes in amino acid transport.[10]

Low and Taylor[13] also examined the interactions between the extracellular matrix (ECM), integrins, and the cytoskeleton as components of a mechanochemical transduction system for signaling cell volume changes in rat skeletal muscle (using the same type of cells and osmolalities). To determine the role of integrin-substratum interactions, the integrin-binding peptide GRGDTP (which inactivates integrin-substratum interactions) was compared with the inactive peptide GRGESP as a control. Neither GRGDTP nor GRGESP significantly affected basal glutamine uptake (0.05 mM; 338 ± 58 pmol min^{-1} $(mg\ protein)^{-1}$), but GRGDTP specifically prevented the hypo-osmotic increase (71%) and hyperosmotic decrease (39%) in glutamine uptake 13. The role of the cytoskeleton was assessed by disrupting the cytoskeleton with either colchicine or cytochalasin D. Colchicine and cytochalasin D prevented the increase and decrease in glutamine uptake in response to changes in external osmolality. They also increased basal glutamine uptake by 59 ± 19 and $85 \pm 16\%$, respectively, via a wortmannin-sensitive pathway. The results indicated that the ECM-integrin-mediated cell adhesion and the cytoskeleton are involved in the mechanochemical transduction of cell volume changes to chemical signals modulating glutamine transport in skeletal muscle. This anabolic pathway involves PI_3, which may act in a permissive fashion to maintain integrins in an active conformation, promoting cell adhesion.

In addition to research examining the effects of hydration state on cell volume and glutamine uptake, other studies examined the effects of hydration state on glucose metabolism glycogen synthesis.[9,10,14] Using skeletal muscle cells from the thigh muscles of 1-day-old neonatal rats, the effects of hyposmotic media (170 mOsm/kg^{-1}), isosmotic control (300 mOsm/kg^{-1}), and hyperosmotic media (430 mOsm/kg^{-1}) on [14C]glucose incorporation into glycogen (glycogen synthesis) were compared. Sixty minutes of exposure to hyposmotic media increased glycogen synthesis (by 75%, $P < 0.01$) relative to isosmotic control values, while hyperosmotic media decreased glycogen synthesis (by 31%, $P < 0.05$). Myotube 2-deoxy-D-glucose (0.05 mM) uptake was unaffected by changes in external osmolality. The PI_3 inhibitor, wortmannin, decreased basal glycogen synthesis by 28%, whereas rapamycin, the $p70^{S6}$ inhibitor, had no effect. Both wortmannin and rapamycin blocked the changes in glycogen synthesis resulting from hypo- and hyperosmotic exposure. These results provide evidence that myotube glycogen synthesis is modulated by volume changes independently of changes in glucose uptake. The role of this phenomenon is speculated to be physiologically important in promoting glycogen storage during circumstances of myofibrillar swelling, e.g., after feeding or exercise.[14]

The involvement of ECM-integrin interactions in glycogen synthesis were also investigated using the previous study design (in terms of cells and hydration states).[9] The integrin binding peptide GRGDTP was used to disrupt integrin actions and the inactive analogue GRGESP served as a control, while glycogen synthesis was measured by the D-[14C]glucose incorporation into glycogen. Glycogen synthesis was increased by hyposmolality (77%) and decreased (34%) by hyperosmolality. Both volume-stimulated changes were prevented by GRGDTP, but not GRGESP, and neither affected glucose transport. The cytoskeletal disruptors cytochalasin D and colchicine prevented changes in glycogen synthesis induced by osmolality. The osmotically induced modulation of mus-

cle glycogen synthesis involves ECM-integrin interactions and cytoskeletal elements, possibly as components of a cell-volume 'sensing' mechanism.[9]

The effects of hyperosmolarity on adipose tissue have also been studied.[15–17] In vitro studies have shown that the addition of NaCl to an incubation solution decreases the rate of fatty acid mobilization or lipolysis.[15,18] These effects are not mediated by impairments in the hormone-receptor interactions, as the ability of ACTH to increase cAMP levels in adipocytes is enhanced by hyperosmolarity.[16] Despite the increased accumulation of cAMP in adipocytes, lipolysis was decreased (it would be expected to increase). Therefore, the mechanism of inhibition of lipolysis must have occurred after the hormone-receptor, binding-initiated, intracellular signaling events that led to increased cAMP levels. The effects of glucagon on cAMP levels are also enhanced during hyperosmolarity, although to a lesser degree than ACTH.[16] Other in vitro models are used to better understand the impairment of glucose utilization in diabetics during the hyperosmolar state.[17] Rat epididymal fat pads and diaphragms were used to evaluate the effects of hyperosmolality on basal and insulin-dependent glucose uptake. NaCl-induced hyperosmolality (400 mOsm/kg^{-1}) diminished basal and insulin-stimulated glucose uptake by 35 and 90%, while urea (500 mOsm/kg^{-1}) decreased the same parameters by 29 and 68%. The in vitro data support the clinical contention that a hyperosmolal state, which corresponds to a loss of fluid in excess of solutes, is able to impair basal glucose use and hormone action on glucose metabolism.[16,17]

Although the focus of this chapter is the effects of hydration on protein synthesis in skeletal muscle and body composition, the effects of hydration on other tissues should not be overlooked. Numerous cell types and tissues have been the focus of research on hydration-induced volume changes.[6] Erythrocytes, lymphocytes, renal epithelia, nervous, mesenchymal, cardiovascular, and gastrointestinal tissues have been studied. On the whole, this indicates the potential far-reaching consequences of hydration state on the health of the individual. It should be noted that the changes in cell volume in vivo occur in an isosmotic environment. It is the differences between intra- and extracellular concentrations of osmotic particles that determines the osmotic forces the cell is exposed to. Returning to the original focus of this chapter, the previous data set up a role for hydration state (as determined by changes in osmolality) to influence muscle cell size. Several amino acid transporters in skeletal muscle (and heart) have been identified. These "systems" include A, ASC, N^m, L, and ^{X-}AG.[19–22] Of these systems, the amino acid transporters A and N^m appear to play a role in cell volume regulation. System A is downregulated by a cell volume increase (swelling) and may serve as a regulatory volume decrease mechanism.[14] System N^m is upregulated by swelling and acts as a component of a positive feedback (or feedforward) mechanism, promoting anabolism in proportion to nutrient supply.[14] System N^m is important to study in more detail because of its greater role in anabolism.

Most of the research thus far has used rat skeletal muscles cells to study cell volume changes and system N^m, so similarities and differences between the rat system N^m and the human system N^m should be addressed. In both rats and humans, these transporters are substrate specific for glutamine, asparagine, histidine, and 3-methyl histidine. Both are also Na^+ dependent, tolerant of Li^+-for-Na^+ substitution, rheogenic, stimulated by insulin to take up substrate, and stimulated by corticosteroid to efflux substrate.[19–23] Kinetic differences between these transporters distinguish rat and human system N^m. The human counterpart is pH sensitive, has Na^+-independent glutamine uptake, and has a K_m value (Michaelis constant—the substrate concentration at which an enzyme-catalyzed reaction proceeds at one-half maximum velocity) closer to plasma glutamine concentrations.[22] Glutamine transport kinetics also differ between tissues, possibly due to differences in fiber types or intracellular glutamine concentrations. The practical significance of near-plasma glutamine concentrations for the K_m of glutamine indicates that the intramuscular glutamine pool may be modulated by changes in human plasma glutamine concentrations.

Looking at the literature on hydration status and protein synthesis, a number of similarities is noted between different cell types.[6,24,25] Liver cells have received a great deal of attention, revealing that hydration can influence protein turnover,[26] glycogen synthesis,[27,28] and lipogenesis.[29] Protein synthesis in mammary tissue is also acutely regulated by hydration state.[30] These functional similarities in response to alterations of the hydration state are often mirrored by activation of similar intracellular signaling pathways. Caution should be taken when applying pathways identified in one cell type with other cell types. Nevertheless, to understand the potential ways in which cell volume may be altered in skeletal muscle cells, a brief review of the different identified signaling pathways is necessary.

Cell swelling leads to dilution of macromolecules, while cell shrinkage leads to concentration (crowding) of macromolecules. The macromolecular crowding theory postulates that the thermodynamic activity of proteins in a solution in which unreactive macromolecules are present exceeds the activity of that species at an identical concentration in an uncrowded fluid.[31–35] The cell volume-sensing role for macromolecular crowding is based upon the presence of large molecules and the cytoskeleton crowding the intracellular environment and that changes in the thermodynamic activity of enzymes (i.e., effector proteins) can alter the transport and/or permeability of targeted transporters and/or channels.[36] Testing of this theory has yet to be reported for human skeletal muscle; however, there is published information for barnacle muscle.[37] The researchers chose this preparation because it

allowed them to study the effects of changes in intracellular macromolecular concentration and size on the cell volume while maintaining constant ionic strength, membrane stretch, and osmolality. The results demonstrated that isotonic replacement of large macromolecules by smaller molecules induced volume decreases proportional to the initial macromolecular concentration and size, as well as to the magnitude of the concentration reduction. Although the results tend to support the various contentions of the theory, it should be noted that while large macromolecules may exert an effect on cell volume at physiological concentrations, smaller molecules are ineffective even at concentrations many times greater than the physiological range.[37]

Cell swelling or shrinkage can affect the cytoskeletal architecture. A variety of cell types have been studied, at the exclusion of skeletal muscle.[25] In general, actin filaments are found to depolarize after cell swelling.[38,39] This effect may be due to increased intracellular Ca^{++} concentrations after osmotic swelling leading to binding of Ca^{++} to gelsolin and resulting in actin depolymerization.[40] Actin filaments may be also be depolymerized by phosphatidylinositol 4,5-bisphosphate, an inhibitor of depolymerization, by interacting with profilin.[41,42] Transient depolymerization of actin may lead to polymerization of actin filaments, as in the case of hepatocytes.[43,44] Alterations in actin or other cytoskeletal elements may affect volume-regulatory elements. These cytoskeletal elements may regulate specific Na^+ [45,46] and K^+ [47] channels, insert cell volume regulatory channels into the plasma membrane,[48,49] regulate kinases[50,51] and phospholipids,[52] activate anion channels,[53,54] regulate activity of the Na^+–H^+ exchanger,[55,56] and mediate gene expression.[57] While many of these cytoskeletal signaling elements have been identified in cardiac muscle, confirmation of these potential pathways in skeletal muscle is necessary. For a more detailed review of cytoskeletal mechnotransduction the reader is referred to a review by Ingber.[58]

Other intracellular signaling pathways involve cell membrane stretch, cell membrane potential, cytosolic pH, Ca^{++}, G proteins, protein phosphorylation, Cl^-, Mg^{++}, eicosanoids, pH changes in cellular compartments, and gene expression.[25] As in the case of the cytoskeletal signaling elements, confirmation of these potential pathways in skeletal muscle is necessary, but speculated to exist based upon functional similarities between skeletal muscles cells and other cells (i.e., liver and cardiac).

Animal Studies

Various in vitro studies have shown the role of hydration and the nutritional state to influence proteolysis in liver cells.[1,24,59–63] Data from in vivo studies on the effects of hydration on protein synthesis are limited to the rat liver.[64] The effects of amino acids, glucagon, insulin, and cell volume during development (development versus 7 days versus 21 day versus adult) and after an overnight fast were studied. After feeding, glucagon levels were highest in suckling animals and gradually declined in older rats, whereas the insulin concentrations increased during development. Liver and plasma amino acid concentrations declined during the suckling period to in vitro levels that are permissive for the induction of autophagic proteolysis. Fasting was associated with a drop in hepatic protein content and significant decrease in hepatocellular volume and insulin concentrations for all of the age groups investigated. In perinatal and suckling animals, fasting decreased glucagon and many of the amino acids in plasma and liver. This response became blunted at weaning and disappeared in adult animals. These findings suggest that insulin and/or hepatocellular volume may be more important short-term physiological regulators of the hepatic nitrogen balance than glucagon or amino acids, and that cell volume is the more important factor.[64] The results also indicated that to maintain hepatic protein synthesis and minimize proteolysis, suckling animals have to be fed throughout a daily interval.

The similarities between the human transport system N^m (in skeletal muscle) and the rat system N (in liver),[22] and the fact that both are the predominant cell volume–regulated amino acid transporters in their respective tissues, suggests a similar effect of hydration in these tissues. Logically, from all the in vitro data on changes in the hydration state, it would make sense to maximize the hydration state of skeletal muscle for performance. To date, there are no in vivo animal data on the effects of hydration on skeletal muscle and/or performance. One could speculate that given the positive effects of an increased hydration state on hepatic tissue, increased hydration of skeletal muscle would result in increased recovery from the stress of resistance, sprint, and endurance exercise.

The ability to oxidize fatty acids for fuel is important in terms of both exercise and body composition. The effects of hyperosmolality on lipolysis were studied using mongrel dogs.[65] An injection of 50 mL of 20% sterile NaCl solution (171 mE/l Na^+ and 171 mE/l Cl^-) was administered to three dogs, elevating the mean plasma Na^+ concentrations from 149 mE/l to 160–170 mE/l. Mean plasma osmolality increased from 310 mOsm/kg^{-1} to 347 mOsm/kg^{-1}. Prior to the injection, plasma levels of free fatty acids (FFAs) were constant. After the injection, FFA plasma levels declined for the succeeding 2 hours. In another experiment reported in the same paper, six dogs received a 5 µg/kg/min noradrenaline (norepinephrine) infusion to enhance the rate of lipolysis and increase the concentration of free fatty acids in the blood. This increased plasma FFAs from about 0.3 mE/l to 2–3 mE/l. Three of the dogs received an injection of the NaCl solution described earlier and, for 2 hours postinjection, their FFA levels decreased sharply. The other three dogs received a constant infusion of hypertonic 20% NaCl. FFA levels

declined in response to the constant infusion, although more gradually than after the 50-mL injection. Collectively, these experiments demonstrate that induced hyperosmolality depresses norepinephrine-induced lipolysis. The data do not allow for the distinction between the effects of hypertonic saline versus hyperosmolality in general. They do, however, indicate that during periods of hyperosmolality, normal fat metabolism may be depressed, forcing the body to resort to other fuel sources, such as protein.

Data from perfused cat calf muscle indicate that increases in plasma volume induced by hypertonic fluids may come entirely at the expense of cell volume, not interstitial volume.[66] Combined with the animal data above, the effects of increased osmolality (i.e., hyperosmolality) in the blood result in decreased cell volumes leading to increased proteolysis and decreased lipolysis. These effects are exactly the opposite of what most athletes are hoping to achieve in terms of improved body composition and performance. They also raise serious questions regarding the prudence of weight reduction strategies used in weight class sports, in which extreme calorie restriction and dehydration are often used to make weight.

Human Studies

A close relationship between whole-body nitrogen balance and cellular hydration state of skeletal muscle was reported for healthy subjects and patients.[1] The authors postulated that protein wasting in critically ill patients was due in part to decreased cellular hydration in skeletal muscle and liver. The profound loss of body protein that occurs in critically ill patients is triggered and maintained by cell shrinkage secondary to cellular dehydration. While the pathogenetic mechanisms of cell volume control may be heterogeneous and multifactorial in nature, the cellular hydration state represents a unique and potentially useful target for influencing whole-body protein synthesis. This has broad potential applications not only in the clinical realm where it was initially discussed, but also in improving health and performance in the nonclinical settings.

Changes in intracellular water, total body protein, total body potassium, and intracellular potassium were measured in patients receiving intensive care for blunt trauma or sepsis.[67] Patients from an intensive care unit (9 with multiple blunt traumas and 11 with severe sepsis) were studied for 21 days. Total body water was assessed using tritium dilution and extracellular water was assessed using bromide dilution. The difference between the two and bioimpedance spectroscopy were used to calculate intracellular water. Whole-body neutron activation analysis was used to measure total body protein and whole-body counting was used to measure total body potassium. Over the 21-day study period, intracellular water decreased by 15–20%, total body protein by 15%, and total body potassium by about 20%. Intracellular potassium concentration did not change, and was similar to that in healthy adult volunteers. Sequential measurements of the ratio of potassium to protein in the lost tissue indicated that cells were losing water in quantities greater than would be expected from protein losses in these patients. In major trauma or sepsis, the loss of protein and potassium from body stores is accompanied by progressive cellular dehydration. Limiting the loss of body protein in critically ill patients is important to maintaining health. These data support the findings[1] that hydration state is an important determinant of health during disease.

Thus far, only the effects of disease-induced decreases in hydration state have been investigated in humans. These data indicate the importance of maintaining the cellular hydration state during disease, but does not indicate what happens during an increase in hydration state. Approaching the effects of hydration state from another perspective, how can osmolality influence protein and glucose metabolism in healthy people? To address this question, 10 male subjects were studied during conditions of hyperosmolality, isosmolality, and hyposmolality. (See Research Review—Hyposmolality To Build A Better Body?) This study is the first to examine the acute effects of osmolality on whole-body protein and glucose metabolism in humans. Hyposmolality conditions resulted in normal protein synthesis rates and a decrease in protein breakdown, thus indicating a net protein synthesis. No differences were noted for an effect of hyperosmolality on protein metabolism. Baseline measurements for protein metabolism calculations were obtained after a 5-hour fast, while treatment measurements were obtained after a 12-hour fast. It is conceivable that the different fasting periods influenced the study results. In addition, although changes in net water balance were induced by the hyposmolar treatment, no changes in water balance were found during the hyperosmolality treatment. Endogenous glucose production was increased by hyperosmolality and decreased during hyposmolality. Exogenous glucose clearance was decreased during hyposmolality, indicating decreased insulin sensitivity of peripheral glucose metabolism. The decrease in insulin sensitivity may have masked increases in protein synthesis and/or allowed increases in fatty acid oxidation. Lipolysis was increased during hyposmolality, despite no changes in catecholamine levels. Glycerol, acetoacetate, and β-hydroxybutyrate levels were significantly elevated during hyposmolality. An increase in the oxidation of lipid substrates and ketone body concentrations may induce a protein-sparing effect.[68] The 17-hour study did not measure cell volume, so the direct effects of changes in osmolality on cell volume could not be assessed. The authors concluded that hyposmolality exerts a protein and glucose-sparing effect with increased use of fat.[69]

The effects of osmolality on lipolysis were investigated in another study from the same group using a similar experimental design.[70] Changes in extracellular osmolality are assumed to alter the cellular hydration state and appear to directly influence cell metabolism. The metabolic changes associated with cell swelling lead to the inhibition of glycogenolysis, glycolysis, and proteolysis. Because of the close interrelationship between carbohydrate and fat metabolism, the investigators speculated that adipose tissue lipolysis and fatty acid oxidation are regulated by changes in extracellular osmolality. The intravenous administration of desmopressin, the liberal ingestion of water, and an infusion of hypotonic (0.45%) saline solution induced hyposmolality in seven healthy young men. Lipolysis was assessed using a stable-isotope method (2-[13C]-glycerol infusion). The glycerol rate of appearance, reflecting whole-body lipolysis, was higher under hyposmolar (2.35 ± 0.40 μmol/kg/min) compared with isosmolar conditions (1.68 ± 0.21 μmol/kg/min, $P = .03$). Hyperinsulinemia and euglycemic clamping resulted in a more pronounced suppression of lipolysis (0.90 ± 0.08 versus 0.61 ± 0.03 μmol/kg/min, respectively, $P = .002$). Indirect calorimetry measurements of plasma free fatty acids, glycerol, ketone bodies, insulin and glucagon concentrations, and carbohydrate and lipid oxidation revealed no significant effects of hyposmolality. Surprisingly, plasma norepinephrine concentrations were lower under hyposmolar conditions ($P = 0.01$ versus control). The investigators concluded that in vivo hyposmolality results in increased whole-body lipolysis, which is not due to changes in major hormones regulating lipolysis.[70]

This study reported similar changes in plasma Na^+ and osmolality in the subjects as the previous study. In the Berneis et al. study, hyposmolality increased plasma concentrations of glycerol, acetoacetate, and β-hydroxybutyrate while lowering insulin. In the present study, no changes were found in these plasma variables after hyposmolality. The rate of appearance of glycerol increased and the plasma concentration of norepinephrine decreased. The low number of subjects (10 in the Berneis et al. study, 7 in the Bilz et al. study) may have skewed the results in either study, thus making interpretation of the results more difficult. Both studies conclude that hyposmolality increases lipolysis, although the basis for each conclusion is derived from different variables (increased glycerol and ketones versus increased glycerol rate of appearance).

In another study by a different lab, the acute effects of graded increases in plasma volume (PV) on substrate turnover and oxidation during exercise were studied.[71] In this experiment, dextran, a plasma expander, was used. Eight untrained males cycled for 2 hours at approximately 46% of VO_{2peak} on three occasions in a randomized order, after plasma volume expansions of 0, 14, and 21%. Glucose turnover was measured using primed continuous infusions of [6,6-2H2]glucose. Glycerol turnover was measured using primed continuous infusions of [2H5]glycerol. The glycerol rate of appearance was measured as a relative index of whole body lipolysis. Glucose, glycerol rate of appearance, and glycerol rate of disappearance were similar after all plasma volume increases. The effects were consistent at rest and during exercise. Total lipolysis during exercise was reduced during the 14% increase in plasma volume. An increase of plasma volume to 21% had no additional effect on whole-body lipolysis. No effect of hypervolemia was observed on whole-body fat or carbohydrate oxidation. The researchers concluded that acute PV expansion could alter whole-body lipolysis, possibly via a reduction in catecholamine secretion.[71]

Blood osmolality levels in this study and plasma volume levels in the previous studies were not reported; therefore, comparison between them is difficult. Differences in the use of hydration agents (desmopressin versus dextran), plasma osmolality, and/or plasma volume may explain the discrepancies in lipolysis results. Increases in plasma volume through the use of dextran have resulted in reduced muscle lactate during prolonged exercise[72] and improved cycling performance.[73] The improvements in exercise performance appear to be related to the increase in plasma volume as opposed to the use of dextran.[73] However, exercise-induced plasma volume expansion is associated with a catabolic state due to a decrease in intracellular water and increase in extracellular fluid.[74] Assuming treatment with dextran does not also decrease intracellular fluid, it would appear to have an advantage over exercise-induced plasma expansion by increasing performance without increasing protein catabolism. The interrelationships between plasma volume, plasma osmolarity, substrate turnover, body composition, physical performance, and in vivo changes in cell volume will provide exciting research opportunities in the coming years.

Safety and Toxicity

Adequate fluid consumption without the use of plasma-expanding agents is the first approach to improving performance. Because the renal system is efficient and capable of regulating blood volume levels, there are no safety or toxicity concerns and liberal fluid ingestion should be encouraged. In the event that hydrating agents are used,

Current Controversy:
Cell Volume Regulation

Magazine readers are bombarded by advertisements for gaining muscle via cell volume regulation. Creatine, glutamine, taurine, alpha lipoic acid, and many other supplements are touted to increase cell size. Human studies have shown favorable effects of creatine on body composition, exercise performance, and/or nitrogen balance. However, in vivo data are lacking for most of the other supplements. Supplement companies rely on in vitro data and weak relationships to support their advertising claims. At the heart of these claims is the contention that all of these supplements increase cell volume or swelling. Cell volume regulation is currently a hot topic in research. Numerous factors have been shown to influence cell volume. In general, most of the published studies focused on the use of a single agent to alter the swelling state of skeletal muscle or other cells. For example, Low et al. studied the effects of cell volume on glutamine uptake. They did not study the combined effects of glutamine and taurine or glutamine and alpha lipoic acid. This is important to note because one common assumption is that the simultaneous intake of a variety of supplements will result in a synergistic effect, leading to greater increases in cell swelling. Several flaws exist with this assumption. The first is that the swelling is permanent. Most in vitro studies on cell swelling have been for 2 hours or less,

hardly sufficient to indicate if the effects are permanent. Second, and perhaps more important, is the substrate specificity of the transporter. As discussed in the section on in vitro studies, transporters are fairly specific and differentially influenced by cell swelling. Although an increase in cell volume may trigger glutamine uptake via system N[m] in skeletal muscle, system A is downregulated. The transport of alanine and methionine may be decreased. While the intracellular concentration of amino acids may increase during cell swelling and initiate protein synthesis, downregulation of transporters and ion channels may result in rate-limiting amounts of other ingredients. So, although research on the potential to influence the cell volume of skeletal muscle is exciting right now, realize that there are safety valves to prevent the uncontrolled swelling that would result in cell lysis.

Low SY, Rennie MJ, et al. Modulation of glycogen synthesis in rat skeletal muscle by changes in cell volume. J Physiol (Lond) 1996;495:299–303.

Low SY, Rennie MJ, et al. Signaling elements involved in amino acid transport responses to altered muscle cell volume. FASEB J 1997;11:1111–1117.

Low SY, Taylor PM. Integrin and cytoskeletal involvement in signalling cell volume changes to glutamine transport in rat skeletal muscle. J Physiol (Lond) 1998;512:481–485.

such as excessive Na^+, desmopressin, glycerol, or dextran, there would be some potential safety and toxicity concerns. Excessive fluid retention could lead to edema if uncontrolled, with particular concern for effects on the brain.

Plasma volume increases from dextran have resulted in increased left ventricular end diastolic volume, increased stroke volume, and increased cardiac output.[75,76] Central venous pressure was noted to increase by 2.1–3.0 mm Hg.[75] Given the cardiovascular effects, hypertensive

individuals, and those exposed to states of increased cardiovascular load (i.e., pregnancy, edema) should contact a physician before attempting to alter their hydration state. Additionally, the swelling of muscle cells may result in the release of enzymes or other important cellular factors by making the cell membrane more permeable.[77] This last concern may be more dependent on the concentration gradient for the specific cellular factor as opposed to swelling in general.

SUMMARY

In the past few years, the importance of cell volume for the regulation of cell function, including substrate metabolism, has been established. To survive, cells have to avoid excessive alterations of cell volume that jeopardize their structural integrity and the constancy of their intracellular milieu. Even at constant extracellular osmolarity, volume constancy of any mammalian cell is permanently challenged by the transport of osmotically active substances across the cell membrane and the formation or disappearance of cellular osmolarity by metabolism. Cell swelling inhibits proteolysis, glycolysis, and glycogenolysis and stimulates protein synthesis and glycogenesis. Conversely, cell shrinkage stimulates proteolysis and inhibits protein synthesis. A decrease in cell volume correlates with catabolic states in a variety of diseases. Thus, cell volume constancy requires the continued operation of cell volume regulatory mechanisms, including ion transport across the cell membrane, as well as the accumulation or disposal of organic osmolytes and metabolites. The functions of

cellular proteins appear specifically sensitive to dilution and concentration. The various cell volume regulatory mechanisms are triggered by a multitude of intracellular signaling events, including alterations of cell membrane potential and of intracellular ion composition, various second-messenger cascades, phosphorylation of diverse target proteins, and altered gene expression. Hormones exploit the influence of cell volume on metabolism to exert their effects. Thus, cell volume may be considered a second message in the transmission of hormonal signals. Accordingly, alterations of cell volume and volume-regulatory mechanisms participate in a variety of cellular functions, including substrate metabolism. Recent research has shown the potential of plasma osmolality to influence protein, carbohydrate, and lipid metabolism, with conflicting results reported for lipolysis. Other studies have reported that increases in plasma volume improve cycling performance by decreasing the amount of time to reach the goal.

AUTHOR'S RECOMMENDATIONS

Certainly, adequate hydration is important for a variety of reasons. Focusing more on the topics reviewed in this chapter, we find that states of hyperhydration can potentially increase whole-body net protein synthesis, whole-body lipolysis, and cycling performance. The question is how can we achieve these effects safely without putting ourselves at risk? It seems that the addition of glutamine to a commercial sports drink may be beneficial. I would also speculate at this time (based on data not reviewed in this chapter) that ribose and branched-chain amino acids should be included in this drink. Glycerol and Na^+ are the two most readily available hydrating agents. The long-term consumption of excessive Na^+ is a concern for long-term blood

pressure control. Although I think glycerol ingestion can have some acute benefits for bodybuilders and athletes, I am hesitant to recommend it for long-term consumption. There are not enough data on the effects of glycerol or dextran-induced hyperhydration on protein synthesis. The acute research available so far indicates that glycerol, dextran, and desmopressin are safe, but longer-term studies are needed to verify that there are no functional impairments in renal function or other side effects. For now I recommend a drink that contains glucose, Na^+, K^+, and glutamine. The more ambitious athletes can add branched-chain amino acids, taurine, glycerol, creatine, and ribose.

FUTURE RESEARCH

The in vitro studies examining the effects of osmolarity on skeletal muscle cell volume have used cells from rats and barnacles. Additionally, the osmolality of the extracellular environment used to induce cell volume changes in myocytes is often beyond normal human physiological ranges. Many of the in vitro studies kept extracellular conditions constant for an extended period of time (i.e., 60 minutes), which is not representative of in vivo conditions. Muscle cells from healthy humans (or at least healthy skeletal muscle tissue) would allow for more pertinent research to be performed. The use of perfusion preparations where the osmolarity of the extracellular environment could be altered according to in vivo conditions (i.e., postprandial states) may allow for more applicable information to be obtained.

The explanations given for cell volume alterations are often mergers of research from different cell lines (i.e., hepatocytes, red blood cells, white blood cells, skeletal muscle cells, and smooth muscle cells). The in vitro work has yet to demonstrate an increase in contractile protein synthesis. Future work using markers and/or inhibitors for intracellular signaling agents should be applied to a single cell type (i.e., human skeletal muscle cells).

Recent research has shown the potential of plasma osmolality to influence protein, carbohydrate, and lipid metabolism, with conflicting results reported for lipolysis. Future research should address differences in the effects of hydrating agents (i.e., glycerol, dextran, desmopressin, Na^+), incorporate larger numbers of subjects, and assess the direct effects of hydration status on skeletal muscle and physical performance. Long-term data on renal function and data on endogenous androgen, estrogen, and growth hormone production are lacking. Studies addressing these shortcomings in the literature can increase the current body of knowledge and add to the understanding of the interactions between cell volume and hormone function.

REFERENCES

1. Haussinger D, Roth E, et al. Cellular hydration state: an important determinant of protein catabolism in health and disease. Lancet 1993;341:1330–1332.
2. Beyenbach KW. Cell volume regulation. Basel: Karger, 1990.
3. Strange K. Cellular and molecular physiology of cell volume regulation. Boca Raton: CRC Press, 1994.
4. Lang F. Cell volume regulation. Basel: Karger, 1998.
5. Okada, Y. Cell volume regulation: the molecular mechanism and volume sensing machinery. In: Proceedings of the 23rd Taniguichi Foundation Biophysics Symposium held in Okazaki, Japan, 17–21 November, 1997. Amsterdam: Elsevier, 1998.
6. O'Neill WC. Physiological significance of volume-regulatory transporters. Am J Physiol 1999;276:C995–C1011.
7. Low SY, Taylor PM, et al. Responses of glutamine transport in cultured rat skeletal muscle to osmotically induced changes in cell volume. J Physiol (Lond) 1996;492:877–885.
8. Tadros LB, Taylor PM, et al. Characteristics of glutamine transport in primary tissue culture of rat skeletal muscle. Am J Physiol 1993;265:E135–E144.
9. Low SY, Rennie MJ, et al. Involvement of integrins and the cytoskeleton in modulation of skeletal muscle glycogen synthesis by changes in cell volume. FEBS Lett 1997;417:101–103.
10. Low SY, Rennie MJ, et al. Signaling elements involved in amino acid transport responses to altered muscle cell volume. FASEB J 1997;11:1111–1117.
11. Kajstura J, Cheng W, et al. The IGF-1 receptor system modulates myocyte proliferation but not myocyte cellular hypertrophy in vitro. Exp Cell Res 1994;215:273–283.
12. Fang CH, Li BG, et al. The anabolic effects of IGF-1 in skeletal muscle after burn injury are not caused by increased cell volume. J Parenter Enteral Nutr 1998;22:115–119.
13. Low SY, Taylor PM. Integrin and cytoskeletal involvement in signalling cell volume changes to glutamine transport in rat skeletal muscle. J Physiol (Lond) 1998;512:481–485.
14. Low SY, Rennie MJ, et al. Modulation of glycogen synthesis in rat skeletal muscle by changes in cell volume. J Physiol (Lond) 1996;495:299–303.
15. Kuzuya T, Samols E, et al. Stimulation by hyperosmolarity of glucose metabolism in rat adipose tissue and diaphragm in vitro. J Biol Chem 1965;240:2277–2283.
16. Wada M, Akanuma Y, et al. Effects of hyperosmolarity on the cyclic AMP concentration and lipolysis of the adipocyte stimulated by adrenocorticotropic hormone. Endocrinology 1976;98:84–90.
17. Komjati M, Kastner G, et al. Detrimental effect of hyperosmolality on insulin-stimulated glucose metabolism in adipose and muscle tissue in vitro. Biochem Med Metab Biol 1988;39:312–318.
18. Jeanrenaud B. Adipose tissue dynamics and regulation, revisited. Ergeb Physiol 1968;60:57–140.
19. Hundal HS, Rennie MJ, et al. Characteristics of L-glutamine transport in perfused rat skeletal muscle. J Physiol (Lond) 1987;393:283–305.
20. Hundal HS, Rennie MJ, et al. Characteristics of acidic, basic and neutral amino acid transport in the perfused rat hindlimb. J Physiol (Lond) 1989;408:93–114.
21. Ahmed A, Gibson JN, et al. Isolation of human skeletal muscle sarcolemmal vesicles for the investigation of glutamine transport. Biochem Soc Trans 1990;18:1238–1239.
22. Ahmed A, Maxwell DL, et al. Glutamine transport in human skeletal muscle. Am J Physiol 1993;264: E993–1000.
23. Ahmed A, Taylor PM, et al. Characteristics of glutamine transport in sarcolemmal vesicles from rat skeletal muscle. Am J Physiol 1990;259:E284–291.
24. Haussinger D, Lang F, et al. Regulation of cell function by the cellular hydration state. Am J Physiol 1994;267:E343–355.
25. Lang F, Busch GL, et al. Functional significance of cell volume regulatory mechanisms. Physiol Rev 1998;78:247–306.
26. Stoll B, Gerok W, et al. Liver cell volume and protein synthesis. Biochem J 1992;287:217–222.
27. al-Habori M, Peak M, et al. The role of cell swelling in the stimulation of glycogen synthesis by insulin. Biochem J 1992;282:789–796.
28. Peak M, al-Habori M, et al. Regulation of glycogen synthesis and glycolysis by insulin, pH and cell volume: interactions between swelling and alkalinization in mediating the effects of insulin. Biochem J 1992;282:797–805.
29. Baquet A, Lavoinne A, et al. Comparison of the effects of various amino acids on glycogen synthesis, lipogenesis and ketogenesis in isolated rat hepatocytes. Biochem J 1991;273:57–62.
30. Millar ID, Barber MC, et al. Mammary protein synthesis is acutely regulated by the cellular hydration state. Biochem Biophys Res Commun 1997;230:351–355.
31. Minton AP, Wilf J. Effect of macromolecular crowding upon the structure and function of an enzyme: glyceraldehyde-3-phosphate dehydrogenase. Biochemistry 1981;20:4821–4826.
32. Wilf J, Minton AP. Evidence for protein self-association induced by excluded volume: myoglobin in the presence of globular proteins. Biochim Biophys Acta 1981;670:316–322.

33. Minton AP. The effect of volume occupancy upon the thermodynamic activity of proteins: some biochemical consequences. Mol Cell Biochem 1983;55:119–140.

34. Minton AP. Macromolecular crowding and molecular recognition. J Mol Recognit 1993;6:211–214.

35. Zimmerman SB, Minton AP. Macromolecular crowding: biochemical, biophysical, and physiological consequences. Annu Rev Biophys Biomol Struct 1993;22:27–65.

36. Minton AP, Colclasure GC, et al. Model for the role of macromolecular crowding in regulation of cellular volume [published erratum appears in Proc Natl Acad Sci USA 1993 Feb 1;90(3):1137]. Proc Natl Acad Sci USA 1992;89:10504–10506.

37. Summers JC, Trais L, et al. Role of concentration and size of intracellular macromolecules in cell volume regulation. Am J Physiol 1997;273:C360–370.

38. Cornet M, Isobe Y, et al. Effects of anisoosmotic conditions on the cytoskeletal architecture of cultured PC12 cells. J Morphol 1994; 222:269–286.

39. Cornet M, Lambert IH, et al. Relation between cytoskeleton, hypoosmotic treatment and volume regulation in Ehrlich ascites tumor cells. J Membr Biol 1993;131:55–66.

40. Weber K, Osborn M. Cytoskeleton: definition, structure and gene regulation. Pathol Res Pract 1982;175:128–145.

41. Lassing I, Lindberg U. Specific interaction between phosphatidylinositol 4,5-bisphosphate and profilactin. Nature 1985;314:472–474.

42. Lassing I, Lindberg U. Specificity of the interaction between phosphatidylinositol 4,5-bisphosphate and the profilactin complex. J Cell Biochem 1988;37:255–267.

43. Schulz WA, Eickelmann P, et al. Increase of beta-actin mRNA upon hypotonic perfusion of perfused rat liver. FEBS Lett 1991;292:264–266.

44. Theodoropoulos PA, Stournaras C, et al. Hepatocyte swelling leads to rapid decrease of the G-/total actin ratio and increases actin mRNA levels. FEBS Lett 1992;311:241–245.

45. Berdiev BK, Prat AG, et al. Regulation of epithelial sodium channels by short actin filaments. J Biol Chem 1996;271:17704–17710.

46. Ismailov, II, B. K. Berdiev, et al. Role of actin in regulation of epithelial sodium channels by CFTR. Am J Physiol 1997;272:C1077–1086.

47. Grinstein S, Cohen S, et al. Induction of 86Rb fluxes by Ca2+ and volume changes in thymocytes and their isolated membranes. J Cell Physiol 1983;116:352–362.

48. Lewis SA, de Moura JL. Incorporation of cytoplasmic vesicles into apical membrane of mammalian urinary bladder epithelium. Nature 1982;297:685–688.

49. Foskett JK, Spring KR. Involvement of calcium and cytoskeleton in gallbladder epithelial cell volume regulation. Am J Physiol 1985;248:C27–36.

50. Watson PA. Accumulation of cAMP and calcium in S49 mouse lymphoma cells following hyposmotic swelling. J Biol Chem 1989;264: 14735–14740.

51. Tilly BC, van den Berghe N, et al. Protein tyrosine phosphorylation is involved in osmoregulation of ionic conductances. J Biol Chem 1993;268:19919–19922.

52. Song D, O'Regan MH, et al. Amino acid release during volume regulation by cardiac cells: cellular mechanisms. Eur J Pharmacol 1998;341:273–280.

53. Tseng GN. Cell swelling increases membrane conductance of canine cardiac cells: evidence for a volume-sensitive Cl channel. Am J Physiol 1992;262:C1056–1068.

54. Yamamoto Y, Suzuki H. Two types of stretch-activated channel activities in guinea-pig gastric smooth muscle cells. Jpn J Physiol 1996; 46:337–345.

55. Wakabayashi S, Bertrand B, et al. Growth factor activation and "H(+)-sensing" of the Na+/H+ exchanger isoform 1 (NHE1): evidence for an additional mechanism not requiring direct phosphorylation. J Biol Chem 1994;269:5583–5588.

56. Wakabayashi S, Fafournoux P, et al. The Na+/H+ antiporter cytoplasmic domain mediates growth factor signals and controls "H(+)-sensing." Proc Natl Acad Sci USA 1992;89:2424–2428.

57. Shoemaker SD, Ryan AF, et al. Transcript-specific mRNA trafficking based on the distribution of coexpressed myosin isoforms. Cells Tissues Organs 1999;165:10–15.

58. Ingber DE. Tensegrity: the architectural basis of cellular mechanotransduction. Annu Rev Physiol 1997;59:575–599.

59. Hallbrucker C, vom Dahl S, et al. Control of hepatic proteolysis by amino acids: the role of cell volume. Eur J Biochem 1991;197:717–724.

60. Haussinger D, Hallbrucker C, et al. Cell volume is a major determinant of proteolysis control in liver. FEBS Lett 1991;283:70–72.

61. Poso AR, Hirsimaki P. Inhibition of proteolysis in the liver by chronic ethanol feeding. Biochem J 1991;273:149–152.

62. Lang F, Ritter M, et al. The biological significance of cell volume. Ren Physiol Biochem 1993;16:48–65.

63. Vom Dahl S, Haussinger D. Nutritional state and the swelling-induced inhibition of proteolysis in perfused rat liver. J Nutr 1996; 126:395–402.

64. Blommaart PJ, Charles R, et al. Changes in hepatic nitrogen balance in plasma concentrations of amino acids and hormones and in cell volume after overnight fasting in perinatal and adult rat. Pediatr Res 1995;38:1018–1025.

65. Eklund J, Hallberg D. Hyper-osmolality and lipolysis: I. An experimental study with reference to hypernatremia in burned patients. Acta Chir Scand 1970;136:91–93.

66. Hamilton MT, Ward DS, et al. Effect of plasma osmolality on steady-state fluid shifts in perfused cat skeletal muscle. Am J Physiol 1993; 265:R1318–1323.

67. Finn PJ, Plank LD, et al. Progressive cellular dehydration and proteolysis in critically ill patients. Lancet 1996;347:654–656.

68. Nair KS, Welle SL, et al. Effect of beta-hydroxybutyrate on whole-body leucine kinetics and fractional mixed skeletal muscle protein synthesis in humans. J Clin Invest 1988;82:198–205.

69. Berneis K, Ninnis R, et al. Effects of hyper- and hypoosmolality on whole body protein and glucose kinetics in humans. Am J Physiol 1999;276:E188–195.

70. Bilz S, Ninnis R, et al. Effects of hypoosmolality on whole-body lipolysis in man. Metabolism 1999;48:472–476.

71. Phillips SM, Green HJ, et al. Effect of acute plasma volume expansion on substrate turnover during prolonged low-intensity exercise. Am J Physiol 1997;273:E297–304.

72. Green HJ, Grant SM, et al. Reduced muscle lactate during prolonged exercise following induced plasma volume expansion. Can J Physiol Pharmacol 1997;75:1280–1286.

73. Luetkemeier MJ, Thomas EL. Hypervolemia and cycling time trial performance. Med Sci Sports Exerc 1994;26:503–509.

74. Lehmann M, Huonker M, et al. Serum amino acid concentrations in nine athletes before and after the 1993 Colmar ultra triathlon. Int J Sports Med 1995;16:155–159.

75. Kanstrup IL, Marving J, et al. Acute plasma expansion: left ventricular hemodynamics and endocrine function during exercise. J Appl Physiol 1992;73:1791–1796.

76. Grant SM, Green HJ, et al. Effects of acute expansion of plasma volume on cardiovascular and thermal function during prolonged exercise. Eur J Appl Physiol 1997;76:356–362.

77. Diederichs F, Muhlhaus K, et al. On the mechanism of lactate dehydrogenase release from skeletal muscle in relation to the control of cell volume. Enzyme 1979;24:404–415.

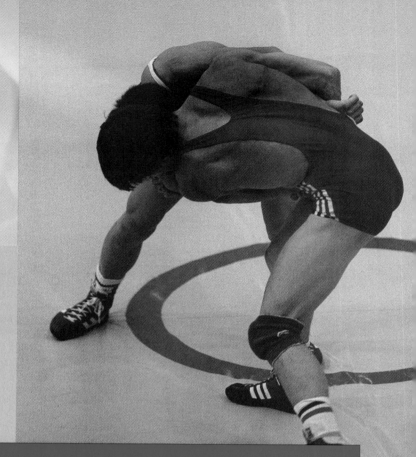

CHAPTER

11

Recovery

Conrad Earnest and Chuck Rudolph

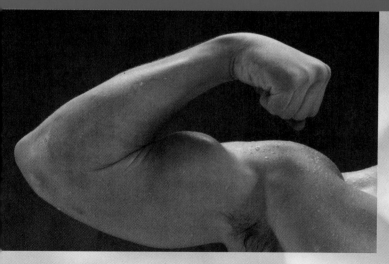

Research Review

Supplements Affect Hormonal Milieu

To examine the effect of carbohydrate and/or protein supplements on the hormonal state of the body after weight-training exercise, nine experienced male weightlifters were given water (Control) or an isocaloric carbohydrate (CHO; 1.5 g/kg body weight), protein (PRO; 1.38 g/kg), or carbohydrate-protein (CHO/PRO; 1.06 g carbohydrate/kg and 0.41 g protein/kg) supplement immediately and 2 hours after a standardized weight-training workout. Venous blood samples were drawn before and immediately after exercise and during 8 hours of recovery. Exercise-induced changes in plasma lactate, glucose, testosterone, and growth hormone were measured. CHO and CHO/PRO stimulated higher insulin concentrations than PRO and Control.

CHO/PRO led to an increase in growth hormone 6 hours post-exercise that was greater than PRO and Control. Supplements had no effect on insulin-like growth factor, but caused a significant decline in testosterone. The decline in testosterone, however, was not associated with a decline in luteinizing hormone. This would indicate that there was an increased clearance of testosterone after supplementation. Thus, nutritive supplements after weight-training exercise can produce a hormonal environment during recovery that may be favorable to muscle growth by increasing insulin and growth hormone concentrations. However, it should be noted that alterations in blood do not indicate what is occurring within skeletal muscle cells.

Chandler RM, Byrne HK, Patterson JG, Ivy JL. Dietary supplements affect the anabolic hormones after weight-training exercise. J Appl Physiol 1994;76(2):839–845.

Introduction

In reasonable doses, exercise has many profound health benefits. However, when physical limits and adequate recovery periods are surpassed, work output and subsequent training efforts are compromised for a variety of reasons. These include poor macronutrient replenishment strategies that ultimately affect muscle energetics, tissue injury, overtraining syndromes, and compromises to immune function. Whether presented alone or in combination, the advent of these maladies often results in an overall decrease in participation time and sport performance. Although time and healing are necessary for complete return to activity, nutritional support may help expedite recovery. Ultimately, however, the concept of *recovery* is an umbrella term comprised of many factors such as acute trauma, chronic overuse or overtraining, and the acute recovery following exhaustive exercise so that an adequate training stimulus can ensue on the following day. As it pertains to energetics, the mechanism(s) for recovery are largely macronutrient based. When it comes to injury, the recovery process entails a relationship that stems from local inflammatory responses to the injured area, subsequent mechanisms to control inflammation, and compromises in immune status that are relative to the extent of injury (i.e., tissue damage) and the allotted time necessary for healing.

Although nutritional support may attenuate the amount of time necessary for adequate healing and recovery, the paradox involved in a blanket prescription is complicated by the lack of a common denominator between sports. Trauma induced by accidents (e.g., musculoskeletal) is as debilitating as is the extent of musculoskeletal involvement. Thus, on a very simplistic scale, a grade one ankle sprain is easier to recover from than is the debilitation associated with the *unhappy triad* of the knee injury that involves the medial meniscus, anterior cruciate ligament, and the medial collateral ligament. Similarly, the needs of an athlete who is fatigued from the pre-season two-a-day practice schedule is also different than those needs associated with the athlete who practices once per day or who is chronically overtrained following months of heavy work.

The etiology of injuries subsequent to exercise may be related to eccentric exercise, stress fractures and overuse injuries, oxidative stress, and even the anti-inflammatory drugs used to control injury response.[1-7] Perhaps the one common thread among all injuries is that regardless of the cause, inflammatory responses and potential compromises in immune function are usually involved in the events following injury. This response involves a complex cascade of cellular events (see Chapter 8 by Dr. Kohut).

The Immune System and Injury

Injuries are caused by bacteria, trauma, chemicals, heat, or multiple factors that result in dramatic secondary changes in the tissues. Once initiated, vasodilatation of the local blood vessels occurs. This causes excess local blood flow followed rapidly by increased capillary permeability and leakage of large quantities of fluid into the interstitial spaces. Subsequently, the clotting of the fluid in interstitial spaces due to excessive amounts of fibrinogen and other proteins leaking from the capillaries soon occurs. As the process continues, the migration of large numbers of

Table 11-1 Inflammation and Immune System Markers

Prostaglandin	A group of lipids that are modified fatty acids. They are found in many tissues where they act as messengers involved in reproduction, and in the inflammatory response to infection.
Interleukins	**IL-I**—chemical mediator released by macrophages—large, tissue-bound phagocytic specialists that are stimulated by the presence of bacteria and microbes; enhanced by interferon (family of proteins released from cells invaded by a virus and protect noninvaded cells from these viruses). They are activated by helper T cells; stimulated by antibodies on the surface of foreign material. It is released in the presence of microbes and enhances the growth and differentiation of B & T cells.
	IL-2—lymphokine (chemical mediator, other than antibodies, secreted by lymphocytes, including B & T cells) secreted by helper T cells; released by the presence of macrophage-presented antigen; stimulated by IL-1; augmented activity of all T cells.
Cytokines	Proteins secreted by many different cell types, which regulate the intensity and duration of immune responses and are involved in cell-to-cell communication. They are involved in mediating immunity and regulating lymph activity. They promote allergic reactions and because T cell function is boosted by cytokines, these proteins are used to evaluate immune activity.
Leukotrienes	Leukotrienes are biologically active compounds formed from arachidonic acid and other polyunsaturated fatty acids. They are of importance in host defense reactions and have a pathophysiological role in inflammation and allergic reactions.
T-Cell Lymphocyte	**T-cell lymphocytes**—white blood cells; activated by macrophage-presented antigen; stimulated by interferon, IL-1, and helper T cells; responsible for cell-mediated immunity (kills cells through nonphagocytic means).
	Cytotoxic T cells—destroy host cells bearing foreign antigen, such as body cells invaded by viruses.
	Helper T cells—enhance the development of antigen-stimulated B cells into antibody-secreting cells; enhance activity of the appropriate cytotoxic and suppressor T cells and activate macrophages.
	Suppressor T cells—suppress both B cell antibody production and cytotoxic and T helper cell activity.
Immunoglobulin Markers	**IgM**—immunoglobulin that serves as the B cell (antibody-mediated immunity) surface receptor for antigen attachment and is secreted in the early stages of plasma-cell response.
	IgG—most abundant immunoglobulin in the blood; is produced copiously upon the body's subsequent exposure to the same antigen.
	IgM and IgG—antibodies responsible for most specific immune responses against bacterial invaders and a few types of viruses.
	IgE—antibody mediator for common allergic responses such as hay fever, asthma, and hives.
	IgA—immunoglobulins are found in secretions of the digestive, respiratory, and genitourinary systems, as well as in milk and tears.
	IgD—is present on the surface of many B cells, but its function is not clear.

granulocytes and monocytes occurs into the tissue, leading to swelling of the tissue cells. These reactions are caused by a host of mechanisms that may involve histamine, bradykinin, serotonin, prostaglandins, different reaction products, the blood-clotting system, and multiple hormonal substances (e.g., lymphokines) that are released by T cells. Following this response, the macrophage system is activated within a few hours so as to eliminate damaged tissues. This defense mechanism is believed to occur to block injury to surrounding tissues as fibrinogen clots form within spaces (TABLE 11-1).

When activated by the products of infection and inflammation, the first effect is a rapid enlargement of macrophages. These macrophages break loose from their attachments and become mobile, forming the first line of defense against infection in the first hour or so. Soon after, large numbers of neutrophils begin to invade the inflamed area from the blood. In a migratory pattern, the release products from the inflamed tissues cause the alteration of the capillary endothelium, causing neutrophils to stick to the capillary walls in the inflamed area. When this occurs, endothelial cells within the capillaries and small venules separate easily, allowing openings large enough for neutrophils to pass into the tissue spaces. Thus, within several hours after tissue damage begins, the area becomes well supplied with neutrophils. The number of neutrophils might increase four to five times from a normal concentration of 4000–5000 to 15,000–25,000 neutrophils per microliter (i.e., neutrophilia).

After several days, macrophages converge in the damaged area to help remove damaged tissue. Moreover, macrophages act as a source of growth factors that increase the activity of various cytokines, platelet-activating factors, and leukotrienes and which can act as direct growth factors, stimulate lymphocytes, induce free radical production in neutrophils, induce adherence molecules on endothelial cells and leukocytes, and cause pain and edema.[8–15] All of these responses are essential to the acute healing response, yet *normal* healing can also be impeded by excessive inflammation. When this occurs, additional damage may occur via free radical production caused by the interleukin-8 family and related cytokines, tumor necrosis factor-α (TNF-α), leukotrienes, and platelet-activating factors.[12,16,17]

Along with the invasion of neutrophils, monocytes from the blood enter the inflamed tissue and enlarge to become macrophages. However, the number of monocytes in the circulating blood is low; also, the storage pool of monocytes in the bone marrow is much less than that of neutrophils. Therefore, the buildup of macrophages in the inflamed tissue area is much slower than that of neutrophils, requiring several days to become effective. Yet after several days to several weeks, the macrophages finally come to dominate the phagocytic cells of the inflamed area because of greatly increased bone marrow production of monocytes, as explained below.

Although many other factors have been implicated in the control of the macrophage-neutrophil response to inflammation, the top five are 1) tumor necrosis factor (TNF), 2) interleukin-1 (IL-1), 3) granulocyte-monocyte colony stimulating factor (GM-CSF), 4) granulocyte colony stimulating factor (G-CSF), and 5) monocyte colony stimulating factor (M-CSF). It is this combination of TNF, IL-1, and colony stimulating factors, along with other important factors that provides a powerful feedback mechanism that begins with tissue injury and inflammation. As injury recovery begins immediately following the injurious event, tissue preservation is also facilitated by aggregated platelet release, platelet-derived growth factor, insulin-like growth factor, epidermal growth factor, and transforming growth factor to help stem the tide of tissue preservation and repair.[10,17–20] Another mediating factor in recovery is via prostaglandins.[21]

Prostaglandins comprise any of a group of components derived from unsaturated 20 carbon fatty acids, primarily arachidonic acid, via the cyclooxygenase pathway and are extremely potent mediators of a diverse group of physiologic processes (Table 11-1). The abbreviation for prostaglandin is PG and the individual designates for each compound are designated by adding one of the letters A through I. Furthermore, a subscript[1–3] is then added to indicate the number of double bonds in the hydrocarbon skeleton (e.g., PGE_2). Most prostaglandins have two double bonds and are synthesized from arachidonic acid. All of the prostaglandins act by binding to specific cell surface receptors, causing an increase in the level of the intracellular second messenger cAMP. PGs have a variety of important roles in regulating cellular activities, especially in the inflammatory response in which they may act as vasodilators in the vascular system.

Prostaglandins of the E series downregulate the activity and cytokine production of many cells including macrophages and lymphocytes.[22,23] PGEs are also released concomitantly with other prostaglandins, leukotrienes, and inflammatory cytokines upon stimulation of macrophages and other cells by endotoxin or cytokines. Cytokines also stimulate the hypothalamic-pituitary-adrenocortical (HPA) axis, resulting in marked elevation of plasma ACTH and corticosteroid levels within 1 hour.[24] Arachidonic acid metabolites, prostaglandins, and leukotrienes also have inflammatory effects.[25] Thus, nonsteroidal anti-inflammatory drugs (NSAIDs) act by interfering with arachidonic acid metabolism.[26,27] The interesting paradox in this sequence of events is that inflammation signals immune system activation. Yet, anti-inflammatory measures can be immunosuppressive. For example, serum and tissue fluids from patients with severe trauma or burn injuries show inhibited lymphocyte stimulation, suppressed cellular immunity, and impaired antibody response.[25,28]

In response to inflammation, the capacity for cells to repair themselves is facilitated by heat shock proteins, which are induced by oxidative stress.[29] These proteins assist in protein formation and are assisted by free radical scavengers such as superoxide dismutase. Heat shock proteins also inhibit the TNF-induced activation of phospholipase A2, an enzyme that acts at the beginning of platelet-activating factor and eicosanoid production. To this end, nutritional status and serum levels of antioxidative vitamins E, A, and C (free radical scavengers), zinc, and iron may aid the healing process.[30–33] Inflammation is also controlled via cytokines as increased serum levels of IL-2 that are followed by an elevation of IL-2 receptor, which neutralizes the biological activity of the cytokine in surgery patients.[34] Cortisone has potent antiproliferative effects on many cellular systems, one mechanism being a downregulation of cytokines with growth factor activity.[35]

Strenuous Exercise and Tissue Injury

As it pertains to exercise, acute exhaustive or eccentric exercise can also induce muscle soreness, weakness, pain, and signs of inflammation that may negatively influence productive training.[36] For example, exercise involving a high percentage of eccentric work can lead to skeletal myofiber damage (i.e., tearing or streaming of Z-bands and myofibrils).[37,38] Complicating the recovery process, of course, is previous injury, poor fitness, hypoxia, cold temperatures, and inadequate nutrition. Although the factors that most strongly influence this response are not fully understood, several have been proposed. These include the loss of intramuscular energy stores, accumulated ammonium and lactate, impaired circulation, the activation of proteases by an accumulation of calcium ions in the cytosol, and the release of lysosomal proteases leading to intracellular degradation.[39–41]

Other studies via skeletal muscle biopsy data have shown an accumulation of neutrophils, as well as the accumulation of macrophages and lymphocytes, phagocytic cell proliferation, platelet activation, humoral coagulation factors, cytokines, and prostaglandins.[42–48] Also, there is evidence that strenuous exercise leads to free radical production which could be influenced by plasma antioxidant status.[30,31,49,50] These observations do not appear to be without sequelae in that strenuous exercise may increase susceptibility to viral and recurrent infections, which is likely influenced by training intensity.[51–54] In this regard, Neiman et al.[53] have reported a J-shaped curve between moderate and strenuous exercise. As with other paradoxes, moderate exercise yields mild but significant increases in immunoglobulin levels and enhanced natural killer cell activity, whereas strenuous exercise may unfavorably alter several immune reactions.[32,53,55]

T cells also serve an important function during exercise as they promote cytokine production and facilitate B-cell antibody production. Reduced numbers of T cells have been described in elite athletes, though it is not clear what impact this has on the risk of infection.[56] Furthermore, strenuous exercise has been shown to reduce the mitogen-dependent proliferation of T cells, while 1 minute of maximal effort has shown to decrease the T-cell cell surface glycoproteins in trained subjects only.[57] This suppression of T-cell function may be mediated in part by elevated cortisol and epinephrine levels.[35,53] Whether these responses have clinical implications still needs to be determined. However, athletes with a high volume and/ or high-intensity training schedule may at times be of increased susceptibility to accumulate enough alterations in immune-altering parameters to make a significant difference to health and performance.

Nutrient Support

One of the keys of nutrient support to aid recovery and facilitate immune competence largely depends on replacing lost energy stores coupled with measures that will ensure adequate immune support. When injury does occur, steps to aid tissue repair are also required. Regarding macronutrient replacement, contemporary nutrient replacement entails adequate carbohydrate, protein, and essential fatty acids as replacement strategies. However, limitations should not be placed on macronutrient replacement alone. Therefore, this chapter will also examine the use of glutamine, glucosamine/chondroitin sulfate, various proteins, and certain over-the-counter medications.

During intense exercise, there is a net breakdown of body protein as well as an increase in the catabolic hormones adrenocorticotropic hormone (ACTH) and cortisol. ACTH is released by the pituitary gland in response to the fiber damage caused by intense exercise. This increase in ACTH ignites a release of cortisol to help suppress inflammation and trigger the release or breakdown of

muscle to amino acids for post-exercise protein synthesis. Though cortisol might assist in the provision of fuel, it also has catabolic properties that may delay recuperation after intense exercise.

Overall, protein synthesis increases in response to insulin, growth hormone, testosterone, and adequate amounts of amino acids, but decreases in response to cortisol, glucocorticoids, glucagon, exercise, and inadequate amount of amino acids.[58–60] Because insulin and growth hormone play a dominant role in everyday protein metabolism, it seems essential to provide an environment for recuperation that promotes either or both of these hormones following exercise. Despite the *carbohydrate paranoia* that sometimes exists in the world of strength development, a combination of carbohydrate *and* protein supplementation immediately after intense exercise significantly increases plasma insulin and growth hormone levels and helps to draw the body back into an anabolic state necessary for protein synthesis. Although the direct actions of growth hormone are not fully understood, it is believed that growth hormone facilitates protein synthesis by increasing amino acid transport through plasma membranes, stimulating RNA formation, or activating cellular ribosomes, both of which increase protein synthesis. Insulin acts by inhibiting protein breakdown. Both hormones are essential for skeletal muscle protein accretion.[61,62]

Following high-intensity exercise, the body begins to replenish blood glucose and muscle and liver glycogen stores. In addition, the body commences the healing of muscle tissue that is damaged or injured during training. To accomplish this, the timing of carbohydrate and protein intake is extremely important. Some have posited that it is the consumption of these macronutrients immediately following exercise that leads to increased rates of muscle glycogen resynthesis and an augmentation of net muscle protein accretion. Ultimately, this would result in a more rapid recovery, thus allowing an athlete to return to his or her training.

Using Carbohydrates for Post-Exercise Recovery

During prolonged endurance exercise, if one's carbohydrate stores become significantly depressed, protein becomes an active substrate, accounting for about 12–15% of oxidized fuel.[63–66] How much protein used differs from workout to workout and depends on 1) the length of exercise, 2) the intensity of exercise, and 3) the frequency of training. One could view all of these factors as what some scientists refer to as 4) training volume.

Intense aerobic[65] and anaerobic training[64,66] have been shown to use protein as a fuel, though not to the same extent as carbohydrates or fat. Without proper nutrient intervention, this negative balance leads to the potential for decreased muscle mass and an increased injury risk.[67]

Currently, the literature suggests that intensive and/or high-volume aerobic and weight-training exercise increases the need for specific protein/amino acids.[63,66,68–73] Thus, one must attempt to ameliorate the hypoglycemia that is initially caused by low muscle glycogen concentrations[74] but is also exacerbated by chronic overwork, overtraining, and poor nutrition.[75]

In active individuals, protein intake above the RDA[63,66,76–78] is necessary and can range from 1.2 to 2.2 g/kg of body weight.[65,66,68,69,77] This extra protein is needed for the repair of damaged muscle fibers, the provision of additional amino acids for muscle protein accretion (vis-a-vis heavy resistance training), and as an additional fuel source during prolonged endurance exercise. Additionally, post-exercise recovery includes the following variables: normalization of blood glucose levels and restoration of skeletal muscle and liver glycogen stores.

The main substrate for muscle glycogen resynthesis is blood glucose, derived from liver glycogen breakdown as well as from exogenous carbohydrate ingestion before, during, and especially after exercise. Various studies have looked at the timing, amount, and the type of carbohydrate needed to increase muscle glycogen resynthesis following exercise. One study looked at the time of ingestion of a carbohydrate supplement on muscle glycogen resynthesis after exercise. Twelve male cyclists exercised at 68% of VO_{2max} for 70 minutes with six 2-minute intervals at 88% VO_{2max} on two occasions. At the conclusion of the exercise test, a carbohydrate solution was ingested immediately post-exercise or 2 hours post-exercise. They found that delaying carbohydrate intake post-exercise for 2 hours reduces the rate of muscle glycogen resynthesis.[79] Thus, the immediate consumption of carbohydrates post-exercise is critical for muscle glycogen repletion.

Another study looked at the rate of muscle glycogen resynthesis during the initial hours of recovery following prolonged lower body exercise. It was noted that muscle glycogen resynthesis occurs at a rate approximating 1–2 mmol/kg wet wt^{-1} if no carbohydrate is ingested. However, when carbohydrate is ingested immediately post-exercise, muscle glycogen resynthesis increases to 7–10 mmol/kg wet wt^{-1}.[80] The time required for complete muscle glycogen resynthesis after prolonged exercise is generally considered to be 24 hours provided carbohydrate intake is adequate (500–700 g); however, the first 2 hours after exercise is when muscle glycogen resynthesis is the highest.[81] Thus, carbohydrate ingested *immediately* after exercise restores muscle glycogen nearly *three times faster* than waiting for 2 hours.

A multitude of factors affects post-exercise muscle glycogen restoration. In addition to the type of exercise performed, the type of carbohydrate consumed is critical regarding glycogen repletion.[82,83] Carbohydrates that elicit a high blood-glucose response upon ingestion are considered to have a *high glycemic index*, whereas those carbohydrate foods evoking a small blood glucose response are considered to have a *low glycemic index*.[84] Post-exercise carbohydrate intake should then consist of high glycemic foods versus low glycemic foods, thus eliciting a high blood-glucose response to increase muscle glycogen resynthesis. Thus, the ingestion of glucose or sucrose, which are simple carbohydrates with high glycemic indexes, is best used for muscle glycogen resynthesis, in which liver glycogen resynthesis is better assisted with the ingestion of a complex carbohydrate or fructose (low glycemic index).

It is well known that carbohydrate consumption post-exercise increases plasma insulin and growth hormone levels. Increasing these hormones promotes muscle protein accretion.[85] A recent publication noted that carbohydrate supplementation in excess of 1.0 g/kg body weight should be consumed immediately following intense exercise. It also noted that the best type of carbohydrate to consume was of a high glycemic index. Glucose or glucose polymers were most effective in muscle glycogen resynthesis, whereas fructose or low glycemic index carbohydrate were better used for liver glycogen resynthesis. This study not only validates the importance of carbohydrate intake after intense exercise, but also indicates that the addition of protein may increase the rate of glycogen resynthesis stimulating the secretion of insulin.[86]

With regard to training, the maintenance of blood glucose levels is important for energy. When blood glucose levels become low, there is an increase in plasma ACTH, cortisol, and growth hormone and a decreased insulin concentration. Although this is essential for continued energy production, many immune-modulating effects occur as blood glucose concentrations are decreased.[24,32,35,44,87–108] While many of these findings exist for prolonged endurance activity, similar data regarding strength and power events are not widely available.[54,56,109–111]

Adequate carbohydrate intake should attenuate increases in stress hormones, and thereby diminish changes in immune function as well. In a study involving marathon runners, a 6% carbohydrate fluid given before, during, and after 2.5 hours of running attenuated the rise in both cortisol and neutrophil/lymphocyte ratios. Similar findings have also been noted in both cycling and running.[112,113] Furthermore, post-exercise monocytes and lymphocytes were higher in the placebo conditions, with lymphocytes falling from 1.5 to 3 hours post-exercise.[112] Further analysis of these results also show an elevated neutrophil/lymphocyte ratio in the placebo conditions for both modes of exercise as well as an increase in NK cell activity.[112,113] As it may pertain to strength training, eccentric muscle activity is associated with a higher IL-6 response than concentric exercise.[89] As with many factors related to exercise, these responses are related to intensity, volume, and duration of exercise. Thus, carbohydrate intake may affect immune parameters as well (TABLE 11-2).

Neutrophilia and lymphopenia induced by high plasma cortisol

Increased in blood granulocyte and monocyte phagocytosis

Decreased nasal neutrophil phagocytosis

Decreased mitogen-induced lymphocyte proliferation

Decrease in ex vivo production of cytokines (IFN-γ, IL-1, and IL-6) in response to mitogens and endotoxin

Decreased in granulocyte oxidative burst activity

Decreased nasal mucociliary clearance

Decreased natural killer cell cytotoxic activity

Increased plasma concentrations of pro- and anti-inflammatory cytokines

Decreased nasal and salivary IgA concentration

Data from Nieman DC. Influence of carbohydrate on the immune response to intensive, prolonged exercise. Exerc Immun Rev 1998:4:64–76.

Using Protein for Post-Exercise Recovery

Various studies have investigated the effects of a carbohydrate-protein combination after exercise. Carbohydrate and protein meals produce significantly greater plasma levels of insulin than do carbohydrate and protein meals alone. In one study, scientists investigated the effects of carbohydrate, protein, and carbohydrate plus protein supplementation during the recovery period following intense exercise on muscle glycogen resynthesis. During this trial, nine male subjects cycled for 2 hours on three separate occasions to deplete muscle glycogen stores. Immediately and 2 hours after each exercise bout, they ingested carbohydrate (112 g), protein (40.7 g), or carbohydrate plus protein (112 g + 40.7 g). During the recovery period, plasma glucose response was greater for carbohydrate than carbohydrate plus protein, but the plasma insulin response of carbohydrate plus protein was significantly greater than the carbohydrate treatment. Both carbohydrate plus protein and carbohydrate treatments produced greater insulin response than the protein treatment alone. The rate of muscle glycogen resynthesis during the carbohydrate plus protein treatment was significantly greater (35.5 ± 3.3 [SE] μmol/g/hr) than during the carbohydrate treatment (25.6 ± 2.3 μmol/g/hr). Both conditions were greater than protein treatment alone (7.6 ± 1.4 μmol/g/hr). The results suggest that post-exercise muscle glycogen resynthesis may be enhanced with a carbohydrate plus protein supplement as a result of the interaction of carbohydrate and protein on insulin secretion.[114]

In a similar study, experienced weight-lifters were given water (control), isocaloric carbohydrate (1.5 g/kg), protein (1.38 g/kg), or carbohydrate plus protein (1.06 g/kg + 0.41 g/kg) supplement immediately and 2 hours after weight training. Carbohydrate and carbohydrate plus protein stimulated higher plasma insulin levels than protein and control. It was also noted 6-hours post–weight training that carbohydrate plus protein increased growth hormone levels greater than carbohydrate and protein alone. The supplements had no effect on IGF-1, whereas testosterone levels decreased. The decrease in testosterone was not associated with a decline in luteinizing hormone, suggesting an increased clearance of testosterone. These results propose that carbohydrate plus protein supplementation after weight-training exercise may increase plasma insulin and growth hormone levels, thus producing a hormonal milieu favorable to muscle growth (TABLE 11-3).[115]

Protein Quality and Immunoenhancement

Similar to carbohydrates, protein might have positive immunomodulating effects. One must remain cognizant of the fact that proteins differ in *quality* and that this might impact your choice of a post-exercise protein source. Protein quality is usually measured in one of three ways: 1) the Protein Efficiency Ratio (PER), 2) Biological Value (BV), and 3) the Protein Digestibility Corrected Amino Acid Score (PDCAAS). The PER uses a procedure in which immature rats are fed a measured amount of protein and weighed over a given time. The PER is then calculated by dividing the weight gain by the protein intake. Based on a recent study in Fisher, 344 weanling rats, the corrected PER and the foods with the best protein quality, were egg (3.24), beef sirloin (3.16), and chicken breast (3.07), all of which were significantly different from milk powder (2.88) and casein (2.50).[116]

Biological value measures the amount of protein retained per gram of protein absorbed. If a given protein provides all the essential amino acids in the correct proportions and is readily absorbed, the BV score will approach 100. On the other hand, if the protein is deficient in one essential amino acid, then its BV score will be much lower. The newest measure of protein quality is the PDCAAS. This method takes into consideration the advancements made in amino acid analysis and protein digestibility, the availability of data on digestibility of protein, the individual amino acids found in a variety of foods, and the reliability of human amino acid requirements and scoring patterns. The PDCAAS is a simple approach for evaluating the protein quality of foods and has been validated based on metabolic balance studies in humans. Proteins are rated on a scale of 0.0–1.0.[117] The scores derived from this method rate egg white, casein, and soy protein isolates at 1.0, with beef closely behind. Moreover, high-quality protein can be found in

Table 11-3 **Carbohydrate and Protein Recovery Requirements Following Training**

Protein needs per day*

Athlete	g/kg/day
Strength Athletes	1.4–1.8
Interval Type Training	1.6–1.8
Aerobic Athletes	1.2–1.4

*Use the upper range for 3–4 weeks when first starting to train and/or when beginning a new training phase.

Post-exercise Carbohydrate: Protein Replacement Strategy Following Training

(1) Ingest 1 g of carbohydrate per kg of body weight within 15 min of exercise cessation.

(2) Add adequate protein so as to ingest a 3:1, CHO:PRO ratio

Post Exercise Carbohydrate and Protein Replacement in 3:1 Ratio*

Weight (kg)	Weight (lbs.)	CHO (g)	PRO (g)
40	88	40	13
45	99	45	15
50	110	50	17
55	121	55	18
60	132	60	20
65	143	65	22
70	154	70	23
75	165	75	25
80	176	80	27
85	187	85	28
90	198	90	30
95	209	95	32
100	220	100	33
105	231	105	35
110	242	110	37
115	253	115	38
120	264	120	40
125	275	125	42
130	286	130	43
135	297	135	45
140	308	140	47

*All values have been rounded to the nearest whole number.

various foods like eggs, milk, poultry, fish, and lean beef sirloin. There are also many types of high-quality protein supplements on the market such as whey, milk isolates, caseinates, soy isolates, and even some vegetable protein.

Whey Protein

Whey protein is a derivative of milk production with an amino acid profile that is closely related to the amino acids required by the human body.[118] Whey protein also has proportionately more sulfur-containing amino acids and contains a relative surplus of a variety of essential amino acids. This combination would ideally result in an optimal balance of amino acids needed for muscle growth and recovery. Whey is an excellent protein source given its high biological value and amino acid composition.[119] Whey is also a rich source of protein with diverse food properties for nutritional, biological, and functional applications.[120] Because of whey's bioavailability and ease of dispersion in solution, it is looked upon as being the superior protein supplement for athletes to use as a post-workout meal.

Studies have indicated whey protein also has immune-enhancing properties.[121] In a study by Bounous (1989), the authors indicated that whey protein contains essentially more of the amino acid cysteine than casein. This is important because the amino acid cysteine is considered to be a rate-limiting substrate for the synthesis of glutathione (a major antioxidant of the body that is necessary for lymphocyte proliferation).[122] In a comparison study of whey and casein on glutathione production in critically ill patients, whey protein (cysteine levels reported at 2.0–2.5%) increased glutathione concentrations well above those displayed by casein (cysteine levels reported at 0.3%).[123] There is also evidence that mitochondrial function and the glutathione-dependent antioxidant system are important for the maintenance of proper structure and function of muscles. Exercise puts much stress not only on the muscles, bones, and joints, but it also stresses the body's defense mechanisms, which is indicated by changes in glutathione status in plasma during intense exercise. Strenuous exercise also increases the production of free radicals[124] and is characterized by an increased oxygen consumption and derangement of intracellular pro-oxidant/antioxidant homeostasis.[125] These free radicals can be potentially injurious to genes, membranes, and other cell structures and may impede normal daily metabolic responses.[126] Adequate antioxidants and foods that help manage oxidative stress and support the immune system may benefit athletes during and after exercise. In addition to the unique amino acid profile of whey protein, it also features one of the highest percentages of branched-chain amino acids and is rich in vitamins and minerals. Diets high in branched-chain amino acids (BCAAs) demonstrate greater signs of muscle preservation when the body is in a catabolic state. This is due to the ability of BCAAs to improve nitrogen balance and serve as an energy source for skeletal muscle.[127] Severe metabolic stresses such as sepsis, surgery, burns, and strenuous exercise are associated with accelerated requirements for BCAAs.

Casein

Casein is also a derivative of milk production and possesses some unique biological properties that affect human protein metabolism as well. Casein is an easily digested protein that supplies the body with essential amino acids, along with various minerals and bioactive peptides. Caseinates are salts of casein (calcium caseinate or sodium caseinate) and are made by dissolving acid casein in a suitable hydroxide, then drying it to make a water-soluble product. Many protein supplements use caseinates because of the high quality of protein. Caseinates have a PDCAAS of 1.0, giving it a very high standard for protein quality. Caseinates are also low in fat and cholesterol and may contain varied amounts of sodium and/or calcium based on the form used.

A recent study that looked at the absorption and plasma amino acid content of whey and casein showed that casein induced a prolonged elevation of plasma amino acids, probably because of slower gastric emptying, whereas whey protein induced a faster, but shorter increase of plasma amino acids. Casein was also noted to inhibit whole-body protein breakdown yet whey had no effect on protein catabolism. However, whey protein increased protein synthesis at twice the rate of casein.[128] Thus, it appears that the benefits of both whey and casein may be applicable to athletes during the recovery phase. Both are of high quality and render all of the essential amino acids in adequate and identifiable proportions for the body. Caseinates are easily digested, as are whey proteins. Both increase plasma amino acid concentrations to a varying degree, eliciting different hormonal and metabolic responses.

Egg Protein

Egg protein is considered to be a high-quality protein source and is usually the standard against which other proteins are compared. In comparison to casein and whey, egg protein is higher in sodium and most egg supplements contain levels of sodium per serving exceeding 300 mg. Thus, if some athletes are "sodium sensitive," an abundance of egg whites might not be the best source for satisfying protein needs. However, when recuperating from intense physical exercise, egg protein is a great source of essential amino acids that will serve as the building blocks for damaged muscle fibers.

Soy Protein

Soy proteins provide a high quality of protein and are free from cholesterol and very low in saturated fat. The PDCAAS of 1.0 gives soy protein a quality equivalent to casein and various animal proteins. Soy also contains high amounts of glutamine and arginine. Although available in supplement form, glutamine deficiencies have been related to intense, strenuous exercise, "overtraining syndromes," increased infection, suppressed immunity, and critical illness. Supplementation has been shown to be beneficial against these conditions.[129,130] The functional role of glutamine is in its role as the primary nitrogen carrier to skeletal muscle and other vital tissues. It is also the main source of energy for the lining of the gut and the intestines and can promote increases in growth hormone and elicit immune-enhancing properties.[129,131–133] Arginine has been shown to play a vital role in stimulating the release of growth hormone and IGF-1.[134–136] Arginine has also been investigated for supporting the immune system and enhancing wound healing.[137–140] What soy is lacking are the sulfur-containing amino acids, particularly methionine and cysteine. It is the sulfur-containing amino acids that are important for glutathione synthesis. A 1983 study examined the protein nutritional value of an isolated soy protein in comparison to beef in healthy young men. The studies indicated that no differences in nitrogen balance, digestibility, or net protein use were observed when the soy protein replaced beef.[141] Another study investigated the protein nutritional value of two isolated soy proteins compared with dried skim milk proteins in healthy young men and it was concluded that well-processed isolated soy proteins are indistinguishable from milk as a protein source for maintenance of short-term nitrogen balance in adult human nutrition.[142] The evaluation of the protein quality of an isolated soy protein in young men and the relative nitrogen requirements and effect of methionine supplementation was looked at again in 1984. The results suggested that, for healthy adults, isolated soy protein is of high nutritional quality, comparable to that of animal protein sources, and that the methionine content is not limiting for adult protein maintenance. A more recent study also investigated the quality of soy protein in comparison to food proteins of animal origin. These findings clarified that well-processed soy protein isolates and soy-protein concentrates are essentially equivalent to those of animal proteins. During normal usage of soy protein, methionine supplementation is not necessary. Soy proteins have also been found to be of good quality, well tolerated, and of good acceptability.[143]

As for immune status, a 1998 study performed at Ohio State University examined 20 healthy males during a vigorous exercise regimen that was supplemented with soy protein isolate or whey protein. The tests' subjects who were fed soy protein isolate showed an increase in plasma antioxidants, whereas the whey protein–supplemented group did not experience an increase in total plasma antioxidants. Isoflavones, which naturally occur in soy protein isolate, were suggested as possibly being responsible for the reduced free radical

Does the Addition of Protein or Amino Acids Augment Muscle Glycogen Restoration?

According to Carrithers et al., the addition of protein or amino acids has no effect on muscle glycogen restoration after an exhaustive bout of cycling. In this study, 7 male cyclists (age, 26 yrs; VO$_{2peak}$—4.20 L/min) performed three trials separated by 1 week. In essence, they underwent glycogen-depleting exercise followed by the consumption of 1)100% glucose, 2) 70% carbohydrate—20% protein—10% fat, or 3) 86% carbohydrate—14% amino acids. All feedings had the same number of calories. Needless to say, after a 4-hour period of feeding (equivalent to 1 g/kg body weight per hour of carbohydrate), they found no difference in muscle glycogen stores.

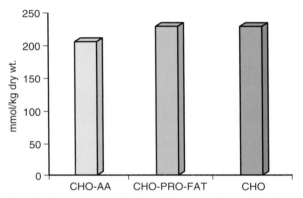

Muscle glycogen concentrations 4 hours post-exercise. Thus, one could surmise that it is the total energy intake, and not necessarily the carbohydrate intake that is the most important factor governing muscle glycogen restoration. CHO-AA indicates carbohydrates plus amino acids; CHO-PRO-FAT, carbohydrates, protein, and fat; CHO, carbohydrates only. There were no significant differences between treatments. *Data from* Carrithers JA, Williamson DL, Gallagher PM, et al. Effects of postexercise carbohydrate-protein feedings on muscle glycogen restoration. J Appl Physiol 2000;88:1976–1982.

production.[144] It would appear that soy protein is beneficial because of its antioxidant and immune-enhancing properties.

Glutamine

Given its metabolic properties as a glucose precursor and abundance in plasma and skeletal muscle,[145] the value of glutamine is likely understated. It has been posited that

the decreased plasma glutamine concentration observed post-exercise is an important factor regarding immune system regulation. Several studies have tried to link the changes in the immune system induced by exercise or other stress situations to changes in plasma glutamine concentration.[146–149] Severe metabolic stress (e.g., exercise, surgery, trauma, injury, burns, etc.) places high demands on muscles and organs, thereby compromising immunity.[109,150] This compromise takes place because glutamine is an important energy source for lymphocytes and macrophages.[109,151,152] Some have suggested that the cells of the immune system in essence *borrow* glutamine from skeletal muscle[153,154]; thus, skeletal muscle, which is the major site of glutamine production, plays a vital role in maintaining the rate of glutamine use by cells of the immune system.

Taken up by the intestine at high rates, small amounts of glutamine enter the circulation leaving the skeletal muscle, kidneys, liver, lungs, and heart, with skeletal muscle likely being the most important site for glutamine synthesis.[109,155] Glutamine is also produced from glutamate and ammonia, via glutamine synthase and protein degradation, the combination of 2-oxoglutarate (a citric cycle intermediate) and branched-chain amino acids via branched-chain amino acid transaminase, or from glutamate that is taken up from the circulation. Ammonia can be obtained from the free pool of ammonia or donated from the branched-chain amino acid via deamination. Both glutamine synthase and branched-chain amino acid transaminase are present in high quantities in skeletal muscle. Glutamine also plays a major role in overall nitrogen metabolism and transports nitrogen in a nontoxic form between various organs.[156]

As it pertains to recovery, glutamine is essential to a variety of mammalian cells, including cells of the immune system.[157–159] Glutamine appears to be a key nutrient by itself, whereas other amino acids (i.e., glutamate and leucine) cannot substitute for glutamine.[160,161] This is an interesting observation as many product manufacturers often substitute glutamate into supplement formulae because of its cheaper price. In humans, glutamine can also influence the *in vitro* proliferation of lymphocytes.[160,162] Several *in vitro* studies have shown that strenuous exercise is followed by numerous changes in blood mononuclear cells. These include a depressed lymphocyte count in the blood, impaired function of natural killer and B cells, and inhibited mucosal immunity.[163] Although mononuclear cells have a high intracellular activity of glutaminase, they do not have the ability to synthesize glutamine because they appear to have no glutamine synthase activity.[160,161] Because of this, lymphocytes must be supplied with glutamine in the plasma.

In this regard, the concentration of free glutamine in plasma has been reported to decline during catabolic conditions such as trauma, sepsis, and burns.[158] Of interest to athletic populations are several studies showing that

Maintaining Muscle Cell Energy: The Possible Role of D-Ribose

Jeffrey R. Stout, PhD, CSCS

High-energy phosphates (ATP, ADP, and AMP) that are stored in skeletal muscle cells or fibers serve as fuel that drives many metabolic functions. The ratio of these adenine nucleotides in healthy muscle cells remains quite stable over a range of physiological conditions. The stability of this ratio is vitally important for maintaining cellular function. For example, scientists believe that the energy charge of a muscle cell is one of the primary factors regulating protein synthesis (i.e., muscle protein accretion and repair of damaged muscle fibers). Also, scientists have suggested that a decrease in adenine nucleotide (i.e., ATP) content would decrease muscle protein synthesis. Thus, if a muscle cell is low on ATP (i.e., altered energy charge) it would take longer to repair itself and be almost impossible to build new muscle.

The concept of energy charge in muscle cells was first introduced by Dr. Atkinson, who determined that the overall energy status of the cell is best expressed in terms of the concentration ratio between the ATP-ADP-AMP. For example, if all the adenine nucleotide in the cell is ATP (a condition that does not occur naturally) the *energy charge* equals 1.0 and reflects a system that is completely filled with high-energy phosphates. On the other hand, if the muscle cell were to contain only ADP, the energy charge would equal 0.5 and, and in the extreme, if AMP were the only adenine nucleotide present, the energy charge would equal 0.0, because no high-energy phosphate bonds would be available to fuel cellular function. Typically, energy charge tends to vary little from 0.85 and is tightly controlled by the muscle cell. Deviations below this level indicate loss of energy potential and levels below 0.80 indicate significant energy depletion.

By performing muscle biopsies or using a noninvasive technique (pNMR), energy charge of the cell can be easily calculated for any given set of concentrations of adenine nucleotides by the equation:

$$\text{Energy Charge} = 0.5([\text{ADP}] + 2[\text{ATP}]/[\text{ATP}] + [\text{ADP}] + [\text{AMP}])$$

Many regulatory enzymes in both the catabolic (breaking down) and anabolic (building up) pathways are sensitive to AMP, ADP, and/or ATP as modulators. Therefore, Dr. Atkinson has suggested that the regulation of metabolic pathways that produce and use high-energy phosphates is a function of the energy charge of the cell.

Effects of Exercise on the Muscle Cell Energy Charge

Under normal physiological conditions, cells are highly efficient at maintaining steady state. However, under conditions of physiological stress, such as hypoxia (reduced oxygen supply) caused by ischemia or strenuous exercise, the energy balance can be disrupted and the functional integrity of the cell can be compromised. In these conditions, ATP concentrations fall, which leads to increases in ADP and AMP levels. In an attempt to maintain energy balance the first response of both heart and skeletal muscle cells is to break down AMP, leading to an increase in cellular IMP concentration. If ATP use continues to exceed the rate of regeneration, energy charge is further depressed. The ultimate result is catabolism of IMP to inosine and then hypoxanthine, and AMP to adenine. Hypoxanthine and adenine are lost from the cell and the concentration of total adenine nucleotides is depressed. As such, a fall in energy charge below physiological limits of the cell is prevented and it takes several days for the concentration of adenine nucleotides to return to normal.

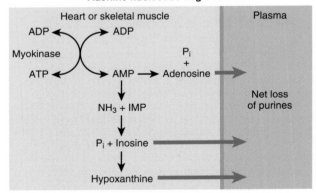

Adenine nucleotide degradation

Data from Tullson and Terjung, 1990 and Pasque and Wechsler, 1984.

Possible Ergogenic Effect of Ribose?

The time-consuming process of replacing lost adenine nucleotides follows two metabolic processes, the *de novo* synthesis of nucleotides and the *salvage* of nucleotide precursors before they are lost from the cell. The salvage pathways take less time because they take advantage of substrates already present and do not require synthesis of new compounds. Both processes require adequate supply of 5-phosphoribosyl-1-pyrophosphate (PRPP) to function.

PRPP is formed in the cell from ribose-5-phosphate synthesized in the pentose phosphate pathway (PPP) from

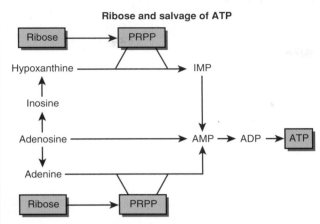

Ribose and salvage of ATP

Data from Pasque and Wechsler, 1984.

conditions, ADP and AMP concentrations rise and energy charge falls. As ATP use continues to surpass ATP generation, nucleotides are lost from the cell in its attempt to control ATP-ADP-AMP ratios. Research has shown that in heart and skeletal muscle several days are required to replace lost nucleotides and restore pool levels to normal—which means that not only are you low on energy, but the speed at which you repair muscle fibers or gain added muscle protein may be dramatically reduced.

Supplemental D-ribose allows the cell to significantly increase adenine nucleotide salvage and *de novo* synthesis. As a result, adenine nucleotide pools are preserved, concentrations of ADP and ATP increase, and energy charge is restored to baseline more quickly, allowing the cell to maintain normal, maximal functional capacity.

glucose-6-phosphate. In heart and skeletal muscle, the PPP is limited by the activity of glucose-6-phosphate dehydrogenase and 6-phosphogluconate dehydrogenase, enzymes found to be in short supply in muscle tissue. The effect of supplemental ribose to circumvent the PPP in heart tissue has been well researched. By bypassing the rate-limiting enzymes of the PPP, ribose goes directly to PRPP production, allowing the cell to increase nucleotide salvage and speed the *de novo* synthetic rate.

The effect of ribose in skeletal muscle has been less well studied; however, research by Brault and Terjung, and Tullson and Terjun has shown that supplemental ribose increases the salvage and *de novo* synthetic rates, respectively, in skeletal muscle at rest and during exercise. In these studies, addition of ribose to skeletal muscle perfusate increased adenine nucleotide salvage up to six-fold and *de novo* synthesis up to 4.3-fold. Additional studies are underway and preliminary results confirm these findings.

In summary, the energy charge of the cell is normally controlled to within tight limits by regulating the ratio of adenine nucleotides. However, under certain physiological conditions, such as high-intensity exercise or tissue ischemia, ATP is used by the cell at a rate exceeding its regeneration. Under these

Atkinson, DE. The energy charge of the adenylate pool as a regulatory parameter: interaction with feedback modifiers. Biochem 1968;7:4030–4034.

Brault J, Terjung RL. Purine Salvage Rates Differ Among Skeletal Muscle Fiber Types and are Limited by Ribose Supply. Presentation to American College of Sports Medicine, June 1999.

Bylund-Fellenius A, et al. Protein synthesis versus energy state in contracting muscles of perfused rat hindlimb. Am J Physiol 1984;246:E297.

Hellsten-Westing Y, Norman B, Balsom PD, Sjodin B. Decreased resting levels of adenine nucleotides in human skeletal muscle after high-intensity training. J Appl Physiol 1993;74(5):2523–2528.

Pasque MK, Wechsler AS. Metabolic intervention to affect myocardial recovery following ischemia. Ann Surg 1984;200:1–12.

Tullson PC, Terjung RL. Adenine nucleotide synthesis in exercising and endurance-trained skeletal muscle. Am J Physiol 1991;261:C342–C347.

Ward HB, St. Cyr JA, Cogordan JA, et al. Recovery of adenine nucleotide levels after global myocardial ischemia in dogs. Surgery 1984;96(2):248–255.

Zimmer HG. Regulation of and intervention into the oxidative pentose phosphate pathway and adenine nucleotide metabolism in the heart. Mol Cell Biochem 1996;160/161:101–109.

Zimmer HG. Significance of the 5-phosphoribosyl-1-pyrophosphate pool for cardiac purine and pyrimidine nucleotide synthesis: studies with ribose, adenine, inosine, and orotic acid in rats. Cardiovasc Drugs Ther 1998;12:179–187.

plasma glutamine concentration decreases in relation to intense sustained exercise and may be the result of either net overuse[147,148,164–166] or an increased rate of glutamine used by the kidneys and cells of the immune system.[109] During long-term exercise or in chronically overtrained athletes, another theory suggests that these conditions interfere with the rate of glutamine release from muscles and thus could be responsible for the decrease in plasma glutamine concentration.[109] Furthermore, changes in glutamine concentration vary depending on the type, duration, and intensity of the exercise. However, most of the studies concerning changes in glutamine in relation to exercise indicate a transient decrease in the period following acute exercise and in the overtraining

syndrome, with the largest decrease reported after major burns.[109,110,130,148,149,167]

Studies on rats have shown that addition of glutamine to TPN suppressed biliary IgA and may offer protection against bacterial transfer from the gut.[168] Yoshida et al.[169] showed that the rate of hepatic regeneration following partial hepatectomy in rats was increased due to increased protein synthesis in the liver and increased DNA synthesis in hepatocytes when glutamine was added to standard TPN. In septic rats it was shown that glutamine-supplemented TPN diminished the increase of urea production, partially prevented the decrease in lymphocyte blastogenesis, and increased the phagocytic index as compared to standard TPN.[170] However, these results may be less profound in humans.[171] A recent study by Shewchuk et al.[172] evaluated the influence of regular exercise and dietary glutamine supplementation in rats and found no effect of glutamine supplementation on immune function. Still, a decline in plasma glutamine has been correlated to the decline in LAK cell activity and CD41 cells, which reflect immune status.[165,173]

In humans, Castell et al.[146] supplemented runners participating in ultramarathons, marathons, 10-km races, or 15-mile training sessions as well as rowers undertaking circuit training for 1 hour or 5-km ergometer rowing. After consuming two drinks, containing either glutamine or placebo after exercise, the percentage of athletes reporting no infections was considerably higher in the glutamine group (81%, n = 72) than in placebo (49%, n = 79, p < 0.001). In contrast, Mackinnnon et al.[110] found no significant difference in glutamine levels between subjects who did or did not develop upper respiratory tract infections in a study on the effect of intensified training on swimmers. Furthermore, it was shown that the plasma glutamine concentration did not necessarily decrease during periods of intensified training.

In another placebo-controlled study, Castell et al.[132] showed that glutamine supplementation in runners after a marathon race did not influence the lymphocyte distribution or the plasma concentration of IL-6, IFN-γ, or CRP. In a blind crossover, randomized, placebo-controlled study by Rohde et al.,[166] well-trained athletes undergoing repeated bicycle-ergometer exercise were supplemented with glutamine. The athletes performed 60, 45, and 30 minutes of exercise at 75% of maximal oxygen consumption separated by 2-hour rest periods. Glutamine (100 mg/kg body weight) was supplemented 30 minutes before the end, at the end, and again 30 minutes after each exercise bout. Arterial plasma glutamine concentration declined from 508 ± 35 (pre-exercise) to 402 ± 38 pM (2 hrs after the last exercise bout) in the placebo trial. Glutamine was maintained above pre-exercise level at all times in the glutamine supplementation trial, yet no differences between the two trials in the concentration of lymphocytes, leukocyte subpopulations, lymphocyte proliferation, LAK activity, or NK activity existed. Others have also shown similar results.[174] Nonetheless, increased levels of plasma glutamine during prolonged exercise have been shown in several studies and attributed to skeletal muscle release.[175-177] This response is mirrored by a decrease in muscle glutamine concentrations during exercise.[145,177] Therefore, it has been proposed that the decrease in plasma glutamine concentration after exercise is a result of increased use by the cells of the immune system.[109,150] Although the data are not abundantly clear regarding its utility as a supplement, it does appear that its usefulness may be *depletion dependent* and hence useful during training cycles that are heavy, intense, and chronic in nature.

Glucosamine and Chondroitin Sulfate

The management of joint repair is often facilitated by cryotherapy and nonsteroidal anti-inflammatory drugs (NSAIDs); these types of interventions often contribute to joint repair via secondary mechanisms (i.e., decreased inflammation). However, an increased knowledge of joint disease and injury pathophysiology may provide treatment modalities with better long-term application. This is especially true as current medications may be complicated by intolerance and toxicity. In this regard, any therapeutic agent that potentially offers greater symptomatic relief with less overall toxicity is desired. At present, the leading contenders to fulfill this role are glucosamine and chondroitin sulfate. Although their onset of action is slower, a review of the literature reveals that several short-term studies suggest that these agents have the effectiveness equal to nonsteroidal anti-inflammatory drugs or NSAIDs.[178-194]

Currently, no drugs are available that reverse the structural or biochemical abnormalities of joint tissue damage, although some chondroprotective agents are being studied in animal models.[195] Traditionally, nonopioid analgesics and NSAID therapy have been the choice for treatment. Unfortunately, this form of therapy often includes side effects.[196] Although the adverse effects of therapeutic doses of acetaminophen up to 4000 mg/day are generally believed to be mild, acetaminophen has been linked to liver toxicity in patient populations consuming excessive amounts of alcohol.[197] Moreover, renal failure during the long-term ingestion of acetaminophen and NSAIDs have been noted.[198,199]

In addition to over-the-counter drugs (e.g., aspirin, ibuprofen, and naproxen), several forms of prescriptive NSAIDs are also currently available.[200,201] Though the toxicity and effectiveness appears to be comparable, nonacetylated salicylates have less renal toxicity and antiplatelet effects, while low-dose ibuprofen (<1600 mg/day) may have less serious gastrointestinal toxicity.[202,203] However, among persons 65+, 20–30% of all hospitalizations and deaths due to peptic ulcer disease have been attributed to NSAID therapy.[202] Although these risk factors are compounded by history of peptic ulcer disease, upper GI bleeding, concomitant use of oral corticosteroids and anticoagulants, and, possibly, smoking and alcohol consumption,[204] they are important to note given the potential for harm with chronic usage starting in younger populations.

Chemical Structure

Glucosamine is an aminomonosaccharide that is found in human tissues, including cartilage, and is produced in the body by the addition of an amino group to glucose. The primary components of the structure are glycosaminoglycans

(GAGs), which form the matrix of all connective tissues. Subsequently, this molecule is then acetylated to acetyl glucosamine. Thus, various joint structure components such as hyaluronan, keratan sulfate, and heparan sulfate are composed, in part, of repeating units of acetyl glucosamine. By itself, glucosamine has a molecular weight of 179.17. Glucosamine sulfate, the form most often studied, has a molecular weight of 456.42 and is the sulfate, or salt moiety of glucosamine which plays an important role in the synthesis of proteoglycans because the constituent glycosaminoglycans (GAGs) are highly sulfated. In addition to glucosamine sulfate, other over-the-counter glucosamine products take various forms including hydrochloride, N-acetyl, and a dextrorotatory isomer. These distinctions become important with regard to usage. Unlike glucosamine sulfate and glucosamine hydrochloride, glucosamine does not appear to have active intestinal transport; it may be digested by intestinal bacteria and is excreted in the feces. On the other hand, the hydrochloride and N-acetyl forms lack the sulfate group, which also appears to be important for therapeutic effect.

Pharmacokinetics and Tissue Effects

The pharmacokinetics of glucosamine sulfate have been investigated after intravenous, intramuscular, and oral administration in dogs, rats, and humans. Findings from these studies suggest that following intravenous administration labeled (C14), glucosamine sulfate has a radioactive half-life in the plasma of about 0.28 hours. Subsequent incorporation into plasma proteins begins after 1–2 hours, peaks by about 10 hours, and then declines over a 70-hour period.[205–207] Results obtained after administration of glucosamine sulfate in humans shows results not that much different than in dogs and that oral administration results in similar results to those of intravenous administration; however, oral concentrations are five times lower because of the liver.[205–207] Overall, it has been estimated that about 8–12% is retained in the tissues and, as delineated by animal studies, ^{14}C-labeled glucosamine may appear in cartilage 4 hours after ingestion.[208] Until recently, glucosamine has been characterized as a slow-acting treatment of osteoarthritis with improvements in symptoms but not demonstrated in vivo chondroprotective affects. However, in in vitro evidence using damaged human chondrocytes, glucosamine increases proteoglycan synthesis, human chondrocyte gene expression, and steady-state levels of perlecan and aggrecan mRNA.[209,210]

Anti-Inflammatory Effects

In rat models, glucosamine has shown anti-inflammatory activity that appears to be different from that of NSAIDs. Although NSAIDs act primarily through inhibition of cyclooxygenases, glucosamine is more related to stimulation of proteoglycan biosynthesis, the reduction of superoxide radicals by macrophages, and inhibition of lysosomal enyzmes. Combined, these mechanisms may stabilize cell membranes, resulting in decreased inflammation.[194] Moreover, when combined with NSAID therapy, the combination allows for a substantial decrease in the NSAID consumption.[211]

In one of the earliest trials involving glucosamine sulfate, 80 patients with established osteoarthritis (OA) were treated with placebo or 1.5 g of glucosamine sulfate daily for 30 days. During this trial, a 72% decrease in symptom score in the glucosamine sulfate group was compared to a 36% decrease in the placebo group. In addition, the time it took to achieve relief from joint pain improved after 7 days. After 14 days, tenderness, swelling, and active range of motion improved while passive range of motion increased after 21 days. All of these effects persisted for 30 days.[212] In other studies performed during the 1980s, similar findings have also been noted as when compared with a placebo.[181,188,193,213]

Regarding drug comparisons and more traditional lines of therapy, Vaz[193] treated 40 patients with unilateral knee OA with glucosamine at 1.5 g/day while using 400 mg of ibuprofen as the control for 8 weeks. During this trial, pain scores improved in both groups, but improvement was more rapid in the ibuprofen group. Pain scores, however, continued to improve in the glucosamine group throughout the 8-week period and, by the end of the 8-week period, were more pronounced in the glucosamine group. These results are partially supported by Tapadinhas et al.[214] in a trial involving 1208 patients examined in an open-label trial using 1.5 g of glucosamine sulfate daily. During this investigation, patients' pain at rest, standing, and during exercise showed that active motion not only improved, but was sustained for up to 12 weeks after discontinuation of the treatment. Physician-rated improvement was also reported as "good" in 59% of patients and "sufficient" in 35% in the glucosamine group. Overall, patients rated glucosamine as significantly better than their previous NSAIDs. What this trial suggests is that glucosamine may have more prolonged treatment effects, possibly owing to a tissue saturating of the active treatment.

More recent investigations in larger cohorts confirm these earlier findings when examined versus a placebo or versus traditional drug treatments.[186,187,215,216] For example, 200 ambulatory patients with OA of the knee who received 1500 mg/day of glucosamine or 1200 mg/day of ibuprofen for 4 weeks showed no difference for indices of pain at night, after immobility, after standing, and after getting up from a chair. Furthermore, no differences were noted for activities of daily living, which included stair walking and squatting. As per previous trials, the time course of the response differed between the two treatment groups as 48% of the patients on ibuprofen responded by 1 week versus 28% taking glucosamine who responded after 2 weeks. After 4 weeks however, 52% of the ibuprofen-treated patients and 48% of those on glucosamine had responded with fewer adverse events occurring in the glucosamine group (6%) as compared to the ibuprofen group (35%).[186]

In a more involved trial, Rovati[216] randomized 329 patients to receive 1) 1500 mg of glucosamine, 2) 20 mg of piroxicam, 3) glucosamine and piroxicam, or d) placebo. All subjects were treated for 90 days and were then followed for 60 days after treatment was discontinued. As a result, the Lequesne index decreased by 4.8 points in the glucosamine group, 4.6 points in the glucosamine/piroxicam group, 2.9 points in the piroxicam only group, and 0.8 point in the placebo group. Statistically, the glucosamine response was better than that for placebo or piroxicam (P = 0.001). Sixty days after discontinuation of treatment, the Lequesne index had risen only 0.4 point in the glucosamine group but 1.7 points in the piroxicam group (P = 0.001). In the one trial using glucosamine hydrochloride, 89 patients with knee OA were treated with glucosamine hydrochloride (500 mg) three times a day (n = 41) and compared in double-blind fashion with a placebo group (n = 48). In this 8-week study, pain indices revealed significant improvement with glucosamine hydrochloride, relative to placebo (P < 0.005), after 3 to 4 weeks of treatment.

In the most recent trial, Reginster showed that glucosamine sulfate significantly reduced progression of knee osteoarthritis over 3 years.[217] During this trial, 212 patients with knee OA were randomly assigned, in a double-blind fashion, to continuous treatment with oral glucosamine sulfate, 1500 mg once-a-day, or placebo for 3 years. Weightbearing, anteroposterior radiographs of each knee were taken at enrollment and after 1 and 3 years to assess total mean joint space width of the medial compartment of the tibio-femoral joint. Symptomatology was also assessed at each 4-month visit by the (total) WOMAC index. Data were analyzed separately according to a per-protocol (PP) approach on 3-year completers, or on an intention-to-treat (ITT) basis including all randomized patients by the last-observation-carried-forward. Results of this trial showed that the placebo-treated patients had an average joint space narrowing of approximately 0.08–0.1 mm/yr, while no narrowing occurred in the glucosamine sulfate group. In addition, a slight worsening in symptoms was evident at the end of treatment with placebo, compared with the improvement observed after glucosamine sulfate.

Nutraceutical Hype?

On March 15, 2000, the Journal of the American Medical Association published a meta-analysis which concluded: "Trials of glucosamine and chondroitin preparations for OA symptoms demonstrate moderate to large effects, but quality issues and likely publication bias suggest that these effects are exaggerated. Nevertheless, some degree of efficacy appears probable for these preparations." An accompanying editorial concluded: "As with many nutraceuticals that currently are widely touted as beneficial for common but difficult-to-treat disorders, the promotional enthusiasm often far surpasses the scientific evidence supporting clinical use. Until high-quality studies, such as the National Institutes of Health study, are completed, work such as [the meta-analysis] is the best hope for providing physicians with information necessary to advise their patients about the risks and benefits of these therapies."

http://www.quackwatch.com/01QuackeryRelatedTopics/DSH/glucosamine.html

McAlindon TE, LaValley MP, Gulin JP, Felson DT. Glucosamine and chondroitin for treatment of osteoarthritis: a systematic quality assessment and meta-analysis. JAMA 2000;283(11): 1469–1475.

Editors' Note: Certainly, the JAMA editors raise legitimate points that are also relevant to "conventional medicine." As with any nutraceutical, glucosamine and chondroitin (if they do what their proponents claim), would ultimately put a dent in the medical industry where it hurts most (i.e., their pocketbooks). It is always a good practice to be skeptical of nutraceutical as well as conventional medical claims.

Chondroitin Sulfate

In a similar fashion to glucosamine, preparations of chondroitin sulfate have also been examined. The two most widely used chondroitin materials used today contain principally chondroitin-4 sulfate and chondroitin-6 sulfate. In addition, the absorption from the gastrointestinal tract of chondroitin is limited as more than 90% of glucosamine is absorbed, whereas less than 10% of chondroitin sulfate is absorbed. Although early studies using chondroitin sulfate administered the molecule parenterally, it is now more commonly administered orally.

Clinical Trials

In one study,[184] 120 patients were treated with chondroitin sulfate in a placebo-controlled study of 3 months in which patients were allowed to continue their use of NSAIDs and then were followed for 2 months after treatment. Those taking chondroitin sulfate used significantly less NSAIDs than the placebo group, had a lower incidence of joint pain, as measured on a visual analog scale (Lequesne index), and patient and physician global assessments all showed significant improvement (P < 0.05) in the chondroitin sulfate–treated group.

Others have also reported treatment effectiveness.[178,182,185] For example, 56 patients with knee OA were enrolled in a 1-year double-blind placebo-controlled study comparing 800 mg of chondroitin sulfate with placebo. Forty-seven patients (25 chondroitin sulfate–treated, 22 placebo) completed 1 year of investigation. Results showed better mobility, and decreased joint effusion, swelling, and supportive drug use (e.g., Paracetamol) during chondroitin treatment. These results have been supported by similar studies.[179,184]

In a larger study,[185] 146 patients with knee OA were evaluated. Of these patients, 74 received 400 mg of chondroitin sulfate three times per day for 3 months, followed by 3 months of no treatment. In comparison, 72 patients were treated with 50 mg of diclofenac three times a day for 1 month, followed by 5 months of no treatment. Those treated with diclofenac had a decrease in joint pain after 10 days, which disappeared shortly after the discontinuation of treatment. Those treated with chondroitin sulfate had a significant response at 30 days, which lasted for 3 months after discontinuation of the drug. Through the use of the Lequesne index, the chondroitin sulfate treatment was 78% lower after 3 months than at baseline, whereas with the diclofenac it was 62.6% lower. Three months after discontinuation of chondroitin sulfate, the Lequesne index remained 64.4% lower than the pretreatment level. Three months after discontinuation of

diclofenac, however, the index was only 29.7% lower than at baseline. Thus, the effects of chondroitin sulfate treatment persisted longer after discontinuation than those of traditional NSAID therapy.

Two studies have attempted to evaluate the effects of chondroitin sulfate on the progression of radiographic changes of OA. A computerized technique was used to measure medial tibiofemoral joint space in patients treated with 800 mg/day of chondroitin sulfate or with placebo.[191] After 1 year, tibiofemoral joint space width had decreased significantly in placebo-treated patients ($P < 0.05$ versus treated patients) but had not changed from the baseline value in the chondroitin sulfate treatment group.

In a similar trial, Verbruggen evaluated hand radiographs from 119 patients with OA for 3 years.[194] Results in 34 patients receiving chondroitin sulfate (400 mg t.i.d.) were compared with the results of 85 patients who received placebo. During treatment, the chondroitin sulfate–treatment group showed a significant decrease in the number of patients with new erosive OA (i.e., 8.8% of patients with classic or loss of joint space developed erosions in the chondroitin sulfate–treatment group versus 29.4% in the placebo group).

SUMMARY

Over time, most athletes will experience some form of debilitation during sport participation. How this will occur in each participant will differ and likely depend on the sports modality chosen. Endurance athletes will suffer overuse and overtraining syndromes, although strength athletes involved in combatant-type sports are more likely to encounter traumatic injuries, which often cannot be helped regardless of preparation. Currently, there is some evidence to suggest that nutrient intervention will reduce the likelihood of overuse and overtraining maladies. Still, the most potent cure lies in prevention. Overall, imparting a proper training stimulus that is matched by a proper recovery period best suits prevention. Currently, the best evidence available involves proper caloric and macro/micronutrient intake. Regarding energetics, the strength athlete will benefit most by the adequate intake of carbohydrates and protein immediately following exercise. These measures not only appear to enhance the necessary nutrient stores for future energy needs and tissue repair following training, but they also appear to positively affect overall immune function. Although these qualities are difficult to assess in short trials lasting 2–3 months, their cumulative benefits

may be more striking over longer periods of time that involve yearly training cycles. Supplementation may also improve the aforementioned parameters, as athletes do not always use the quality eating habits that scientific inquiry and allied health practice have bestowed onto them as *necessary*. Thus, supplementation may prove most beneficial merely as a means of improving overall nutrient intake. As it pertains to biological efficiency, several protein supplements offer good quality protein alternatives. Despite popular marketing hype, there is no clear *best*. Certainly, the combination of several sources should be entertained. When injury of any type does occur, proper time and healing are necessary for complete return to activity. Initially, the healing response is predicated on the immediate imparting of standard first aid measures. Following closely, and in conjunction with such intervention, is the use of NSAIDs as a means of anti-inflammation. Although the use of glucosamine may have similar benefits, the onset of action may be too long for the athlete desiring to return to competition rapidly. Combining them may thus be the best alternative as NSAIDs have the ability to promote rapid anti-inflammatory effects while glucosamine and chondroitin have more profound joint tissue effects. Additionally, because prolonged NSAID use may be complicated by some minor, yet irritating side effects, early co-administration, followed by NSAID withdrawal after 6–8 weeks may prove to be an attractive alternative.

This may be especially true given that NSAIDs have an acute effect that ceases once removed. Alternatively, glucosamine and chondroitin appear to have more prolonged effects as once they saturate the tissue, relief continues with either smaller or withdrawn dosing.

AUTHORS' RECOMMENDATIONS

As with many nutritional supplements, most of the issues related to product efficiency involve marketing wars aimed at determining product superiority. Seldom, however, do these marketing efforts involve true science. Perhaps the largest offender of this strategy involves protein supplementation. As has been outlined above, the disparity between protein quality and biological value is relatively small. The primary factor that regulates immune competence is the consumption of adequate dietary energy (i.e., calories). When injury does occur, steps to aid tissue repair are also required. Regarding macronutrient replacement, nutrient replacement entails adequate carbohydrate and protein replacement strategies. Overall, protein synthesis increases in response to insulin, growth hormone, testosterone, and adequate amounts of amino acids, but decreases in response to cortisol, glucocorticoids, glucagon, exercise, and inadequate amount of amino acids.[58–60] As insulin and growth hormones play a dominant role in everyday protein metabolism, it seems essential to provide a nutrient-facilitated environment for recuperation that promotes either or both of these hormones following exercise. Despite the *carbohydrate paranoia* that sometimes exists in the world of strength development, a combination of carbohydrate and protein supplementation is required to create a hormonal milieu that is favorable to muscle recovery and protein synthesis. The time period immediately following intense training could be the most critical for beginning nutritional support and recuperation. To accomplish this, the timing of carbohydrate plus protein intake is extremely important, as is their consumption immediately following exercise that leads to increased rates of muscle glycogen resynthesis and increased anabolic hormones needed for enhanced protein synthesis. Several overall factors appear to play a dominant role during this time. First, muscle glycogen resynthesis after high-intensity exercise ranges from 7.5 to 15 times faster than after prolonged or endurance-oriented exercise provided that adequate carbohydrate is consumed. In comparison to high-intensity exercise, general resistance training factors in at about half of that for the high-intensity exercise group. Therefore, "high intensity" may not be the group that best represents the strength athlete overall. Instead, the training response, relative to strength training, may be largely influenced by the training cycle. What is clear is that the more intense the training, the greater the requirement for nutrient replacement. This is most likely due to the broader extent of glycogen use during heavy and more intense training cycles. How much carbohydrate and protein are actually needed following exercise really depends on how hard (intensity) and how long (volume) one trains. It will also vary on how naïve one is to the training stimulus. Thus, new training cycles and/or new training programs may require slightly greater protein needs, whereas the latter part of a training cycle in which adaptation has taken place may require less.

As it pertains to protein requirements, the restoration of nitrogen balance can be enhanced in several ways. First, athletes must allow the body to adapt to a new training stimulus. Second, intensity will change relatively as the body adapts and gets stronger. Third, the timing of nutrient intake is essential following a training stimulus. Lastly, the type of protein ingested will always be a source of controversy among strength-training athletes. However, as there is no definitive consensus regarding protein type, the jury is still out. Whey protein is beneficial due to its high BCAA and immunoglobulin content. This may be especially beneficial during post-workout nutrient replacement strategies. However, casein may be beneficial as well as casein, which also shows an adequate release of amino acids that is slower than whey. Thus, latter meal supplementation with casein may show equal effectiveness. Soy also has its benefits when ingested as a food. This is likely due to the high isoflavone content of whole soy foods. Powdered soy may be somewhat questionable as a supplement due to a reduction in isoflavones associated with processing techniques. Regardless of choice, the addition of glutamine might prove advantageous to athletes, particularly with intense periods of training. Ribose is a relatively *new* supplement that has an interesting theoretical basis for an ergogenic effect.

One might surmise that ribose could delay fatigue in repeated, high-intensity, intermittent work bouts (e.g., repeated sprints, multiple sets on a weight-lifting exercise, etc.). Future work will hopefully provide answers to this.

FUTURE RESEARCH

The role of recovery post-exercise is an oft-neglected aspect of many athletes' training programs. Certainly, it would behoove athletes and coaches to monitor recovery with the same diligence as training itself. However, with regard to the scientific study of recovery per se, it is not a simple task. For instance, it would seem sensible that adequate protein and carbohydrate intake could, over an extended period of time, confer benefits regarding general musculoskeletal health, fitness, and perhaps athletic performance. However, this is not a phenomenon that one would likely observe in the multitude of short-term trials (6–12 weeks) seen in the exercise science literature. Thus, to adequately answer questions related to recovery, longer treatment durations are of necessity. For instance, if one were to assess if glutamine supplementation impacted the health (e.g., as measured by the incidence of upper respiratory tract infections) of collegiate cross-country runners, it would be wise to follow these athletes over the course of several months, perhaps up to a year. Only then could one answer with any semblance of confidence if the treatment actually improved health and therefore recovery from exercise. Also, is there a superior protein source for gains in lean body mass? That question cannot adequately be answered in a short-term exercise/diet intervention. Nor could it be answered via an acute intervention that examines changes in protein synthesis and degradation; longer trials are needed. Regardless, there is more research needed (in general) regarding the supplements mentioned in this chapter as it pertains to recovery or otherwise.

REFERENCES

1. Balnave CD, Thompson MW. Effect of training on eccentric exercise-induced muscle damage. J Appl Physiol 1993;75(4):1545–1551.
2. O'Reilly KP, Warhol MJ, Fielding RA, et al. Eccentric exercise-induced muscle damage impairs muscle glycogen repletion. J Appl Physiol 1987;63(1):252–256.
3. Rodenburg JB, Bar PR, De Boer RW. Relations between muscle soreness and biochemical and functional outcomes of eccentric exercise. J Appl Physiol 1993;74(6):2976–2983.
4. Weiler JM. Medical modifiers of sports injury: the use of non-steroidal anti-inflammatory drugs (NSAIDs) in sports soft-tissue injury. Clin Sports Med 1992;11(3):625–644.
5. Gerster H. Function of vitamin E in physical exercise: a review. Z Ernahrungswiss 1991;30(2):89–97.
6. Almekinders LC. Anti-inflammatory treatment of muscular injuries in sports. Sports Med 1993;15(3):139–145.
7. Meyer SA, Saltzman CL, Albright JP. Stress fractures of the foot and leg. Clin Sports Med 1993;12(2):395–413.
8. Adams DO, Hamilton TA. The cell biology of macrophage activation. Annu Rev Immunol 1984;2:283–318.
9. Sun X, Hsueh W, Torre-Amione G. Effects of in vivo "priming" on endotoxin-induced hypotension and tissue injury: the role of PAF and tumor necrosis factor. Am J Pathol 1990;136(4):949–956.
10. Baggiolini M, Moser B, Clark-Lewis I. Interleukin-8 and related chemotactic cytokines. The Giles Filley Lecture. Chest 1994;105(3 suppl):95S–98S.
11. Dijkmans R, Van Damme J, Cornette F, et al. Bacterial lipopolysaccharide potentiates gamma interferon-induced cytotoxicity for normal mouse and rat fibroblasts. Infect Immunol 1990;58(1):32–36.
12. Ferrante A, Kowanko IC, Bates EJ. Mechanisms of host tissue damage by cytokine-activated neutrophils. Immunol Ser 1992;57:499–521.
13. Lowry SF. Cytokine mediators of immunity and inflammation. Arch Surg 1993;128(11):1235–1241.
14. Menger MD, Lehr HA, Messmer K. Role of oxygen radicals in the microcirculatory manifestations of postischemic injury [published erratum appears in Klin Wochenschr 1990;69(24):1185]. Klin Wochenschr 1991;69(21–23):1050–1055.
15. Smith CW, Marlin SD, Rothlein R, et al. Cooperative interactions of LFA-1 and Mac-1 with intercellular adhesion molecule-1 in facilitating adherence and transendothelial migration of human neutrophils in vitro. J Clin Invest 1989;83(6):2008–2017.
16. Ward PA, Warren JS, Johnson KJ. Oxygen radicals inflammation and tissue injury. Free Radic Biol Med 1988;5(5–6):403–408.
17. Venable ME, Zimmerman GA, McIntyre TM, Prescott SM. Platelet-activating factor: a phospholipid autacoid with diverse actions. J Lipid Res 1993;34(5):691–702.
18. Assoian RK, Grotendorst GR, Miller DM, Sporn MB. Cellular transformation by coordinated action of three peptide growth factors from human platelets. Nature 1984;309(5971):804–806.
19. Bennett NT, Schultz GS. Growth factors and wound healing: Part II. Role in normal and chronic wound healing. Am J Surg 1993;166(1):74–81.
20. Schmid P, Kunz S, Cerletti N, et al. Injury induced expression of TGF-beta-1 mRNA is enhanced by exogenously applied TGF-beta-s. Biochem Biophys Res Commun 1993;194(1):399–406.
21. Antoniades HN, Galanopoulos T, Neville-Golden J, et al. P53 expression during normal tissue regeneration in response to acute cutaneous injury in swine. J Clin Invest 1994;93(5):2206–2214.

22. Kelly CJ, Zurier RB, Krakauer KA, et al. Prostaglandin E1 inhibits effector T cell induction and tissue damage in experimental murine interstitial nephritis. J Clin Invest 1987;79(3):782–789.

23. Takayama TK, Miller C, Szabo G. Elevated tumor necrosis factor-alpha production concomitant to elevated prostaglandin E-2 production by trauma patients' monocytes. Arch Surg 1990;125(1):29–35.

24. Northoff H, Weinstock C, Berg A. The cytokine response to strenuous exercise. Int J Sports Med 1994;15(suppl 3):S167–S171.

25. Rivkind AI, Siegel JH, Guadalupi P, Littleton M. Sequential patterns of eicosanoid platelet and neutrophil interactions in the evolution of the fulminant post-traumatic adult respiratory distress syndrome. Ann Surg 1989;210(3):355–372.

26. Bestit C, Alvarez A, Carrillo JP, et al. Double-blind multicenter trial of a new anti-inflammatory spray, fepradinol, in soft-tissue injuries. Curr Ther Res 1989;45(1):53–62.

27. Simpson R, Phillis JW. The use of nonsteroidal anti-inflammatory drugs in sports medicine. Ann Sports Med 1990;5(2):107–109.

28. Meakins JL, Pietsch JB, Bubenick O, et al. Delayed hypersensitivity: indicator of acquired failure of host defenses in sepsis and trauma. Ann Surg 1977;186(3):241–250.

29. Jaattela M. Overexpression of major heat shock protein hsp70 inhibits tumor necrosis factor-induced activation of phospholipase A-2. J Immunol 1993;151(8):4286–4294.

30. Amelink GJ, Van der Wal WAA, Wokke JHJ, et al. Exercise-induced muscle damage in the rat: the effect of vitamin E deficiency. Pfluegers Arch 1991;419(3–4):304–309.

31. Cannon JG, Orencole SF, Fielding RA, et al. Acute phase response in exercise: interaction of age and vitamin E on neutrophils and muscle enzyme release. Am J Physiol 1990;259(6 pt 2):R1214–R1219.

32. Nieman DC, Nehlsen-Cannarella SL. The effects of acute chronic exercise on immunoglobulins. Sports Med 1991;11(3):183–201.

33. Lauffer RB. Exercise as prevention: do the health benefits derive in part from lower iron levels? Med Hypotheses 1991;35(2):103–107.

34. Lahat N, Shtiller R, Zlotnick AY, Merin G. Early IL-2/sIL-2R surge following surgery leads to temporary immune refractoriness. Clin Exper Immunol 1993;92(3):482–486.

35. Cupps TR, Fauci AS. Corticosteroid-mediated immunoregulation in man. Immunol Rev 1982;65:133–155.

36. Armstrong RB. Muscle damage and endurance events. Sports Med 1986;3(5):370–381.

37. Friden J. Muscle soreness after exercise: implications of morphological changes. Int J Sports Med 1984;5(2):57–66.

38. Friden J, Kjorell U, Thornell LE. Delayed muscle soreness and cytoskeletal alterations: an immunocytological study in man. Int J Sports Med 1984;5(1):15–18.

39. Salminen A. Lysosomal changes in skeletal muscles during the repair of exercise injuries in muscle fibers. Acta Physiol Scand Suppl 1985;539:1–31.

40. Furuno K, Goldberg AL. The activation of protein degradation in muscle by calcium or muscle injury does not involve a lysosomal mechanisms. Biochem J 1986;237(3):859–864.

41. Armstrong RB. Initial events in exercise-induced muscular injury. Med Sci Sports Exerc 1990;22(4):429–435.

42. Fielding RA, Manfredi TJ, Ding W, et al. Acute phase response in exercise III: Neutrophil and IL-1-beta accumulation in skeletal muscle. Am J Physiol 1993;265(1 pt 2):R166–R172.

43. Camus G, Pincemail J, Ledent M, et al. Plasma levels of polymorphonuclear elastase and myeloperoxidase after uphill walking and downhill running at similar energy cost. Int J Sports Med 1992;13(6):443–446.

44. Dufaux B, Order U. Plasma elastase-alpha 1-antitrypsin, neopterin, tumor necrosis factor, and soluble interleukin-2 receptor after prolonged exercise. Int J Sports Med 1989;10(6):434–438.

45. Hansen JB, Wilsgard L, Olsen JO, Osterud B. Formation and persistence of procoagulant and fibrinolytic activities in circulation after strenuous physical exercise. Thromb Haemost 1990;64(3):385–389.

46. Hasson SM, Daniels JC, Divine JG, et al. Effect of ibuprofen use on muscle soreness, damage, and performance: a preliminary investigation. Med Sci Sports Exerc 1993;25(1):9–17.

47. Jones DA, Newham DJ, Round JM, Tolfree SEJ. Experimental human muscle damage: morphological changes in relation to other indices of damage. J Physiol (Lond) 1986(375):435–448.

48. Round JM, Jones DA, Cambridge G. Cellular infiltrates in human skeletal muscle exercise induced damage as a model for inflammatory muscle disease? J Neurol Sci 1987;82(1–3):1–12.

49. Maughan RJ, Donnelly AE, Gleeson M, et al. Delayed-onset muscle damage and lipid peroxidation in man after a downhill run. Muscle Nerve 1989;12(4):332–336.

50. Camus G, Felekidis A, Pincemail J, et al. Blood levels of reduced/oxidized glutathione and plasma concentration of ascorbic acid during eccentric and concentric exercises of similar energy cost. Archives Internationales de Physiologie de Biochimie et de Biophysique (Liege) 1994;102(1):67–70.

51. Fitzgerald L. Overtraining increases the susceptibility to infection. Int J Sports Med 1991;12(suppl 1):S5–S8.

52. Hoffman-Goetz L, Pedersen BK. Exercise and the immune system: a model of the stress response? Immunol Today 1994;15(8):382–387.

53. Nieman D. Exercise, upper respiratory tract infection, and the immune system. Med Sci Sports Exerc 1994;26(2):128–139.

54. Nieman DC, Miller AR, Henson DA, et al. Effects of high- vs moderate-intensity exercise on natural killer cell activity. Med Sci Sports Exerc 1993;25(10):1126–1134.

55. Pedersen BK, Ullum H. NK cell response to physical activity: possible mechanisms of action. Med Sci Sports Exerc 1994;26(2):140–146.

56. Nieman DC, Henson DA, Johnson R, et al. Effects of brief heavy exertion on circulating lymphocyte subpopulations and proliferative response. Med Sci Sports Exerc 1992;24(12):1339–1345.

57. Gray AB, Smart YC, Telford RD, et al. Anaerobic exercise causes transient changes in leukocyte subsets and Il-2r expression. Med Sci Sports Exerc 1992;24(12):1332–1338.

58. Tawa NE, Jr., Goldberg AL. Suppression of muscle protein turnover and amino acid degradation by dietary protein deficiency. Am J Physiol 1992;263(2 pt 1):E317–325.

59. Watt PW, Corbett ME, Rennie MJ. Stimulation of protein synthesis in pig skeletal muscle by infusion of amino acids during constant insulin availability. Am J Physiol 1992;263(3 pt 1):E453–460.

60. Marshall S, Monzon R. Amino acid regulation of insulin action in isolated adipocytes: selective ability of amino acids to enhance both insulin sensitivity and maximal insulin responsiveness of the protein synthesis system. J Biol Chem 1989;264(4):2037–2042.

61. Rooyackers OE, Nair KS. Hormonal regulation of human muscle protein metabolism. Ann Rev Nutr 1997;17:457–485.

62. Umpleby AM, Russell-Jones DL. The hormonal control of protein metabolism. Baillieres Clin Endocrinol Metab 1996;10(4):551–570.

63. Dohm GL, Kasperek GJ, Tapscott EB, et al. Protein metabolism during endurance exercise. Fed Proc 1985;44(2):348–352.

64. Lemon PW, Nagle FJ. Effects of exercise on protein and amino acid metabolism. Med Sci Sports Exerc 1981;13(3):141–149.

65. Friedman JE, Lemon PW. Effect of chronic endurance exercise on retention of dietary protein. Int J Sports Med 1989;10(2):118–123.

66. Lemon PW. Protein and exercise: update 1987. Med Sci Sports Exerc 1987;19(5 suppl):S179–190.

67. Stone MH, Keith R, Kearney JT, et al. Overtraining: a review of the signs and symptoms of overtraining. J Appl Sports Res Sci Res 1991;5(1):35–50.

68. Tarnopolsky MA, Atkinson SA, MacDougall JD, et al. Evaluation of protein requirements for trained strength athletes. J Appl Physiol 1992;73(5):1986–1995.

69. Tarnopolsky MA, MacDougall JD, Atkinson SA. Influence of protein intake and training status on nitrogen balance and lean body mass. J Appl Physiol 1988;64(1):187–193.

70. Pivarnik JM, Hickson JF, Jr., Wolinsky I. Urinary 3-methylhistidine excretion increases with repeated weight training exercise. Med Sci Sports Exerc 1989;21(3):283–287.

71. Lemon PW, Tarnopolsky MA, MacDougall JD, et al. Protein requirements and muscle mass/strength changes during intensive training in novice bodybuilders. J Appl Physiol 1992;73(2):767–775.

72. Dohm GL, Williams RT, Kasperek GJ, van Rij AM. Increased excretion of urea and N tau-methylhistidine by rats and humans after a bout of exercise. J Appl Physiol 1982;52(1):27–33.

73. Evans WJ, Meredith CN, Cannon JG, et al. Metabolic changes following eccentric exercise in trained and untrained men. J Appl Physiol 1986;61(5):1864–1868.

74. Lemon PW, Mullin JP. Effect of initial muscle glycogen levels on protein catabolism during exercise. J Appl Physiol 1980;48(4):624–629.

75. Stone MH. Muscle conditioning and muscle injuries. Med Sci Sports Exerc 1990;22(4):457–462.

76. Brooks GA. Amino acid and protein metabolism during exercise and recovery. Med Sci Sports Exerc 1987;19(5 suppl):S150–156.

77. Butterfield GE. Whole-body protein utilization in humans. Med Sci Sports Exerc 1987;19(5 suppl):S157–165.

78. Wolfe RR. Does exercise stimulate protein breakdown in humans? Isotopic approaches to the problem. Med Sci Sports Exerc 1987;19(5 suppl):S172–178.

79. Ivy JL, Katz AL, Cutler CL, et al. Muscle glycogen synthesis after exercise: effect of time of carbohydrate ingestion. J Appl Physiol 1988;64(4):1480–1485.

80. Robergs RA. Nutrition and exercise determinants of post-exercise glycogen synthesis. Int J Sports Nutr 1991;1(4):307–337.

81. Friedman JE, Neufer PD, Dohm GL. Regulation of glycogen resynthesis following exercise: dietary considerations. Sports Med 1991;11(4):232–243.

82. Blom PC, Vollestad NK, Costill DL. Factors affecting changes in muscle glycogen concentration during and after prolonged exercise. Acta Physiol Scand Suppl 1986;556:67–74.

83. Pascoe DD, Gladden LB. Muscle glycogen resynthesis after short-term, high-intensity exercise and resistance exercise. Sports Med 1996;21(2):98–118.

84. Walton P, Rhodes EC. Glycemic index and optimal performance. Sports Med 1997;23(3):164–172.

85. Conley MS, Stone MH. Carbohydrate ingestion/supplementation or resistance exercise and training. Sports Med 1996;21(1):7–17.

86. Ivy JL. Glycogen resynthesis after exercise: effect of carbohydrate intake. Int J Sports Med 1998;19 suppl 2:S142–S145.

87. Weinstock C, Konig D, Harnischmacher R, et al. Effect of exhaustive exercise stress on the cytokine response. Med Sci Sports Exerc 1997;29(3):345–354.

88. Berk LS, Nieman DC, Youngberg WS, et al. The effect of long endurance running on natural killer cells in marathoners. Med Sci Sports Exerc 1990;22(2):207–212.

89. Bruunsgaard H, Galbo H, Halkjaer-Kristensen J, et al. Exercise-induced increase in serum interleukin-6 in humans is related to muscle damage. J Physiol (Lond) 1997;499(Pt 3):833–841.

90. Bruunsgaard H, Hartkopp A, Mohr T, et al. In vivo cell-mediated immunity and vaccination response following prolonged, intense exercise. Med Sci Sports Exerc 1997;29(9):1176–1181.

91. Bury TB, Pirnay F. Effect of prolonged exercise on neutrophil myeloperoxidase secretion. Int J Sports Med 1995;16(6):410–412.

92. Bury TB, Louis R, Radermecker MF, Pirnay F. Blood mononuclear cells mobilization and cytokines secretion during prolonged exercises. Int J Sports Med 1996;17(2):156–160.

93. Drenth JP, Van Uum SH, Van Deuren M, et al. Endurance run increases circulating IL-6 and IL-1ra but downregulates ex vivo TNF-alpha and IL-1 beta production. J Appl Physiol 1995;79(5):1497–1503.

94. Evans WJ, Cannon JG. The metabolic effects of exercise-induced muscle damage. Exerc Sport Sci Rev 1991;19:99–125.

95. Gabriel H, Muller HJ, Kettler K, et al. Increased phagocytic capacity of the blood, but decreased phagocytic activity per individual circulating neutrophil after an ultradistance run. Eur J Appl Physiol 1995;71(2–3):281–284.

96. Mackinnon LT, Hooper S. Mucosal (secretory) immune system responses to exercise of varying intensity and during overtraining. Int J Sports Med 1994;15 suppl 3:S179–S183.

97. Nieman DC, Berk LS, Simpson-Westerberg M, et al. Effects of long-endurance running on immune system parameters and lymphocyte function in experienced marathoners. Int J Sports Med 1989;10(5):317–323.

98. Nieman DC, Fagoaga OR, Butterworth DE, et al. Carbohydrate supplementation affects blood granulocyte and monocyte trafficking but not function after 2.5 h or running. Am J Clin Nutr 1997;66(1):153–159.

99. Nieman DC, Simandle S, Henson DA, et al. Lymphocyte proliferative response to 2.5 hours of running. Int J Sports Med 1995;16(6):404–409.

100. Papanicolaou DA, Petrides JS, Tsigos C, et al. Exercise stimulates interleukin-6 secretion: inhibition by glucocorticoids and correlation with catecholamines. Am J Physiol 1996;271(3 pt 1):E601–E605.

101. Pedersen BK, Ostrowski K, Rohde T, Bruunsgaard H. The cytokine response to strenuous exercise. Can J Physiol Pharmacol 1998;76(5):505–511.

102. Sato H, Abe T, Kikuchi T, et al. [Changes in the production of reactive oxygen species from neutrophils following a 100-km marathon]. Nippon Eiseigaku Zasshi 1996;51(2):612–616.

103. Shinkai S, Kurokawa Y, Hino S, et al. Triathlon competition induced a transient immunosuppressive change in the peripheral blood of athletes. J Sports Med Phys Fitness 1993;33(1):70–78.

104. Smith JA, Pyne DB. Exercise, training, and neutrophil function. Exerc Immunol Rev 1997;3:96–116.

105. Sprenger H, Jacobs C, Nain M, et al. Enhanced release of cytokines, interleukin-2 receptors, and neopterin after long-distance running. Clin Immunol Immunopathol 1992;63(2):188–195.

106. Suzuki K, Naganuma S, Totsuka M, et al. Effects of exhaustive endurance exercise and its one-week daily repetition on neutrophil count and functional status in untrained men. Int J Sports Med 1996;17(3):205–212.

107. Suzuki K, Sato H, Kikuchi T, et al. Capacity of circulating neutrophils to produce reactive oxygen species after exhaustive exercise. J Appl Physiol 1996;81(3):1213–1222.

108. Ullum H, Haahr PM, Diamant M, et al. Bicycle exercise enhances plasma IL-6 but does not change IL-1 alpha, IL-1 beta, IL-6, or TNF-alpha pre-mRNA in BMNC. J Appl Physiol 1994;77(1):93–97.

109. Newsholme EA. Biochemical mechanisms to explain immunosuppression in well-trained and overtrained athletes. Int J Sports Med 1994;15 Suppl 3:S142–S147.

110. Mackinnon LT, Hooper SL. Plasma glutamine and upper respiratory tract infection during intensified training in swimmers. Med Sci Sports Exerc 1996;28(3):285–290.

111. Pyne DB, Baker MS, Fricker PA, et al. Effects of an intensive 12-wk training program by elite swimmers on neutrophil oxidative activity. Med Sci Sports Exerc 1995;27(4):536–542.

112. Henson DA, Nieman DC, Blodgett AD, et al. Influence of exercise mode and carbohydrate on the immune response to prolonged exercise. Int J Sports Nutr 1999;9(2):213–228.

113. Nieman DC, Nehlsen-Cannarella SL, Fagoaga OR, et al. Influence of mode and carbohydrate on the cytokine response to heavy exertion. Med Sci Sports Exerc 1998;30(5):671–678.

114. Zawadzki KM, Yaspelkis BBd, Ivy JL. Carbohydrate-protein complex increases the rate of muscle glycogen storage after exercise. J Appl Physiol 1992;72(5):1854–1859.

115. Chandler RM, Byrne HK, Patterson JG, Ivy JL. Dietary supplements affect the anabolic hormones after weight-training exercise. J Appl Physiol 1994;76(2):839–845.

116. Hernandez M, Montalvo I, Sousa V, Sotelo A. The protein efficiency ratios of 30:70 mixtures of animal: vegetable protein are similar or higher than those of the animal foods alone [see comments]. J Nutr 1996;126(2):574–581.

117. Sarwar G, McDonough FE. Evaluation of protein digestibility-corrected amino acid score method for assessing protein quality of foods. J Assoc Anal Chem 1990;73(3):347–356.

118. Rigo J, Salle BL, Picaud JC, et al. Nutritional evaluation of protein hydrolysate formulas. Eur J Clin Nutr 1995;49 suppl 1:S26–S38.

119. Barth CA, Behnke U. [Nutritional physiology of whey and whey components]. Nahrung 1997;41(1):2–12.

120. Smithers GW, Ballard FJ, Copeland AD, et al. New opportunities from the isolation and utilization of whey proteins. J Dairy Sci 1996;79(8):1454–1459.

121. Wong CW, Watson DL. Immunomodulatory effects of dietary whey proteins in mice. J Dairy Res 1995;62(2):359–368.

122. Bounous G, Batist G, Gold P. Immunoenhancing property of dietary whey protein in mice: role of glutathione. Clin Invest Med 1989;12(3):154–161.

123. Rowe B, Kudsk K, Borum P, et al. Effects of whey and caseine based diets on glutathione and cysteine metabolism in ICU patients. J Am Coll Nutr 1994;254:535.

124. McBride JM, Kraemer WJ, Triplett-McBride T, Sebastianelli W. Effect of resistance exercise on free radical production. Med Sci Sports Exerc 1998;30(1):67–72.

125. Ji LL, Leeuwenburgh C, Leichtweis S, et al. Oxidative stress and aging: role of exercise and its influences on antioxidant systems. Ann N Y Acad Sci 1998;854:102–117.

126. Jenkins RR. Exercise, oxidative stress, and antioxidants: a review. Int J Sports Nutr 1993;3(4):356–375.

127. MacLean DA, Graham TE, Saltin B. Stimulation of muscle ammonia production during exercise following branched-chain amino acid supplementation in humans. J Physiol (Lond) 1996;493(pt 3): 909–922.

128. Boirie Y, Dangin M, Gachon P, et al. Slow and fast dietary proteins differently modulate postprandial protein accretion. Proc Natl Acad Sci USA 1997;94(26):14930–14935.

129. Tremel H, Kienle B, Weilemann LS, et al. Glutamine dipeptide-supplemented parenteral nutrition maintains intestinal function in the critically ill [see comments]. Gastroenterology 1994;107(6): 1595–1601.

130. Newsholme EA, Calder PC. The proposed role of glutamine in some cells of the immune system and speculative consequences for the whole animal. Nutrition 1997;13(7–8):728–730.

131. Newsholme EA. Biochemical control logic and the metabolism of glutamine [editorial]. Nutrition 1994;10(2):178–179.

132. Castell LM, Poortmans JR, Leclercq R, et al. Some aspects of the acute phase response after a marathon race, and the effects of glutamine supplementation. Eur J Appl Physiol 1997;75(1):47–53.

133. Castell LM, Newsholme EA. Glutamine and the effects of exhaustive exercise upon the immune response. Can J Physiol Pharmacol 1998;76(5):524–532.

134. Ghigo E, Procopio M, Boffano GM, et al. Arginine potentiates but does not restore the blunted growth hormone response to growth hormone-releasing hormone in obesity. Metab Clin Exper 1992; 41(5):560–563.

135. Bode-Boger SM, Boger RH, Loffler M, et al. L-arginine stimulates NO-dependent vasodilation in healthy humans–effect of somatostatin pretreatment. J Investig Med 1999;47(1):43–50.

136. Korbonits M, Trainer PJ, Fanciulli G, et al. L-arginine is unlikely to exert neuroendocrine effects in humans via the generation of nitric oxide [see comments]. Eur J Endocrinol 1996;135(5):543–547.

137. Barbul A, Lazarou SA, Efron DT, et al. Arginine enhances wound healing and lymphocyte immune responses in humans. Surgery 1990;108(2):331–337.

138. Barbul A, Sisto DA, Wasserkrug HL, Efron G. Arginine stimulates lymphocyte immune response in healthy human beings. Surgery 1981;90(2):244–251.

139. Imoberdorf R. Immuno-nutrition: designer diets in cancer. Support Care Cancer 1997;5(5):381–386.

140. Reynolds JV, Daly JM, Zhang S, et al. Immunomodulatory mechanisms of arginine. Surgery 1988;104(2):142–151.

141. Wayler A, Queiroz E, Scrimshaw NS, et al. Nitrogen balance studies in young men to assess the protein quality of an isolated soy protein in relation to meat proteins. J Nutr 1983;113(12): 2485–2491.

142. Scrimshaw NS, Wayler AH, Murray E, et al. Nitrogen balance response in young men given one of two isolated soy proteins or milk proteins. J Nutr 1983;113(12):2492–2497.

143. Young VR. Soy protein in relation to human protein and amino acid nutrition. J Am Diet Assoc 1991;91(7):828–835.

144. Rossi A, Disilvestro RA, Blostein-Fujii A. Effects of soy consumption on exercise-induced acute muscle damage and oxidative stress in young adult males. FASEB J 1998;12(5):A653.

145. Rennie MJ, Edwards RH, Krywawych S, et al. Effect of exercise on protein turnover in man. Clin Sci 1981;61(5):627–639.

146. Castell LM, Poortmans JR, Newsholme EA. Does glutamine have a role in reducing infections in athletes? Eur J Appl Physiol 1996;73(5):488–490.

147. Keast D, Arstein D, Harper W, et al. Depression of plasma glutamine concentration after exercise stress and its possible influence on the immune system. Med J Aust 1995;162(1):15–18.

148. Parry-Billings M, Budgett R, Koutedakis Y, et al. Plasma amino acid concentrations in the overtraining syndrome: possible effects on the immune system. Med Sci Sports Exerc 1992;24(12):1353–1358.

149. Parry-Billings M, Evans J, Calder PC, Newsholme EA. Does glutamine contribute to immunosuppression after major burns? Lancet 1990;336(8714):523–525.

150. Newsholme EA, Newsholme P, Curi R. The role of the citric acid cycle in cells of the immune system and its importance in sepsis, trauma and burns. Biochem Soc Symp 1987;54:145–162.

151. Ardawi MS, Newsholme EA. Glutamine metabolism in lymphocytes of the rat. Biochem J 1983;212(3):835–842.

152. Ardawi MS, Newsholme EA. Intracellular localization and properties of phosphate-dependent glutaminase in rat mesenteric lymph nodes. Biochem J 1984;217(1):289–296.

153. Newsholme EA, Board M. Application of metabolic-control logic to fuel utilization and its significance in tumor cells. Adv Enzyme Regul 1991;31:225–246.

154. Newsholme EA, Crabtree B, Ardawi MS. The role of high rates of glycolysis and glutamine utilization in rapidly dividing cells. Biosci Rep 1985;5(5):393–400.

155. Windmueller HG, Spaeth AE. Uptake and metabolism of plasma glutamine by the small intestine. J Biol Chem 1974;249(16):5070–5079.

156. Bulus N, Cersosimo E, Ghishan F, Abumrad NN. Physiologic importance of glutamine. Metabolism 1989;38(8 suppl 1):1–5.

157. Reitzer LJ, Wice BM, Kennell D. Evidence that glutamine, not sugar, is the major energy source for cultured HeLa cells. J Biol Chem 1979;254(8):2669–2676.

158. Smith RJ. Glutamine metabolism and its physiologic importance. JPEN J Parenter Enteral Nutr 1990;14(4 suppl):40S–44S.

159. Zielke HR, Ozand PT, Tildon JT, et al. Reciprocal regulation of glucose and glutamine utilization by cultured human diploid fibroblasts. J Cell Physiol 1978;95(1):41–48.

160. Rohde T, MacLean DA, Klarlund Pedersen B. Glutamine, lymphocyte proliferation and cytokine production. Scand J Immunol 1996; 44(6):648–650.

161. Ardawi MS, Newsholme EA. Maximum activities of some enzymes of glycolysis, the tricarboxylic acid cycle and ketone-body and glutamine utilization pathways in lymphocytes of the rat. Biochem J 1982;208(3):743–748.

162. Juretic A, Spagnoli GC, Hoerig H, et al. Glutamine requirements in the generation of lymphokine-activated killer cells. Clin Nutr 1994;13(1):42–49.

163. Mackinnon LT, Chick TW, van As A, Tomasi TB. The effect of exercise on secretory and natural immunity. Adv Exp Med Biol 1987: 869–876.

164. Keast D, Cameron K, Morton AR. Exercise and the immune response. Sports Med 1988;5(4):248–267.

165. Rohde T, MacLean DA, Hartkopp A, Pedersen BK. The immune system and serum glutamine during a triathlon. Eur J Appl Physiol 1996;74(5):428–434.

166. Rohde T, MacLean DA, Pedersen BK. Effect of glutamine supplementation on changes in the immune system induced by repeated exercise. Med Sci Sports Exerc 1998;30(6):856–862.

167. Rowbottom DG, Keast D, Morton AR. The emerging role of glutamine as an indicator of exercise stress and overtraining. Sports Med 1996;21(2):80–97.

168. Burke DJ, Alverdy JC, Aoys E, Moss GS. Glutamine-supplemented total parenteral nutrition improves gut immune function. Arch Surg 1989;124(12):1396–1399.

169. Yoshida S, Yunoki T, Aoyagi K, et al. Effect of glutamine supplement and hepatectomy on DNA and protein synthesis in the remnant liver. J Surg Res 1995;59(4):475–481.

170. Yoshida S, Kaibara A, Yamasaki K, et al. Effect of glutamine supplementation on protein metabolism and glutathione in tumor-bearing rats. JPEN J Parenter Enteral Nutr 1995;19(6):492–497.

171. Buchman AL, Moukarzel AA, Bhuta S, et al. Parenteral nutrition is associated with intestinal morphologic and functional changes in humans. JPEN J Parenter Enteral Nutr 1995;19(6):453–460.

172. Shewchuk LD, Baracos VE, Field CJ. Dietary L-glutamine does not improve lymphocyte metabolism or function in exercise-trained rats. Med Sci Sports Exerc 1997;29(4):474–481.

173. Hack V, Weiss C, Friedmann B, et al. Decreased plasma glutamine level and CD4+ T cell number in response to 8 wk of anaerobic training. Am J Physiol 1997;272(5 pt 1):E788–795.

174. Ostrowski K, Rohde T, Asp S, et al. Pro- and anti-inflammatory cytokine balance in strenuous exercise in humans. J Physiol (Lond) 1999;515(pt 1):287–291.

175. Eriksson LS, Broberg S, Bjorkman O, Wahren J. Ammonia metabolism during exercise in man. Clin Physiol 1985;5(4):325–336.

176. MacLean DA, Graham TE. Branched-chain amino acid supplementation augments plasma ammonia responses during exercise in humans. J Appl Physiol 1993;74(6):2711–2717.

177. Sahlin K, Katz A, Broberg S. Tricarboxylic acid cycle intermediates in human muscle during prolonged exercise [published errata appear in Am J Physiol 1995 Feb;268(2 pt 1):section C following table of contents and 1995 Jun;268(6 pt 3):section C following table of contents]. Am J Physiol 1990;259(5 pt 1):C834–841.

178. Bourgeois P, Chales G, Dehais J, et al. Efficacy and tolerability of chondroitin sulfate 1200 mg/day vs chondroitin sulfate 3 × 400 mg/day vs placebo. Osteoarthritis Cartilage 1998;6(suppl)A: 25–30.

179. Bucsi L, Poor G. Efficacy and tolerability of oral chondroitin sulfate as a symptomatic slow-acting drug for osteoarthritis (SYSADOA) in the treatment of knee osteoarthritis. Osteoarthritis Cartilage 1998; 6(suppl)A:31–36.

180. Crolle G, D'Este E. Glucosamine sulphate for the management of arthrosis: a controlled clinical investigation. Curr Med Res Opin 1980;7(2):104–109.

181. D'Ambrosio E, Casa B, Bompani R, et al. Glucosamine sulphate: a controlled clinical investigation in arthrosis. Pharmatherapeutica 1981;2(8):504–508.

182. Fleisch AM, Merlin C, Imhoff A. A one-year randomized, double-blind, placebo-controlled study with oral chondroitin sulfate in patients with osteoarthritis. Osteoarthritis Cartilage 1997;5:70.

183. Houpt JB, McMillan R, Wein C, Paget-Dellio SD. Effect of glucosamine hydrochloride in the treatment of pain of osteoarthritis of the knee [In Process Citation]. J Rheumatol 1999;26(11):2423–2430.

184. Mazieres B, Loyau G, Menkes CJ, et al. [Chondroitin sulfate in the treatment of gonarthrosis and coxarthrosis: 5-months result of a multicenter double-blind controlled prospective study using placebo]. Rev Rhum Mal Osteoartic 1992;59(7–8):466–472.

185. Morreale P, Manopulo R, Galati M, et al. Comparison of the anti-inflammatory efficacy of chondroitin sulfate and diclofenac sodium in patients with knee osteoarthritis. J Rheumatol 1996;23(8):1385–1391.

186. Muller-Fabbender H, Bach GL, Haase W, et al. Glucosamine sulfate compared to ibuprofen in osteoarthritis of the knee. Osteoarthritis Cartilage 1994;2:61–69.

187. Noack W, Fischer M, Forster KK, et al. Glucosamine sulfate in osteoarthritis of the knee. Osteoarthritis Cartilage 1994;2:51–59.

188. Pujalte JM, Llavore EP, Ylescupidez FR. Double-blind clinical evaluation of oral glucosamine sulphate in the basic treatment of osteoarthrosis. Curr Med Res Opin 1980;7(2):110–114.

189. Reichelt A, Forster KK, Fischer M, et al. Efficacy and safety of intramuscular glucosamine sulfate in osteoarthritis of the knee: a randomised, placebo-controlled, double-blind study. Arzneimittelforschung 1994;44(1):75–80.

190. Uebelhart D, Zhang J, Thonar EJ, et al. Acute degeneration of articular cartilage in the rabbit: protective effect of chondroitin 4 and 6 sulfate. Osteoarthritis Cartilage 1997;5:68.

191. Uebelhart D, Thonar EJ, Delmas PD. Chondroitin 4 and 6 sulfate: a symptomatic slow-acting drug for osteoarthritis does also have structural modifying properties. Osteoarthritis Cartilage 1997;5:70.

192. Valverde Garcia J, Nolla Sole JM, Juanola Roura X. [Salazopyrine and reactive arthritis (letter)]. Med Clin (Barc) 1987;89(10):442.

193. Vaz A. Double-blind clinical evaluation of the relative efficacy of ibuprofen and glucosamine sulfate in the management of osteoarthritis of the knee in out-patients. Curr Med Res Opin 1982;8:145.

194. Verbruggen G, Goemaere S, Veys EM. Chondroitin sulfate: S/DMOAD (structure/disease modifying anti-osteoarthritis drug) in the treatment of finger joint OA. Osteoarthritis Cartilage 1998;6(suppl)A:37–38.

195. Brandt KD. Toward pharmacologic modification of joint damage in osteoarthritis [editorial]. Ann Intern Med 1995;122(11):874–875.

196. Brandt KD. Should nonsteroidal anti-inflammatory drugs be used to treat osteoarthritis? Rheum Dis Clin North Am 1993;19(1):29–44.

197. Denison H, Kaczynski J, Wallerstedt S. Paracetamol medication and alcohol abuse: a dangerous combination for the liver and the kidney. Scand J Gastroenterol 1987;22(6):701–704.

198. Sandler DP, Burr FR, Weinberg CR. Nonsteroidal anti-inflammatory drugs and the risk for chronic renal disease [see comments]. Ann Intern Med 1991;115(3):165–172.

199. Perneger TV, Whelton PK, Klag MJ. Risk of kidney failure associated with the use of acetaminophen, aspirin, and nonsteroidal anti-inflammatory drugs [see comments]. N Engl J Med 1994;331(25): 1675–1679.

200. Brooks PM, Day RO. Nonsteroidal anti-inflammatory drugs—differences and similarities [published erratum appears in N Engl J Med 1991 Sep 5;325(10):747] [see comments]. N Engl J Med 1991;324(24):1716–1725.

201. Furst DE. Are there differences among nonsteroidal anti-inflammatory drugs? Comparing acetylated salicylates, nonacetylated salicylates, and nonacetylated nonsteroidal anti-inflammatory drugs [see comments]. Arthritis Rheum 1994;37(1):1–9.

202. Griffin MR, Piper JM, Daugherty JR, et al. Nonsteroidal anti-inflammatory drug use and increased risk for peptic ulcer disease in elderly persons. Ann Intern Med 1991;114(4):257–263.

203. Griffin MR, Brandt KD, Liang MH, et al. Practical management of osteoarthritis: integration of pharmacologic and nonpharmacologic measures. Arch Fam Med 1995;4(12):1049–1055.

204. Lichtenstein DR, Syngal S, Wolfe MM. Nonsteroidal anti-inflammatory drugs and the gastrointestinal tract: the double-edged sword. Arthritis Rheum 1995;38(1):5–18.

205. Setnikar I, Giacchetti C, Zanolo G. Pharmacokinetics of glucosamine in the dog and in man. Arzneimittelforschung 1986; 36(4):729–735.

206. Setnikar I, Palumbo R, Canali S, Zanolo G. Pharmacokinetics of glucosamine in man. Arzneimittelforschung 1993;43(10):1109–1113.

207. Setnikar I, Pacini MA, Revel L. Antiarthritic effects of glucosamine sulfate studied in animal models. Arzneimittelforschung 1991; 41(5):542–545.

208. Van der Kraan PM, De Vries BJ, Vitters EL, et al. Inhibition of glycosaminoglycan synthesis in anatomically intact rat patellar cartilage by paracetamol-induced serum sulfate depletion. Biochem Pharmacol 1988;37(19):3683–3690.

209. Bassleer C, Reginster JY, Franchinmont P. Effects of glucosamine on differential human chondrocytes cultivated in clusters. Rev Esp Reumatol 1993;20(suppl 1):95.

210. Deal CL, Moskowitz RW. Nutraceuticals as therapeutic agents in osteoarthritis. Rheum Dis Clin North Am 1999;25(2):379–395.

211. Zupanets IA, Drogovoz SM, Bezdetko NV, et al. Influence of glucosamine on the antioxidative effect of nonsteroidal anti-inflammatory drugs. Farmakologiya i Toksikologiya (Moscow) 1991;54(2):61–63.

212. Drovanti A, Bignamini AA, Rovati AL. Therapeutic activity of oral glucosamine sulfate in osteoarthrosis: a placebo-controlled double-blind investigation. Clin Ther 1980;3(4):260–272.

213. Vajaradul Y. Double-blind clinical evaluation of intra-articular glucosamine in outpatients with gonarthrosis. Clin Ther 1981;3(5): 336–343.

214. Tapadinhas MJ, Rivera IC, Bignamini AA. Oral glucosamine sulphate in the management of arthrosis: report on a multi-centre open investigation in Portugal. Pharmatherapeutica 1982;3(3): 157–168.

215. Pipitone VR. Chondroprotection with chondroitin sulfate. Drugs Exp Clin Res 1991;17(1):3–7.

216. Rovati LC. Clinical research in osteoarthritis: design and results of short-term and long-term trials with disease-modifying drugs. Int J Tissue React 1992;14(5):243–251.

217. Reginster JY, Deroisy R, Paul I, et al. Glucosamine sulfate significantly reduces progression of knee osteoarthritis over 3 years: a large, randomised, placebo-controlled, double-blind, prospective trial. Arthritis Rheum 1999;42(9 suppl):S400.

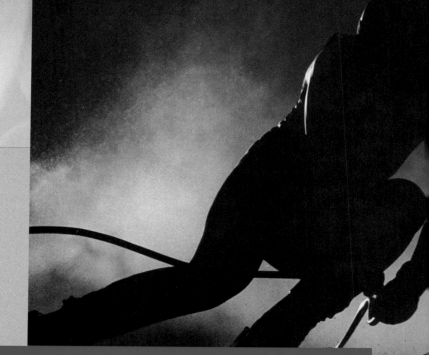

Antioxidant Supplementation and Exercise

Lonnie M. Lowery, John M. Berardi, and Tim N. Ziegenfuss

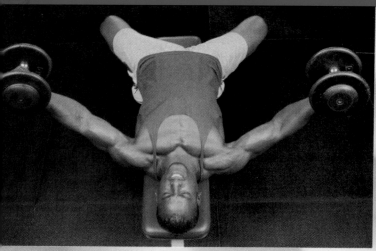

Research Review

Vitamin E and Skeletal Muscle

Vitamin E is well recognized for its antioxidant properties; furthermore, there is evidence that suggests a possible role of vitamin E in maintaining skeletal muscle. To wit: In a study performed at Penn State University, 12 weight-trained men were divided into two groups: one group received 1200 IUs of vitamin E once per day for 2 weeks while the control group received a cellulose-based placebo pill. They subsequently performed some typical resistance exercises such as the bench press, military press, calf raise, leg press, rows, bicep curls, and squat.

Creatine kinase (CK), an indirect marker of muscle fiber injury, is known to increase after a bout of unaccustomed or intense exercise(s). In this study, plasma CK levels increased significantly in both groups after 24 and 48 hours; however, the increase in CK was less in the vitamin E–supplemented group than it was in the placebo group at 24 hours. In essence, this would suggest that the degree of injury caused by lifting heavy weights was much less in the vitamin E–supplemented group versus the placebo group.

Though vitamin E has been touted as an agent that might decrease the incidence of cardiovascular disease, it could also aid in skeletal muscle recovery post-exercise. Certainly, the evidence is intriguing.

McBride JM, Kraemer WJ, Triplett-McBride T. Effect of resistance exercise on free radical production. Med Sci Sports Exerc 1998; 30:67–72.

Introduction

Living in an oxygen-rich environment presents an enigma for principally aerobic organisms such as human beings. Oxygen (O_2) is an absolute requirement for life, yet paradoxically it also contributes to an "erosion" of the organism over time as metabolism continues. Derivatives of oxygen known as reactive oxygen species (ROS) have been implicated in a number of pathological conditions including cancer, myocardial infarction, inflammatory diseases, and diseases of aging. A listing of the most prevalent reactive oxygen species implicated in such conditions is given in TABLE 12-1. Interestingly, although reactive oxygen species and radicals are implicated in numerous disease states, their presence in small amounts can also be beneficial.

Reactive oxygen species lead to the formation of free radicals, which are atoms or groups of atoms that contain one or more unpaired electrons. Without belaboring this description, atoms with unpaired electrons are extremely volatile and can react with cellular components such as proteins (both enzymatic and structural), membrane lipids, and the nucleotides within DNA and RNA. This places every part of the cell at risk for radical-induced damage. Fortunately, however, humans have well-developed enzymatic and nutritional defenses to protect against such toxic oxygen species (TABLE 12-2). These defense mechanisms help to maintain a favorable pro-oxidant to antioxidant balance and prevent cellular damage. Some conditions, however, such as hypoxia, severe heat stress, septic shock, stretch-induced injury, and intense physical exercise can overwhelm these defenses and lead to

Table 12-1 **Reactive Oxygen Species**	
Oxygen-Containing Radicals	**Oxygen-Containing Nonradicals**
Superoxide O_2^-	Ozone O_3
Hydroxyl $OH^{\bullet}$	Singlet Oxygen $^1O_2$
Hydroperoxyl $HO_2^{\bullet}$	Hypochlorous acid HOCL
Alkoxyl $LO^{\bullet}$ or $RO^{\bullet}$	Hydrogen peroxide H_2O_2
Peroxyl $LO_2^{\bullet}$ or $RO_2^{\bullet}$	

an unfavorable balance in which pro-oxidation and cell damage predominate.[1-4] The interaction between exercise and skeletal muscle oxidative and antioxidative processes are the focus of this chapter; therefore, the remainder of the discussion will primarily deal with exercise-induced free radical production and its impact on skeletal muscle.

Both intense resistance and aerobic exercise have been shown to increase the production of reactive oxygen species and free radicals.[5-7] Although the mechanisms by which this occurs are still under investigation, three main free radical–producing processes are of special concern to individuals who exercise. These three mechanisms are accelerated metabolic (mostly mitochondrial) oxygen processing, ischemic-reperfusion injury, and muscle micro trauma/repair (leukocyte radical production). Accelerated mitochondrial oxygen processing is most associated with endurance training whereas ischemic-reperfusion injury and muscle repair are associated with resistance training. Currently, there is considerable debate

Table 12-2 Endogenous Antioxidant Functions

Endogenous Antioxidants	Cofactors	Function
Enzymatic		
Superoxide Dismutase (SOD)	Copper, Zinc-cytosol Manganese-mitochondria	Dismutases superoxide radicals to hydroperoxides
Glutathione Peroxidase (GPX)	Selenium	Reduces hydrogen peroxide and organic hydroperoxides in the presence of glutathione to water and alcohol
Catalase (CAT)	Iron	Decomposes hydroperoxides to water and oxygen
Nonenzymatic		
Glutathione	—	Assists in the GPX removal of hydroperoxides

as to whether these processes are adaptive and beneficial or whether they are pathological and harmful. Regardless, the impact of free radical production remains the same. Exercise-induced free radical production and damage is capable not only of slowing recovery from strenuous exercise, but also of causing damage to a variety of tissues and organs.[8–11]

Endurance Athletes and Increased Mitochondrial Oxygen Processing

Aerobic athletes produce physical work relatively slowly over long periods of time through the hydrolysis of ATP. The demand for the re-synthesis of ATP to continue muscular work during prolonged exercise is met by the oxidation of fuel (carbohydrates, fats, and some protein) in the mitochondria. Under normal resting conditions the electron transport chain (ETC) of the mitochondria uses oxygen to produce ATP and during aerobic exercise this process is greatly accelerated. In fact, during aerobic exercise, oxygen processing occurs at rates 10–20 fold above resting levels.[7,12] This accelerated oxygen processing contributes to increased free radical formation at the cytochrome level of the electron transport chain, with a two- to threefold increase in free radical levels.[9,12]

Although ETC enzymes have evolved to efficiently process oxygen during the generation of ATP, even with this enzymatic efficiency, an estimated 2–5% of total oxygen flux through the mitochondria can form superoxide radicals at rest.[13] It is speculated that, during exercise, the increased flow of oxygen through the ETC can lead to a significant increase in superoxide radicals beyond resting levels.[14] In addition, at rest, endogenous antioxidants located in the mitochondria can effectively remove super-

oxide radicals but again, during exercise, the increase in oxygen radicals may be more than the endogenous antioxidants can neutralize.

Weight Training and Reperfusion Injury

Ischemia or inadequate blood flow can lead to hypoxic conditions in which there is inadequate blood and oxygen delivery to tissues of the body. The term *ischemia* is usually used in reference to coronary hypoxia such as that seen during myocardial infarction (heart attack). Similarly, weight training can lead to short periods of skeletal muscle ischemia. Weight trainers, while maintaining static contractions (stabilizing a weight, squeezing an isometric repetition, etc.) can develop local hypoxic conditions in the muscle being trained. As blood re-enters the ischemic (pinched-off) skeletal muscle, a state known as reperfusion injury can ensue. Reperfusion injury can occur as a result of the rapid re-oxygenation of the tissue. As ischemic conditions are terminated after a set of contractions and the muscle relaxes, the flow of oxygen to the tissues is returned. This reintroduction of oxygen to ischemic tissue, however, may result in cellular damage through the production of reactive oxygen species from the mitochondria, myoglobin, and hemoglobin.[15] The amount of time that a particular skeletal muscle is suffering from reduced blood flow during these situations is usually minimal when compared with cardiac ischemia. Reperfusion injury in skeletal muscle, although minimal, may still contribute to radical formation and muscle damage.

Although skeletal muscle reperfusion injury may be minimal, of greater concern is the reperfusion injury to visceral organs. During exercise, blood is shunted away from the body's core. As this occurs, the oxygen-rich blood is *robbed* from organs like the intestines and liver

Table 12-3 Distribution of Cardiac Output During Rest (5 L/min) and Maximal Exercise (25 L/min)

Organ	Blood Flow at Rest	Blood Flow During Maximal Exercise
Heart	4–5% 0.2–0.25 L/min	3–4% 0.75–1.0 L/min
Liver and GI	20–25% 1.0–1.25 L/min	1–2% 0.25–0.5 L/min
Kidneys	20% 1.0 L/min	2–4% 0.5–1.0 L/min
Bone	3–5% 0.15–0.25 L/min	0.5–1% 0.125–0.25 L/min
Brain	15% 0.75 L/min	3–4% 0.75–1.0 L/min
Skin	1% 0.05 L/min	5% 1.25 L/min
Skeletal Muscle	15–20% 0.75–1.0 L/min[a]	80–85% 20.0–21.25 L/min[b]

[a]Associated with an O_2 consumption of 0.08 umol/min $\cdot$ g^{-1} wt and ATP turnover of 0.5 μmol/min $\cdot$ g^{-1} wt.
[b]Associated with an O_2 consumption of 6.40 umol/min $\cdot$ g^{-1} wt and ATP turnover of 40.0 μmol/min $\cdot$ g^{-1} wt.

and redistributed to supply the muscle (TABLE 12-3). This decrease in oxygen transport to the internal organs, coupled with the eventual resurgence of blood back into the organ, can damage these tissues via free radical production. The *pump* that is experienced during a weight-training workout illustrates a practical example of this phenomenon. As one develops a thigh pump, for example (localized hyperemia in the quadriceps and related muscles), blood is rerouted from the internal organs, leaving them with much reduced flow. After the training session is terminated, there is a large influx of blood back into the organs. This may also lead to reperfusion injury. Paradoxically, this response is not necessary for energy production; it is principally a response to local chemical mediators that cause vasodilatation within a muscle's vasculature.

However, it would be remiss not to mention that this shunting of blood flow has real advantages and is generally not considered negative. As skeletal muscles are called upon to produce greater amounts of work, their requirements for blood and oxygen increase dramatically. To meet these needs, the body uses (primarily) the sympathetic nervous system to constrict blood vessels of the viscera and dilate those of the working muscles. Without such efficiency, our ancient ancestors would have not been fast enough or have had the necessary endurance to escape predators and you would not be here to read this book. Of course, this increase in cardiac output to skeletal muscle occurs not only when an athlete is *pumped,* but during any situation when muscles are repetitively contracting, as we will see.

Weight Training and Muscle Damage/Repair

Another mechanism involved in the generation of free radicals in weight trainers does not involve the physiological effects of training, but involves the effects of recovery from training; namely, free radical production in damaged muscle. As a result of intense resistance exercise, the skeletal muscle of bodybuilders, power lifters, and Olympic lifters is subjected to both mechanical and oxidative damage. This damage includes the loss of sarcoplasmic reticulum structural integrity, increased lipid peroxidation and membrane perturbations, and the release of both myoglobin and muscle enzymes into circulation.[16] Exercise-induced muscle damage can occur from both concentric and eccentric training, but eccentric contractions, or *negatives,* are known to cause greater structural damage and thereby increased oxidative damage.[17] As mentioned, oxidative stress in resistance training does not come from a dramatically elevated metabolic rate during the exercise bout as in aerobic trainers, but is actually part of the repair process. After muscle damage, including exercise-induced microtrauma, there is a period of neutrophil and monocyte/macrophage infiltration.[18–20] The white blood cells (leukocytes) that are activated in response to muscle damage are mobilized to the damaged area in an attempt to initiate repair. Delayed-onset muscle soreness has been related to this repair process. Although this immune response appears to be proportional to z-band damage, even moderate exercise has been shown to trigger a twofold increase in neutrophil activation.[21] As a consequence of neutrophil activation, these repair processes are well known to use oxygen radicals as a means of clearing away microscopic tissue fragments.[22–25] Again, in this scenario, the *healing* of damaged muscle can lead to further muscle damage due to oxidative stressors brought on by the repair process. In addition to white blood cell infiltration, cell damage can lead to both muscle calcium abnormalities and the disruption of iron-containing proteins, including myoglobin.[26]

One concluding note is necessary to put the concepts of exercise, radical production, and muscle damage into perspective. Although the research is not clear-cut when approaching the question of which came first, the radicals or the damage, it can be speculated that exercise causes a downward spiral situation. Acute bouts of aerobic and resistance exercise both cause increased free radical production, although through different mechanisms (oxygen processing and reperfusion injury). Since these free radicals are known to cause damage to cytoskeletons, membranes, and other cellular components, it can be concluded that post-exercise muscle damage is due, in part, to free radical actions. Once skeletal muscle is damaged, however, leukocyte radical production is initiated to clear away damaged fibers, leading to the subsequent release of more free radicals and further damage. Further research is required to quantify the nature of each step's contribution to the oxidative damage seen is skeletal muscle.

Oxidation: Not Just Bad

Taking a step back, although increased oxygen processing and subsequent radical production seem to be the ultimate villains to exercising individuals, this is not necessarily

Antioxidants/Pro-Oxidants

Although large amounts of oxygen radicals can act as metabolic toxins causing oxidative stress, nontoxic levels of radicals may be beneficial to cellular communication and cellular defense. Many cellular functions are carried out through the use of intracellular messengers such as cAMP, diacylglycerols, and inositol triphosphates. Recently, there has been evidence to support the notion that cellular radicals might also function in similar roles.

One cellular communication role of free radicals may be the regulation of eicosanoid production. Free radical–induced lipid peroxidation can stimulate phospholipase A2, which causes the release of fatty acids from membranes. These fatty acids are involved in the formation of leukotrienes, thromboxanes, and prostaglandins; commonly known as the eicosanoids.

In addition, free radicals can disrupt enzymatic pathways to regulate cell response. In the adrenal cortex, cytochrome P450–derived radicals reduce enzyme activity that controls corticosteroid hormone secretion. In addition, radicals generated from arachidonic acid metabolism can inactivate cyclooxygenase enzyme activity and slow prostaglandin synthesis.

As a defense mechanism, superoxide radicals are produced by neutrophils in response to invading organisms. These radicals are involved in the destruction and clearance of invaders such as bacteria and viruses. During this process, not only do the radicals assist in phagocytosis, but they also stimulate the gathering of more neutrophils to continue cellular defense.

It appears that although an imbalance of pro-oxidants to antioxidants may be linked to pathological conditions, radicals are nonetheless important in cellular communication and defense. This makes them necessary in small, noncytotoxic quantities.

Egan RW, Paxton J, Kuehl FA Jr. Mechanism for irreversible self-deactivation of prostaglandin synthetase. J Biol Chem 1976; 251:7329–7335.

Hornsby PJ. Steroid and xenobiotic effects on the adrenal cortex: Mediation by oxidative and other mechanisms. Free Radic Biol Med 1989;6:103–115.

Sevanian A, et al. Phospholipase A2 dependent release of fatty acids from peroxidized membranes. Free Radic Biol Med 1985;1:263–271.

Winrow VR, Winyard VR, Morris CJ, et al. Free radicals in inflammation: second messengers and mediators of tissue destruction. Br Med Bull 1993;49:506–522.

the case. It's not news to anyone that people need oxygen to survive. This fact is made obvious by traveling to a high altitude, where symptoms quickly arise largely because of the lack of oxygen in the local environment. In an effort to get the oxygen it desperately needs, the body starts adapting to the low-oxygen (hypoxic) conditions immediately. By making more red blood cells (i.e., erythropoiesis) to carry oxygen and by better processing what little oxygen is there, the body starts to look more aerobically oriented—a situation that is advantageous to endurance athletes upon returning to lower elevations.[27] But oxygen is not just for producing physical work; it also combusts our food at rest, supplying energy for numerous metabolic processes and producing body heat. Once again, human beings are principally aerobic animals, even if some choose to focus on primarily anaerobic sports, like weight trainers do.

Furthermore, processes such as lipid peroxidation (cell membrane oxidation by free radicals) are not uniformly pathologic either. This process of breaking down lipids in the cell membrane is one way that the membrane renews itself. In addition, lipid peroxidation can form necessary mediators of inflammation and immune function.[28] Even the leukocyte *oxidative burst* that occurs as a result of cell damage or foreign invaders is part of antigen defense and a necessary clean-up step that precedes new tissue growth (hypertrophy). It is primarily when the pro-oxidant:antioxidant ratio becomes elevated that a detrimental sequelae of events occur, damaging structures like cell and mitochondrial membranes and nuclear material. Chronic elevation of this ratio has, indeed, been implicated in a variety of disease states.[29,30] Thus, although excessive amounts of cell oxidation can be detrimental, without some oxidation humans could not survive. It seems then that one of the nutritional goals of athletes should be to limit the deleterious effects of accelerated oxidation without affecting oxidative processes critical to health and performance. In other words, athletes should seek to find the ideal antioxidant balance.

Do Athletes Need Supplemental Antioxidants?

As a result of training, all of the various oxidative processes are elevated in both aerobic and anaerobic athletes. The magnitude of these elevations depends on the intensity and type of exercise in which one is engaged. Also, some authors have speculated that the oxidative muscle damage associated with exercise may lead to the termination of muscular effort.[31] In light of this knowledge, researchers and lay people alike have speculated that antioxidant supplementation may *level the playing field,* reducing tissue damage and soreness, improving exercise performance, and even prolonging lifespan.[32–26] But do we need nutritional supplements to protect us from oxidative damage?

Or can our bodies handle the stress *naturally* through homeostasis?

Regarding antioxidant homeostasis, most of the research done on endogenous antioxidant enzymes and their adaptation to exercise has been done using endurance protocols. From this research, aerobically trained individuals (including humans and rats) have elevated endogenous (produced within) antioxidant enzyme concentrations and/or activities compared with controls.[3,37–41] As the body adapts to the demands of an increased training load by increasing mitochondrial density, capillarization, stroke volume of the heart, etc., it also defends itself from the increasing amount of oxygen that is delivered and used by the muscle. Because mitochondrial density increases (there are more mitochondria per unit of muscle) in aerobically trained individuals and the antioxidant enzymes are located within the mitochondria, it only stands to reason that antioxidant activity would increase in endurance-trained individuals. Of course, the more mitochondria, the more potential for reactive oxygen species, so the question is whether the increased enzymes can deal with the increased free radicals.

In numerous studies, the activities of the enzymes superoxide dismutase (SOD) and glutathione peroxidase (GPX) were increased in oxidative (type I) skeletal muscle with endurance training. In addition, glutathione levels increase in response to training while oxidative damage is lessened when compared to untrained rats and humans. Although this suggests that trained individuals have a better protection from exercise-induced free radical damage than untrained, it cannot be assumed that the skeletal muscle of these individuals has enzyme levels that completely protect against free radical damage. Nor is it safe to assume that all athletes gain the same degree of antioxidant protection from training. Since enzymatic adaptations occur primarily in slow-twitch muscle fibers (type I), and fast-twitch fibers (type IIB) do not, to a large extent, undergo such changes, athletes with a higher percentage of fast-twitch fibers like bodybuilders, sprinters, and power lifters may be more susceptible to free radical damage.[6]

The knowledge of training-induced endogenous antioxidant upregulation does, in fact, question the need for endogenous antioxidant supplementation. That is, why do athletes need an antioxidant boost when the body naturally adapts to exercise by improving its defenses? Although the antioxidant capacity of the body is increased with endurance training, it appears that even these increases are often not sufficient to neutralize the increase in free radicals generated from long-duration aerobic exercise.[2,3] It is clear that, depending on the type of exercise, free radical formation may supercede the body's ability to protect itself, even in training-adapted individuals. In this case, it would be appropriate to increase the ingestion of exogenous antioxidants.

That said, the next relevant question would address whether the ingestion of foods that are high in bioavailable antioxidants (i.e., dietary antioxidants) would be sufficient to provide for the additional needs of specific

Nutritional Antioxidants and Exercise Performance

Scott K. Powers, PhD, EdD

It is well known that intense or prolonged exercise results in oxidative injury to skeletal muscles, particularly in untrained individuals. Further, there is growing evidence that radicals and other reactive oxygen species contribute to muscular fatigue. Therefore, it is not surprising that there is strong interest in the effects of antioxidant supplements on exercise performance. Numerous animal studies have examined the effects of antioxidants on muscular performance. Many of these experiments have used *in vitro* preparations in which antioxidants (e.g., superoxide dismutase, catalase, etc.) were added to the bathing medium surrounding the muscle. In general, these *in vitro* experiments indicate that the addition of antioxidants results in delayed muscular fatigue. Some *in vivo* animal studies also indicate that the addition of antioxidants can improve muscular performance. Collectively, these experiments suggest that antioxidant supplementation can improve muscular performance by reducing exercise-induced oxidative stress. Nonetheless, most animal studies have used antioxidant treatments that cannot be used in humans. Therefore, results from antioxidant research using animal models cannot always be directly extrapolated to humans.

Research examining the effects of antioxidant supplementation on human performance is in its infancy. At present, limited studies have examined the effects of antioxidant supplementation on muscular endurance in humans. Further, many of the studies suffer experimental design weaknesses and most studies have investigated the effects of a single antioxidant rather than investigating the combined effects of both lipid and water-soluble antioxidants. By far, the most widely studied antioxidant vitamin is vitamin E, whereas few studies have examined the effects of other antioxidants on human performance. Although several human studies have indicated that supplementation with vitamin E and/or vitamin C reduce exercise-induced oxidative stress, there is limited evidence that antioxidant supplementation can improve human performance. However, because of the paucity of research on this topic, many additional studies are required before a firm conclusion can be reached about the effects of antioxidant treatment on human exercise tolerance.

Future studies should examine the potential synergistic effects of several antioxidants on human performance. Further, additional experiments are required to explore the bioavailability of nutritional antioxidants provided in tablet form compared to the bioavailability of these nutrients derived from whole food. This is an interesting area for future research.

populations or whether further antioxidant intake would be necessary. Since intense exercise training leads to the depletion of tissue and plasma concentrations of antioxidants such as coenzyme Q10 or ubiquinone, vitamin C, and vitamin E, this reduction may lead to a decreased antioxidant defense.[42,43] This depletion is evident even in those athletes consuming a "nutritious, well-balanced, and mixed diet." Hence, dietary intake may not provide sufficient amounts of antioxidants to athletes. By increasing tissue and plasma concentrations via antioxidant supplementation, athletes can assist endogenous antioxidant capacity and complement dietary intake to reduce the damage that results from strenuous training. Granted, antioxidants and nutrients seem to be better absorbed and seem to confer greater benefit when consumed as part of whole foods, but when whole food intake is insufficient, additional supplementation is the next best thing.

Research Methods for Assessing Biological Effectiveness

To better understand how researchers make conclusions about the necessity and effectiveness of antioxidant supplements, knowledge of their measurement techniques is required. Basically, three methods are common to assessing the effectiveness of antioxidant compounds in athletes: measurement of the oxidized products or molecules, measurement of tissue damage, and ultimately, measurement of performance itself. Investigators can sample serum, urine, breath, or tissue specimens for oxidized compounds generated as a result of free radical activity. These products include malondialdehyde (MDA), thiobarbituric acid–reactive substances (TBARS), pentane and ethane, conjugated dienes, and lipid hydroperoxides. Of these, high-performance liquid chromatography (HPLC) measurement of lipid hydroperoxides is the most direct assessment of oxidative damage. Because of inconsistencies among these techniques and the variability of oxidized products, the best research takes into account more than one of the oxidation products and may investigate more than one medium (i.e., breath and serum).

In addition to indices of oxidative damage, physiologists interested in muscle damage and recovery also measured damage indirectly through cellular damage markers. Since lipid membrane peroxidation leads to abnormalities in the cell membrane, intracellular enzymes may *leak* from the cell and into the blood plasma with antioxidant damage. These enzymes can be measured in the blood as indirect markers of cell membrane damage. The most frequently measured enzymatic markers of muscle damage in the serum are as creatine kinase (CK), alanine aminotransferase (ALT—formerly known as SGPT), aspartate aminotransferase (AST—formerly SGOT), and lactate

dehydrogenase (LDH). Muscle proteins can also be catabolized as a result of mechanical and oxidative damage; therefore, urinary nitrogen excretion can also be quantified. Taking the nitrogen excretion concept further, nitrogen balance (NBAL) studies and even stable isotope methodology can be used to assess muscle damage via protein breakdown.

Perhaps most pertinent to an athlete's *bottom line* are a variety of exercise performance tests that can be used. These range from treadmill and cycle protocols to strength measurements. Such tests can assess both ergogenic benefits from [antioxidant] supplementation and recovery rate after strenuous bouts of exercise. In essence, the practical effects of antioxidant supplementation can be assessed by the determination of whether performance can be improved or whether a high level of performance can be maintained with repeated bouts of exercise.

When considering the data obtained from the aforementioned measures, often findings are inconsistent. Much of the inconsistent findings in exercise and free radical/antioxidant research may be attributed to the lack of uniformity in study design regarding protocol, especially for performance testing. When evaluating this research, it is important to note the type, intensity, and duration of exercise used as well as the duration of the recovery period between multiple bouts. Since performance testing tends to yield the most inconsistent results in antioxidant research, some authors have criticized the use of performance measures. Physical performance is a multifactorial process, and therefore performance testing may not serve as a good indicator of the effects of antioxidant supplementation.[44] Although exercise testing may not be an extremely sensitive measure, numerous studies have shown positive effects of antioxidant supplementation and therefore, as mentioned earlier, if protocol uniformity is attempted, perhaps the data would show more consistent results in a specific direction.

In addition to protocol concerns, population-specific variables are important to consider. When evaluating the results from antioxidant research, it is important to note the type of population that the subjects were drawn from (i.e., weight lifters, cyclists, runners, old, young, male, female, etc.). Of course, animal ex vivo (pre-treated human cells examined outside the body) or *in vitro* (in a test tube or dish) data are sometimes the only available source of information. In such cases, recognize that humans may react differently but are generally considered similar until proven otherwise.

Antioxidant Supplements and Exercise

Most researchers have tended to focus on more mechanistic measures like the aforementioned parameters and have tended to ignore some of the "practical" effects of

Table 12-4 Antioxidant-Related Vitamins and Minerals

Compound	2000 RDA* (dose/day)	ESADDI (dose/day)	TUL (dose/day)	Food Sources
A (retinol)	1000 μg (3330 IU) (1989 value)	N/A	N/A	Beef liver, sweet potato, carrots, spinach, squash, dandelion greens
Beta-carotene	6000 μg** (1989 value)	N/A	N/A	Carrots, cantaloupe, broccoli, spinach
C	75 mg women 90 mg men	N/A	2000 mg	Fresh fruits, cruciferous vegetables, potatoes
E: alpha-tocopherol	15 mg (22–33 IU)	N/A	1000 mg	Vegetable oils, nuts, whole grains, butter, liver, egg yolk, some fruits and vegetables
E: tocotrienol	N/A	N/A	N/A	
Selenium	55 μg	N/A	400 μg	Grains, meat, poultry, fish, garlic, dairy
Copper	N/A	1.5–3.0 mg (1989 value)	N/A	Liver, shellfish, whole grains, legumes, eggs, meat, fish
Zinc	12 mg women 15 mg men (1989 value)	N/A	N/A	Oysters, wheat germ, beef, liver, poultry, whole grains
Iron	15 mg women 10 mg men (1989 value)	N/A	N/A	Meats, molasses, clams, oysters, nuts, legumes, seeds, green leafy vegetables, grains/breads
Manganese	N/A	2–5 mg (1989 value)	N/A	Wheat bran, legumes, nuts, lettuce, seafood, poultry, meat, blueberries, pineapple

Values presented refer to adult males and females (not lactating or pregnant).
N/A = not applicable or currently available; ESADDI = estimated safe and adequate daily dietary intakes; TUL = tolerable upper limits.
*or 1989 value, if 2000 value has not been established.
**to meet vitamin 1989 A RDA, 6 μg beta-carotene = 1 μg retinol.

antioxidant supplementation on real world performance. A more comprehensive approach may be warranted to assess the health and performance benefits of antioxidant supplementation in athletes. Some of the goals of antioxidant nutrient therapy or *nutritherapy* for athletes have been described by Jan Karlsson in the book *Antioxidants and Exercise*[43] and include the following:

- Less overuse injury and faster recovery from inflammatory process

- Improved immune response and faster recovery after infection

- Less disease in the fitness athlete and a more efficient training program in the elite athlete

- A better quality of life for the fitness athlete and improved sports performance for the elite athlete

Although much of the research has focused on endurance athletes, there are some data in resistance-trained athletes as well. The focus of this review, then, will be to discuss the scientific literature examining both modes of training with respect to the goals specified by Karlsson. Special attention will be paid to the discussion of the research that deals with performance and recovery from intense exercise, although in the absence of such data, a discussion of any other relevant findings will be offered.

To clearly address the plethora of antioxidant supplements that are available to athletes, this review will describe them individually. Vitamins will be listed first, then minerals, and finally, miscellaneous compounds (herbs, etc.) including reported antioxidant effects will be listed. Each antioxidant review will include *in vitro* (in a dish or test tube) data as well as *in vivo* (in a living organism) data on both animals and, if applicable, humans. Epidemiological data regarding intake quantities, occurrence of deficiency, food sources, increased needs in athletes (when appropriate—by type), dose information, and toxicology concerns will be discussed. Finally, some discussion of combined nutrient therapy will be offered (SEE TABLE 12-4).

Vitamins

Vitamin A

The molecules that make up the category "vitamin A" are all part of a group of compounds that exhibit the biological activity of retinol. Most dietary vitamin A is obtained from carotenoids or from animal tissues with high vitamin A content. Being a lipid-soluble vitamin, this nutrient in either large or chronic amounts can concentrate in fatty tissues and cause numerous symptoms of toxicity including headaches, bone pain, weakness, and skin problems, among others. Vitamin A is known to be essential in vision, testicular function, development, bone growth, differentiation, and hematopoiesis. It has also been shown to possess antioxidant properties, offering protection against lipid peroxidation, oxidative modification of proteins, and LDL oxidation.[45–48] Little research has been done examining the effects of vitamin A supplementation in athletes. This is potentially due to a few factors including the fact that vitamin A toxicity is likely at higher doses. In addition, although plasma vitamin A is decreased as a result of exercise in rats, skeletal muscle vitamin A is increased, indicating a homeostatic mechanism for antioxidant balance.[49]

Beta-Carotene

Beta-carotene and lycopene belong to a large class of compounds called carotenoids, some of which can be converted to vitamin A but many of which cannot. Examples of other carotenoids include alpha- and gamma-carotene, canthaxanthin lutein, beta-cryptoxanthin, and crocetin. Acting primarily as the precursor to retinol or vitamin A, beta-carotene is also referred to as "provitamin A." Many carotenoids do not have the provitamin A activity of beta-carotene, and therefore researchers have begun to investigate carotenoids for their vitamin A–independent roles, including free radical quenching, immune enhancement,

and ability to induce detoxification enzymes. In particular, a good deal of research has revolved around beta-carotene and lycopene, much of it focusing on their ability to deter numerous types of cancer and heart disease. The value of carotenoid supplementation alone has not been shown in exercise. With moderate exercise, plasma levels of carotenoids can be reduced.[50] Supplementing a combination of vitamin C, E, and beta-carotene has been shown to decrease the levels of lipid peroxidation at rest and during exercise at different intensities.[51] In addition, it has been reported that this combination of antioxidants has a protective effect on both blood glutathione and muscle damage.[44] No data examine the interaction between lycopene and exercise.

Vitamin C

Vitamin C is known as ascorbic acid and because of its solubility in aqueous environments, is most associated with both intracellular and extracellular fluids (blood). Although there is controversy regarding the proposed correlations between vitamin C and disease such as cancer, heart disease, or stroke, vitamin C is known to be an effective antioxidant. Vitamin C has the unique ability to act

Current Controversy: Vitamin C— Antioxidant or Pro-Oxidant?

Of course thousands of people supplement vitamin C for its antioxidant properties. In fact, many consume several grams per day in an effort to reduce the damage that free radical compounds can cause. But is consuming such high doses beneficial? In addition to the inefficiency of absorption as the vitamin C dose is increased, evidence also exists that large acute doses can result in opposing effects to what is intended. How can this be?

Because of the nature of redox reactions, a substance such as vitamin C could reduce certain cellular components (an antioxidant effect) while oxidizing others. The ability of vitamin C to do this has been reported repeatedly and may be related to dose. Podmore and colleagues (1998) showed that administration of 500 mg/day to healthy humans for 6 weeks induced pro-oxidant effects on particular segments of nuclear material in lymphocytes. This suggests that higher doses actually act in a manner that is opposite to their intended purpose for many people. And in an effort to elucidate a mechanism for vitamin C's pro-oxidant effects, Paolini et al. examined very high dose supplementation

(250 and 500 mg/kg for 4 days) in rats. The researchers showed a dose-response effect on superoxide anion production and an increase in microsomal oxidative enzymes, with the 500 mg/kg dose being substantially *worse*.

As shown in Table 12-1, the new RDA for vitamin C was set by the Institute of Medicine's Food and Nutrition Board to reflect tissue saturation. This 75–90 mg/day recommendation may be exceeded with relative safety up to 2500 mg/day (the "Upper Limit") but this does not ensure a total lack of pro-oxidant effects. To prevent selective oxidation of circulating blood components, it may be prudent to limit the daily dose of vitamin C to below 500 mg/day.

Anonymous. Is too much vitamin C hazardous to your health? Harv Womens Health Watch 1998;5:7.

Bland J. The pro-oxidant and antioxidant effects of vitamin C. Altern Med Rev 1998;3:170.

Levine M, Daruwala RC, Park JB, et al. Does vitamin C have a pro-oxidant effect? Nature 1998;395:231–232.

Podmore I, Griffiths HR, Herbert KE, et al. Vitamin C exhibits pro-oxidant properties. Nature 1998;392:559.

as a primary antioxidant by donating electrons to quench free radicals and reactive oxygen species and as a secondary antioxidant to regenerate vitamin E within the intracellular fluid. In addition to its interaction with vitamin E, oxidized vitamin C is reduced and recycled by glutathione. Due to its nonspecific antioxidant properties, vitamin C is effective in the removal of most reactive oxygen species. In exercise training, vitamin C has been shown to reduce free radical production during and after exercise.[52–54] Also, vitamin C can reduce muscle soreness and improve recovery from muscle damage.[55] In a study examining the eccentric muscle damage, maximum voluntary contractions were greater 24 hours after the damaging exercise when subjects supplemented with vitamin C than when they supplemented with vitamin E or placebo.[56]

Vitamin E

The term *vitamin E* refers to eight similar compounds: alpha, beta, delta, and gamma tocopherol and four tocotrienols of the same designations. The prefixes alpha through gamma refer to the number and position of methyl groups on the aromatic ring on the molecule. The difference is that the tocotrienols have three double bonds along the side chain of the molecule, whereas the tocopherols do not (*tri* means three, of course, and *-ene* refers to a carbon-carbon double bond.) Members of the vitamin E family have direct biological relationships with immunity, aging, exercise, heart disease, and cancer. Although alpha-tocopherol is the most abundant of these compounds in tissues and is the most bioactive and bioavailable, recent marketing attention has been placed on the use of mixed tocopherols and tocotrienol forms. This is due to the research that suggests that different vitamin E derivatives possess increased *in vitro* antioxidant activity as well as unique antioxidant and therapeutic properties.[57–59] The debate, however, continues as many question whether increased *in vitro* antioxidant capacity is beneficial when there is decreased bioavailability of the compounds. This argument is supported by data showing that the *old school* alpha-tocopherol that has been popular for many years has superior biological potency.[60]

Another concern regarding the intake of vitamin E is that because it is present primarily in fats, limiting dietary fat, as many athletes and health-conscious individuals do, will limit its availability. The health and antioxidant benefits of vitamin E have been well documented through numerous trials and have shown that the membrane-bound vitamin E is one of the cell's predominant defense mechanisms against lipid peroxidation. Vitamin E is continuously recycled by numerous other antioxidants including vitamin C, ubiquinone, and glutathione. In terms of exercise performance, Vitamin E is probably the most researched of the antioxidants. As with other antioxidants, improvement in performance trials has not usually been found,[61–64] with the exception of aerobic training at altitude and aerobic training in ozone-rich environments.[65–67] In the studies that did show improvements, vitamin E improved both oxidation status and lactate threshold in mountain climbers; whereas in cyclists, vitamin E supplementation improved pulmonary function and oxidation status in the presence of ozone-rich air. Since ozone (found in polluted air) is a powerful oxidant that reduces lung performance, urban exercisers may benefit from vitamin E's antioxidant characteristics. The benefits would primarily manifest as reduced toxicity rather than actual performance enhancement, however, as pulmonary oxygen provision is not generally considered limiting in aerobic performance.

Although performance may not be greatly impacted by antioxidant supplementation, perhaps the greatest potential benefit that vitamin E can offer athletes is a reduction in exercise-induced tissue damage. Although there are mixed results, the evidence is relatively convincing that vitamin E supplementation can decrease muscle and oxidative damage in response to exercise. First, it has been reported that consuming 800 IU/day of vitamin E can, in fact, elevate serum concentrations of alpha- and gamma-tocopherol by 300% and 74%, respectively. Thus, supplemental regimes with this vitamin are effectively absorbed. Second, these elevations subsequently induce substantial skeletal muscle increases of 53% and 37%, respectively, within 30 days.[68] The results of these increases are encouraging for hard-training athletes. In various studies in humans and in animals, vitamin E supplementation has been shown to decrease plasma levels of the cytosolic enzymes creatine kinase and lactate dehydrogenase.[5,69–71] In addition, markers of lipid peroxidation such as MDA, conjugated dienes, and TBARS have been reduced with vitamin E supplementation.[72–75] Also, reperfusion injury in the quadriceps can be reduced with 600 IU/day of oral vitamin E over 8 days.[76] The effect of vitamin E on protein catabolism needs further work, but in particular studies, vitamin E seems to possess beneficial effects.[75,77,78]

Minerals

Selenium

Selenium is a trace mineral that is a key component in the endogenous antioxidant, glutathione peroxidase (GPX), and it is thought to function as an antioxidant through this role. In research studies, selenium supplementation has been shown to increase GPX levels, but there has been no indication of increased protection or performance.[79,80] Its use then, as an antioxidant, is questionable because even with selenium deficiency, in the presence of adequate vitamin E there is no measurable change in oxidative cell damage.[81] In addition, there is a narrow range between the necessary intake level and the toxic level.

Zinc

Zinc is a trace mineral that has a wide array of functions because of its presence as a component of several enzymes (metalloenzymes). Zinc, along with copper, is a component of the cytosolic antioxidant superoxide dismutase (SOD), but it is thought to have antioxidant properties independent of this role as well. It is not known whether zinc acts directly or indirectly as an antioxidant. These mechanisms, although unclear, are thought to include membrane stabilization, protein (enzyme) stabilization,[82] and the antagonism of transition metals that produce oxidative injury.[83] Zinc is a component of the enzymes of energy metabolism, and deficiency can result in decreased energy supply, altered ability to produce muscle contractions, and decreased immune function.[84] Zinc balance is often unfavorable in athletes because of either altered zinc metabolism or inadequate intake.[85] Research has shown that zinc supplementation during exercise can decrease the production of reactive oxygen species (respiratory burst activity) versus placebo.[86]

Manganese

Manganese is a trace mineral that, like the others mentioned here, functions as either a component of metalloenzymes or as an enzyme activator. The relationship of this mineral to antioxidant status is twofold, like zinc. The first role of manganese in antioxidant status is that it is a component of the mitochondrial antioxidant SOD. Manganese deficiency can decrease SOD activity in the mitochondria,[87] while manganese supplementation can increase mitochondrial lymphocyte SOD activity.[88] In addition, manganese also appears to have antioxidant function independent of SOD activity as it can quench peroxyl radicals.[89] Although there is some dispute regarding whether manganese has pro-oxidant potential, it has been shown to decrease oxidative brain injury, LDL oxidation, and atherosclerosis.[90]

Copper and Iron

Copper and Iron are trace minerals that function as enzyme cofactors, as intermediates in electron transfer, and, in the case of iron, as a component of oxygen transport proteins (hemoglobin and myoglobin). Copper is a component of the cytosolic antioxidant superoxide dismutase, but conversely its function as an intermediate in electron transfer tends to give this mineral the reputation as a pro-oxidant. Iron is a component of the endogenous antioxidant catalase but, like copper, also acts as a pro-oxidant. Metals such as copper and iron, when free in the cell, are easily reduced, making them potent pro-oxidants. In fact, free copper is implicated in the oxidation of LDL and in ischemia-reperfusion injury,[91,92] while iron is implicated in increased risk of cancer and heart disease and attack.[93] Copper deficiency, however, can lead to low cytosolic SOD activity, so it appears that a balance must be achieved between copper as an antioxidant and a pro-oxidant.[94,95]

Miscellaneous

Polyunsaturated Fatty Acids (e.g., corn oil, soybean oil, fish oil)

The human diet contains not only antioxidant compounds, but also pro-oxidants. Perhaps the most obvious example is that of polyunsaturated fatty acids. These common fats are promulgated as beneficial compared with saturated fat (regarding heart disease) but nonetheless can be detrimental when consumed in large quantities. Polyunsaturates are part of cell membranes and are susceptible to peroxidation; the oxidative products of such can be used as markers for oxidative damage.[96] The omega-6 fatty acids (e.g., linoleic acid) are also especially inflammatory, as they also act as a substrate for prostaglandin E2 synthesis. Both the omega-6 and the omega-3 fatty acids seem to alter cellular antioxidant defense and increase the susceptibility to oxidative damage.[97,98] Adequate vitamin E intake has been shown to combat some, but not all of the oxidative effects involving polyunsaturated fatty acids.[99–101] This may be due, in part, to the fact that polyunsaturated fats contain a much less bioavailable vitamin E than other fats.[102] Therefore, an increase in the intake of polyunsaturates might not only lead to increased lipid peroxidation, but may also decrease the intake of vitamin E. Due to greater potential for damage and less potential for defense, polyunsaturates may increase the requirements for supplemental antioxidants. In an effort to combat oxidative damage caused relative to these common oils, dietary lipids that are less susceptible to oxidation and/or act as antioxidants have been researched for their stability as components of membranes. With respect to exercise, the data are inconclusive regarding polyunsaturated fats and performance.[103–105]

Monounsaturated Fatty Acids (e.g., olive oil, canola oil)

These fats do not provide substrate for inflammatory mediators and are more resistant to peroxidation. In fact, rat data exist which document the *in vivo* reduction in markers of tissue oxidation after consumption of an olive oil diet.[106] In addition, research has shown that the addition of monounsaturates to the human diet without changes in saturated or polyunsaturated intake can lead to lower cholesterol and LDL cholesterol as well as may reduce the susceptibility of LDL to oxidative stress.[107] In a comparison of diets containing either 32% of energy from monounsaturates or polyunsaturates, subjects consuming monounsaturates had lower oxidative stress as measured by TBARS.[108] Hence, a simple switch to olive oil from corn oil, soybean oil, and vegetable oil (which is often a blend of the former) may result in favorable changes in tissue and membrane lipids. These changes in fatty acid incorporation into cell membranes may reduce lipid peroxidation. Interestingly, with all the talk regarding vitamin, mineral, and herbal antioxidants, altering the fatty acid composition of the diet may be the most potent diet modification of all for both antioxidant protection and disease prevention.[109–113]

Conjugated Linoleic Acid

CLA is a term describing several geometric and positional isomers of common linoleic acid (an omega-6 fatty acid). CLA, however, has many opposing physiological effects to linoleate, notably in reference to carcinogenesis and inflammation. The unique properties of CLA may in part be due to its postulated antioxidant properties.[114] This mechanism, however, has been questioned.[115] It is more likely that the preliminary positive findings regarding CLA supplementation in athletes[116,117] are due to other mechanisms. This, however, remains to be elucidated.

Co-Enzyme Q10 or Ubiquinone

Ubiquinone is a naturally occurring part of the electron transport chain (ETC) in the mitochondria (*powerhouses*) of cells. It is also found within lipid membranes including the plasma membrane and intracellular membranes. Being a mobile part of the inner mitochondrial matrix where ATP is formed, its biological significance has been well studied. In addition to its role as an electron carrier, it can also prevent oxidative damage to lipids. It has also been suggested that it can help regenerate vitamin E.[118] Muscle concentrations of ubiquinone fall with age, various disease states (e.g., muscular dystrophy, congestive heart failure), and exercise. Thus, there has been research interest in bolstering endogenous levels via dietary means (in the form of vitamin Q). Recent data reveal that supplementary Co-Q10 can increase tissue concentrations in humans after 14 days of supplementation and increase further after 28 days.[119] This research also showed that a combination of 100 IU of vitamin E + Co-Q10 appears to be the best way to maximize its tissue uptake (although vitamin E itself was incorporated in a dose-dependent manner up to 1300 IU). The data are mixed regarding Co-Q10 supplementation and performance with some studies showing benefit,[120–122] some showing no benefit,[123–125] and one showing greater muscular damage with supplementation.[126]

Lipoic Acid

Alpha lipoic acid (ALA) is an antioxidant that has received considerable attention recently, both in the scientific and commercial supplement communities. ALA is present in the mitochondrial proteins necessary for oxidative metabolism. For example, it is a cofactor for dehydrogenase enzymes like PDH, which forms acetyl CoA for the Krebs cycle. In addition, ALA possesses both antioxidant and subchronic glucose disposal activity.[127,128] This compound can scavenge HO_2, HOCL, and O_2 radicals. It is both water- and lipid-soluble, and so may be of benefit to both cellular compartments. Alpha lipoic acid has been shown to combat age-associated decline in metabolism by improving mitochondrial function via increased oxygen consumption, mitochondrial membrane potential, and ambulatory activity. In addition, this research showed decreased oxidative damage as measured by decreases in MDA and increases in ascorbic acid and glutathione.[129] In exercise-induced oxidative stress, lipoic acid decreased lipid peroxidation and increased glutathione levels.[130] Research investigating a lipoic acid + vitamin E combination has revealed evidence of decreased plasma LDL oxidation as well as decreased urinary isoprostanes, which are markers of oxidation.[131] Although these preliminary data are exciting, more research is needed to clarify the exact nature of lipoic acid's beneficial effects as both a glucose disposal agent and an antioxidant.

Polyphenols

Phytochemicals, polyphenols, and their derivatives including the flavonoids, tannins, and catechins discussed herein, are molecules derived from plants that have potential benefit for human health. One of the many proposed benefits of the polyphenols and their derivatives is their potential for antioxidant effects. Due to their structural similarities, the polyphenols act as antioxidants by donating electrons. In addition, like many of the other antioxidant compounds, polyphenols are associated with prevention of diseases such as atherosclerosis and cancer. Listed below are several compounds that contain polyphenolic derivatives. We are unaware of any published data examining the effects of any of the following compounds in exercise-trained individuals or athletes. However, because of the positive results seen in recent research and their popularity as dietary supplements, we have addressed them here.

Milk Thistle

This herb, otherwise known as *Silybum marianum*, contains the active flavonolignans which include the compounds silybin, silydianin, and silychristine. These compounds are collectively known as silymarins. Silymarins are known

Current Controversy: Are Bioflavonoids Poorly Absorbed?

Considerable debate in the dietary supplement community has focused on the human body's ability to absorb bioflavonoid compounds. These substances are present in both foods and dietary supplements and may possess a variety of physiologically relevant properties. Such properties include inhibition of cancer development, inhibition of estrogen formation (*aromitization*), reduction of heart attack risk, prolongation of drug effects, increased bone density, and specific to our discussion here, antioxidant effects. Interestingly, it's the antioxidant capability that seems to be a primary factor in some of these other biological effects. Earlier scientific work on the topic seems to point to a general inability of the human intestines to absorb certain bioflavonoid substances. Newer research, however, seems to be reaching the opposite conclusion—at least when the flavonoids are consumed via whole-food sources.

As an example, the general consensus from current research investigating a grapefruit/onion/apple bioflavonoid, *quercetin,* is that humans absorb about 20% of an oral dose. In contrast, earlier research suggested that less than 1% is absorbed into the bloodstream. Although 20% is not nearly as high as the absorption of macronutrients like protein, carbohydrate, and fat, this percentage is still higher than that of some accepted micronutrients (e.g., non-heme iron). Additionally, the fact that these substances can induce physiological effects in humans is further evidence that they are, indeed, absorbed. Case in point: quercetin was found to be partly responsible for the much-publicized Seldane (an allergy drug) deaths of 1998. Victims were taking their medication as prescribed, yet they were dying of toxic overdoses induced by co-consumption with grapefruit juice.

It needs to be stated that there are thousands of bioflavonoid compounds with widely varying physiological effects. Grapefruit juice is just one example. Soy foods have gained widespread popularity as anti-cancer and anti–heart disease foods; they are even being shown to be potential estrogen replacement alternatives. It

stands to reason then that the bioflavonoids contained therein must be absorbable. Nonetheless, research needs to be done on the extent to which each bioflavonoid is absorbed.

A final point that should be made about the "bioflavonoid absorption controversy" is that consumers and educators must use discretion when reaching conclusions about bioflavonoid research. *In vitro* studies that find impressive effects (e.g., estrogen inhibition) may not translate into equally impressive *in vivo* results. Many factors come into play when a substance is ingested that cannot always be adequately controlled in "test tube studies." Intestinal absorption, gender, hormonal environment, diet, activity level, age, etc., are all factors and thus require population-specific studies on living people to ascertain effectiveness for each person.

In conclusion, although evidence is mounting that bioflavonoids may be important, previously unrecognized nutrients, it is difficult to make blanket statements about their absorption. Finding peer-reviewed, unbiased information on a specific bioflavonoid compound of interest is necessary before making decisions regarding its consumption.

Craig WJ. Health-promoting properties of common herbs. Am J Clin Nutr 1999;70(3 suppl):491S–499S.

Gugler R, Leschik M, Dengler HJ. Disposition of quercetin in man after single oral and intravenous doses. Eur J Clin Pharmacol 1975;9:229–234.

Hackett AM. The metabolism of flavonoid compounds in mammals. In: Cody V, et al. eds. Plant flavonoids in biology and medicine. New York: Alan R. Liss, 1986:177–194.

Hollman PC, Katan MB. Bioavailability and health effects of dietary flavonols in man. Arch Toxicol Suppl 1998;20:237–248.

Hollman PC, Katan MB. Health effects and bioavailability of dietary flavonols. Free Radic Res 1999;31(suppl):S75–S80.

Fuhr U. Drug interactions with grapefruit juice: extent, probable mechanism and clinical relevance. Drug Safety 1998;18:251–272.

Lambson DW, et al. Antioxidants and cancer. Part 3: quercetin. Altern Med Rev 2000;5:196–208.

Scheiber MD, Rebar RW. Isoflavones and postmenopausal bone health: a viable alternative to estrogen therapy? Menopause 1999;6:233–241.

primarily for their hepatoprotective effects including protection against toxins, including acetaminophen, ethanol, carbon tetrachloride, and D-galactosamine; and protection against ischemic injury, radiation, iron toxicity, and viral hepatitis.[132] The hepatoprotective effects of silymarin are thought to include antioxidant action, prevention of lipid peroxidation, enhanced detoxification, and protection against glutathione depletion.[133–137] The improved antioxidant status displayed by hepatic Kupffer cells (which detoxify the blood as it perfuses the liver) with milk thistle supplementation can actually result in improved clinical outcomes in liver disease.

Pine Bark (Pycnogenol)

The French maritime pine, *Pinus maritima*, has been examined for its principal extract, pycnogenol. This extract contains a variety of bioavailable phenolic derivatives (catechins and flavonoids) and investigations have shown that pycnogenol has strong free radical–scavenging activity against reactive oxygen and nitrogen species.[138] In addition it also seems to interact with the cellular antioxidant systems by the regeneration of vitamin C,[139] protecting endogenous vitamin E[137] and glutathione from oxidative stress, and up-regulating intracellular enzymatic and nonenzymatic oxidant scavenging systems. Pycnogenol has been shown to increase cellular glutathione content, SOD, and CAT activities in bovine artery endothelial cells (that line the inner lumen of the vessel), resulting in a concentration-dependent increase in O_2 and H_2O_2 removal.

Grape Seed Extract

Grapes and wine have been receiving much attention lately due to their proposed health benefits, including the reduction of the incidence of mortality and morbidity from coronary heart disease. The polyphenols, which are found in grape seeds, skin, and stems, are thought to serve many favorable biological roles with respect to heart disease. Grape seeds contain the polyphenol, proanthocyanidin, which is thought to have protective properties against free radicals. In one study, grape seed proanthocyanidin was shown to be better than vitamins C and E in scavenging biochemically generated superoxide anions and hydroxyl radicals.[140] In addition, decreases in lipid peroxidation and DNA fragmentation in liver and brain, as well as an inhibition of reactive oxygen species production in peritoneal macrophages has been shown.[141] In this study, grape seed extract was more effective than vitamin C, E, and beta-carotene at similar doses. In another study, grape seed proanthocyanidins were shown to possess a cardioprotective effect against ischemia reperfusion injury. This property was attributed to its ability to directly scavenge peroxyl and hydroxyl radicals and to reduce oxidative stress developed during this state.[142]

Green Tea

The plant *Camellia sinensis* has been the subject of many investigations on the positive health benefits of tea. In epidemiological research, it has been shown that the daily consumption of tea is involved in the prevention of coronary heart disease, artherosclerosis, and some types of cancer. The health benefits of tea are related to the antioxidant effects of its components, namely, its polyphenolic tannins and catechins that are present in highest concentrations in green tea as opposed to other types.[143] Although black tea contains a number of polyphenols as well (i.e., theaflavine gallate, digallate, etc.), the effects of these compounds are not as well researched. The polyphenols in tea appear to act in the prevention of lipid peroxidation and in cellular defense of the reactive oxygen species released during carcinogenesis.[144–146]

Ginkgo Biloba

The leaves and fruit of this plant have been used as therapeutic agents in China for over 5000 years. More recently, ginkgo biloba extracts have been used in western medicine to treat peripheral artery disease and cerebral insufficiency. It has been speculated that the beneficial actions of this extract are due to the antioxidant properties of its ingredients, especially its variety of polyphenols including flavonoids and terpenes. Ginkgo biloba may exert its antioxidant actions by scavenging the superoxide and hydroxyl radicals produced as a result of ischemia-reperfusion injury and inflammation.[147,148] It has been shown *in vivo* that ginkgo biloba is active in the prevention of lipid peroxidation with age, and in the prevention of LDL oxidation.[149–152]

Mechanism for Antioxidant Benefits in Exercise

In the athlete, it appears that the most promising characteristic of antioxidant supplementation regarding performance is the ability to aid recovery. As athletes know, recovery after exercise is vitally important to improved performance. Eccentric contractions (i.e., "negatives") are a necessary part of many types of sport and result in exaggerated myofibrillar disruption, delayed-onset muscle soreness, inflammation, and reduced force generation. Thus, decreasing muscle damage and inflammation (and/or hastening a return to "healthy" status) can allow an athlete to resume training and more rapidly improve in ability. The response to muscle damage can last several days and is hallmarked by increased muscle enzyme release, DOMS, urinary nitrogen excretion, increased metabolic rate, and increased cortisol and interleukin concentrations. Subjects also experience decreased glucose tolerance and strength after eccentric exercise.[153,154] This period of eccentric recovery is in stark contrast to the shorter, less traumatic 24–48 hour recovery period observed after less-damaging concentric exercise.[155] As mentioned earlier, circulating leukocytes (white blood cells) infiltrate traumatized muscle tissue and, in concert with cortisol, prostaglandins, and various cytokines, they induce catabolism, edema, pain, and inflammation. Although this immune response is primarily beneficial, the period of catabolism may be unnecessarily aggressive before growth factors are secreted and tissue growth and/or repair begins.

Think of this scenario as equivalent to a group of janitors arriving to clean up a mess. But, in addition to cleaning up the original mess, these janitors (neutrophils and monocytes) also tend to tear down the walls as they clean. Antioxidant vitamins like vitamin E and vitamin C may combat this aggressive cleaning strategy of the janitors (part of the acute-phase response) both by buffering the reactive oxygen species that are released and by suppressing cell membrane peroxidation and prostaglandin formation, which is partly responsible for the inflammation.[156,157] The next logical question would be: Why would anyone punish themselves with eccentric contractions to

the point of requiring pharmacologic doses of vitamins? The logic behind using repeated, high-intensity eccentric contractions involves the growth response. Because the muscle hypertrophic response is greater, athletes requiring gains in muscular size and/or strength often use *negative* training using resistance exercises and/ or plyometrics.[158] As we have seen, this can aggravate oxidant insult, inducing damage that might only be treated optimally with antioxidant supplementation.

SUMMARY

Sports nutrition and exercise physiology are fields of study that continue to create new information regarding antioxidant supplementation. This knowledge is used routinely by many in the athletic population but is sometimes underemphasized in the presence of *newer* hormonal, herbal, and *specialty* substances that regularly appear. There is generally more research on antioxidants than on other types of ergogenic aids, which makes them a safer bet as an addition to one's training regime. Although existing data are equivocal regarding actual improvements in performance, antioxidants like vitamin C and E do seem to improve recovery and reduce certain detrimental effects that hard training can cause. Because athletes will typically follow strict diets, their discipline can be a problem when it comes to dietary variety, fat intake, and antioxidant intake. In addition, even with varied diets, larger (supra-dietary) amounts of

antioxidants may be required for oxidative protection. As a result, antioxidant vitamins are recommended.

Exercise stressors often mimic other physiological stressors; thus, athletes can learn from diseases having pro-oxidant–related etiologies and apply some of that information to themselves. The pro-oxidant conditions that occur during diseases such as cancer, rheumatoid arthritis, and atherosclerosis are often similar to those induced by intense exercise. Remember that intense exercise generally causes acute, transient injury. During and after intense exercise, the body's antioxidant defenses are overwhelmed. This potentially deleterious state is primarily due to different factors in endurance athletes than in resistance athletes. In both cases, however, supplemental antioxidants are probably helpful, especially in light of the aforementioned dietary constraints that athletes self-impose.

AUTHORS' RECOMMENDATIONS

For all types of athletes (albeit for essentially different reasons), the following are recommendations for decreasing the deleterious effects of oxidative damage:

Dietary Fatty Acids (% of total caloric intake):

5–10% polyunsaturated fat

10% saturated fat

10–15% monounsaturated fat

These recommendations are based on a diet consisting of 30% fat. If desired intake is higher or lower, these recommendations would dictate that 16–33% of total fat should come from polyunsaturated fats, 33% of total fat should come from saturated fats, and 33–50%

of total fat should come from monounsaturated fats. These recommendations take into account the requirements for essential fatty acids and are based on favorable blood lipid profiles. In addition, these recommendations should be sufficient to prevent excessive lipid peroxidation and oxidative damage.

Vitamin C

250–500 mg daily (250 mg, 1–2 times daily)

Taking more at a given time is not advisable, as it increases risk of pro-oxidant effects due to the oxidation of vitamin C, making it a mild reactive species. There may be circulatory benefits to superseding the new RDA of 75–90 mg, which is based on tissue saturation.

Vitamin E

400–800 IU daily (400 IU 1–2 times daily)

With each of these nutrients, overdose is unlikely in individuals not using anticoagulant drugs. Acute and chronic toxicity are not issues at these doses of vitamins C and E. The controversy over synthetic versus natural forms is of secondary importance. Instead of using individual capsules/gelcaps of vitamins C and E, many individuals prefer to simply consume a combination antioxidant 1–3 times daily. Depending on the brand, this usually provides the provitamin beta-carotene as well as selenium and other antioxidant minerals. This approach, however, will likely reduce total vitamin E intake compared with the above recommendation and increase the risk of overconsuming the antioxidant

minerals therein. Consumption of the individual vitamins may be a better approach.

Regarding herbal antioxidants, these compounds can be taken alone or in combination with products that deliver both vitamin and herbal antioxidants like pycnogenol (pine bark), grape seed extract, and ginkgo biloba. Although these phytochemicals have demonstrated potential as potent antioxidants, there seems to be considerable overlap between their effects as well as potential interaction between compounds. Caution should be exercised with products containing multiple ingredients, especially herbs. Each added ingredient increases the risk of nutrient–nutrient interactions that can either negate beneficial effects or induce toxicity. Remember that, contrary to most advertising campaigns, all interactions are not synergistic (or even additive).

FUTURE RESEARCH

Clearly, more research is needed to fully elucidate the possible mechanisms by which antioxidants could improve athletic performance. Though antioxidants may not have a dramatic effect on performance (as seen with creatine monohydrate), we would posit that there is a role that antioxidant supplementation should play in an athlete's dietary repertoire. With that said, we would also implore the

scientific community to perform studies that are of direct relevance to the athletic population. Well-controlled, double-blind, placebo-controlled studies using active or athletic populations would further our understanding in this field. Nonetheless, as scientists and fellow athletes, we are aware that recommendations are often based on incomplete and inconclusive data.

REFERENCES

1. Higuchi M, Carter LJ, Chen M, et al. Superoxide dismutase and catalase in skeletal muscle: adaptive response to exercise. J Gerontol 1985;40:281–286.
2. Machlin LJ. Free radical tissue damage: protective role of antioxidant nutrients. FASEB J 1987;1(6):441–445.
3. Ohno H, Sato Y, Yamashita K, et al. The effect of brief physical exercise on free radical scavenging enzyme systems in human red blood cells. Can J Physiol Pharmacol 1986;64(9):1263–1265.
4. Clanton TL, Zuo L, Klawitter P, et al. Oxidants and skeletal muscle function: physiologic and pathophysiologic implications. Proc Soc Exp Biol Med 1999;222(3):253–262.
5. McBride J, Melady P, Baird A, et al. Effect of resistance exercise on free radical production. Med Sci Sports Exerc 1998;30(1):67–72.
6. Powers SK, Ji LL, Leeuwenburgh C. Exercise training-induced alterations in skeletal muscle antioxidant capacity: a brief review. Med Sci Sports Exerc 1999;31(7):987–997.
7. Alessio HM. Exercise-induced oxidative stress. Med Sci Sports Exerc 1993;25(2):218–224.
8. McBride J, Kraemer WJ, Triplett-McBride T, et al. Effect of resistance exercise on free radical production. Med Sci Sports Exerc 1998;30(1):67–72.
9. Davies KJ, Quintanilha AT, Brooks GA, et al. Free radicals and tissue damage produced by exercise. Biochem Biophys Res Commun 1982;107:1198–1205.
10. Jackson MJ, Jones DA, Edwards RH. Experimental muscle damage: the nature of the calcium-activated degenerative processes. Eur J Clin Invest 1984;14:369–374.
11. Reid MB. Muscle fatigue: mechanisms and regulation. In Sen CS, et al. (eds). Handbook of Oxidants and Antioxidants in Exercise. Amsterdam: Elsevier, 2000:599–630.
12. Sjodin T, Helsten Westing Y, Apple FS. Biochemical mechanisms for oxygen free radical formation during exercise. Sports Med 1990;10:236–254.
13. Boveris A, Chance B. The mitochondrial generation of hydrogen peroxide: general properties and effects of hyperbaric oxygen. Biochem J 1973;134:707–716.
14. Goldfarb AH. Nutritional antioxidants as therapeutic and preventative modalities in exercise induced muscle damage. Can J Appl Physiol 1999;24(3):249–266.
15. Crinnion JN, Homer-Vanniasinkam S, Gough MJ. Skeletal muscle reperfusion injury: pathophysiology and clinical considerations. Cardiovasc Surg 1993;1(4):317–324.
16. Komulainen J, Vihko V. The course of exercise induced skeletal muscle fibre injury. In Reznick AZ, et al. (eds.): Oxidative stress in skeletal muscle. Basel, Switzerland: Birkhauser Verlag 1998:59–73.
17. Clarkson PM, Newham DJ. Associations between muscle soreness, damage, and fatigue. Adv Exp Med Biol 1995;384:457–469.
18. Evans W, Cannon J. The metabolic effects of exercise-induced muscle damage. Exerc Sport Sci Rev 1991:99–119.
19. Fielding RA, Manfredi TJ, Ding W, et al. Acute phase response in exercise. III. Neutrophil and IL-1 beta accumulation in skeletal muscle. Am J Physiol 1993;265(1 pt 2):R166–172.
20. Murakami T, Matsuama T. Appearance of influenza A virus antigenic variants after treatment of infected MDCK cells with human leukocytes. J Gen Virol 1988;69(pt 8):1841–1845.

21. Smith JA, Gray AB, Pyne DB, et al. Moderate exercise triggers both priming and activation of neutrophil subpopulations. Am J Physiol 1996;270(4 pt 2):R838–845.

22. Smith JK, Grisham MB, Ganger DN, et al. Free radical defense mechanisms and neutrophil infiltration in postischemic skeletal muscle. Am J Physiol 1989;256(3 pt 2):H789–793.

23. Kukreja RC, Weaver AB, Hess ML. Stimulated human neutrophils damage cardiac sarcoplasmic reticulum function by generation of oxidants. Biochim Biophys Acta 1989;24;990(2):198–205.

24. Formigli L, Ibba Manneschi L, Tani A, et al. Vitamin E prevents neutrophil accumulation and attenuates tissue damage in ischemic-reperfused human skeletal muscle. Histol Histopathol 1997;12(3):663–669.

25. Ohishi S, Kizaki T, Ookawara T, et al. The effect of exhaustive exercise on the antioxidant enzyme system in skeletal muscle from calcium-deficient rats. Pflugers Arch 1998;435(6):767–774.

26. Jackson MJ. Free radical mechanisms in exercise related muscle damage. In: Reznick AZ, et al. eds. Oxidative Stress in Skeletal Muscle. Basel, Switzerland: Birkhauser Verlag 1998:78–80.

27. Rodriguez FA, Casas H, Casas M, et al. Intermittent hypobaric hypoxia stimulates erythropoiesis and improves aerobic capacity. Med Sci Sports Exerc 1999;31(2):264–268.

28. Meerson FZ. The role of lipid peroxidation in pathogenesis of ischemic damage and the antioxidant protection of the heart. Basic Res Cardiol 1982;77(5):465–485.

29. Deshpande S, et al. Nutritional and health aspects of food antioxidants. In: Food Antioxidants (Madhavi D, Deshpande S, Salunkhe D, Eds.). New York: Marcel Dekker, 1996;361–457.

30. Ji LL. Antioxidants and oxidative stress in exercise. Proc Soc Exp Biol Med 1999;222(3):283–292.

31. Venditti P, Di Meo S. Antioxidants, tissue damage, and endurance in trained and untrained young male rats. Arch Biochem Biophys 1996;331(1):63–68.

32. Dillard CJ. Effects of exercise, vitamin E, and ozone on pulmonary function and lipid peroxidation. J Appl Physiol 1978;45(6):927–932.

33. Meydani SN, Meydani M, Barklund PM, et al. Effect of vitamin E supplementation on immune responsiveness in healthy elderly subjects. Ann NY Acad Sci 1989;570:283–290.

34. Meydani M, Evans WJ, Handelman G, et al. Protective effect of vitamin E on exercise–induced oxidative damage in young and older adults. Am J Physiol 1993;264(5 pt 2):R992–998.

35. Jakemen P, Maxwell S. Effect of antioxidant vitamin supplementation on muscle function after eccentric exercise. Eur J Appl Physiol 1993;67:426–430.

36. Harman D. Aging and oxidative stress. J Int Fed Clin Chem 1998;10(1):24–27.

37. Girten B. Skeletal muscle antioxidant enzyme levels in rats after simulated weightlessness, exercise and dobutamine. Physiologist 1989;32(1 suppl):S59–60.

38. Jenkins RR. Free radical chemistry: relationship to exercise. Sports Med 1988;5:156–170.

39. Kanter MM, Hamlin RL, Unverferth DV, et al. Effect of exercise training on antioxidant enzymes and cardiotoxicity of doxorubicin. J Appl Physiol 1985;59(4):1298–1303.

40. Mena P, Maynar M, Gutierrez JM, et al. Erythrocyte free radical scavenger enzymes in bicycle professional racers: adaptation to training. Int J Sports Med 1991;12(6):563–566.

41. Robertson JD, Maughan RJ, Duthie GG, et al. Increased blood antioxidant systems of runners in response to training load. Clin Sci (Colch) 1991;80(6):611–618.

42. Packer L. Vitamin E, physical exercise, and tissue damage in animals. Med Biol 1984;62:105–109.

43. Karlsson J. Exercise, mixed diets, and nutritherapy. In: Karlsson J, ed. Antioxidants and Exercise. Champaign: Human Kinetics, 1997:108–126.

44. Sen CK, Goldfarb AH. Antioxidants and physical exercise. Sen CK, ed. Handbook of Oxidants and Antioxidants in Exercise. Amsterdam: Elsevier, 2000:297–321.

45. Ciaccio M, Valenza M, Tesoriere L, et al. Vitamin A inhibits doxorubicin-induced membrane lipid peroxidation in rat tissues in vivo. Arch Biochem Biophys 1993;302:103–108.

46. Tesoriere L, Ciaccio M, Valenza M, et al. Effect of vitamin A administration on resistance of rat heart against doxorubin-induced cardiotoxicity and lethality. J Pharmacol Exp Ther 1994;269:430–436.

47. Kartha VN, Krishnamarthy S. Antioxidant function of vitamin A. Int J Vit Nutr Res 1977;47:394–401.

48. Livrea MA, Tesoriere L, Bongiorno A, et al. Contribution of vitamin A to the oxidation resistance of human low density lipoproteins. Free Rad Biol Med 1995;18:401–409.

49. Quiles J, Huertas JR, Manas M, et al. Plasma antioxidants are strongly affected by iron-induced lipid peroxidation in rats subjected to physical exercise and different dietary fats. Biofactors 1998;8(1–2):199–227.

50. Takatsuka N, Kawakami N, Ohwaki A, et al. Frequent hard physical activity lowered serum beta-carotene level in a population study of a rural city of Japan. Tohoku J Exp Med 1995;176(3):131–135.

51. Kanter MM, Nolte LA, Holloszy JD. Effects of an antioxidant vitamin mixture on lipid peroxidation at rest and postexercise. J Appl Physiol 1993;74(2):965–969.

52. Ashton T, Rowlands CC, Jones E, et al. Electron spin resonance spectroscopy, exercise, and oxidative stress: an ascorbic acid intervention study. J Appl Physiol 1998;87(6):2032–2036.

53. Alessio HM, Goldfarb AH, Cao G. Exercise induced oxidative stress before and after vitamin C supplementation. Int J Sports Nutr 1997;7(1):1–9.

54. Vasankari T, Kujala U, Sarna S, et al. Effects of ascorbic acid and carbohydrate ingestion on exercise induced oxidative stress. J Sports Med Phys Fit 1998;38(4):281–285.

55. Kaminski M, Boal R. An effect of ascorbic acid on delayed-onset muscle soreness. Pain 1992;50(3):317–321.

56. Jakeman P, Maxwell S. Effect of antioxidant vitamin supplementation on muscle function after eccentric exercise. Eur J Appl Physiol Occup Physiol 1993;67(5):426–430.

57. Theriault A, et al. Tocotrienol: a review of its therapeutic potential. Clin Biochem 1999;32(5):309–319.

58. Papas AM. Vitamin E: tocopherols and tocotrienols. In: Papas AM, ed. Antioxidant status, diet, nutrition, and health. Boca Raton: CRC Press LLC, 1999:189–210.

59. Watkins TR, et al. Tocotrienols: biological and health effects. In: Papas AM, ed. Antioxidant status, diet, nutrition, and health. Boca Raton: CRC Press LLC, 1999:479–496.

60. Willson R. Free radical protection: why vitamin E, not vitamin C, beta-carotene or glutathione. In: Porter R, Whelan J, eds. Biology of Vitamin E. Ciba Foundation Symposium 101. London: Pitman Books, 1983:19–44.

61. Sharman IM, Down MG, Norgan NG. The effects of vitamin E on physiological function and athletic performance of trained swimmers. J Sports Med 1976;16:215–225.

62. Lawrence JD, Bower RC, Riehl WP, et al. Effects of alpha-tocopherol acetate on the swimming endurance of trained swimmers. Am J Clin Nutr 1975;28:205–208.

63. van der Beek EJ. Vitamin supplementation and physical exercise performance. J Sports Sci 1991;9(spec no):77–90.

64. Takanami Y, Iwane H, Kawai Y, et al. Vitamin E supplementation and endurance exercise: are there benefits? Sports Med 2000;29(2):73–83.

65. Simon-Schnass I, Pabst H. Influence of vitamin E on physical performance. Int J Vit Nutr Res 1988;58:49–54.

66. Grievink L, Jansen SM, van't Veer P, et al. Acute effects of ozone on pulmonary function of cyclists receiving antioxidant supplements. Occup Environ Med 1998;55(1):13–17.

67. Grievink L, Zijlstra AG, Ke X, et al. Double blind intervention trial on modulation of ozone effects on pulmonary function by antioxidant supplements. Am J Epidemiol 1999;15;149(4):306–314.

68. Meydani M, et al. Muscle uptake of vitamin E and its association with muscle fiber type. J Nutr Biochem 1997;8(2):74–78.

69. Jackson MJ, et al. Biology of vitamin E. In: Porter R, et al. eds. Proceedings of a Ciba Foundation Symposium. London: Pittman Medical, 1993:224–239.

70. Cannon JG, Orencole SF, Fielding RA, et al. Acute phase response in exercise: interaction of age and vitamin E on neutrophils and muscle enzyme release. Am J Physiol 1990;259:R1214–R1219.

71. Rokitski L, Logemann E, Huber G, et al. Alpha-tocopherol supplementation in racing cyclists during extreme endurance training. Int J Sport Nutr 1994;4:253–264.

72. Goldfarb AH, McIntosh MK, Boyer BT, et al. Vitamin E effects on indexes of lipid peroxidation in muscle from DHEA treated and exercised rats. J Appl Physiol 1994;76:1630–1635.

73. Meydani M, Evans W. In: Yu B, ed. Free Radicals in Aging. Ann Arbor, M: CRC Press, 1993:184–204.

74. Hartmann A, Niess AM, Grunert-Fuchs M, et al. Vitamin E prevents exercise-induced DNA damage. Mutat Res 1995;346:195–202.

75. Sen CK, Atalay M, Agren J, et al. Fish oil and vitamin E supplementation in oxidative stress at rest and after physical exercise. J Appl Physiol 1997;83:189–195.

76. Novelli G, Adembri C, Gandini E, et al. Vitamin E protects human skeletal muscle from damage from surgical ischemia-reperfusion. Am J Surg 1996;172:206–209.

77. Cannon J, Meydani SN, Fielding RA, et al. Acute phase response in exercise. II. Associations between vitamin E, cytokines, and muscle proteolysis. Am J Physiol 1991;260:R1235–1240.

78. Reznick AZ, Witt E, Matsumoto M, et al. Vitamin E inhibits oxidation in skeletal muscle of resting and exercised rats. Biochem Biophys Res Commun 1992;189:801–806.

79. Tessier F, Margaritis I, Richard MJ, et al. Selenium and training effects on the glutathione system and aerobic performance. Med Sci Sports Exerc 1995;27(3):390–396.

80. Zamora AJ, Tessier F, Marconnet P, et al. Mitochondria changes in human muscle after prolonged exercise, endurance training and selenium supplementation. Eur J Appl Physiol Occup Physiol 1995;71(6):505–511.

81. Brady PS, Brady LJ, Ullrey DE. Selenium, vitamin E and the response to swimming stress in the rat. J Nutr 1979;109(6):1103–1109.

82. Gibbs PN, Gore MG, Jordan PM. Investigation of the effect of metal ions on the reactivity of thiol groups in human 5-aminolaevulinate dehydratase. Biochem J 1985;225(3):573–580.

83. Powell SR. The antioxidant properties of zinc. J Nutr 2000;30(5S suppl):1447S–1454S.

84. Cordova A, Alvarez-Mon M. Behaviour of zinc in physical exercise: a special reference to immunity and fatigue. Neurosci Biobehav Rev 1995;19(3):439–445.

85. Clarkson PM. Minerals: exercise performance and supplementation in athletes. J Sports Sci 1991;9(spec no):91–116.

86. Singh A, Failla ML, Deuster PA. Exercise-induced changes in immune function: effects of zinc supplementation. J Appl Physiol 1994;76(6):2298–2303.

87. Thompson K, et al. Effects of manganese and vitamin E deficiencies on antioxidant enzymes in streptozotocin-diabetic rats. J Nutr Biochem 1993;4:476–481.

88. Davis C, Greger JL. Longitudinal changes of manganese dependent superoxide dismutase and other indexes of manganese and iron status in women. Am J Clin Nutr 1992;55:747–752.

89. Coassin M, Ursini F, Bindoli A, et al. Antioxidant effect of manganese. Arch Biochem Biophys 1992;299:330–333.

90. Sziraki I, Rauhala P, Kok KK, et al. Implications for atypical antioxidative properties of manganese in iron-induced brain lipid peroxidation and copper-dependent low density lipoprotein conjugation. Neurotoxicology 1999;20(2–3):455–466.

91. Patel RP, Darley-Usmar VM. Molecular mechanisms of the copper dependent oxidation of low-density lipoprotein. Free Radic Res 1999;30(1):1–9.

92. Arora AS, Gores GJ. The role of metals in ischemia/reperfusion injury of the liver. Semin Liver Dis 1996;16(1):31–38.

93. Herbert V, Shaw S, Jayatilleke E, et al. Most free-radical injury is iron-related: it is promoted by iron, hemin, holoferritin and vitamin C, and inhibited by desferrioxamine and apoferritin. Stem Cells 1994;p12(3):289–303.

94. Turnlund J, Scott KC, Peiffer GL, et al. Copper status of young men consuming a low copper diet. Am J Clin Nutr 1997;65:72–78.

95. Harris E. Copper as a cofactor and regulator of copper, zinc, superoxide dismutase. J Nutr 1992;123:636–640.

96. Galli C, Marangoni F. Recent advances in the biology of n-6 fatty acids. Nutrition 1997;13(11–12):978–985.

97. D'Aquino M, Benedetti PC, Di Felice M, et al. Effect of fish oil and coconut oil on antioxidant defence system and lipid peroxidation in rat liver. Free Radic Res Commun 1991;12–13(pt 1):147–152.

98. Eritsland J. Safety considerations of polyunsaturated fatty acids. Am J Clin Nutr 2000;71(1 suppl):197S–201S.

99. Laganiere S, Yu BP, Fernandes G. Studies on membrane lipid peroxidation in omega-3 fatty acid-fed autoimmune mice: effect of vitamin E supplementation. Adv Exp Med Biol 1990;262:95–102.

100. Allard JP, Kurian R, Aghdassi E, et al. Lipid peroxidation during n-3 fatty acid and vitamin E supplementation in humans. Lipids 1997;32(5):535–541.

101. Valk EE, Hornstra G. Relationship between vitamin E requirement and polyunsaturated fatty acid intake in man: a review. Int J Vitam Nutr Res 2000;70(2):31–42.

102. Sheppard AJ, et al. Analysis and distribution of vitamin E in vegetable oils and foods. In: Packer L, et al. eds. Vitamin E in Health and Disease. New York: Marcel Dekker, 1993:9–31.

103. Ayre KJ, Hulbert AJ. Dietary fatty acid profile affects endurance in rats. Lipids 1997;32(12):1265–1270.

104. Raastad T, Hostmark AT, Strome SB. Omega-3 fatty acid supplementation does not improve maximal aerobic power, anaerobic threshold and running performance in well-trained soccer players. Scand J Med Sci Sports 1997;7(1):25–31.

105. Aguilaniu B, Flore P, Perrault H, et al. Exercise-induced hypoxemia in master athletes: effects of a polyunsaturated fatty acid diet. Eur J Appl Physiol Occup Physiol 1995;72(1–2):44–50.

106. Mataix J. Tissue specific interactions of exercise, dietary fatty acids, and vitamin E in lipid peroxidation. Free Radic Biol Med 1998; 24(4):511–521.

107. Berry EM, et al. Effects of diets rich in monounsaturated fatty acids on plasma lipoproteins–the Jerusalem Nutrition Study. II. Monounsaturated fatty acids vs carbohydrates. Am J Clin Nutr 1992;56(2):394–403.

108. Berry EM, et al. Effects of diets rich in monounsaturated fatty acids on plasma lipoproteins—the Jerusalem Nutrition Study: high MUFAs vs high PUFAs. Am J Clin Nutr 1991;53(4):899–907.

109. Das UN. Essential fatty acids in health and disease. J Assoc Physicians India 1999 Sep;47(9):906–911.

110. Borlak JT, et al. Health implications of fatty acids. Arzneimittelforschung 1994 Aug;44(8):976–981.

111. Ramirez-Tortosa MC, Suarez A, Gomaz MC, et al. Effect of extra-virgin olive oil and fish-oil supplementation on plasma lipids and susceptibility of low-density lipoprotein to oxidative alteration in free-living spanish male patients with peripheral vascular disease. Clin Nutr 1999;18(3):167–174.

112. Baroni SS, Amelio M, Sangiorgi Z, et al. Solid monounsaturated diet lowers LDL unsaturation trait and oxidisability in hyper-cholesterolemic (type IIb) patients. Free Radic Res 1999;30(4):275–285.

113. Sola R, La Ville, Richard JL, et al. Oleic acid rich diet protects against the oxidative modification of high-density lipoprotein. Free Radic Biol Med 1997;22(6):1037–1045.

114. MacDonald HB. Conjugated linoleic acid and disease prevention: a review of current knowledge. J Am Coll Nutr 2000;19(2 suppl):111S–118S.

115. van den Berg JJ, Cook NE, Tribble DL, et al. Reinvestigation of the antioxidant properties of conjugated linoleic acid. Lipids 1995;30(7):599–605.

116. Lowery L, et al. Conjugated linoleic acid enhances muscle size and strength in novice bodybuilders (abstract). Med Sci Sports Exerc 1998;30(5):S182.

117. Lowery L, et al. Effect of conjugated linoleic acid on physiologic consequences of downhill running. Unpublished doctoral dissertation. Kent State University, 2000.

118. Kagan V, et al. Coenzyme Q: Its role in scavenging and generation of radicals in membranes. In: Cadenas E, et al. ed. Handbook of Antioxidants. New York: Marcel Dekker, 1996:157–202.

119. Lass A, Sohal RS. Effect of coenzyme Q(10) and alpha-tocopherol content of mitochondria on the production of superoxide anion radicals. FASEB J 2000;14(1):87–94.

120. Shimomura Y, Suzuki M, Sagiyama S, et al. Protective effect of coenzyme Q10 on exercise-induced muscular injury. Biochem Biophys Res Commun 1991;15;176(1):349–355.

121. Kamikawa T, Koboyashi A, Yamashita T, et al. Effects of coenzyme Q10 on exercise tolerance in chronic stable angina pectoris. Am J Cardiol 1985;56(4):247–251.

122. Karlsson J, Diamant B, Folkers K, et al. Muscle fibre types, ubiquinone content and exercise capacity in hypertension and effort angina. Ann Med 1991;23(3):339–344.

123. Snider IP, Bazzarre TL, Murdoch SD, et al. Effects of coenzyme athletic performance system as an ergogenic aid on endurance performance to exhaustion. Int J Sports Nutr 1992;2(3):272–286.

124. Zuliani U, Bonetti A, Campana M, et al. The influence of ubiquinone (Co Q10) on the metabolic response to work. J Sports Med Phys Fitness 1989;29(1):57–62.

125. Laaksonen T, Fogelholm M, Himberg JJ, et al. Ubiquinone supplementation and exercise capacity in trained young and older men. Eur J Appl Physiol Occup Physiol 1995;72(1–2):95–100.

126. Malm C, Svesson M, Sjoberg B, et al. Supplementation with ubiquinone-10 causes cellular damage during intense exercise. Acta Physiol Scand 1996;157(4):511–512.

127. Jacob S, Ruus P, Hermann R, et al. Oral administration of RAC-alpha-lipoic acid modulates insulin sensitivity in patients with type-2 diabetes mellitus: a placebo-controlled pilot trial. Free Rad Biol Med 1999;27(3–4):309–314.

128. Khamaisi M, Rudich A, Potashnik R, et al. Lipoic acid acutely induces hypoglycemia in fasting nondiabetic and diabetic rats. Metabolism: Clin Exp 1999;48(4):504–510.

129. Hagen TM, Ingersoll RT, Lykkesfeldt J, et al. (R)–Lipoic acid-supplemented old rats have improved mitochondrial function, decreased oxidative damage, and increased metabolic rate. FASEB J 1999;13:411–418.

130. Khanna S, Atalay M, Laaksonen DE, et al. Alpha-lipoic acid supplementation: tissue glutathione homeostasis at rest and after exercise. J Appl Physiol 1999;864:1191–1196.

131. Marangon K, Deveraj S, Tirosh O, et al. Comparison of the effect of alpha-lipoic acid and alpha-tocopherol supplementation on measures of oxidative stress. Free Radic Biol Med 1999;27(9–10):1114–1121.

132. Luper S. A review of plants used in the treatment of liver disease: part 1. Altern Med Rev 1998;3(6):410–421.

133. Halim AB, el-Ahmady O, Hassab-Allah S, et al. Biochemical effect of antioxidants on lipids and liver function in experimentally-induced liver damage. Ann Clin Biochem 1997;34:656–663.

134. Basaga H, Poli G, Tekkaya C, et al. Free radical scavenging and antioxidative properties of 'silibin' complexes on microsomal lipid peroxidation. Cell Biochem Funct 1997;15:27–33.

135. Bosisio E, Benelli C, Pirola O. Effect of the flavanolignans of Silybum marianum L. on lipid peroxidation in rat liver microsomes and freshly isolated hepatocytes. Pharmacol Res 1992;25:147–154.

136. Campos R, Garrido A, Guerra R, et al. Silybin dihemisuccinate protects against glutathione depletion and lipid peroxidation induced by acetaminophen on rat liver. Planta Med 1989;55:417–419.

137. Cabrera C. Milk thistle: a clinician's report. Medical Herbalism 1996;6:1–5.

138. Packer L, et al. Antioxidant activity and biologic properties of a procyanidin-rich extract from pine (Pinus maritima) bark, pycnogenol. Free Radic Biol Med 1999;27(5–6):704–724.

139. Bors W, Rimbach G, Virgili F. Interaction of flavonoids with ascorbate and determination of univalent redox potential: a pulse radiolysis study. Free Radic Biol Med 1995;19:45–52.

140. Bagchi D, Garg A, Krohn RL, et al. Oxygen free radical scavenging abilities of vitamins C and E, and a grape seed proanthocyanidin extract in vitro. Res Commun Mol Pathol Pharmacol 1997;95(2):179–189.

141. Bagchi D, Garg A, Krohn, RL, et al. Protective effects of grape seed proanthocyanidins and selected antioxidants against TPA-induced hepatic and brain lipid peroxidation and DNA fragmentation, and peritoneal macrophage activation in mice. Gen Pharmacol 1998;30(5):771–776.

142. Sato M, Maulik G, Ray PS, et al. Cardioprotective effects of grape seed proanthocyanidin against ischemic reperfusion injury. J Mol Cell Cardiol 1999;31(6):1289–1297.

143. Serafini M, Ghiselli A, Ferro-Luzzi A. A. In vivo antioxidant effect of green and black tea in man. Eur J Clin Nutr 1996;50:28–32.

144. Vinson JA, Dabbagh YA. Effect of green and black tea supplementation on lipids, lipid oxidation and fibrinogen in the hamster: mechanisms for the epidemiological benefits of tea drinking. FEBS Lett 1998;433(1–2):44–46.

145. Brown MD. Green tea (Camellia sinensis) extract and its possible role in the prevention of cancer. Altern Med Rev 1999;4(5):360–370.

146. Kimori A, Yatsunami J, Okabe S, et al. Anticarcinogenic activity of green tea polyphenols. Jpn J Clin Oncol 1993;23:186–190.

147. Hibatallah J, Carduner C, Poelman MC. In-vivo and in-vitro assessment of the free-radical-scavenger activity of Ginkgo flavone glycosides at high concentration. J Pharm Pharmacol 1999;51(12):1435–1440.

148. Du G, Willet K, Mouithys-Mickaled A, et al. EGb 761 protects liver mitochondria against injury induced by in vitro anoxia/reoxygenation. Free Radic Biol Med 1999;27(5–6):596–604.

149. Sram RJ, et al. Effect of Egb 761 on lipid peroxidation, DNA repair and antioxienzyme activity. In: Ferradini C, et al. eds. Advances in Ginkgo biloba extract research. Paris: Elsevier, 1993:27–38.

150. Clostre F. Ginkgo biloba extract (EGb 761). State of knowledge in the dawn of the year 2000. Ann Pharm Fr 1999;57(suppl)1:1S8–88.

151. Yan LJ, Droy-Lefaix MT, Packer L, et al. Ginkgo biloba extract (EGb 761) protects human low-density lipoproteins against oxidative modification mediated by copper. Biochem Biophys Res Commun 1995;17;212(2):360–366.

152. Maitra I, Marcocci L, Droy-Lefaix MT, et al. Peroxyl radical scavenging activity of Ginkgo biloba extract EGb 761. Biochem Pharmacol 1995;49(11):1649–1655.

153. Asp S, et al. Eccentric exercise decreases maximal insulin action in humans: muscle and systemic effects. J Physiol (Lond) 1996;494 (pt 3):891–898.

154. King DS, Fettmeyer TL, Baldus PJ, et al. Eccentric exercise decreases maximal insulin action in humans: muscle and systemic effects. Effects of eccentric exercise on insulin secretion and action in humans. J Appl Physiol 1993 Nov;75(5):2151–2156.

155. Gibala MJ, MacDougall JD, Tarnopolsky MA, et al. Changes in human skeletal muscle ultrastructure and force production after acute resistance exercise. J Appl Physiol 1995;78(2):702–708.

156. Kuipers H, Keizer HA, Verstappen FT, et al. Influence of a prostaglandin-inhibiting drug on muscle soreness after eccentric work. Int J Sports Med 1995;6(6):336–339.

157. Meydani S, Barklund MP, Liu S, et al. Vitamin E supplementation enhances cell-mediated immunity in healthy elderly subjects. Am J Clin Nutr 1990;52:557–563.

158. Hortobagyi T, Hill JP, Houmard JA, et al. Adaptive responses to muscle lengthening and shortening in humans. J Appl Physiol 1996;80(3):765–772.

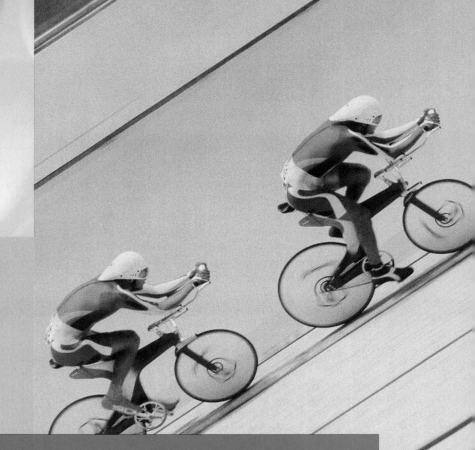

Endurance Performance

Darin Van Gammeren

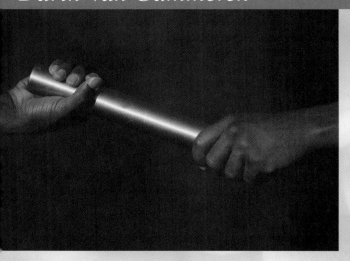

Research Review

Caffeine Increases Running and Cycling Endurance Times

Graham and Spriet examined seven competitive runners (VO_{2max} = 72.6 mL/kg/min) who completed four randomized and double-blind exercise trials at 85% of VO_{2max} (two running and two cycling to exhaustion). The subjects ingested 9 mg/kg body weight of caffeine or a placebo (dextrose) 1 hour before exercise. Endurance times were increased during running with the ingestion of caffeine (71.0 min versus 49.2 min for placebo) and during cycling (59.3 min versus 39.2 min for placebo) (SEE FIGURE). Plasma epinephrine concentrations were also increased with caffeine before running (0.22 to 0.44 nM) and cycling (0.31 to 0.45 nM). Moreover, plasma epinephrine concentrations were increased 15 minutes into exercise with caffeine versus placebo (2.51 and 1.23 nM, respectively, for running; 2.53 and 1.24 nM, respectively, for cycling). The increase in plasma epinephrine concentrations may explain the increase in endurance times

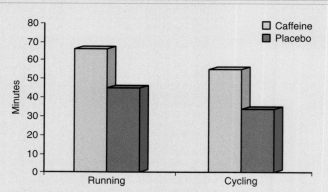

9 mg/kg of caffeine significantly increases running and cycling performance. (Data from Graham TE, Spriet LL. Performance and metabolic responses to a high caffeine dose during prolonged exercise. J Appl Physiol 1991;71:2292–2298.)

with caffeine. Thus, under certain conditions, caffeine can be an effective ergogenic aid.

Graham TE, Spriet LL. Performance and metabolic responses to a high caffeine dose during prolonged exercise. J Appl Physiol 1991;71:2292–2298.

Introduction

Endurance athletes (e.g., marathon runners, triathletes, etc.) are known to use supplements for the purpose of enhancing performance. Of the three energy systems, these athletes' performance depends primarily on oxidative phosphorylation and glycolysis. By increasing the available concentrations of glucose and free fatty acids, some of these so-called endurance supplements may enhance performance. These substances are usually termed nutritional supplements and include carbohydrates and various amino acids. It has been suggested that an average diet may lack certain nutrients that could aid in one's performance.

Other substances such as sodium bicarbonates and phosphates are considered physiological agents.[1] These substances are naturally occurring in the body and aid in exercise performance by changing physiological properties such as blood acidity. Other supplements such as caffeine have been touted as endurance enhancers by stimulating the central nervous system.

This chapter investigates the effect of these and other ergogenic aids on endurance performance. The mechanisms by which each supplement allegedly enhances endurance performance will be investigated. Furthermore, the safety and effectiveness of each supplement will be examined.

Caffeine

Caffeine, a central nervous system stimulant, is one of the most widely used drugs in the world. This substance may improve alertness, concentration, reaction time, and energy levels. In addition, its effect on promoting lipolysis has been touted as a mechanism by which it acts as an endurance ergogenic aid.[1]

Human Studies

One of the first studies conducted on the effects of caffeine and endurance was by Perkins and Williams in 1975.[2] Resting heart rate, submaximal heart rate, maximal heart rate, and ratings of perceived exertion were tested in female subjects before and after a progressive workload to exhaustion on a cycle ergometer. The subjects ingested a placebo, or 4 mg, 7 mg, or 10 mg of caffeine in this double-blind study. There was no significant effect on exercise performance.

Another early study on caffeine was conducted by Costill et al.[3] Nine competitive cyclists exercised until exhaustion on a cycle ergometer at 80% of VO_{2max}. One trial was conducted 1 hour after the ingestion of decaffeinated coffee and the other after the ingestion of coffee containing 330 mg of caffeine. The trial with caffeine resulted in a longer cycling time compared with the trial without caffeine (90.2 versus 75.5 min, respectively). Fat oxidation was significantly higher with the use of caffeine (caffeine = 118 g or 1.31 g/min; placebo = 57 g or 0.75 g/min), and ratings of perceived exertion were significantly lower. The authors concluded that caffeine increased endurance by increasing lipolysis and exerting a positive influence on nerve impulse transmission.

Ivy et al.[4] also conducted a study on caffeine and its effects on endurance in the late 1970s. Nine trained cyclists were used in this study. The subjects ingested 250 mg of caffeine 1 hour before a 2-hour bout of isokinetic cycling at 80 rpm. The subjects also ingested an additional 250 mg of caffeine at 15-minute intervals during the first 90 minutes of exercise. This significantly increased work production and VO_2 by 7.4% and 7.3%, respectively. Fat oxidation was also elevated by 31%; therefore, the increase in work production with the ingestion of caffeine was attributed to an enhanced rate of lipid catabolism.

In a recent study by Cohen et al.,[5] seven competitive road racers (23–51 years of age) performed three, 21-km races in the heat and humidity after randomly ingesting 0, 5, or 9 mg/kg of caffeine. The subjects were allowed to imbibe water at each 5-km interval. They found no improvement in race times for any of the caffeine doses when compared with a placebo.

A study by Wemple et al.[6] also showed no improvements with the use of caffeine. Six subjects performed 3 hours of cycling at 60% VO_{2max}. Also, maximal performance was tested at 85% VO_{2max} following the 3-hour endurance trial. During exercise, the subjects ingested 35 mL of a carbohydrate electrolyte drink with or without 25 mg/dL of caffeine. At rest, the urinary volume was significantly greater during the caffeine trial (1843 mL) versus the placebo (1411 mL), but during exercise there was no difference in urinary volume (398 versus 490 mL for caffeine and placebo, respectively). Conclusively, this study showed no improvement in endurance performance; however, this study also showed that there is not a risk of dehydration with the ingestion of 25 mg/dL of caffeine.

Conversely, most studies conducted on the use of caffeine have shown positive results on endurance performance. Immediately before exercise, six endurance-trained males, who had previously competed in at least two marathons, ingested 10 mg/kg of caffeine or a placebo.[7] The exercise consisted of running on a treadmill at 75% of their VO_{2max} for 45 minutes, and then increasing the speed by two miles per hour until exhaustion. The caffeine trial resulted in a significant increase in the distance run when compared with the placebo (1.9% increase) and control (2.1% increase).

Different dosages of caffeine (0, 5, 9, or 13 mg/kg) were also investigated in nine well-trained cyclists.[8] Encapsulated caffeine was administered 1 hour before the subjects cycled at 80% VO_{2max} until exhaustion. A significant increase in endurance performance was noted during all three trials (endurance time = 58, 59, 58 min for 5, 9,

13 mg/kg, respectively) when compared with the placebo (endurance time = 47 min), but there was not a dose-related response. Also, there was an increase in free fatty acid and glycerol concentrations with the ingestion of caffeine.

In the following study, the effects of caffeine were investigated at different levels of intensity.[9] Eight untrained males cycled until exhaustion at 10% above or below anaerobic threshold after randomly receiving 5 mg/kg of caffeine or a placebo 60 minutes before exercise. There were no differences between trials when the subjects exercised at 10% above anaerobic threshold; however, ratings of perceived exertion were significantly lower (14.1 versus 16.6 for caffeine and placebo, respectively) and time to exhaustion was significantly higher during the caffeine trial (46.54 versus 32.42 min for caffeine and placebo, respectively) at 10% below anaerobic threshold. This may be because the subjects were untrained.

A study was also conducted on the effects of caffeine in coffee or water.[10] Nine fit, young adults performed five trials after ingesting a capsule of caffeine or placebo with water or coffee (decaffeinated coffee, decaffeinated coffee with caffeine added, or regular coffee). The dosage of caffeine was 4.45 mg/kg with 7.15 mL/kg of solution. After 1 hour of rest, the subjects ran at 85% VO_{2max} until exhaustion. Plasma epinephrine was significantly increased with the ingestion of caffeine, and the increase was significantly greater with the capsules when compared with the coffee. Also, endurance performance was only increased during the caffeine capsule trial (7.5- to 10-min increase when compared with the other four trials). The authors speculated that coffee must have a component that moderates the actions of caffeine.

Bell and Jacobs[11] conducted one of the most recent studies done on caffeine. In this field study, nine healthy male recreational runners completed six 3.2-km runs wearing 11 kg of gear (Canadian Forces Warrior Test) after ingesting 325 mg of caffeine and 75 mg of ephedrine. Heart rate was significantly higher in the caffeine and ephedrine trials, and supplementation significantly improved the subjects' time when compared with a control and placebo trial (two caffeine trials = 14.8 and 14.6 min; four placebo trials = 15.4 to 15.5 min; control trial = 15.3 min).

The plethora of data clearly show that there are potential benefits of consuming caffeine before an endurance event. This central nervous system stimulator can increase the release of catecholamines and increase the use of free fatty acids for energy. Dosages as low as 330 mg 1 hour before exercise have been shown to increase an individual's performance time.

Safety and Toxicity

Moderate to high doses of caffeine can result in nervousness, restlessness, insomnia, and tremors. Caffeine is also a diuretic, which might increase the risk of dehydration

Table 13-1 Caffeine Content of Some Common Products

Substance	Caffeine (mg)
28 g (1 oz) baking chocolate	45
57 g (2 oz) chocolate candy	45
237 mL (8 oz) chocolate milk	48
355 mL (12 oz) Mello Yellow	51
355 mL (12 oz) Mountain Dew	54
355 mL (12 oz) cola beverages	32–65
177 mL (6 oz) instant coffee	54–75
177 mL (6 oz) iced tea	70–75
177 mL (6 oz) hot tea (strong)	65–107
Standard dose of some aspirin products	30–128
177 mL (6 oz) automatic perk coffee	125
177 mL (6 oz) automatic drip coffee	181
Standard dose No Doz, Vivarin	100–200
Standard dose Dexatrim, Dietac	200

From Tribole E. Eating on the run. 2nd ed. Champaign, IL: Leisure Press, 1992:442.

and heat-related illness. Caffeine can be addictive and result in severe headaches, fatigue, irritability, and gastrointestinal distress after withdrawal from the substance. In addition, individual differences in caffeine sensitivity may account for the lack of an ergogenic effect.

Also, regarding competitive sports, the International Olympic Committee only permits 12 μg/mL of caffeine in the urine. This is the equivalent of consuming 600 to 800 mg of caffeine within 30 minutes (TABLE 13-1).

Branched-Chain Amino Acids (BCAAs)

Leucine, isoleucine, and valine are essential amino acids and are collectively termed the branched-chain amino acids (BCAAs). BCAAs comprise approximately one-third of muscle protein, and of these three amino acids, leucine has been researched the most extensively. Significant decreases in plasma or serum levels of leucine (11–33%) have been shown to occur after aerobic exercise.[12] Exercise has also been shown to increase the tryptophan/BCAA ratio, which has been touted as support for the central fatigue hypothesis.[13] This hypothesis suggests that an increase in the uptake of tryptophan by the brain will cause an increase in the release of serotonin. This release will ultimately impair endurance performance.

Human Studies

In a study by Blomstrand et al.,[14] BCAAs or a placebo were given to subjects during a 30-km cross-country race or a marathon (42.2 km). The subjects who ran the marathon in 3.05–3.30 hours had a significant improvement in their running time, whereas the faster runners (less than 3.05 hours) showed no improvement in their performance. However, if subjects were grouped together, no significant differences in performance were noted.

Another study by Blomstrand et al.[15] had five male endurance-trained subjects cycle at 75% VO_{2max} until exhaustion. During exercise, the subjects were randomly given a 6% carbohydrate solution with or without 7 g/L of BCAAs or a flavored water solution (placebo). Performance decreased in four out of the five subjects during the flavored water trial when compared with the two carbohydrate periods. However, no differences in performance were seen between the two carbohydrate groups.

In a similar study by van Hall et al.,[16] ten endurance-trained males cycled at 70–75% of their maximum power output and randomly ingested a 6% sucrose solution (control) or a 6% sucrose solution with 3 g/L of tryptophan, 6 g/L of BCAAs, or 18 g/L of BCAAs. Exercise time to exhaustion was not different between the groups.

Moreover, a study by Struder et al.[17] was conducted with ten male subjects. These subjects were required to cycle until exhaustion during four different trials. Subjects ingested a placebo, 20 mg paroxetine, 21 g BCAAs, and 20 g tyrosine separately during the four trials. The results showed that exhaustion was reached earlier during the paroxetine trial, but there were no significant differences among the other trials. When nine well-trained cyclists (VO_{2max} = 63.1 mL/kg/min) ingested glucose, glucose plus BCAA, or a placebo, the results were similar.[18] No differences in performance times were noted in any of the groups after a 100-km cycling test.

Elderly men have also been used as subjects in BCAA studies. Seventeen men, with a mean age of 63 years, were given either BCAA (16, 2, and 2 g of leucine, isoleucine, and valine, respectively) or a placebo.[19] The subjects performed cycling at 75% of their maximum heart rate 1 hour per day, 4 days per week. Maximal oxygen uptake significantly increased by about 5%, but the increase also occurred in the placebo group.

However, when BCAAs were given to subjects in the heat, the results were quite different. Six women and seven men rested in the heat (~34°C) before cycling at 40% of their VO_{2max} until exhaustion. The subjects performed this routine twice while ingesting 5 mL/kg of either a placebo or BCAA drink every 30 minutes. The subjects' times to exhaustion increased significantly during the BCAA trial (~153 versus 137 min).[20]

With a decreased concentration of leucine after aerobic exercise, it would seem probable that the ingestion of supplemental BCAA would increase endurance performance. However, the preponderance of studies shows no effect of BCAA supplementation.

Safety and Toxicity

There are no known toxic side effects of BCAA ingestion.

Carnitine

L-carnitine, a short-chain carboxylic acid, has a potential effect on endurance performance because it is a physiological carrier of activated long-chain fatty acids across the inner mitochondrial membrane. Once inside the mitochondria, the long-chain fatty acids are beta-oxidized and carnitine exports acyl-coenzyme A compounds. The oxidation of fatty acids in the mitochondria is the main fuel source for skeletal muscle. Also, the carnitine shuttle of a muscle controls the efficiency of the use of fatty acids and the activation of branched-chain amino acid oxidation in the muscle.

The ingestion of carnitine has been speculated to enhance fatty acid oxidation and thus spare skeletal muscle glycogen, and this glycogen-sparing effect may aid endurance performance.

Human Studies

Marconi et al.[21] were the first to investigate the use of carnitine supplementation on endurance performance. Six long distance competitive walkers ingested 4 g/day of L-carnitine for 2 weeks. After the 2-week training period, the subjects' VO_{2max} increased 6% (54.5 to 57.8 mL/kg/min). On the other hand, when the subjects walked 120 minutes at 65% of their VO_{2max}, heart rate, pulmonary ventilation, oxygen consumption, and respiratory quotient remained unchanged. The authors concluded that the slight, but significant increase in VO_{2max} was probably due to an activation of substrate flow through the TCA cycle.

In a study by Greig et al.,[22] two groups of untrained individuals were used in a double-blind, crossover designed study. In the first trial, 2 g of L-carnitine were ingested per day for 2 weeks, and in the second trial, the same dose was given for 4 weeks. Maximal and submaximal exercise capacity was assessed with a cycle ergometer at 70 rpm. The results showed no significant increase in VO_{2max} or maximum heart rate.

Gorostiaga et al.[23] conducted a study on ten endurance-trained athletes (VO_{2max} = 62 mL/kg/min). The subjects first performed a control test consisting of 45 minutes of cycling at 66% of VO_{2max} followed by 60 minutes of seated rest. After 28 days of supplementation with 2 g/day of L-carnitine or a placebo (double-blind, crossover design), the subjects performed the same routine. The results showed a lower respiratory quotient in the treatment group, and there were also trends for an improvement in oxygen uptake and heart rate, but no significant improvements in performance were seen.

In a double-blind, crossover design field study, seven male subjects were given 2 g of L-carnitine 2 hours before the start of a marathon and 20 km into the run. The subjects' respiratory exchange ratio (RER) was determined before and after the race, and a submaximal performance test was conducted on a treadmill the morning after the race. Supplementation with L-carnitine showed no significant change in marathon running time or RER. Moreover, there were no changes in the submaximal treadmill test conducted the morning after the run.[24]

One could reasonably conclude at this point that carnitine does not have any consistent effect on endurance performance.

Safety and Toxicity

There are no known toxic side effects of L-carnitine; however, D,L-carnitine is toxic and should not be taken.[25]

Coenzyme Q10

Coenzyme Q10 (CoQ10), sometimes referred to as ubiquinone, is a lipid-soluble coenzyme produced by respiring organisms and some photosynthetic bacteria. CoQ10 aids in the transport of electrons between enzyme complexes of the inner mitochondrial membrane. Through the process of oxidation phosphorylation, CoQ10 also aids in the production of ATP.[26]

Human Studies

The effects of CoQ10 supplementation have been studied using patients with chronic obstructive pulmonary disease (COPD). Eight patients ingested 90 mg/day of CoQ10 for 8 weeks and showed a significant increase in serum CoQ10 levels with a decrease in hypoxemia at rest. Treadmill time tended to increase (12.0–14.0 min) with a significant decrease in heart rate during exercise, whereas lactate production decreased. However, pulmonary function and oxygen consumption during exercise were unaltered.[27]

Studies have also been conducted on elite athletes. Twenty-five Finnish top-level cross-country skiers ingested 90 mg/day of CoQ10 in a double-blind, crossover fashion. Supplementation significantly improved the subjects' VO_{2max} (72.2–75.0 min for group A; 70.3–71.8 min for group B). Also, 94% of the athletes felt their performance and recovery times were improved during the supplementation period versus only 33% during the placebo period.[28]

Conversely, ten male bicycle racers performed graded cycle ergometry before and after supplementation with 100 mg/day of CoQ10 or a placebo for 8 weeks.[29] There was a significant difference in serum CoQ10 levels between groups. Both groups showed improvements in exercise performance, but there were no significant differences between groups.

Snider et al.[30] supplemented 11 highly trained male triathletes with three daily doses of a combination of 100 mg of CoQ10, 500 mg of cytochrome C, 100 mg of inosine, and 200 IU of vitamin E or a placebo for two, 4-week periods. There was a 4-week washout between treatment periods in this double-blind crossover design study. After each treatment period, the subjects ran on a treadmill at 70% VO_{2max} for 90 minutes followed by a period of cycling at 70% VO_{2max} until exhaustion. There were no significant differences between groups for time to exhaustion, blood glucose levels, lactate levels, and free fatty acid concentrations.

Eighteen male road cyclists and triathletes were supplemented with 1 mg/kg/day of CoQ10 or a placebo for 28 days.[31] The subjects were evaluated during and after graded cycling exercise tests. Plasma CoQ10 levels were significantly increased from baseline (0.91–1.97 μg/mL). Nonetheless, CoQ10 had no consistently significant effect on oxygen uptake, anaerobic and respiratory compensation thresholds, blood lactate, glucose and triglyceride kinetics, heart rate, or blood pressure during and following the exercise protocol.

In 1996, Malm et al.[32] conducted research on CoQ10 using 15 healthy males. The results showed that CoQ10 might actually cause cell damage under intense exercise conditions. Malm et al.[33] also conducted a follow-up study on CoQ10. Subjects ingested CoQ10 for 22 days while performing aerobic exercise, except on days 11 through 14, the subjects performed high-intensity anaerobic training. The results showed that during an anaerobic cycling test, the placebo group performed significantly better than the CoQ10 group on day 14 of supplementation (9.7 versus 9.3 W/kg for the placebo and CoQ10 groups, respectively). Furthermore, the CoQ10 group had a significantly lower increase in total work performed. Overall, there were no significant differences between the groups in VO_{2max}, rate of perceived exertion (RPE), respiratory quotient, blood lactate concentration, or heart rate.

CoQ10 may aid in the transportation of electrons within the mitochondria and also aid in the production of ATP. However, it probably does not enhance endurance performance.

Safety and Toxicity

Studies have been conducted on the safety and effectiveness of CoQ10 supplementation in patients who suffer from heart failure. These studies showed an improvement in the patient's health status.[34,35] However, the results from a study using 15 healthy males showed that supplementation with CoQ10 may cause some cell damage in the intramembrane compartment of the mitochondria.[36]

Dimethylglycine (DMG)

N, N, dimethylglycine (DMG) was discovered in 1943 and marketed under the name *pangamic acid* or *vitamin B15*. This substance was touted as a cure for various ailments such as cancer and glaucoma. Since then, it is the belief that supplementation with DMG could increase performance.

Marketers of DMG have made various claims such as an increased use of oxygen and increased mental alertness with the use of DMG. A review of DMG has shown an increase in tissue oxygen uptake and increased exercise performance[37]; however, most of these studies were highly criticized.[38,39]

Animal Studies

In a crossover study by Rose et al.,[40] 1.2 mg/kg of DMG or a placebo paste were orally administered to six thoroughbred horses (body weight = 424–492 kg) twice per day for 5 days. The horses exercised at 40–50% VO_{2max} for 2 minutes followed by 1 minute of exercise at 60, 70, 80, 90, and 100% of VO_{2max}. Values of VO_2, carbon dioxide production, heart rate, arterial blood and plasma lactate concentration, arterial blood gases, and pH were measured during the last 5 seconds of each stage. Also, muscle biopsy specimens were taken from the middle gluteal muscle before and immediately after exercise to determine muscle lactate concentrations. The results showed no significant differences between the groups for any of the parameters measured.

Human Studies

A study by Pipes[41] was conducted using 12 male track athletes (18–21 years of age). The subjects received 5 mg of pangamic acid or a placebo for 1 week. Performance was measured by having the subjects run on a treadmill at a 7.5% grade and 9.0 mph. The speed was increased 1.5 mph every minute until exhaustion. The subjects receiving pangamic acid improved their running times significantly (23.6%) when compared with the placebo group (0.9%). There was also a significant increase in VO_{2max} in the treatment group (27.5%) when compared with the placebo (3.3%). Pangamic acid also significantly improved performance in a study by Kemp[42]; however, neither one of these studies involved subject or investigator blinding.

The effect of pangamic acid on treadmill performance was determined using 16 male track athletes.[43] The athletes ingested six, 50-mg tablets per day of pangamic acid or a placebo for 3 weeks in this double-blind study. Before and after supplementation, the subjects performed a Bruce treadmill protocol to determine maximal heart rate, treadmill time, recovery heart rate (1 and 3 min), blood glucose levels, and lactate levels. The results showed no significant difference between groups for any of the parameters.

Black and Sucec[44] also showed no improvement with the ingestion of DMG. They had 18 physically active men perform an inclined treadmill test after the ingestion of six 50-mg tablets of calcium pangamate (two per meal) or a placebo for 2 weeks. The results showed no significant improvement in VO_{2max} or 15-minute running performance time.

A study by Bishop et al.[45] was conducted using 16 trained runners. The results showed no significant improvement in ventilation, oxygen uptake, heart rate, or total run time when compared with a placebo. These results were similar to a study done by Girandola et al.[46]

DMG has been proposed to increase oxygen use by skeletal muscle. This should lead to an increase in endurance performance. Regardless, DMG has not shown much potential as an endurance enhancement.

Safety and Toxicity

Studies have been conducted on the effects of DMG using rabbit models.[47] When testing for the immunomodulating capacity of DMG, no toxic or adverse side effects occurred. Also, when DMG (300–600 mg/day) was administered to patients with epilepsy to control seizure frequency, no toxicity was noted.[48]

Ginseng

Ginseng is a popular herbal remedy traditionally used by the Chinese. The mechanism of action of this herb is unclear; nonetheless, many studies have been conducted on ginseng's effect on the central nervous system, neuroendocrine function, carbohydrate and lipid metabolism, immune function, and the cardiovascular system. Much of the research is equivocal. One possible reason for this is that the ginsenoside content of the ginseng root can differ due to the method of extraction and even the season in which the root is harvested.[49]

A recent study has shown that treatment with ginseng significantly increased plasma free fatty acid levels and maintained plasma glucose levels during exercise. Also, glycogen levels in the liver and skeletal muscle were slightly higher in the ginseng-supplemented group. This indicates that the use of ginseng may increase endurance performance by altering the body's choice of fuel (i.e., free fatty acids used preferentially over glucose).[50]

Animal Studies

Banerjee and Izquierdo[51] administered Panax ginseng to Swiss albino mice. The ginseng was chronically administered in drinking water for 16–18 days as well as by acute injection 30–60 minutes before the experiments. The ginseng treatment proved to be effective in increasing endurance time and decreasing fatigue time in both the male and female mice (swim time ~350 versus 270 min for males given ginseng and placebo, respectively; swim time ~375 versus 340 min for females given ginseng and placebo, respectively). Other studies conducted on mice have also shown an improvement in endurance performance (swimming time) with ginseng when compared with a control.[52,53] Also, a 4-day treatment of 10 and 20 mg/kg/day of ginseng saponin were given to nontrained rats and

significantly prolonged their aerobic endurance at approximately 70% VO_{2max}.[54]

Two separate studies were later performed by Ferrando et al.[55,56] In both studies, male Winstar rats were given 50 mg/kg of Panax ginseng extract for 12 weeks. After 24 hours of inactivity, the hindlimb muscles were removed. The results showed an increase in the capillary density and mitochondrial content in the red gastrocnemius muscle of the rats given ginseng. The increase in capillary density and oxidative capacity was evidence towards a greater potential in aerobic performance. However, these results were similar in the group of rats that participated in exercise only. The evidence showed a clear physiological response to ginseng. However, there were no synergistic effects of exercise and ginseng together in either study.

Human Studies

Fifty male sports teachers (21–47 years of age) were used as subjects in a double-blind, randomized, crossover study on ginseng.[57] The subjects ingested two capsules per day containing a combination of ginseng extract, dimethylaminoethanol bitartrate, vitamins, minerals, and trace elements or a placebo for 6 weeks. The subjects performed a treadmill test at an increasing workload before and after supplementation. The subjects in the treatment group experienced a significant increase in total workload (before treatment = 12,796 kg*m, after placebo = 13,167 kg*m, after ginseng = 16,265 kg*m) and maximal oxygen consumption (before treatment = 51.54 mL/kg/min, after placebo = 52.23 mL/kg/min, after ginseng = 56.57 mL/kg/min). Also, the ingestion of ginseng resulted in a significant decrease in oxygen consumption, plasma lactate levels, ventilation, carbon dioxide production, and heart rate. These results were greater in the subjects with a lower VO_{2max} (<60 mL/kg/min) than the subjects with a higher VO_{2max} (>60 mL/kg/min).

However, studies conducted on ginseng 5 years later showed different results. In the first study, 36 men participated in a randomized, double-blind, placebo-controlled trial on ginseng.[58] These subjects ingested 200 or 400 mg/day of ginseng for 8 weeks. With 31 subjects completing the study, the results showed no significant changes in oxygen consumption, respiratory exchange ratio, minute ventilation, blood lactic acid concentration, heart rate, or perceived exertion.

Another study done on ginseng also showed no improvement in endurance performance.[59] Twenty young men and eight young women were given 200 mg/day of ginseng for 3 weeks in a double-blind, randomized fashion. Before and after supplementation, subjects performed a graded exercise test on a Schwinn Airdyne cycle ergometer. No significant changes were discovered between groups for VO_2, exercise time, workload, plasma lactate and hematocrit at peak levels, or heart rate and rate of perceived exertion at 150 watts, 200 watts, and peak.

An investigation by Ziemba et al.[60] had the same results as the previous two. Fifteen soccer players (mean age, 19 years) were randomly assigned to receive 350 mg of ginseng per day for 6 weeks or a placebo. Before and after treatment, the subjects performed an incremental bicycle ergometer test with the workload increasing 50 watts every 3 minutes until exhaustion. There were no significant improvements in either group for VO_{2max} or lactate threshold.

Early studies on ginseng with animal models showed some potential with the use of ginseng. Nevertheless, studies using human models have not shown the same potential.

Safety and Toxicity

Long-term administration of ginseng has not shown any toxicity.[61] A study by Scaglione et al.[62] was done to determine the safety and effectiveness of ginseng extract. Two-hundred and twenty-seven subjects ingested 100 mg of ginseng for 12 weeks. Laboratory values for 24 safety parameters showed no significant differences between pre- and post-values. Ginseng is generally considered a safe herbal supplement.

Pyruvate

Pyruvate is the end product of glycolysis. When individuals are supplemented with pyruvate, the Krebs cycle has been speculated to perform more efficiently. This would lead to an increased rate of ATP production, therefore improving endurance performance. Also, studies performed on rats have shown that supplementation with pyruvate lowers the animals' respiratory exchange ratio.[63] This would also lead to an increase in performance. Many studies have been done on pyruvate supplementation and weight loss, but few have been performed on pyruvate's effect on endurance performance.

Human Studies

The effect of pyruvate on endurance was studied by Stanko et al.[64] Ten physically active males substituted 25 g of pyruvate and 75 g of dihydroxyacetone for the same amount of carbohydrate in a standard diet (55% carbohydrate, 15% protein, 30% fat; 35 kcal/kg) for 7 days. An isocaloric glucose polymer solution was used as a placebo. After supplementation, the subjects performed arm ergometry at 60% VO_{2max} until exhaustion. Glycogen levels at rest were significantly higher during the pyruvate trial. Whole arm arteriovenous glucose difference was greater at rest and after 60 minutes of exercise, but did not differ at exhaustion for the supplemented trial

versus the placebo. Therefore, glucose extraction was presumed to account for the significant increase in arm endurance during the pyruvate trial versus the placebo (160 versus 133 min, respectively).

In a similar study, the effects of pyruvate leg endurance were evaluated by Stanko et al.[65] Eight untrained subjects consumed a high-carbohydrate diet (70% carbohydrate, 18% protein, 12% fat; 35 kcal/kg) for 7 days with 100 g of polycose (placebo) or dihydroxyacetone (75 g) and pyruvate (25 g) substituted for a portion of carbohydrate. After the diet, cycle ergometer was performed at 70% VO_{2max} until exhaustion. Muscle glycogen at rest and exhaustion did not differ between trials. Whole leg arteriovenous glucose difference was greater during the pyruvate trial when compared with the placebo at rest and after 30 minutes of exercise, but not at exhaustion. Estimated total glucose oxidation during exercise was significantly greater in the pyruvate group when compared with the placebo. This led to a significant increase in leg endurance for the pyruvate trial when compared with the placebo (79 versus 66 min, respectively).

Conversely, the most recent study on pyruvate was conducted by Morrison et al.[66] Nine recreationally active subjects (8 women and 1 man) ingested 7, 15, or 25 g of pyruvate and were monitored for the next 4 hours. The pyruvate showed no elevation in blood pyruvate, and had no effect on indexes of carbohydrate (blood glucose and lactate) or lipid metabolism (blood glycerol and plasma free fatty acids). Also, in a randomized, double-blind, crossover fashion, 7 g of pyruvate or a placebo were ingested for 1 week by seven, well-trained male cyclists (VO_{2max} = 62.32 mL/kg/min). When the subjects cycled at 74–80% of their VO_{2max}, there were no significant differences in performance between the trials (placebo = 91 min; pyruvate = 88 min) (FIG. 13-1).

An increased production of ATP would be expected after supplementation of pyruvate since endogenous pyruvate leads to the production of ATP. Early, high-dose studies showed positive results; however, the most recent study using 7 g showed no improvement in endurance time. More studies on pyruvate supplementation and endurance performance are warranted.

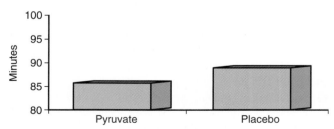

Figure 13-1. Pyruvate does not improve cycling performance. (*Data from* Morrison MA, Spriet LL, Dyck DJ. Pyruvate ingestion for 7 days does not improve aerobic performance in well-trained individuals. J Appl Physiol 2000;89:549–556.)

Current Controversy: Pyruvate—High Doses Needed?

Pyruvate has been touted as a weight loss aid and an endurance enhancer. Its use as a weight-loss supplement has been researched, but its effectiveness as an endurance performance aid has been sparsely investigated. Earlier studies were conducted on pyruvate supplementation in combination with dihydroxyacetone. When subjects were given 25 g of pyruvate and 75 g of dihydroxyacetone, arm and leg endurance performance increased. Conversely, Morrison et al. conducted a two-part study on pyruvate supplementation. When subjects ingested 7, 15, or 25 g of pyruvate, there were no increases in blood pyruvate, lactate, glucose, glycerol, or plasma free fatty acids. In the second part of the study, 7 g of pyruvate (for 7 days) were ingested in this randomized, double-blind, placebo-controlled study. The results showed no significant increase in endurance performance.

At this point, it is not clear if pyruvate can consistently affect muscular endurance. Also, the feasibility of an individual ingesting 25 g of pyruvate is questionable. When 25 g of pyruvate are encapsulated, it would require a large number of capsules to obtain this quantity. Furthermore, the bitterness (and bad taste) of pyruvate would preclude its use in a powder form.

Morrison MA, Spriet LL, Dyck DJ. Pyruvate ingestion for 7 days does not improve aerobic performance in well-trained individuals. J Appl Physiol 2000;89:549–556.

Stanko RT, Robertson RJ, Galbreath RW, et al. Enhanced leg exercise endurance with a high carbohydrate diet and dihydroxyacetone and pyruvate. J Appl Physiol 1990;69:1651–1656.

Stanko RT, Robertson RJ, Spina RJ, et al. Enhancement of arm exercise endurance capacity with dihydroxyacetone and pyruvate. J Appl Physiol 1990;68:119–124.

Safety and Toxicity

Supplementation with pyruvate has been shown to have minimal side effects; however, borborygmus (bowel rumbling), flatus, and diarrhea were reported by Stanko et al.[67–69] Nonetheless, these side effects were mild and usually did not affect performance. Also, in the same studies, vital functions, blood count, and biochemical profiles were not affected.

Polylactate

Polylactate is semisoluble amino acid/lactate salt and has been developed as a carbohydrate supplement for increasing endurance performance. It has been proposed that polylactate will increase pH and bicarbonate levels, therefore increasing the body's ability to buffer lactate in the blood. This could delay the onset of fatigue during exercise.

Human Studies

Five trained, fasted male cyclists performed at 50% of VO_{2max} for 180 minutes on a cycle ergometer three times.[70] The subjects consumed a solution containing polylactate (80% polylactate and 20% sodium lactate in 7% solution

with water), glucose polymer (maltodextrin in 7% solution with water), or a control (water sweetened with aspartame) 5 minutes before exercise and at 20-minute intervals during exercise. Polylactate and the glucose polymer produced similar results, except that the polylactate increased pH and bicarbonate levels. There were no differences between treatments in perceived exertion, sodium, potassium, chloride, lactate, heart rate, oxygen consumption, or temperature. The authors stated that polylactate may help maintain blood glucose and enhance blood buffering capacity during endurance exercise.

A few years later, Swensen et al.[71] conducted a randomized, double-blind study on polylactate using five subjects. The subjects consumed a glucose polymer solution alone or with polylactate at a rate of 0.3 g of carbohydrate per kg of body weight in a 7% solution every 20 minutes until exhaustion. The glucose polymer/polylactate solution was mixed at a ratio of 6.25 g of glucose polymer to 0.75 g of polylactate per 100 mL of water. The subjects exercised to exhaustion at 70% VO_{2max} before and after supplementation. VO_2, respiratory exchange ratio, heart rate, and perceived exertion were measured at 20-minute intervals. Serum glucose, insulin, free fatty acids, glycerol, whole blood lactate, and pH were measured at 30-minute intervals. The results showed no significant physiological or performance effects with the addition of polylactate.

Safety and Toxicity

Few studies have been done on the use of polylactate supplementation and even fewer on the issue of safety. In a study by Swenson et al.,[72] when subjects ingested polylactate at concentrations greater than 2.5%, they experienced severe gastrointestinal efflux. Polylactate ingestion was only tolerable in concentrations less than 0.75%.

Phosphates

Numerous mechanisms have been proposed by which phosphates increase endurance performance. Phosphates may increase extra- and intracellular levels of phosphate, thereby increasing the amount of phosphate available for oxidative phosphorylation and phosphocreatine synthesis. Phosphates are also thought to increase the production of 2,3-diphosphoglycerate (2,3-DPG) in red blood cells (RBCs). 2,3-DPG aids the release of oxygen from hemoglobin on RBCs. The increase in 2,3-DPG concentrations shifts the oxygen-hemoglobin curve to the right, allowing for more oxygen to be delivered to skeletal muscles.[73]

The final proposed mechanism of action for phosphates is the notion that phosphates are buffers, which supposedly decreases the accumulation of hydrogen ions that can inhibit glycolysis. This may ultimately lead to a decrease in energy production. This may also decrease force production by impairing the cross-bridge formation between myofilaments.

Human Studies

Duffy and Conlee[74] had 11 male subjects ingest 1.24 g of sodium acid phosphate and potassium phosphate 1 hour before exercise (acute) and 3.73 g/day of the phosphate combination for 6 days before exercise (chronic). Treadmill endurance time, after 15 minutes of recovery from the first exercise, and oxygen uptake during the treadmill exercise, were measured. Running times ranged from 172–183 seconds during the first run and 145–152 seconds during the second run. Oxygen uptake averaged 52 mL/kg/min during all conditions. The results showed no significant effect of acute or chronic ingestion of a combination of phosphates.

Bredle et al.[75] conducted a double-blind, crossover experiment with 11 male runners. The subjects ingested 176 mmol/day of calcium phosphate or a placebo for 4 days. On day 3, subjects performed an incremental VO_{2max} test on a treadmill, and on day 4, subjects ran on the treadmill at 70% VO_{2max} until exhaustion. On day 4, plasma phosphate levels were significantly higher than in controls, but erythrocyte phosphate, 2,3-DPG, and oxygen half-saturation pressure of hemoglobin were unchanged. Also, neither VO_{2max} nor submaximal run time to exhaustion was changed by the treatment.

Treatment with phosphate increased the arteriovenous oxygen difference. The authors concluded that phosphates improve some cardiovascular functions, but do not have an effect on aerobic power.

Thirty endurance-trained males (age = 23–26 years; maximum oxygen uptake = 65 mL/kg/min) were studied for 364 days.[76] Ten control subjects exercised 14.4 km/day at 10,000 steps/day. The other 20 subjects exercised less than 2.9 km/day (3000 walking steps/day) with half of them consuming phosphate, fluid, and salt. The results showed that hyperhydration and phosphate supplementation could minimize phosphate loss in endurance-trained subjects during periods of low exercise routines.

Conversely, when ten well-trained distance runners were given a phosphate load or a placebo for 3 days, the results were different.[77] Pre- and post-measures included plasma phosphate concentration, RBC 2,3-DPG, hematocrit and hemoglobin concentrations, VO_{2max}, and degree of lactic acidemia. Blood samples for the control condition were drawn before and after a warm-up, after treadmill exercise at a 10% grade, and after the completion of the VO_{2max} determination. Serum phosphate and RBC 2,3-DPG levels were significantly increased after the ingestion of phosphate. Also, VO_{2max} was significantly increased and correlated with the rise in RBC 2,3-DPG (r = 0.81).

Next, eight trained cyclists participated in three cycle ergometer tests after consuming phosphate, placebo, or no supplement.[78] VO_{2max}, time to exhaustion, serum 2,3-DPG, and serum phosphate levels were measured before and after treatment. Serum phosphate levels did not change in any group, but there were increases in 2,3-DPG during phosphate supplementation. There was also a significant difference in VO_{2max} (control = 48.54 mL/kg/min, placebo = 47.83 mL/kg/min, phosphate = 53.36 mL/kg/min) and time to exhaustion (control = 9.86 min, placebo = 10.6 min, phosphate = 12.29 min).

Moreover, Krieder et al.[79] had seven male competitive runners (VO_{2max}, 73.9 mL/kg/min) participate in a two-session, placebo-controlled, double-blind study on phosphate loading. Oxygen uptake, ventilatory anaerobic threshold, and 5-mile performance were randomly tested on day 3 or day 6 after supplementation with tribasic sodium phosphate four times per day for 6 days. Phosphate loading significantly increased resting and post-exercise serum phosphate concentrations and also significantly increased maximum oxygen uptake (4.77–5.18 L/min) and ventilatory anaerobic threshold (3.74–4.18 L/min). Five-mile run times were different between sessions, but not significantly; however, mean performance run oxygen uptake was significantly lower (3.87–3.80 L/min) with the ingestion of phosphate.

Two years later, Kreider et al.[80] had six male cyclists and triathletes consume 1 g of tribasic sodium phosphate or a glucose placebo four times per day for 3 days before exercise. The exercise consisted of an incremental maximal cycling test or a simulated 40-km time trial on a computerized race simulator. The subjects continued supplementation for 1 extra day, and performed the same exercise again. Metabolic data were collected during 15-second intervals and venous blood samples were collected during each stage of the cycling test and every 8 km during the run. The results showed that the phosphates increased anaerobic threshold, myocardial ejection fraction and fractional shortening, VO_{2max} (69.3 versus 75.4 mL/kg/min for placebo and phosphate groups, respectively).

A fair amount of data have been collected on the use of phosphates as an endurance enhancer. With proposed mechanisms such as increasing oxidative phosphorylation, phosphocreatine synthesis, 2,3-DPG production, and also decreasing blood pH, it would seem plausible that phosphates would increase endurance performance. Currently, the data are mixed, with some studies showing an improvement in endurance performance and others showing no improvement. Phosphates do seem to have some potential as an ergogenic aid, but more studies are needed to prove this.

Safety and Toxicity

There are no known toxic side effects of phosphate ingestion; however, there is currently an insufficient amount of data on phosphate loading. More studies are needed on the toxic effects of phosphate loading.

Sodium Bicarbonate (NaHCO₃)

Bicarbonates are an important factor in the body's buffering system, which allows the maintenance of the fluid's acid-base balance. Sodium bicarbonate ($NaHCO_3$), usually in the form of baking soda, can increase blood pH, therefore making blood less acidic. In theory, this would allow a greater concentration of lactate in the blood, thus increasing time to fatigue.

Human Studies

Eight lean men exercised to exhaustion at 80% VO_{2max} on a cycle ergometer.[81] This exercise was performed with the infusion of 1.5 L of a 1.3% mixture of $NaHCO_3$, a 0.9% mixture of sodium chloride (NaCl), or with no infusion. Arterialized venous blood and breath-by-breath analysis of expired gases were collected. The hydrogen ion concentration (H+) (46.5 nmol/L) and HCO_3 (19.9 nmol/L) were similar in the control and NaCl group, but remained unchanged in the $NaHCO_3$ group (38.4 and 24.8 nmol/L, respectively). At exhaustion, VO_2, VCO_2, respiratory exchange ratio, heart rate, systolic blood pressure, free fatty acids, glycerol, insulin, norepinephrine, and epinephrine

were not different between any of the trials. Time to exhaustion was significantly longer in the $NaHCO_3$ (30.9 min) and NaCl (31.8 min) groups when compared with the control (19.0 min). Plasma glucose levels were higher in the control condition when compared with the other two conditions at exhaustion, and lactate was higher in the $NaHCO_3$ trial than in the other two conditions. Therefore, $NaHCO_3$ increased endurance performance, but the increase could not be explained by $NaHCO_3$'s effects on the acid-base balance of blood or any other metabolic changes.

McNaughton et al.[82] had 10 well-trained male cyclists (mean VO_{2max} = 67.3 mL/kg/min) randomly perform a 1-hour maximum cycle ergometer test after the ingestion of 300 mg/kg of $NaHCO_3$, a placebo, or no supplement. Blood samples were taken at 10-minute intervals during exercise and at 1, 3, 5, and 10 minutes post-exercise. Blood was sampled for lactate, partial pressure of carbon dioxide and oxygen, pH, and plasma HCO_3 concentrations. The $NaHCO_3$ did increase blood HCO_3 concentrations before exercise, and also allowed the subjects to perform significantly more work (950.9 kJ) when compared with the placebo (839.0 kJ) and control groups (835.5 kJ) (FIG. 13-2).

On the other hand, in a study by Housh et al.,[83] 18 men (mean age = 23 years) randomly ingested 0.3 g/kg of ammonium chloride or sodium bicarbonate over a 3-hour period. In the first experiment, the subjects performed a discontinuous incremental cycle ergometer test until the onset of fatigue after the ingestion of the supplement. In the second experiment, the subjects performed a continuous exercise until the onset of fatigue. Neither experiment showed an increase in time until fatigue.

Moreover, six endurance athletes performed two successive cycle ergometer tests after the ingestion of a normal diet, or a fatty meal either with or without $NaHCO_3$.[84] Relationships between ventilation, plasma potassium concentration, and plasma pH were examined. The plasma free fatty acid concentration was significantly increased in both of the fatty meal trials. During the $NaHCO_3$

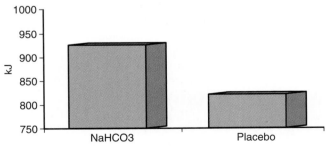

Figure 13-2. Sodium bicarbonate increases total work performed on a cycle ergometer. (*Data from* McNaughton L, Dalton B, Palmer G. Sodium bicarbonate can be used as an ergogenic aid in high-intensity, competitive cycle ergometry of 1 h duration. Eur J Appl Physiol 1999;80:64–69.)

trial, plasma pH was significantly higher compared with the other two trials. Nonetheless, ventilation and plasma potassium concentrations were the same during all trials. The authors concluded that changes in ventilation and plasma potassium ion concentrations are not affected by plasma free fatty acids or plasma pH and the changes were independent of changes in plasma pH or plasma HCO_3 concentrations.

A similar result was found in a study by Potteiger et al.[85] Seven male runners (mean $VO_{2max} = 61.7$ mL/kg/min) performed three, 30-minute treadmill runs at lactate threshold followed by a run to exhaustion at 110% of lactate threshold. The exercise was performed after randomly ingesting 0.3 g/kg of $NaHCO_3$, 0.5 g/kg of sodium citrate, or a placebo. Concentrations of lactate, bicarbonate, and levels of pH were obtained via venous blood samples at 5, 15, and 25 minutes during the run and immediately after. When compared with the placebo, pH levels were significantly higher during exercise in both treatment trials, but not post-exercise. During exercise the lactate concentrations were significantly higher in the sodium citrate trial when compared with the placebo, and the concentrations were higher for both treatment periods post-exercise. Blood HCO_3 concentrations were significantly higher during the $NaHCO_3$; however, exercise time to exhaustion was not significantly different between the groups. The authors commented that even though the $NaHCO_3$ produced a more favorable metabolic condition for exercise, the performance times still did not change.

$NaHCO_3$ is probably one of the older supplements used to enhance performance. As another blood buffer, it would seem feasible that the ingestion of $NaHCO_3$ would increase performance. Nevertheless, most of the data show that $NaHCO_3$ supplementation does not improve endurance performance.

Safety and Toxicity

High doses of $NaHCO_3$ have been known to cause gastrointestinal discomfort, including diarrhea, cramps, and bloating. This may be prevented by ingesting extra amounts of water and dividing the dosage of at least 300 mg/kg into five equal parts within a 1- to 2-hour time period.[86] Studies have also shown that sodium citrate may have the same buffering capacity without the gastrointestinal problems.[87,88]

Medium-Chain Triglycerides (MCTs)

MCTs are a family of triglycerides containing mostly caprylic (8 carbon) and capric (10 carbon) fatty acids with lower amounts of caproic (6 carbon) and lauric (12 carbon) fatty acids. Studies have shown that increasing free fatty acids during exercise may spare muscle glycogen due to the increased use of free fatty acids for fuel. MCTs are easily hydrolyzed by lipase in the stomach and in the intestines. Once MCTs are broken down into medium-chain fatty acids (MCFAs), they can be transported directly to the liver. These MCFAs are oxidized as quickly as glucose because they can easily cross the double membrane of the hepatocyte and enter the mitochondria for beta-oxidation. This may provide an alternative carbon source for skeletal muscles during endurance exercise.[89,90]

Human Studies

Nine subjects participated in a study by Satabin et al.[91] These subjects cycled on an ergometer at 60% VO_{2max} until exhaustion four separate times, 2 hours after ingesting 400 kcal of glucose, MCTs, long-chain triglycerides (LCTs), or after a night of fasting. Oxidation of the nutrients was 80% for glucose, 45% for MCTs, and 9% for LCTs. The average work time was the same for all trials (116 ± 11 min). The MCT trial also resulted in an increase in ketones.

Jeukendrup et al.[92] had nine trained athletes cycle four separate times for 180 minutes at 57% VO_{2max}. Subjects consumed 4 mL/kg at the start and 2 mL/kg every 20 minutes during exercise of 150 g/L carbohydrate solution, an equicaloric, 70% energy from carbohydrates, 30% from MCT suspension containing 29 g of MCTs, or 150 g/L of carbohydrate solution plus 20 g of MCTs. The fourth trial was a control. Muscle biopsy specimens were taken from the quadriceps muscle to determine glycogen levels. Breath samples were taken during exercise to determine exogenous and endogenous carbohydrate oxidation. The results showed no significant differences between trials in glycogen breakdown or respiratory exchange ratio during exercise. There were no differences between trials for exogenous or endogenous carbohydrate oxidation. Plasma ketones were the only parameter significantly elevated during the MCT trial.

Jeukendrup et al.[93] conducted a second study on MCTs a couple of years later. Seven well-trained cyclists exercised during four separate trials, for 2 hours, at 60% VO_{2max}, followed by a simulated time trial of approximately 15 minutes. Subjects ingested either a) 10% carbohydrate solution (170 ± 6 g of glucose), b) 10% carbohydrate electrolyte solution with 5% MCTs (85 g of MCT), c) a 5% MCT solution, or d) colored and flavored water (placebo). The ingestion of carbohydrates and carbohydrates plus MCTs did not have any effect on performance when compared with the placebo, whereas the MCTs actually decreased performance (time to complete preset amount of work was 14.18 min, 14.02 min, 17.33 min, and 14.43 min for the carb, carb plus MCT, MCT, and placebo groups, respectively). MCTs did not affect fat or carbohydrate oxidation, or exogenous and endogenous carbohydrate use.

Similar results were seen in a study by Angus et al.[94] Investigators had eight endurance-trained men (VO_{2max} = 4.71 L/min) complete 35 kJ/kg of work as quickly as possible while ingesting 250 mL every 15 minutes of a 6% carbohydrate solution, a 6% carbohydrate plus 4.2% MCT solution, or a sweet placebo. Time to complete the work also decreased during both treatment periods when compared to the placebo (carbohydrate only = 166 min, carbohydrate plus MCT = 169 min, placebo = 178 min).

A study by Horowitz et al.[95] had seven well-trained men cycle for 30 minutes at 84% VO_{2max}. One hour before exercise, the subjects consumed carbohydrate (0.72 g of sucrose/kg) or carbohydrate plus MCT (0.72 g of sucrose/kg plus 0.36 g of tricaprin/kg). Muscle biopsies were extracted from the vastus lateralis muscle of the quadriceps before and after exercise to detect changes in glycogen. The change in muscle glycogen and glycogen oxidation was not different between groups. Carbohydrate plus MCT did increase rate of glucose disappearance from plasma at rest, but not during exercise.

Moreover, 2 hours postprandial (after lunch), nine endurance-trained cyclists performed cycle ergometry for 2 hours at 63% of VO_{2max}, and then performed a simulated 40-km time trial.[96] The subjects ingested either a) 10% glucose, b) 10% glucose plus 1.72% MCT, or c) 10% glucose plus 3.44% MCT solutions. The subjects consumed 400 mL at the start and 100 mL every 10 minutes during exercise. MCT ingestion raised serum free fatty acid and beta-hydroxybutyrate concentrations; however, this did not affect fuel oxidation for endurance performance.

On the other hand, Van Zyl et al.[97] had six endurance-trained cyclists ride for 2 hours at 60% VO_{2max} and then performed a simulated 40-km time trial. During exercise, the subjects ingested 2 L of 10% glucose, 4.3% MCT, or 10% glucose plus 4.3% MCT. Replacing the glucose with MCT significantly decreased performance (i.e., took longer to complete the 40 km; 66.8–72.1 min), but adding the MCT to the glucose significantly improved the time trial (66.8–65.1 min). The glucose plus MCT trial had an increased final circulating concentration of free fatty acids and ketones with a decreased final circulating concentration of glucose and lactate. Adding MCT to glucose also reduced the total carbohydrate oxidation rate.

MCTs are easily hydrolyzed and converted into glucose, thereby sparing muscle glycogen. However, the preponderance of the data reviewed showed either no change or a decrease in performance with MCT supplementation.

Safety and Toxicity

A study has been conducted on MCTs and their toxic effects on the central nervous system in dogs.[98] Dogs

received three different infusion doses of MCTs. During the highest infusion rate, the results showed an increase in ketone body concentrations and production. Also, at the highest infusion rate, there was an increase in plasma lactate (1.3–4.3 mmol/L). The authors concluded that there is significant dose-related central nervous system toxicity in dogs. This study is consistent with human studies also showing an increase in ketone bodies with the ingestion of MCTs.[99–101]

Another side effect that has been reported is gastrointestinal problems such as cramping. When subjects in the study by Jeukendrup et al.[102] ingested 85 g of MCT, the subjects reported gastrointestinal distress, which may have led to a decrease in performance. A look into the use of structured triglycerides (which contain both MCTs and LCTs) as a performance enhancer may be warranted because they seem to be safe and well tolerated.

Glycerol

Glycerol is released from the breakdown of triglycerides. In a study by Ohkuwa et al.[103] blood glycerol levels were measured in trained long distance runners. The results showed that the concentrations of glycerol in the blood might be a reflection of the subjects' performance. Therefore, it would seem probable that the ingestion of glycerol may increase performance. One way in which this may occur is by creating a state of hyperhydration. The increased levels of hydration should lead to an increase in athletic performance. The mechanism by which this will occur may be due to the reduced volume of urine excreted after the ingestion of glycerol. Another way in which glycerol ingestion may improve performance is by reducing the use of muscle and liver glycogen stores. These hypotheses have been tested in animals and humans, but not extensively.

Animal Studies

Schott et al.[104] conducted a study on the effects of electrolytes and glycerol supplementation on recovery from endurance exercise. In this study, six Arabian horses completed a 60-km treadmill test after 12, 24, 48, and 72 hours of recovery. The horses were given a) 2.4 mL/kg of water (W), b) 0.2 g/kg of potassium chloride and 0.4 g/kg of sodium chloride in 2.4 mL/kg of water (E), or c) 0.2 g/kg of potassium chloride and 0.4 g/kg of sodium chloride in 2.4 mL/kg of glycerol (GE). The W group had a greater amount of water loss after exercise (3.2%) compared with the E (1.0%) and GE groups (0.9%). However, by 24 hours, the E and GE groups continued to lose water (2.2 and 2.1%, respectively) while the W group remained unchanged from post-exercise. The authors concluded that glycerol had no physiological benefit and actually increased urine electrolyte loss when compared to the electrolytes alone.

Also, in a study by Dusterdieck et al.,[105] the exact same supplementation and exercise protocol was used. These results also showed no improvements in the amount of water imbibed by the horses in the GE group when compared with the E group.

Human Studies

Six men exercised until exhaustion on a cycle ergometer at 73% of VO_{2max} after ingesting glycerol, glucose, or a placebo.[106] Exercise time until exhaustion was longer for the glucose trial compared to the glycerol trial (108.8 versus 86.0 min). There were no differences between the glycerol and placebo trials. The ingestion of 1 g/kg of glycerol 45 minutes before exercise increased blood glycerol concentrations by 340-fold immediately before exercise, but did not have an effect on blood glucose or plasma insulin levels. On the other hand, blood glucose levels were up to 14% higher in the later stages of exercise and post-exercise during the glycerol trial when compared with the glucose and placebo trials. Nonetheless, these rises in blood glucose did not transfer to an improvement in performance; in fact, the glycerol trial actually had a significantly lower time to exhaustion when compared with the glucose group (FIG. 13-3).

Likewise, Inder et al.[107] conducted a study on 1 g/kg of glycerol using eight male triathletes (19–23 years of age). The athletes completed an exercise protocol three times, which involved 60 minutes of exercise at 70% VO_{2max} followed by an incremental increase in workload every 2 minutes until exhaustion. The results showed that glycerol does not enhance athletic performance or produce hyperhydration.

The concentrations of glycerol in the blood were thought to be a reflection of an individual's performance. Therefore, the ingestion of exogenous glycerol should increase endurance performance. The data, however, clearly show no improvement in performance.

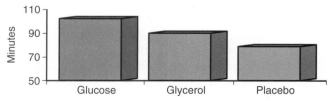

Figure 13-3. Glucose improves cycling endurance performance while glycerol does not. (*Data from* Gleeson M, Maughan RJ, Greenhaff PL. Comparison of the effects of pre-exercise feeding of glucose, glycerol and placebo on endurance and fuel homeostasis in man. Eur J Appl Physiol 1986;55:645–653.)

Safety and Toxicity

No adverse side effects have been noted with the supplementation of glycerol; however, studies have not been extensively done on the use of this supplement.

Carbohydrates

Carbohydrates are the primary macronutrient ingested in most athletes' diets. When carbohydrates are ingested, they are broken down into glucose and enter the bloodstream. The body uses blood glucose and stored muscle glycogen for energy during exercise. As the duration of exercise increases, more blood glucose and less muscle glycogen is used for energy. This is why it may be important to ingest carbohydrates before and/or during exercise. As the carbohydrates are broken down into glucose, the body can use them for energy. The body's use of blood glucose depends on the type, intensity, and duration of exercise. Numerous studies have been conducted on the use of carbohydrate supplementation with different types of carbohydrates, different timing of the ingestion of carbohydrates, and different duration of the exercise performed.

Human Studies

Langenfeld et al.[108] had 14 trained cyclists ride at their own pace for 80 miles on two separate occasions during a simulated time trial. The trials were preceded by a prescribed diet with a final feeding 3 to 4 hours before exercise. After every 10 miles, subjects ingested either a noncaloric placebo or a carbohydrate maltodextrin supplement (5% maltodextrin and 2% fructose). Glucose levels were significantly higher after 40 miles and free fatty acid levels were significantly lower after the completion of the race with the carbohydrate supplementation. Carbohydrate oxidation was significantly higher with carbohydrate supplementation and these riders could sustain a higher average intensity with significantly faster times (241.0 versus 253.2 min for placebo and carbohydrate groups, respectively).

Next, seven well-trained male cyclists exercised at either 45% or 75% VO_{2max} while receiving a placebo, 10% liquid carbohydrate supplement (3×18 g/h), or a solid carbohydrate supplement (2×25 g/h).[109] The subjects performed this exercise for 124 minutes and then a second set for 190 minutes followed by a ride to exhaustion at 80% VO_{2max}. Plasma glucose and insulin responses were significantly greater in the liquid carbohydrate trial when compared with the placebo. The time to exhaustion for the liquid (233.4 min) and solid carbohydrate (223.9 min) trials did not differ, but both were significantly greater than the placebo (202.4 min).

A study of carbohydrate use in U.S. National Field Hockey Team members also showed positive results.[110] Seven members of the team and seven team counterparts were given a carbohydrate drink containing 1 g/kg of carbohydrate four times per day while the other group ingested a placebo for 7 days of intense training. The results showed a significant pre- to post-change in maximal time to exhaustion (carb group increased 0.38 min; placebo group decreased 0.31 min) and less psychological fatigue in the carbohydrate-supplemented group.

Tsintzas et al.[111] had 11 male subjects run on a treadmill at 70% VO_{2max} until exhaustion three times separated by a week. During the first two occasions, a carbohydrate-electrolyte solution (5.5% or 6.9%) was ingested for the first hour of exercise while water was ingested for the remaining time. On the third occasion, water was ingested throughout the entire run. There were no differences between the two carbohydrate trials, but the time to exhaustion was greater in the 5.5% carbohydrate trial when compared to the water trial (water trial = 109.6 min, 5.5% carb trial = 124.5 min, 6.9% carb trial = 121.4 min). Overall, the average performance times for the two carbohydrate trials were significantly longer than the water trial.

Another study showing positive results of carbohydrate supplementation was done by Tarnopolsky et al.[112] Supplementation trials were a) 177 kcal of 81% carbohydrate and 19% protein consumed during the 3-day pretest and less than 10 minutes after exercise plus 600 mL 8% glucose polymers/fructose 1 hour before and the same supplementation during testing, b) placebo during 3-day pretest plus the remainder the same as trial A, c) placebo at all points, or d) same as trial B with 8% glucose 1 hour before the test and the same supplementation during the test. With this complex supplementation protocol, the results showed a greater time to fatigue at 85% VO_{2max} (9.6 versus 7.8 min for group A and placebo, respectively) and total carbohydrate oxidation for trial A versus the placebo trial. Plasma glucose concentrations were higher for trials A and B versus the placebo. Overall, these results show that 3 days of carbohydrate and protein supplementation followed by 1-hour pre- and during-exercise supplementation with mixed carbohydrates increases time to fatigue and carbohydrate oxidation.

A study on carbohydrates with or without BCAAs has shown positive results.[113] Eight subjects drank carbohydrate drinks 1 hour before (5 mL/kg, 18% carbohydrate) and during exercise (2 mL/kg, 6% carbohydrate), the same carbohydrate solutions with BCAAs, or a placebo. The subjects ran longer when fed either carbohydrate solution when compared to the placebo (9.66, 9.00, and 6.36 min for the carb, carb plus BCAAs, and placebo, respectively), but there were no differences between the carbohydrate groups.

Next, McConell et al.[114] conducted a study on eight endurance-trained men cycling to exhaustion at 69% VO_{2max}. The subjects ingested an 8% carbohydrate solution or a placebo. No differences were noted in oxygen uptake, heart rate, or respiratory exchange ratio during exercise; however, time to exhaustion was 30% greater when the carbohydrates were ingested.

Moreover, the effects of carbohydrate supplementation before and during exercise were examined using five moderately trained subjects.[115] A high-intensity exercise test (90% VO_{2max}) was performed for 60 minutes under the following conditions: a) pre-exercise glucose polymer and placebo during exercise, b) glucose polymer before and during exercise, or c) placebo before and during exercise. The subjects ingested 300 mL of a placebo or 10% glucose solution immediately before and every 15 minutes during exercise. There were no differences in power output in the groups for the first 40 minutes, but power output was greater with glucose during the final 20 minutes (total power output = 619 kJ for the glucose/placebo, 599 kJ for the glucose/glucose, and 560 kJ for the placebo). VO_2 followed a similar pattern, and the authors concluded that the ingestion of glucose before exercise results in less of a decline in power output, but no further benefit is seen with the ingestion of glucose during exercise.

Other studies have shown that carbohydrate ingestion increases performance to a greater degree than a combination of carbohydrate, fat, and protein. Six highly trained endurance cyclists rode for 330 minutes at 50% peak power output while ingesting a sports bar containing 7 g of fat, 14 g of protein, and 19 g of carbohydrate or an equicaloric amount of carbohydrate before performing a time trial.[116] Rates of fat oxidation were greater after exercise during the combination trial compared to the carbohydrate trial. However, two subjects could not complete the time trial after they ingested the combination of fat, protein, and carbohydrates, while all of the subjects completed the time trial after the ingestion of just carbohydrate. The authors concluded that the combination of fat, protein, and carbohydrate can increase fat metabolism during prolonged exercise, but may impair subsequent high-intensity performance.

On the other hand, a study by Madsen et al.[117] showed no improvement in performance with carbohydrate ingestion. Nine well-trained cyclists (VO_{2max} = 63.1 mL/kg/min) cycled 100 km as fast as possible after ingesting glucose, glucose plus BCAAs, or a placebo. The results showed no significant differences between groups for performance time.

Another recent study by Burke et al.[118] also showed no difference in endurance performance. Six well-trained cyclists consumed 2 g/kg of carbohydrate of either high glycemic index (GI) (potato), low GI (pasta), or a low-energy jelly (control) 2 hours before exercise. The exercise consisted of 2 hours of cycling at 70% VO_{2max}, followed by a performance ride at 300 kJ. Also, immediately before and during exercise, the subjects consumed 10 g/100 mL

Carbohydrate Loading Does Not Improve Cycling Performance in a Double-Blind, Placebo Controlled Study

Seven well-trained cyclists performed a 100-km time trial 3 days after ingesting 9 g/kg/day (carbohydrate loading) or 6 g/kg/day (placebo) in this crossover design study. A carbohydrate breakfast was consumed 2 hours before the time trial, and 1 g of carbohydrate/kg/hr of a carbohydrate drink was consumed during exercise. During the time trial, there were four, 4-km sprints and five 1-km sprints. Muscle glycogen concentrations were significantly increased with carbohydrate loading; however, muscle glycogen use, time to complete the trial, and mean power output were not significantly different between the trials (SEE FIGURE). Therefore, this study shows that carbohydrate loading does not improve endurance performance. This is in contrast to many studies done on carbohydrate loading; however, the use of a blinded approach was not incorporated in previous studies. Furthermore, this study raises the possibility that carbohydrate loading might confer a beneficial effect via a placebo effect or from higher pre-exercise liver glycogen stores that could delay the onset of hypoglycemia during prolonged exercise. Thus, it would seem sensible to use carbohydrate ingestion during exercise; this would likely negate any effect

of carbohydrate loading as it relates to ameliorating exercise-induced hypoglycemia.

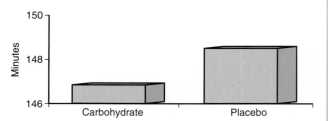

Sidebar Figure 1. Total time to complete 100-km time trial is not improved with carbohydrate loading. (*Adapted from* Burke LM, Hawley JA, Schabort EJ, et al. Carbohydrate loading failed to improve 100-km cycling performance in a placebo-controlled trial. J Appl Physiol 2000;88:1284–1290.)

Burke LM, Hawley JA, Schabort EJ, et al. Carbohydrate loading failed to improve 100-km cycling performance in a placebo-controlled trial. J Appl Physiol 2000;88:1284–1290.

of a glucose solution (total = 24 mL/kg). The results showed no significant differences between any of the trials for carbohydrate oxidation or time to complete the performance ride.

Carbohydrates are the most frequently used endurance enhancer. With the ingestion of carbohydrates before and/or during exercise, there will be more glucose available for energy. This should result in an increase in endurance performance.

Safety and Toxicity

One might suffer abdominal cramping or gastrointestinal problems after ingesting too great of an amount of carbohydrate before and/or during exercise. The use of a liquid carbohydrate solution may prevent this.

Beta-hydroxy-beta-methylbutyrate (HMB)

HMB is a metabolite of the essential amino acid leucine. HMB is usually promoted as a muscle-building supplement. It has been claimed to increase strength and lean body mass via an antiproteolytic effect. Recently,

HMB has been touted as an endurance enhancer. However, the literature on HMB and endurance performance is scant.

Human Studies

A recent study was conducted by Knitter et al.[119] on the effects of HMB on muscle damage after a prolonged run. Thirteen subjects randomly received 3 g/day of HMB or a placebo for 6 weeks. After the training period, all subjects completed a 20-km run. Creatine phosphokinase and lactate dehydrogenase (LDH) activities were measured before and after the prolonged run to assess muscle damage. The placebo group had a significantly greater increase in creatine phosphokinase activity when compared with the HMB-supplemented group. Also, LDH activity was significantly lower in the HMB-supplemented group. These results suggest that supplementation with HMB may prevent exercise-induced muscle damage. However, it is not clear if this could translate into an enhanced endurance performance.

Safety and Toxicity

The use of HMB has been reported to be safe. A summary of safety data was collected in nine studies in which humans were ingesting 3 g of HMB per day.[120] The duration of the studies lasted from 3 to 8 weeks and included young and old, male and female, and exercising and nonexercising subjects. HMB supplementation did not affect any markers of tissue health and function. Furthermore, HMB resulted in a significant decrease in total cholesterol (5.8%), LDL cholesterol (7.3%), and systolic blood pressure (4.4 mm Hg).

SUMMARY

Caffeine is perhaps the most extensively researched endurance ergogenic aid. By stimulating the central nervous system, caffeine can enhance the release of catecholamines (epinephrine and norepinephrine) and increase the use of fatty acids for energy. Research has shown an increase in fat oxidation and free fatty acid concentrations with the use of caffeine,[121–123] therefore sparing muscle glycogen. Also, plasma epinephrine concentrations have been shown to be elevated with the ingestion of caffeine.[124] A third way in which caffeine may increase performance is by decreasing an individual's rate of perceived exertion at a given workload.[125,126] The combination of these three factors can significantly increase an individual's endurance performance. Some studies have shown no improvements in performance with the use of caffeine, but most studies have shown positive results.

BCAAs were thought to increase performance because plasma and serum levels of leucine (one of the three BCAAs) were significantly lowered after aerobic exercise.[127] Two studies did show some improvements in endurance performance with BCAA supplementation[128,129]; nonetheless, most studies have shown no improvement.

As a conditionally essential amino acid, carnitine is a physiological carrier of activated long-chain fatty acids. Carnitine aids in the transport of these fatty acids into the mitochondria for oxidation. It is the oxidation of fatty acids that supplies the body with energy. The use of fatty acids for energy will spare muscle glycogen. This is why carnitine has been proposed as an ergogenic aid for endurance performance. Nonetheless, studies have not been able to show an improvement in endurance performance with the use of carnitine.

As a metabolite of leucine, HMB is normally used as a muscle-building supplement. The mechanism by which HMB may influence skeletal muscle growth or enhance endurance performance is unknown. Currently, no studies have been conducted on HMB and its influence on endurance; however, one study showed no increase in creatine phosphokinase activity and a decrease in LDH activity after a prolonged run with HMB supplementation. These changes suggest that HMB may help ameliorate skeletal muscle damage after exercise. HMB may help increase performance because it can decrease muscle damage, but more studies are needed.

CoQ10 aids in the transport of electrons within the mitochondria and aids in the production of ATP. Studies have shown that the ingestion CoQ10 significantly increases serum concentrations of CoQ10; nevertheless, these studies did not show any improvements in endurance performance. In fact, one study showed that the use of CoQ10 actually decreased performance,[130] and another study by the same investigator showed that CoQ10 might cause some cell damage.[131]

Dimethylglycine (DMG) has also been touted as an endurance enhancer by increasing oxygen use and mental alertness. A couple of studies have shown improvements in performance with DMG; however, these studies were highly criticized for various reasons such as not having blinding for either the subjects or the investigators. Most of the more recent studies on DMG have not shown positive results. The basis by which DMG supposedly works has little merit.

The herbal supplement, ginseng, is widely used to enhance performance and aid in various health-related issues. Early studies conducted on ginseng and its effect on endurance in mice showed positive results. These studies showed an increase in performance time, swim time, capillary density, and mitochondrial content with ginseng supplementation. At least one human study has also shown an improvement in endurance performance with ginseng; nonetheless, the bulk of human data on ginseng have not shown an improvement in endurance.

On the other hand, the use of pyruvate on endurance performance has shown some encouraging results. When pyruvate is ingested, it will apparently enhance the efficiency of the Krebs cycle, thereby producing more ATP for energy. Although many studies have been performed on pyruvate's effect on weight loss, few have been conducted on its effectiveness in endurance performance. Two of the studies conducted on pyruvate have shown that it can aid in performance; then again, these studies used 25 g of pyruvate combined with 75 g of dihydroxyacetone. To ingest this extremely high dose, you would be consuming more capsules than the average individual would care to. Also, the most recent study on low doses of pyruvate (7 g) showed no improvement in endurance performance. Moreover, the use of pyruvate has resulted in some mild side effects including flatus and diarrhea.

Polylactate has been shown to increase blood pH, thereby allowing a greater lactic acid buildup before fatigue. The few studies that have been conducted on polylactate have not shown an increase in endurance performance. Also, individuals ingesting polylactate at a concentration greater than 2.5% had severe gastrointestinal efflux. The sparse data available do not show much hope for this supplement.

Phosphates are a blood buffer that might also increase the production of 2,3 DPG, thereby increasing the amount of oxygen delivered to skeletal muscles. The research conducted on phosphates is mixed, with slightly more data showing an increase in endurance performance with phosphates. Thus far, studies have not shown any toxic side effects of phosphates, but few studies have tested for them.

Another blood buffer, sodium bicarbonate, has also had mixed results. The data are basically split with approximately half of the studies showing an improvement in performance, while the other half showed no improvement. Also, sodium bicarbonate has been known to cause severe gastrointestinal discomfort depending on the individual.

Many studies have been conducted on the use of medium-chain triglycerides (MCTs) and their effects on endurance performance. MCTs are oxidized as easily as glucose, and therefore they may have a glucose-sparing effect. Out of the numerous studies conducted on MCT, only one has shown an increase in endurance performance. Also, most of these studies have shown an increase in ketone bodies, and some gastrointestinal problems have also resulted.

Moreover, glycerol concentrations in the blood may be a reflection of an athlete's performance. Therefore, it would be feasible that ingesting exogenous glycerol may help increase performance. Nevertheless, of the few animal and human studies conducted on glycerol and performance, none have shown an increase in performance, and some have shown a significant decrease in performance.

Finally, the most likely and frequently used supplement in endurance athletics is carbohydrates. Numerous studies support an ergogenic role of carbohydrates under the proper conditions. Carbohydrates are readily broken down into glucose and used for energy; therefore, ingestion of extra carbohydrates before and/or during exercise should increase endurance performance.

AUTHOR'S RECOMMENDATIONS

Few supplements have sufficient evidence to support their role as an ergogenic aid for endurance athletes. The first substance that may improve performance would be one of the three blood buffers. Polylactate does not show any potential, but phosphates and sodium bicarbonate may have some benefits. The data are mixed on both supplements, and more research is needed; however, it is the author's opinion that phosphates have the best potential of increasing endurance without the unwanted side effects of sodium bicarbonate ingestion. More work is needed on phosphates, but its use looks promising.

Another effective ergogenic aid would be caffeine. This supplement has been clearly shown to improve endurance performance. Five mg/kg of body weight (i.e., 400 mg for an 80-kg individual) 30 minutes before exercise should suffice. However, some individuals may become too nervous and jittery with caffeine to perform well. Finally, because caffeine is a diuretic it may cause dehydration. Hence, exercising in the heat while using caffeine should be accompanied with plenty of fluids.

Finally, the best endurance supplement would be carbohydrates. There is a plethora of data on the positive effects of carbohydrate supplementation. Perhaps the best use of carbohydrates is during a prolonged endurance event, (i.e., >1 h); in this case, the ingestion of carbohydrate may aid in performance because the body will have used most of its glucose and glycogen during the first hour and the ingested glucose could serve as an additional fuel source. It has been recommended that you should ingest 0.5–1 g/kg (i.e., 40–80 g for an 80-kg individual) in a 6–8% solution. This may vary from individual to individual. You will need to experiment with the dosage to determine your personal needs (L. Burke, personal communication, October, 2000). With regards to carbohydrate loading, however, the most recent study showed that carbohydrate loading for 3 days before exercise did not increase endurance performance.[132]

FUTURE RESEARCH

The use of caffeine and carbohydrates and their effect on endurance performance has been extensively studied; however, some of the other supplements reviewed have not been so extensively researched. Certainly, HMB merits further examination as a potential endurance aid. The study by Knitter et al.[133] showed significant increases in creatine phosphokinase activity in the placebo group and significant decreases in lactate dehydrogenase activities in the HMB group; therefore, HMB might reduce exercise-induced muscle damage. To the author's knowledge no studies have been conducted on the effects of HMB on endurance time and/or performance. This may be a viable research project that should be conducted in the future.

High doses of pyruvate in combination with dihydroxyacetone have shown a significant improvement in arm and leg endurance performance. On the other hand, the low doses of pyruvate (seen on various over-the-counter supplements) have not been shown to have any beneficial effects. This particular supplement will need to be further researched to verify whether it increases endurance performance. Moreover, the practicality of the dosages administered should be taken into consideration.

Lastly, the effects of phosphates and sodium bicarbonate warrant more research. The current literature is mixed for both of these supplements. Phosphates apparently increase the production of 2,3-DPG and also decrease the acidity of blood, both resulting in an improved performance. Sodium bicarbonate is also a blood buffer, therefore allowing a greater amount of lactic acid buildup before hampering performance. Both supplements show great potential as an endurance enhancer, but more research is needed to clearly show an improvement.

REFERENCES

1. Wilmore JH, Costill DL. Ergogenic aids and performance. In: Physiology of Sport and Exercise. Champaign, IL: Human Kinetics, 1999:409–449.
2. Perkins R, Williams MH. Effect of caffeine upon maximal muscular endurance of females. Med Sci Sports 1975;7:221–224.
3. Costill DL, Dalsky GP, Fink WJ. Effects of caffeine ingestion on metabolism and exercise performance. Med Sci Sports 1978;10:155–158.
4. Ivy JL, Costill DL, Fink WJ, Lower RW. Influence of caffeine and carbohydrate feedings on endurance performance. Med Sci Sports 1979;11:6–11.
5. Cohen BS, Nelson AG, Prevost MC, et al. Effects of caffeine ingestion on endurance racing in the heat and humidity. Eur J Appl Physiol Occup Physiol 1996;73:358–363.
6. Wemple RD, Lamb DR, McKeever KH. Caffeine vs caffeine-free sports drinks: effects on urine production at rest and during prolonged exercise. Int J Sports Med 1997;18:40–46.
7. French C, McNaughton L, Davies P, Tristram S. Caffeine ingestion during exercise to exhaustion in elite distance runners. Revision. J Sports Med Phys Fitness 1991;31:425–432.
8. Pasman WJ, van Baak MA, Jeukendrup AE, de Haan A. The effects of different dosages of caffeine on endurance performance time. Int J Sports Med 1995;16:225–230.
9. Denadai BS, Denadai ML. Effects of caffeine on time to exhaustion in exercise performed below and above the anaerobic threshold. Braz J Med Biol Res 1998;31:581–585.
10. Graham TE, Hibbert E, Sathasivam P. Metabolic and exercise endurance effects of coffee and caffeine ingestion. J Appl Physiol 1998;85:883–889.
11. Bell DG, Jacobs I. Combined caffeine and ephedrine ingestion improves run times of Canadian Forces Warrior Test. Aviat Space Environ Med 1999;70:325–329.
12. Mero A. Leucine supplementation and intensive training. Sports Med 1999;27:347–358.
13. Davis JM. Carbohydrates, branched-chain amino acids, and endurance: the central fatigue hypothesis. Int J Sports Nutr 1995;5:S29–S38.
14. Blomstrand E, Hassmen P, Ekblom B, Newsholme EA. Administration of branched-chain amino acids during sustained exercise—effects on performance and on plasma concentration of some amino acids. Eur J Appl Physiol Occup Physiol 1991;63:83–88.
15. Blomstrand E, Andersson S, Hassmen P, et al. Effect of branched-chain amino acid and carbohydrate supplementation on the exercise-induced change in plasma and muscle concentration of amino acids in human subjects. Acta Physiol Scand 1995;153:87–96.
16. van Hall G, Raaymakers JS, Saris WH, Wagenmakers AJ. Ingestion of branched-chain amino acids and tryptophan during sustained exercise in man: failure to affect performance. J Physiol 1995;486:789–794.
17. Struder HK, Hollmann W, Platen P, et al. Influence of paroxetine, branched-chain amino acids and tyrosine on neuroendocrine system responses and fatigue in humans. Horm Metab Res 1998;30:188–194.
18. Madsen K, MacLean DA, Kiens B, Christensen D. Effects of glucose, glucose plus branched-chain amino acids, or placebo on bike performance over 100-km. J Appl Physiol 1996;81:2644–2650.
19. Freyssenet D, Berthon P, Denis C, et al. Effect of a 6-week endurance training program and branched-chain amino acid supplementation on histomorphometric characteristics of aged human muscle. Arch Physiol Biochem 1996;104:157–162.
20. Mittleman KD, Ricci MR, Bailey SP. Branched-chain amino acids prolong exercise during heat stress in men and women. Med Sci Sports Exerc 1998;30:83–91.
21. Marconi C, Sassi G, Carpinelli A, Cerretelli P. Effects of L-carnitine loading on the aerobic and anaerobic performance of endurance athletes. Eur J Appl Physiol 1985;54:131–135.
22. Greig C, Finch KM, Jones DA, et al. The effect of oral supplementation with L-carnitine on maximum and submaximum exercise capacity. Eur J Appl Physiol Occup Physiol 1987;56:457–460.
23. Gorostiaga EM, Maurer CA, Eclache JP. Decrease in respiratory quotient during exercise following L-carnitine supplementation. Int J Sports Med 1989;10:169–174.
24. Colombani P, Wenk C, Kunz I, et al. Effects of L-carnitine supplementation on physical performance and energy metabolism of endurance-trained athletes: a double-blind crossover field study. Eur J Appl Physiol Occup Physiol 1996;73:434–439.
25. McArdle WD, Katch FI, Katch VL. Sports & Exercise Nutrition. Baltimore: Lippincott Williams & Wilkins, 1999.
26. Horton HR, Moran LA, Ochs RS, et al. Electron transport and oxidative phosphorylation. In: Principles of Biochemistry, 2nd ed. Upper Saddle River, NJ: Prentice-Hall, 1996:411–434.
27. Fujimoto S, Kurihara N, Hirata K, Takeda T. Effects of coenzyme Q10 administration on pulmonary function and exercise performance inpatients with chronic lung diseases. Clin Investig 1993;71:S162–166.
28. Ylikoski T, Piirainen J, Hanninen O, Penttinen J. The effect of coenzyme Q10 on the exercise performance of cross-country skiers. Mol Aspects Med 1997;18:S283–290.
29. Braun B, Clarkson PM, Freedson PS, Kohl RL. Effects of coenzyme Q10 supplementation on exercise performance, VO2 max, and lipid peroxidation in trained cyclists. Int J Sports Nutr 1991;1:353–365.

30. Snider IP, Bazzarre TL, Murdoch SD, Goldfarb A. Effects of coenzyme athletic performance system as an ergogenic aid on endurance performance to exhaustion. Int J Sports Nutr 1992;2:272–283.
31. Weston SB, Zhou S, Weatherby RP, Robson SJ. Does exogenous coenzyme Q10 affect aerobic capacity in endurance athletes? Int J Sports Nutr 1997;7:197–206.
32. Malm C, Sversson M, Sjoberg B, et al. Supplementation with ubiquinone-10 causes cellular damage during intense exercise. Acta Physiol Scand 1996;157:511–512.
33. Malm C, Sversson M, Ekblom B, Sjodin B. Effects of ubiquinone-10 supplementation and high intensity training on physical performance in humans. Acta Physiol Scand 1997;161:379–384.
34. Baggio E, Gandini R, Plancher AC, et al. Italian multicenter study on the safety and efficacy of coenzyme Q10 as adjunctive therapy in heart failure. CoQ10 Drug Surveillance Investigators. Mol Aspects Med 1994;15:287–294.
35. Folkers K, Langsjoen P, Langsjoen PH. Therapy with coenzyme Q10 of patients in heart failure who are eligible or ineligible for a transplant. Biochem Biophys Res Commun 1992;182:247–253.
36. Malm C, Sversson M, Sjoberg B, et al. Supplementation with ubiquinone-10 causes cellular damage during intense exercise. Acta Physiol Scand 1996;157:511–512.
37. Stackpoole PW. Pangamic acid (Vitamin B15). Wld Rev Nutr Diet 1977;27:145–163.
38. Herbert V. Pangamic acid ("Vitamin B15"). Am J Clin Nutr 1979; 32:1534–1540.
39. Gray ME, Titlow LW. B15: Myth or miracle. Phys Sports Med 1982;10:107–112.
40. Rose RJ, Schlierf HA, Knight PK, et al. Effects of N,N-dimethylglycine on cardio respiratory function and lactate production in thoroughbred horses performing incremental treadmill exercise. Vet Rec 1989; 125:268–271.
41. Pipes TV. The effects of pangamic acid on performance in trained athletes. Med Sci Sports Exerc 1980;12:98.
42. Kemp GL. A clinical study and evaluation of pangamic acid. JAOA 1959;58:714–718.
43. Gray Me, Titlow LW. The effects of pangamic acid on maximal treadmill performance. Med Sci Sports Exerc 1982;14:424–427.
44. Black DG, Sucec AA. Effects of calcium pangamate on aerobic and endurance parameters, a double blind study. Med Sci Sports Exerc 1981;13:93.
45. Bishop PA, Smith JF, Young B. Effects of N, N-Dimethylglycine on physiological response and performance in trained runners. J Sports Med 1987;27:53–56.
46. Girandola RN, Wiswell RA, Bulbulian. Effects of pangamic acid (B-15) ingestion on metabolic response to exercise. Biochem Med 1980;24:218–222.
47. Reap EA, Lawson JW. Stimulation of the immune response by dimethylglycine, a nontoxic metabolite. J Lab Clin Med 1990;115: 481–486.
48. Gascon G, Patterson B, Yearwood K, Slotnick H. N, N-dimethylglycine and epilepsy. Epilepsia 1989;30:90–93.
49. Gillis CN. Panax ginseng pharmacology: a nitric oxide link? Biochem Pharmacol 1997;54:1–8.
50. Wang LC, Lee TF. Effect of ginseng saponins on exercise performance in non-trained rats. Planta Med 1998;64:130–133.
51. Banerjee U, Izquierdo JA. Antistress and antifatigue properties of Panax ginseng: comparison with piracetam. Acta Physiol Lat Am 1982;32:277–285.
52. Grandhi A, Mujumdar AM, Patwardhan B. A comparative pharmacological investigation of Ashwagandha and Ginseng. J Ethnopharmacol 1994;44:131–135.
53. Singh A, Saxena E, Bhutani KK. Adrenocorticosterone alterations in male, albino mice treated with Trichopus zeylanicus, Withania somnifera and Panax ginseng preparations. Phytother Res 2000; 14:122–125.
54. Wang LC, Lee TF. Effect of ginseng saponins on exercise performance in non-trained rats. Planta Med 1998;64:130–133.
55. Ferrando A, Vila L, Voces JA, et al. Effects of ginseng extract on various haematological parameters during aerobic exercise in the rat. Planta Med 1999;65:288–290.
56. Ferrando A, Vila L, Voces JA, et al. Effects of standardized Panax ginseng extract on the skeletal muscle of the rat: a comparative study in animals at rest and under exercise. Planta Med 1999;65:239–244.
57. Pieralisi G, Ripari P, Vecchiet L. Effects of a standardized ginseng extract combined with dimethylaminoethanol bitartrate, vitamins, minerals, and trace elements on physical performance during exercise. Clin Ther 1991;13:373–382.
58. Engels HJ, Wirth JC. No ergogenic effects of ginseng (Panax ginseng C.A. Meyer) during graded maximal aerobic exercise. J Am Diet Assoc 1997;97:1110–1115.
59. Allen JD, McLung J, Nelson AG, Welsch M. Ginseng supplementation does not enhance healthy young adults' peak aerobic exercise performance. J Am Coll Nutr 1998;17:462–466.
60. Ziemba AW, Chmura J, Kaciuba-Uscilko H, et al. Ginseng treatment improves psychomotor performance at rest and during graded exercise in young athletes. Int J Sports Nutr 1999;9:371–377.
61. Aphale AA, Chhibba AD, Kumbhakarna NR, et al. Subacute toxicity study of the combination of ginseng (Panax ginseng) an ashwagandha (Withania somnifera) in rats: a safety assessment. Indian J Physiol Pharmacol 1998;42:299–302.
62. Scaglione F, Cattaneo G, Alessandria M, Cogo R. Efficacy and safety of the standardized Ginseng extract G115 for potentiating vaccination against the influenza syndrome and protection against the common cold. Drugs Exp Clin Res 1996;22:65–72.
63. Stanko RT, Adibi SA. Inhibition of lipid accumulation and enhancement of energy expenditure by the addition of pyruvate and dihydroxyacetone to a rat diet. Metabolism 1986;35:182–186.
64. Stanko RT, Robertson RJ, Spina RJ, et al. Enhancement of arm exercise endurance capacity with dihydroxyacetone and pyruvate. J Appl Physiol 1990;68:119–124.
65. Stanko RT, Robertson RJ, Galbreath RW, et al. Enhanced leg exercise endurance with a high carbohydrate diet and dihydroxyacetone and pyruvate. J Appl Physiol 1990;69:1651–1656.
66. Morrison MA, Spriet LL, Dyck DJ. Pyruvate ingestion for 7 days does not improve aerobic performance in well-trained individuals. J Appl Physiol 2000;89:549–556.
67. Stanko RT, Robertson RJ, Galbreath RW, et al. Enhanced leg exercise endurance with a high carbohydrate diet and dihydroxyacetone and pyruvate. J Appl Physiol 1990;69:1651–1656.
68. Stanko RT, Tietze DL, Arch JE. Body composition, energy utilization, and nitrogen metabolism with a severely restricted diet supplemented with dihydroxyacetone and pyruvate. Am J Clin Nutr 1992;55:771–776.
69. Stanko RT, Tietze, DL, Arch JE. Body composition, energy utilization, and nitrogen metabolism with a 4.25-MJ/d low-energy diet supplemented with pyruvate. Am J Clin Nutr 1992;56:630–635.
70. Fahey TD, Larsen JD, Brooks GA, et al. The effects of ingesting polylactate or glucose polymer drinks during prolonged exercise. Int J Sports Nutr 1991;1:149–156.
71. Swensen T, Crater G, Bassett DR Jr, Howley ET. Adding polylactate to a glucose polymer solution does not improve endurance. Int J Sports Med 1994;15:430–434.
72. Swensen T, Crater G, Bassett DR Jr, Howley ET. Adding polylactate to a glucose polymer solution does not improve endurance. Int J Sports Med 1994;15:430–434.
73. Wilmore JH, Costill DL. Ergogenic aids and performance. In: Physiology of sport and exercise. Champaign, IL: Human Kinetics, 1999:409–449.
74. Duffy DJ, Conlee RK. Effects of phosphate loading on leg power and high intensity treadmill exercise. Med Sci Sports Exerc 1986; 18:674–647.
75. Bredle DL, Stager JM, Brechue WF, Farber MO. Phosphate supplementation, cardiovascular function, and exercise performance in humans. J Appl Physiol 1988;65:1821–1826.
76. Zorbs YG, Federenko YF, Naexu KA. Phosphate-loading test influences on endurance-trained volunteers during restriction of muscular activity and chronic hyperhydration. Biol Trace Elem Res 1995;48:51–65.
77. Cade R, Conte M, Zauner C, et al. Effects of phosphate loading on 2,3-diphosphoglycerate and maximal oxygen uptake. Med Sci Sports Exerc 1984;16:263–268.
78. Stewart I, McNaughton OL, Davies P, Tristram S. Phosphate loading and the effects on VO_2 max in trained cyclists. Res Q Exerc Sport 1990;61:80–84.
79. Kreider RB, Miller GW, Williams MH, et al. Effects of phosphate loading on oxygen uptake, ventilatory anaerobic threshold, and run performance. Med Sci Sports Exerc 1990;22:250–256.

80. Kreider RB, Miller GW, Schenck D, et al. Effects of phosphate loading on metabolic and myocardial responses to maximal and endurance exercise. Int J Sports Nutr 1992;2:20–47.

81. Mitchell TH, Abraham G, Wing S, et al. Intravenous bicarbonate and sodium chloride both prolong endurance during intense cycle ergometer exercise. Am J Med Sci 1990;300:88–97.

82. McNaughton L, Dalton B, Palmer G. Sodium bicarbonate can be used as an ergogenic aid in high-intensity, competitive cycle ergometry of 1 h duration. Eur J Appl Physiol Occup Physiol 1999;80:64–69.

83. Housh TJ, deVries HA, Johnson GO, et al. The effect of ammonium chloride and sodium bicarbonate ingestion on the physical working capacity at the fatigue threshold. Eur J Appl Physiol Occup Physiol 1991;62:189–192.

84. Busse MW, Scholz J, Maassen N. Plasma potassium and ventilation during incremental exercise in humans: modulation by sodium bicarbonate and substrate availability. Eur J Appl Physiol Occup Physiol 1992;65:340–346.

85. Potteiger JA, Webster MJ, Nickel GL, et al. The effects of buffer ingestion on metabolic factors related to distance running performance. Eur J Appl Physiol Occup Physiol 1996;72:365–371.

86. Linderman J, Fahey TD. Sodium bicarbonate ingestion and exercise performance: an update. Sports Med 1991;11:71–77.

87. Kowalchuk JM, Maltais SA, Yamaji K, Hughson RL. The effect of citrate loading on exercise performance, acid-base balance and metabolism. Eur J Appl Physiol 1989;58:858–864.

88. McNaughton LR. Sodium citrate and anaerobic performance: Implications of dosage. Eur J Appl Physiol 1990;61:392–397.

89. Bering JR. The role of medium-chain triglycerides in exercise. Int J Sports Nutr 1996;6:121–133.

90. Calabrese C, Myer S, Munson S, et al. A cross-over study of the effects of a single oral feeding of medium chain triglyceride oil vs. canola oil on post-ingestion plasma triglyceride levels in healthy men. Altern Med Rev 1999;4:23–28.

91. Satabin P, Portero P, Defer G, et al. Metabolic and hormonal responses to lipid and carbohydrate diets during exercise in man. Med Sci Sports Exerc 1987;19:218–223.

92. Jeukendrup AE, Saris WH, Brouns F, et al. Effects of carbohydrate (CHO) and fat supplementation on CHO metabolism during prolonged exercise. Metabolism 1996;45:915–921.

93. Jeukendrup AE, Thielen JJ, Wagenmakers JM, et al. Effect of medium-chain triacylglycerols and carbohydrate ingestion during exercise on substrate utilization and subsequent cycling performance. Am J Clin Nutr 1998;67:397–404.

94. Angus DJ, Hargreaves M, Dancey J, Febbraio MA. Effect of carbohydrate or carbohydrate plus medium-chain triglyceride ingestion of cycling time trial performance. J Appl Physiol 2000;88:113–119.

95. Horowitz JF, Mora-Rodriguez R, Byerley LO, Coyle EF. Pre-exercise medium-chain triglyceride ingestion does not alter muscle glycogen use during exercise. J Appl Physiol 2000;88:219–225.

96. Goedecke JH, Elmer-English R, Dennis SC, et al. Effects of medium-chain triacylglycerol ingested with carbohydrate on metabolism and exercise performance. Int J Sports Nutr 1999;9:35–47.

97. Van Zyl CG, Lambert EV, Hawley JA, et al. Effects of medium-chain triglyceride ingestion on fuel metabolism and cycling performance. J Appl Physiol 1996;80:2217–2225.

98. Miles JM, Cattalini M, Sharbrough FW, et al. Metabolic and neurologic effects of an intravenous medium-chain triglyceride emulsion. JPEN 1991;15:37–41.

99. Jeukendrup AE, Saris WH, Brouns F, et al. Effects of carbohydrate (CHO) and fat supplementation on CHO metabolism during prolonged exercise. Metabolism 1996;45:915–921.

100. Satabin P, Portero P, Defer G, et al. Metabolic and hormonal responses to lipid and carbohydrate diets during exercise in man. Med Sci Sports Exerc 1987;19:218–223.

101. Van Zyl CG, Lambert EV, Hawley JA, et al. Effects of medium-chain triglyceride ingestion on fuel metabolism and cycling performance. J Appl Physiol 1996;80:2217–2225.

102. Jeukendrup AE, Thielen JJ, Wagenmakers JM, et al. Effect of medium-chain triacylglycerols and carbohydrate ingestion during exercise on substrate utilization and subsequent cycling performance. Am J Clin Nutr 1998;67:397–404.

103. Ohkuwa T, Miyamura M, Andou Y, Utsuno T. Sex differences in lactate and glycerol levels during maximal aerobic and anaerobic running. Eur J Appl Physiol Occup Physiol;1987;57:746–752.

104. Schott HC II, Dusterdieck KF, Eberhart SW, et al. Effects of electrolyte and glycerol supplementation on recovery from endurance exercise. Equine Vet J Suppl 1999;30:384–393.

105. Dusterdieck KF, Schott HC II, Eberhart SW, et al. Electrolyte and glycerol supplementation improve water intake by horses performing a simulated 60 km endurance ride. Equine Vet J Suppl 1999;30:418–424.

106. Gleeson M, Maughan RJ, Greenhaff PL. Comparison of the effects of pre-exercise feeding of glucose, glycerol and placebo on endurance and fuel homeostasis in man. Eur J Appl Physiol Occup Physiol 1986;55:645–653.

107. Inder WJ, Swanney MP, Donald RA, et al. The effect of glycerol and desmopressin on exercise performance and hydration in triathletes. Med Sci Sports Exerc;1999;30:1263–1269.

108. Langenfeld ME, Seifert JG, Rudge SR, Bucher RJ. Effect of carbohydrate ingestion on performance of non-fasted cyclists during a simulated 80-mile time trial. J Sports Med Phys Fitness 1994;34:263–270.

109. Yaspelkis BB III, Patterson JG, Anderla PA, et al. Carbohydrate supplementation spares muscle glycogen during variable-intensity exercise. J Appl Physiol 1993;75:1477–1485.

110. Kreider RB, Hill D, Horton G, et al. Effects of carbohydrate supplementation during intense training on dietary patterns, psychological status, and performance. Int J Sports Nutr 1995;5:125–135.

111. Tsintzas OK, Williams C, Wilson W, Burrin J. Influence of carbohydrate supplementation early in exercise on endurance running capacity. Med Sci Sports Exerc 1996;28:1373–1379.

112. Tarnopolsky MA, Dyson K, Atkinson SA, et al. Mixed carbohydrate supplementation increases carbohydrate oxidation and endurance exercise performance and attenuates potassium accumulation. Int J Sport Nutr 1996;6:323–336.

113. Davis JM, Welsh RS, Volve KL, Alderson NA. Effects of branched-chain amino acids and carbohydrate on fatigue during intermittent, high-intensity running. Int J Sports Med 1999;20:309–314.

114. McConell G, Snow RJ, Proietto J, Hargreaves M. Muscle metabolism during prolonged exercise in humans: influence of carbohydrate availability. J Appl Physiol 1999;87:1083–1086.

115. Anantaraman R, Carmines AA, Gaesser GA, Weltman A. Effects of carbohydrate supplementation on performance during 1 hour of high-intensity exercise. Int J Sports Med 1995;16:461–465.

116. Rauch HG, Hawley JA, Woodey M, et al. Effects of ingesting a sports bar versus glucose polymer on substrate utilization and ultra-endurance performance. Int J Sports Med 1999;20:252–257.

117. Madsen K, MacLean DA, Kiens B, Christensen D. Effects of glucose, glucose plus branched-chain amino acids, or placebo on bike performance over 100-km. J Appl Physiol 1996;81:2644–2650.

118. Burke LM, Claassen A, Hawley JA, Noakes TD. Carbohydrate intake during prolonged cycling minimizes effect of glycemic index of pre-exercise meal. J Appl Physiol 1998;85:2220–2226.

119. Knitter AE, Panton L, Rathmacher JA, et al. Effects of beta-hydroxy-beta-methylbutyrate on muscle damage after a prolonged run. J Appl Physiol 2000;89:1340–1344.

120. Nissen S, Sharp RL, Panton L, et al. Beta-hydroxy-beta-methylbutyrate (HMB) supplementation in humans is safe and may decrease cardiovascular risk factors. J Nutr 2000;130:1937–1945.

121. Costill DL, Dalsky GP, Fink WJ. Effects of caffeine ingestion on metabolism and exercise performance. Med Sci Sports 1978;10:155–158.

122. Ivy JL, Costill DL, Fink WJ, Lower RW. Influence of caffeine and carbohydrate feedings on endurance performance. Med Sci Sports 1979;11:6–11.

123. Pasman WJ, van Baak MA, Jeukendrup AE, de Haan A. The effects of different dosages of caffeine on endurance performance time. Int J Sports Med 1995;16:225–230.

124. Graham TE, Hibbert E, Sathasivam P. Metabolic and exercise endurance effects of coffee and caffeine ingestion. J Appl Physiol 1998;85:883–889.

125. Costill DL, Dalsky GP, Fink WJ. Effects of caffeine ingestion on metabolism and exercise performance. Med Sci Sports 1978;10:155–158.

126. Denadai BS, Denadai ML. Effects of caffeine on time to exhaustion in exercise performed below and above the anaerobic threshold. Braz J Med Biol Res 1998;31:581–585.

127. Mero A. Leucine supplementation and intensive training. Sports Med 1999;27:347–358.

128. Blomstrand E, Hassmen P, Ekblom B, Newsholme EA. Administration of branched-chain amino acids during sustained exercise—effects on performance and on plasma concentration of some amino acids. Eur J Appl Physiol Occup Physiol 1991;63:83–88.

129. Mittleman KD, Ricci MR, Bailey SP. Branched-chain amino acids prolong exercise during heat stress in men and women. Med Sci Sports Exerc 1998;30:83–91.

130. Malm C, Sversson M, Ekblom B, Sjodin B. Effects of ubiquinone-10 supplementation and high intensity training on physical performance in humans. Acta Physiol Scand 1997;161:379–384.

131. Malm C, Sversson M, Sjoberg B, et al. Supplementation with ubiquinone-10 causes cellular damage during intense exercise. Acta Physiol Scand 1996;157:511–512.

132. Burke LM, Hawley JA, Schabort EJ, et al. Carbohydrate loading failed to improve 100-km cycling performance in a placebo-controlled trial. J Appl Physiol 2000;88:1284–1290.

133. Knitter AE, Panton L, Rathmacher JA, et al. Effects of beta-hydroxy-beta-methylbutyrate on muscle damage after a prolonged run. J Appl Physiol 2000;89:1340–1344.

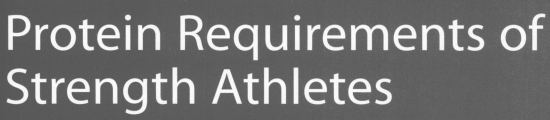

CHAPTER

14

Protein Requirements of Strength Athletes

Peter W.R. Lemon

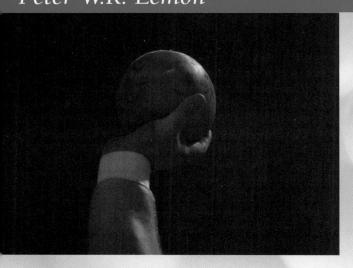

Research Review

Whole-Body Protein Synthesis for Strength Athletes

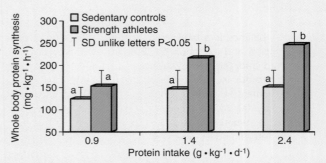

According to the expert committee responsible for the US dietary guidelines, any increased need for protein induced by strength exercise does not exceed the safety buffer included in the current recommended dietary allowance (RDA) (0.8 g protein/kg/day). However, it is important to realize that this opinion is somewhat speculative as the recommendation is based on experiments completed on subjects who did not engage in regular strength exercise. A study conducted by Tarnopolsky and colleagues addressed this issue by comparing measured rates of whole-body protein synthesis for strength athletes in regular training with sedentary controls while both groups consumed protein at each of three different protein intakes (0.9, 1.4, and 2.4 g/kg/day). Although increasing protein intake did not affect protein synthetic rates in the controls, increasing from 0.9 to 1.4 g/kg/day produced a significant increase in protein synthesis in the strength athletes (SEE FIGURE). This is a significant observation because over time this acute increase in protein synthesis would be expected to result in increased muscle size and strength. Consequently, this is objective evidence supporting the athletes' opinions (i.e., dietary protein in excess of the RDA in combination with strength training can enhance muscle growth). However, of equal importance was a second finding of this study. The consumption of even greater amounts of protein (2.4 g/kg/day) did not further increase the protein synthetic rate in the strength athletes. These data suggest that a *ceiling* exists for protein intake and

Effect of quantity of dietary protein on whole body protein synthetic rate. Note that increasing dietary protein above the requirement for sedentary individuals ($0.8 \text{ g} \cdot \text{kg}^{-1} \cdot \text{d}^{-1}$) had no effect on protein synthesis; however, increasing from 0.9 to $1.4 \text{ g} \cdot \text{kg}^{-1} \cdot \text{d}^{-1}$ in the strength athletes led to an increase in protein synthesis. Over time this should increase both muscle mass and size. Note also that a further increase in protein intake (to $2.4 \text{ g} \cdot \text{kg}^{-1} \cdot \text{d}^{-1}$) did not increase protein synthesis any further indicating that this was more dietary protein than needed. (*Data from* Tarnopolsky MA, Atkinson SA, MacDougall JD, et al. Evaluation of protein requirements for trained strength athletes. J Appl Physiol 1992;73:1986–1995.)

muscle growth with strength training. This means that for those engaged in a regular strength-training program, protein intake of approximately 50% more than the current recommendations appear to be advantageous for muscle development but that even greater intakes provide no additional benefit.

Tarnopolsky MA, Atkinson SA, MacDougall JD, et al. Evaluation of protein requirements for trained strength athletes. J Appl Physiol 1992;73:1986–1995.
US Food and Nutrition Board. Recommended Dietary Allowances. Washington, DC: National Academy Press, 1989.

Introduction

Dietary protein requirements have been debated for at least the past 150 years[1] yet there is still little consensus on this issue.[2,3] For most of the 20th century, nutritional scientists believed that protein requirements were not substantially affected by regular exercise.[4] However, during this same time, athletes, especially those engaged in bodybuilding exercise, remained convinced that their dietary protein needs were dramatically greater than sedentary individuals. These opposing views raise several obvious questions—including why the discrepancy, and which opinion is actually correct? The answer to the first question seems to be straightforward because each group appears to have come to its conclusion independently using

different information. The scientists have used laboratory data collected under controlled conditions (using nitrogen balance experiments primarily) while the athletes have formed their opinion using performance data and a trial and error approach. Although it is easy to dismiss the latter as too subjective, the fact remains that it is based on a tremendous amount of experimentation and, despite its nonscientific origin, has been replicated many times. Moreover, the scientific view could be flawed because, although objective, the laboratory data may have little relationship to athletic performance. For example, it might be possible to maintain nitrogen balance at protein intakes below what is necessary to maximize muscle performance. If so, the athletes' opinion could have merit. As a result, the correct viewpoint on protein needs for strength/power athletes remains debatable.

Nitrogen Balance

Nitrogen balance is a laboratory technique by which both consumption and excretion of all nitrogen is meticulously quantified and the net difference calculated. On average, dietary protein is 16% nitrogen so protein retention or loss is calculated by multiplying this net nitrogen difference by 6.25, i.e., 100/16. The amount of protein necessary to elicit balance, i.e., when intake and excretion are exactly equal, can be determined (Y intercept in FIGURE) by measuring

nitrogen excretion at a variety of different protein intakes. This quantity of protein is thought to be the dietary requirement. Although this technique has been called nitrogen balance traditionally, the terminology is somewhat unfortunate because it results in the nonsensical nitrogen balance descriptors *positive* (when intake exceeds excretion) and *negative* (when excretion exceeds intake). The term *nitrogen status* is more accurate and, therefore, recommended.

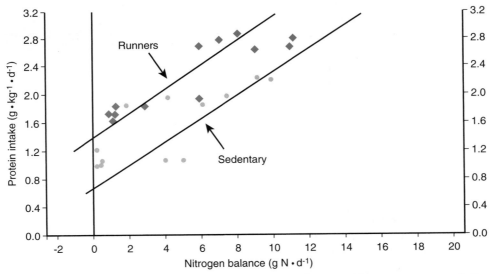

Effect of quantity of dietary protein on nitrogen balance in sedentary subjects versus runners. Notice that nitrogen retention is linearly related to protein intake and that the runners' data are above and to the left of those of the sedentary subjects (Y intercept is greater in runners) indicating that the dietary protein requirement is increased by a regular running program. (*Data from* Tarnopolsky MA, MacDougall JD, Atkinson SA. Influence of protein intake and training status on nitrogen balance and lean body mass. J Appl Physiol 1988;64:187–193.)

About 35 years ago, scientists began to study the effects of acute and chronic exercise on a more systematic basis.[5] Although definitive protein intake recommendations for various athletes must await the completion of additional experimentation, several of these recent studies suggest that regular intense exercise (both strength and endurance) increases dietary protein need. The purpose of this chapter is to review these recent data, especially those experiments that involve strength exercise.

Protein Requirements

Skeletal muscle makes up about 40–50% of total body mass, i.e., 28–35 kg in a 70-kg individual. The main constituents of skeletal muscle include water (~75%) and protein

(~20%). Of this 20%, the majority is contractile protein (myofilaments) (~11%) with smaller amounts of sarcoplasmic (~6%) and connective tissue (~3%) protein. Of the 20 amino acids that are the component parts of protein, only approximately 50% can be produced in the body—the remainder are called indispensable (or essential) because they must be consumed in the diet or the ability to form body protein (both structural and enzymatic) is compromised. Consequently, the supply of amino acid (type and quantity of protein) in the diet plays a critical role in muscle growth. Historically, as mentioned above, the adequacy of dietary protein has been assessed using the nitrogen balance technique. This involves quantifying nitrogen intake (food protein is ~16% nitrogen) and excretion (urine, feces, sweat, and miscellaneous) as accurately as possible (FIG. 14-1). Dietary protein requirement is determined as

Essential (or Indispensable) Amino Acids

Essential (or indispensable) amino acids are those amino acids that must be present in one's diet or the body's ability to synthesize protein is compromised. These amino acids include histidine, isoleucine, leucine, lysine, methionine, phenylalanine, threonine, tryptophan, and valine. Recently, other amino acids have been suggested to be conditionally indispensable, meaning that under stressful conditions (including exercise training) their need can exceed the maximal rate at which the body can synthesize them. Examples of these include but may not be limited to glutamine, arginine, cysteine, glycine, and serine (see Chapter 5). If correct, dietary intake of these particular amino acids would need to be greater than it would for sedentary individuals.

the quantity of protein in which nitrogen intake exactly matches nitrogen excretion, i.e., when the individual is at nitrogen balance.

Classically, the daily RDA for protein has been determined by measuring the requirement in a sample that is representative of the population of interest and adding a safety buffer equal to two standard deviations of the mean. Statistically, this should mean that when this quantity of protein is consumed, the vast majority (>95%) of individuals from the representative population would receive

an adequate supply of amino acids. This safety buffer is necessary because requirements can vary somewhat among individuals. Many experiments have been completed over the years and, at least in sedentary individuals, it is clear that the requirement for protein is about 0.6 g/kg/day. When the safety buffer is included, the recommendation for protein intake is slightly higher (0.8 g/kg/day).[4,6] Logically, it would seem that for those attempting to build muscle mass or maintain an increased muscle mass additional protein might be necessary. In fact there are data that support this idea (RESEARCH REVIEW FIGURE AND FIG. 14-2), but there is still little consensus on this topic.[3,4,7] Further complicating the issue is that the nitrogen status (balance) technique is rather labor intensive and has several other limitations—the major one being its *black box* approach, i.e., it cannot distinguish whether changes in balance are due to effects on protein degradation/synthesis, or amino acid oxidation, etc.

Another way to investigate the dietary protein requirements involves the use of metabolic tracers which make it possible to see into the "nitrogen status black box" by assessing which components of protein metabolism are affected by an exercise or dietary treatment. This is an improvement when compared with the nitrogen status

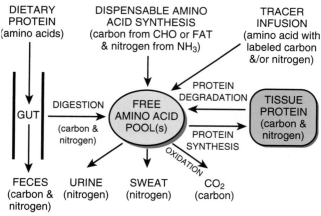

Figure 14-1. Simplified schematic of the major processes involved in protein metabolism. Nitrogen balance experiments involve quantifying the overall net effect (nitrogen intake minus excretion) while tracer studies allow investigators to quantify amino acid oxidation, tissue protein synthesis, tissue protein degradation, etc. (*Data from* Lemon PWR. Effects of exercise on dietary protein requirements. Int J Sports Nutr 1998;8:426–447.)

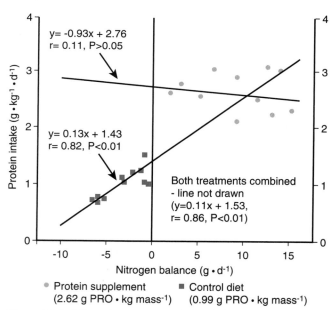

Figure 14-2. Effect of quantity of dietary protein on nitrogen balance in novice bodybuilders. Note that for protein intakes around 1.0 $g \cdot kg^{-1} \cdot d^{-1}$ (solid squares) the Y intercept (dietary protein requirement) is 1.43 $g \cdot kg^{-1} \cdot d^{-1}$ (more than double the sedentary requirement). Note also that with high protein intakes (~2.6 $g \cdot kg^{-1} \cdot d^{-1}$, filled circles) the linear relationship between nitrogen retention and protein intake does not hold up. (*Data from* Lemon PWR, Tarnopolsky MA, MacDougall JD, et al. Evaluation of protein requirements for trained strength athletes. J Appl Physiol 1992;73:1986–1995.)

Metabolic Tracer Technique

This technique is a laboratory approach in which a representative amino acid (tracer) is tagged (in humans usually with ^{13}carbon, ^{2}hydrogen, or ^{15}nitrogen) and infused or ingested until its concentration in the body reaches a steady state, i.e., the rate of appearance of unlabelled tracee equals its disappearance. In other words, the injected/ingested tracer is diluted by the tracee such that its concentration (isotopic enrichment) remains constant over the experimental measurement period. Using measures of exhaled breath carbon dioxide (for carbon tracing), urine (for nitrogen tracing), and blood it is possible to calculate rates of whole body amino acid oxidation, protein degradation, and/or synthesis (SEE FIG. 14-1). Further, if one quantifies the concentration of a representative labelled amino acid in skeletal muscle (via needle biopsy) at two time points it is even possible to determine the protein synthetic rate in a specific muscle (amount of incorporation per unit time/volume of muscle).

Tipton KD, Ferrando AA, Phillips SM. Postexercise net protein synthesis in human muscle from orally administered amino acids. Am J Physiol 1999;276:E628–E634.

Wolfe RR. Radioactive and Stable Isotope Tracers in Biomedicine: Principles and Practice of Kinetic Analysis. New York: Wiley-Liss, 1992.

Factors That Affect Dietary Protein Need

Dietary Energy

Although frequently overlooked, it has been known for approximately 50 years that insufficient energy intake can lead to a negative nitrogen status[11] presumably because when energy intake becomes borderline or worse, both dietary and body protein can be used by the body to compensate for the energy deficit. As a result, decreases in protein synthesis and/or increases in protein degradation

Body Composition

The most accurate method to assess body composition involves chemical analysis of the body. However, as this can be done only after death, it is of limited value in the assessment of body composition in the living. Fortunately, several indirect methods for assessment have been developed for estimation in living subjects. The most common are densitometry (underwater weighing or air displacement) anthropometry (measures of body girths, breaths, and/or skinfold thickness), and bioelectrical impedance (measures of opposition to a weak electrical current introduced into the body). Of these, densitometry is considered the most accurate because its estimation is based on results obtained from direct chemical analysis of cadavers. However, it cannot be exact for given individuals because most will differ somewhat from the cadavers that were analyzed. Consequently, there will always be a small absolute error (perhaps 2–3%) that must be considered when these measures are used. This, of course, is of little concern when relative measures are compared, i.e., in a study in which before and after measures are compared, because the error is constant. Typically, anthropometry and bioimpedance methods involve more absolute error, as their estimations are based on results from densitometric analyses, i.e., they are estimates of an estimate. However, they are widely used because they are easy and the necessary equipment is both portable and relatively inexpensive. Other more sophisticated body composition measures are possible including magnetic resonance imaging and dual energy X-ray absorptiometry but are primarily used in research settings as the equipment necessary is expensive. For a more comprehensive review on body composition techniques, see Wagner and Heyward.

Wagner DR, Heyward VH. Techniques of body composition assessment: a review of laboratory and field methods. Res Q Exerc Sport 1999;70(2):135–149.

technique. Some recent data that were obtained using this technique[8,9] suggest that current amino acid requirements (determined using the nitrogen status technique) may underestimate resting need by 40–90% but these new data remain controversial.[10] In addition, some studies (to be discussed below) indicate that strength athletes can benefit from protein intakes that exceed the current RDA (note: in the US this recommendation was last updated in 1989). Recent experiments using both metabolic tracers and nitrogen balance methodologies indicate that the protein requirement for strength athletes is likely about 1.5 g/kg/day, i.e., almost twice the current RDA (SEE RESEARCH REVIEW FIGURE AND FIG. 14-2). When two standard deviations are added, the protein RDA for strength athletes could be as high as 1.7–2.0 g/kg/day.[7] Despite this, it is unlikely that protein deficiencies will be rampant in athletes because it is not difficult to obtain this quantity of protein in one's diet given the high energy intake of most athletes. For example, even if only 10% of the energy in a 21,000 kJ (5000 kcal) diet is protein, an 80-kg individual consuming this diet would receive 1.6 g of protein/kg/day (21,000 kJ/day × 0.10/16.7 kJ/g/80 kg = 1.6 g/kg/day). Typically, the percentage of protein in a US diet is closer to 12–15%.

would occur. Consequently, protein intake recommendations should be even greater for those who restrict food intake (dieters) or who have extremely high-energy expenditures (athletes). This may be especially important for female athletes whose energy intake is frequently insufficient relative to their energy expenditures. Recommendations for energy intake (kJ/kg) have been established (about 185 and 105 for young men and young women, respectively) but these are for individuals who are essentially sedentary.[6] Obviously, regular exercise increases energy requirements.[12] For strength athletes energy requirements may be 40–50% greater.[13] This means that recommended energy intake (kJ/kg) should be about 275 for young male and about 155 for young female strength athletes. However, large individual differences can occur so it must be understood that these are only guidelines. Consequently, gains in body mass should be monitored closely and regular assessments of muscle growth versus gains in body fat content are recommended to fine-tune these recommendations on an individual basis.

Dietary Carbohydrate

Although stored fat can provide significant energy for prolonged and/or moderate-intensity exercise, it is well established that carbohydrate is the major muscle fuel—particularly when exercise is intense such as would occur with strength training. The underlying reason relates to the maximal rate at which energy for muscle contraction (adenosine triphosphate [ATP]) can be regenerated. Oxidative energy delivery takes several minutes to be fully used and has a maximal ATP delivery rate of about 2.5 mmol/kg dry matter/sec. This is much less than anaerobic energy delivery that is instantaneous and can deliver in excess of 11 mmol/kg dry matter/sec.[14] During situations in which carbohydrate stores are depleted, i.e., starvation and/or prolonged exercise, body protein can be mobilized to help meet the energy need[15] and/or to optimize aerobic energy production by increasing the concentration of tricarboxylic acid cycle intermediates via the alanine aminotransferase reaction (anaplerotic role).[16] Both situations would be disadvantageous for strength athletes as they would lead to decreases in muscle mass and strength. As a result, carbohydrate intake is critical for strength athletes and daily intake should be at least 5–6 g/kg—for some, even higher.

Dietary Protein Quality

A variety of methods have been used to assess the quality of food protein including biological value, net protein utilization, protein efficiency ratio, and protein digestibility-corrected amino acid score (PDCAAS). Perhaps the best one of these is the latter because it evaluates the amino acid content of a food relative to human requirements.[17]

For strength athletes, the best way to ensure adequate protein intake is to consume daily a variety of protein foods totaling about 1.5–2.0 $g \cdot kg^{-1}$ together with sufficient total energy. Although vegetarians can obtain this quantity of dietary protein, it is more difficult as grains, vegetables, and fruits are typically lacking one or more of the indispensable amino acids. This suggests that vegetarian strength athletes may experience less than optimal mass/strength gains and some recent data support this possibility at least in men aged 59–69 years.[18]

Whether consuming certain protein types might be advantageous for strength athletes is intriguing, but the available data are far too inconclusive to make definitive recommendations. Recently, whey protein (isolates or hydrolyzed peptides) have become a popular sports supplement. Clearly, whey protein has high bioavailability

Protein Quality Evaluation Methods

Biological Value (%) is calculated as retained nitrogen/absorbed nitrogen × 100. To illustrate how this provides an evaluation of protein quality, consider a scenario in which all amino acids in a protein are used for protein synthesis. Here, retained and absorbed nitrogen would be equal and the biological value would equal 100%. Conversely, if some indispensable amino acids are not available in the protein source, protein synthesis is impaired and some unused nitrogen is excreted from the body, i.e., retained nitrogen decreases relative to absorbed and the biological value drops below 100%. Consequently, some foods such as complete protein foods (e.g., milk) have high biological values (95%), while incomplete protein foods are much lower (i.e., corn [60%]). Note: It is not possible to have a biological value >100%. Net Protein Utilization is a similar measure but involves a direct measure of retained nitrogen, i.e., destruction and analysis of the body, and therefore is only used with animal studies. Protein Efficiency Ratio is determined as body mass gain/protein intake and, although a useful measure when used in growing animals, has little value for humans for two reasons. First, this method is not used in human experiments because, ethically, human subjects cannot be deprived of necessary nutrients. Second, the difference in species growth rates, i.e., lower in humans versus rats, results in errors when animal data are used to estimate human needs. Protein Digestibility-Corrected Amino Acid Score is based on the amino acid content of a food corrected for digestibility. The score reflects the limiting indispensable amino acids (those amino acids that humans cannot synthesize) in a food. The reference value used is the requirement for a 2–5-year-old individual. This provides a built-in safety buffer because protein needs of this age group are greater than for adults.

and its content of several important amino acids (gluta-mine, leucine, isoleucine, and valine) makes it a high-quality protein. However, whether its effects on strength gains surpass those of other protein sources is contro-versial. One recent study suggests whey supplementation for 3 months can help promote positive changes in both muscle performance and body fat.[19] However, at least in overweight subjects on a strength training program con-suming a hypo-energy diet, supplementation with casein (1.5 g/kg/day) produced greater gains in muscle strength and greater losses in fat mass when compared with whey supplementation.[20] In another study, isoenergetic supp-lementation with whey, soy, casein, or maltodextrin (0.7 g/kg/day) combined with a strength training program in young men produced similar gains in muscle size and strength.[21] These latter data fail to support the idea that one protein type is superior to another, but also because the maltodextrin group responded as well as the protein groups did, it could be that the protein content of the subjects' typical diet (1.4–1.6 g/kg/day) provided suffi-cient amino acids to maximally stimulate protein synthe-sis. Combining several dietary proteins may be the best approach to promote muscle mass and strength gains with training because of differences in digestibility (i.e., casein is absorbed more slowly than whey protein).[22] Therefore, a mixture of proteins could provide the nec-essary building blocks (i.e., amino acids) for muscle over a more prolonged period of time, which, when combined with the anabolic stimulus of regular strength training could enhance muscle gains, at least theoreti-cally. However, to date, this theory has not been tested experimentally.

Evidently, some amino acids are more important than are others. Obviously, the indispensable amino acids are likely candidates, as they cannot be produced in the body. Of these, the branched-chain amino acids (leucine, isoleucine, and valine) are most often implicated (see Chapter 5). Branched-chain amino acid supplementation has been reported to minimize nitrogen losses associ-ated with short-term bed rest.[23] However, this and other studies that examine protein synthesis during catabolic situations (starvation, burn/surgery patients, individuals exposed to microgravity, etc.) must be interpreted with caution because minimizing a catabolic situation may be mechanistically different than stimulating an already enhanced protein synthetic rate, which is the case with strength training. Recently, as little as 6 g of indispensable amino acids (leucine, lysine, phenylalanine, threonine, valine, histidine, isoleucine, methionine at 1.12, 0.93, 0.93, 0.88, 0.7, 0.65, 0.6, 0.19 g, respectively) and 35 g of sucrose ingested 1 or 3 hours following a strength session enhanced the muscle protein synthetic response of the exercise alone (FIG. 14-3).[24] This response is likely medi-ated by both insulin and amino acids acting in concert. It remains to be seen whether this represents the optimal combination of amino acids to maximize muscle growth

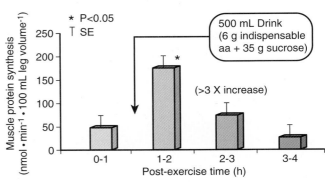

Figure 14-3. Effect of ingesting an amino acid–sucrose mixture fol-lowing a strength-training session on muscle protein synthetic rate. Note the large increase in protein synthesis following nutrient inges-tion, suggesting that the anabolic effect of strength exercise might be significantly enhanced with appropriate post-exercise nutrition. (*Data from* Rasmussen BB, Tipton KD, Miller SL, et al. An oral essential amino acid-carbohydrate supplement enhances muscle protein anabolism after resistance exercise. J Appl Physiol 2000;88:386–392.)

or if other combinations are superior. For example, leucine was the largest single amino acid in the mixture and some data indicate that by itself leucine is a potent stimulator of protein synthesis.[25,26] Moreover, oral administration of leucine, phenylalanine, and arginine or leucine, pheny-lalanine, and wheat protein hydrolysate can produce a large insulin release[27] which, when combined with ade-quate carbohydrate, increases muscle glycogen synthesis when compared to carbohydrate alone.[28] Similarly, this mixture would be expected to increase protein synthetic rates assuming an adequate supply of amino acids is avail-able. Unfortunately, many of these types of supplement studies include several compounds in a cocktail, mak-ing mechanistic determinations difficult. For example, branched-chain amino acid plus arginine and ornithine supplementation have been shown to enhance hormonal responses that may contribute to the hypertrophic response.[29] Moreover, branched-chain amino acids and glutamine combined with whey protein supplementation may enhance fat-free mass gains with strength training when compared with the same program and whey alone.[30] Finally, a variety of potential benefits of glutamine sup-plementation for athletes (including positive effects on immune function, muscle hypertrophy, and insulin sensi-tivity) have recently been published.[31]

Exercise Intensity, Type, Duration, and Training

Exercise Intensity

Several early studies indicated that at least with aerobic-type exercise, the contribution of amino acids to exer-cise energy production was linearly related to exercise intensity.[32–35] The branched-chain amino acids (leucine, isoleucine, and valine) are the major ones oxidized and the mechanism responsible is thought to be an exercise intensity–dependent activation of the limiting enzyme (branched-chain oxoacid dehydrogenase activity) in their oxidation pathway.[35,37]

Exercise Type

Apparently any increased protein need for strength exercise does not involve this exercise intensity mechanism (above) because, despite the intense nature of this type of exercise, amino acid oxidation remains unchanged (FIG. 14-4).[37] Likely, this is a result of the large anaerobic component of strength exercise. Consequently, if bodybuilders need large amounts of protein it is not to provide auxiliary exercise fuel (carbohydrate provides that) but rather because sufficient amino acids must be available to maximize any increase in muscle synthetic rate produced by the exercise stimulus. Several studies indicate that there may be some truth to this commonly held belief.[38–40] However, the optimal intake would appear to be 1.5–2.0 g/kg/day. This is an amount far less than what many strength athletes consume on a regular basis. Several possibilities might explain this apparent contradiction. Obviously, the athletes could be incorrect, i.e., they may have been influenced by a powerful placebo effect.

Alternatively, some other constituent(s) in high-protein foods might, in combination with the surplus supply of amino acids, be responsible for a muscle-building effect. Several candidates are possible including creatine, a nitrogen compound found in meat and fish that has been studied recently.[41] Although not all studies report positive effects with creatine supplementation, many demonstrate significant ergogenic effects (10% or more), especially during intense brief efforts. Such exercise-enhancing effects combined with a training program might accelerate further the normal gains observed with strength training indirectly via a super training effect.[42] Moreover, some data exist indicating that creatine has anabolic effects on muscle,[43–45] which could also play a role. Finally, although associated with a variety of adverse health effects, some compounds (i.e., anabolic steroids) are known to be anabolic[46] and it is possible that the high-protein intakes consumed by some strength athletes are only advantageous when combined with these agents.

Exercise Duration

With exercise duration, energy use from amino acids increases likely due to the decreased availability of carbohydrate as the body's stores of this important fuel can be depleted in a single exercise bout.[5,14] A similar response occurs with starvation, i.e., protein can be used for energy once the limited carbohydrate stores are exhausted.[47] This may play some role for strength athletes if training sessions are prolonged.

Training History

In endurance exercise training, it appears that amino acid oxidation both at rest and during exercise increases[48–50] perhaps due to training-induced changes in branched-chain oxoacid dehydrogenase activity.[50] Yet, this possibility remains controversial as the data from one study disagree[51] and no obvious explanation to explain the discrepancy is available. The data with strength training are also somewhat unclear. It has been suggested that protein needs of novice bodybuilders might exceed those of more experienced strength trainers.[52] Although this is consistent with the well-known observation of greater gains in muscle growth of novice strength trainers, several other studies indicate protein needs remain at similar levels for more experienced strength athletes.[39,40] A recent study with acute eccentric exercise demonstrated similar increases in protein synthesis between resistance-trained and untrained subjects but that protein breakdown was greater in the latter.[53] This observation may explain why prior eccentric exercise reduces subsequent muscle damage and pain,[54] and because eccentric exercise is part of most training programs this may indicate that the magnitude of increased protein needs induced by strength training could be reduced as one becomes more experienced. However, at this point in time, this question cannot be answered conclusively. More study of the protein needs of novice versus experienced strength trainers is definitely needed.

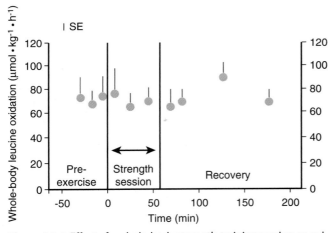

Figure 14-4. Effect of a whole-body strength-training session on oxidation of the amino acid leucine. Note that both during and for several hours following the exercise there is no change in oxidation of this representative amino acid. These data indicate that if increased dietary protein is beneficial for strength athletes it is not because of a need for additional amino acids to provide fuel for exercise. (*Data from* Tarnopolsky MA, Atkinson SA, MacDougall JD, et al. Whole body leucine metabolism during and after resistance exercise in fed humans. Med Sci Sports Exerc 1991;23:326–333.)

Gender

Despite the popularity of strength training among women in recent years, there has been little scientific study of specifically how women respond to this type of exercise. With endurance exercise, some data suggest that women use less protein for energy than men perhaps as a result of differences in fat use induced by gender-specific hormonal responses.[55–60] Rodent data indicate that estradiol is protective for muscle cell membranes and, consequently, part of this response may be due to less exercise-induced damage to the muscle membrane in women.[61–63] Moreover, there is some evidence that protein need with endurance exercise may even vary across the menstrual cycle.[64] Unfortunately, the effects of strength training on protein requirements in females have not been investigated extensively. Based on the observed gender differences in metabolism and the known differences in hormonal responses, it is quite possible that women respond to strength exercise somewhat differently than men. As a result, detailed study of how strength exercise training is influenced by dietary protein in women is needed.

Age

Muscle mass is dramatically reduced in both men and women with advancing age. Called sarcopenia, this phenomenon has considerable significance because it leads to a decreased quality of life, and often, major health care expenses for the associated medical/nursing care. Moreover, these costs represent only a fraction of what is likely to come over the next 20–30 years as the post-war baby boom generation enters the age range in which sarcopenia begins to affect them. Clearly, the effects of aging on the body's ability to respond undoubtedly play a role in this response—it has been reported that myofibrillar protein synthesis is reduced by 30% in individuals over 60 years of age[65] (FIG. 14-5); however, inactivity must always be a factor. Indeed, strength training has been shown to augment muscle function in both men and women even in the 10th decade of life.[66] Further, this type of functional improvement is not the result of neurological changes alone as muscle protein synthesis can be increased with 3 months of strength exercise even in frail 76–92-year-old men and women.[67] Some data indicate that as little as 10 days of energy and protein supplementation can enhance protein synthesis and fat-free (lean) mass at least in poorly nourished 60–90-year-old men and women.[68] As nutrient intake is frequently less than ideal in the elderly and energy and macronutrient needs are increased with strength exercise (as discussed above) it is logical to assume that nutrient supplementation would enhance the response of muscle to strength exercise. One study observed that a supplement containing 60% carbohydrate, 23% fat, and 17% protein (1500 kJ/day) given to 72–98-

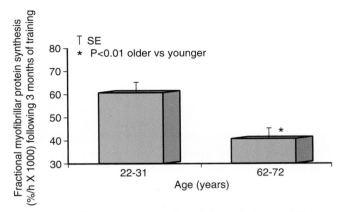

Figure 14-5. Effect of age on muscle protein synthetic rate following 3 months of strength training. Although both age groups increase, note the 30% decreased response observed in the older subjects compared to the younger. (*Data from* Welle S, Thornton CA. High-protein meals do not enhance myofibrillar synthesis after resistance exercise in 62- to 75-year-old men and women. Am J Physiol 1998;274:E677–E683.)

year-old men and women who participated in a 10-week strength training program produced significant increases in muscle strength and size than the same training alone (FIG. 14-6).[69] Although increasing dietary protein intake from 0.6 to 1.2 to 2.4 g/kg did not alter myofibrillar protein synthesis in elderly men and women, these data do not necessarily implicate energy as the causative factor because this latter study only involved 1 day of supplementation and a brief (3-day) strength program.[70] As discussed above, acute versus chronic exercise could be a significant factor in determining nutrient need. Further,

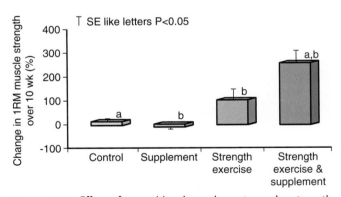

Figure 14-6. Effect of a nutritional supplement, regular strength exercise, and regular strength exercise combined with the nutritional supplement over 10 weeks on strength gains (one repetition maximum) in elderly men and women (72–98 yrs). Note the significant effect of the combined treatment. Although not shown here, percent muscle size gains followed the same trend (Control, −16.1, −14.2; Supplement, −2.8, −0.4; Strength Exercise, +4.6, −11.5; Strength Exercise & Supplement, +12.8, +10.1 for type I and type II fiber types, respectively). (*Data from* Fiatarone Singh MA, Ding W, Manfredi TJ, et al. Insulin-like growth factor I in skeletal muscle after weight lifting exercise in frail elders. Am J Physiol 1999;277:E135–E143.)

length of time on the dietary treatment is likely critical. Finally, at least in older women, there is some evidence that quantity of the protein per intake may affect subsequent protein synthetic rate. Over a 14-day interval in older women (60–73 years), when the protein intake was divided equally into four aliquots (0800, 1200, 1600, 2000 h) fat-free mass gain was significantly less when compared with a situation in which most of the protein was consumed a large bolus (79% at 1200 h, 7% at 0800 h, and 14% at 2000 h).[71] However, the bolus protein-feeding pattern had no such effect in younger (26 ± 1 yr) women.[72] Although clearly more study is necessary before these data can be explained fully, mass of protein consumed and/or timing of intake throughout the day may be critical to the protein synthetic response. Finally, the latter two studies were conducted on sedentary subjects and it is likely that these factors become even more important when combined with chronic strength exercise.

Due to the increased requirements of the growth process, protein intake is also important for young children and adolescents.[4,73] Although not well studied, it is quite likely that regular strength training could lead to even greater requirements in this population.[74–76] Moreover, from a practical perspective, this is likely to be of increasing importance in the future as strength training is becoming more of an essential component of almost all sporting endeavors. For the same reason, women who are pregnant who continue to exercise would be another group likely to benefit from additional dietary protein.

Timing of Intake Relative to Training Sessions

It is well understood by the athletic community that increased carbohydrate intake (loading) can significantly enhance exercise performance in situations in which muscle glycogen stores are limiting. Less well known, but of critical importance is that there is a brief window of opportunity perhaps 60 minutes or so following exercise in which the muscle glycogen synthetic rate is significantly greater than at any other time during the day.[77,78] Similarly, it is becoming clear that strength exercise causes disruptions in both muscle protein synthesis (FIG. 14-7) and degradation, resulting over time in substantial muscle growth.[79–81] Perhaps, nutrient supplementation postexercise might optimize muscle growth. For example, this overall growth response could be limited by energy and/or amino acid availability. If so, providing either or both could enhance muscle growth/repair via increasing protein synthesis or decreasing protein degradation. Some evidence for this possibility can be found in Figure 14-3.[8,24,82,83] Combining carbohydrate and amino acids may be the best approach because the insulin released in response to the carbohydrate stimulates amino acid uptake by muscle, leading, at least potentially, to enhanced protein synthetic

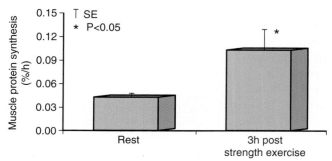

Figure 14-7. Effect of a strength-training session on muscle protein synthesis. Note the significant increase following the exercise session. Although the exact onset and the duration of this effect remain to be mapped out it is clear that strength training is a powerful stimulator of muscle growth. (*Data from* Biolo G, Maggi SP, Williams BD, et al. Increased rates of muscle protein turnover and amino acid transport after resistance exercise in humans. Am J Physiol 1995; 268:E514–E520.)

rates (FIGS. 14-3 AND 14-8).[8,24,27,28,82–84] As mentioned above, some amino acids are also powerful stimulators of insulin release.[24,27] Moreover, other hormones important for positive training adaptations could be involved.[29] It appears that the essential amino acids are the most critical and that only small amounts may be necessary.[24] As further study clarifies the details of the effects of strength training on net protein balance in muscle it should become possible to prescribe precise recommendations regarding type, amounts, and timing of nutrient supplementation to maximize the anabolic stimulus following strength training. If so, this information would be of considerable benefit not only to the athletic community but also to any group of individuals who have lost muscle function due to disease or disuse (i.e., post-surgery, injuries, elderly, zero-gravity environment, etc.).

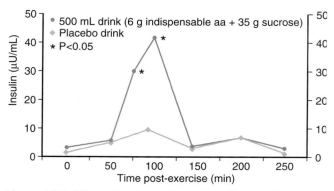

Figure 14-8. Effect of amino acid–sucrose ingestion following a strength-training session on plasma insulin concentration. Note the significant increase in plasma insulin that would be expected to enhance both muscle amino acid uptake and muscle protein synthetic rate. (*Data from* Rasmussen BB, Tipton KD, Miller SL, et al. An oral essential amino acid-carbohydrate supplement enhances muscle protein anabolism after resistance exercise. J Appl Physiol 2000;88:386–392.)

High-Protein Intake—Is It Safe?

Chris Street, MS, CSCS

Excess protein has been considered by many nutritional experts to be hazardous to the health of athletes. According to research from the Medlantic Research Foundation, "Protein intake is more than adequate in the USA and further increases could have negative effects on the prevalence of renal disease and osteoporosis." Certainly, there is little evidence in active, athletic individuals that high-protein consumption is harmful to one's health.

Because of the kidney's role in processing and ridding the body of nitrogenous waste, this organ could be particularly susceptible to damage from being overworked. Theoretically, large amounts of nitrogen from a high-protein diet may become toxic. Despite its role in nitrogen excretion, there are presently no data in the peer-reviewed scientific literature demonstrating the normal kidney will be damaged by the increased demands of protein consumed in quantities above the RDA. Furthermore, *real world* examples support this contention as kidney problems are nonexistent in the bodybuilding community in which high-protein has been the norm for over half a century.

Researchers Poortmans and Dellalieux from the Department of Physiological Chemistry, Institute of Physical Education and Kinesiotherapy at Free University in Brussels, Belgium, studied the effects of a high- and medium-protein intake in bodybuilders and other well-trained athletes. Subjects underwent blood and urine sampling in addition to keeping a 7-day record of their food intake. Data demonstrated that despite higher plasma concentrations of uric acid and calcium, the group of bodybuilders on the high-protein diet had normal renal clearance of creatinine, urea, and albumin. Interestingly, the nitrogen balance for both groups became positive when daily protein intake exceeded 1.26 g/kg. Researchers concluded that protein intake under 2.8 g/kg/day does not impair renal function in well-trained athletes.

Animal data enforce the belief that a high-protein diet does not damage the mammalian kidney. This lack of toxicity is present even at extremely high amounts for prolonged periods of time. Zaragoza and colleagues fed rats a dietary regimen in which protein constituted 80% of their energy intake for more than half of their life span. In spite of the amount of protein and the time of administration, no deleterious effects were noted.

High-protein diets may increase the excretion of calcium, a particular concern to women at risk for osteoporosis. However, work by Orwell and Porter & Johnson suggest that increased protein intake is often beneficial and associated with anabolic processes in bone. In a study published in *Calcified Tissue International,* Cooper et al. studied bone density (dual-photon absorptiometry in the lumbar spine and proximal femur and single-photon absorptiometry in the distal and mid-radius) in 290 women ranging from 30 to 94 years of age. Dietary information on calcium, phosphorus, vitamin D, protein, fat, and total energy were obtained from a 7-day food record. Among the 72 premenopausal women studied, there was a statistically significant positive association between protein intake and bone mineral content in the distal radius and proximal femur. Postmenopausal women showed no relationship between protein and bone mineral content. From the food record, all of the women studied consumed a mean of 75 g/day of protein. These results suggest that dietary protein consumption may be a determinant of the peak bone mass attained by premenopausal white women. They further commented that the finding of a positive association between protein consumption and bone mineral content was a surprise because animal and human studies on calcium metabolism show excess urinary excretion of the mineral as protein intake increases. According to work by Freudenheim et al., it is possible that the hypercalciuric effect of protein is offset by a hypocalciuric effect of phosphorus, which is present in substantial quantities in diets high in meat protein. In women who engage in strength training, any hypercalciuric effect of protein may be offset by the strong effect this mode of exercise has on increasing bone density. There may be further benefits on bone from a high-protein diet and weight training via increased insulin-like growth factor-1, which has been shown to have a positive effect on bone mass. Levels of this peptide hormone have been shown to increase in strength-trained subjects after a protein-carbohydrate supplement and in those who consume a protein supplement after hip fracture.

Atherogenic effects of high-protein diets have been overstated, especially in regards to athletic populations. In the past, strength athletes and football players (especially offensive and defensive linemen) were known for consuming protein sources that were high in saturated fat such as various forms of fast food, whole milk, and fatty cuts of beef. Today, athletes have access to protein sources that contain minimal amounts of fat like chicken breast without skin, fish, lean cuts of beef, and egg whites. Protein supplements available today contain little to no fat. To consider a diet high in protein that is also high in fat is an outdated concept. With the variety of lean, whole-food sources of protein and the multitude of protein supplements available, some athletes may need to be advised to consume additional fat in an effort to get sufficient calories to meet their daily requirement.

Brown WV. Dietary recommendations to prevent coronary heart disease. Ann N Y Acad Sci 1990;598:376–388.

Cooper C, Atkinson EJ, Hensrund DD, et al. Dietary protein intake and bone mass in women. Calcif Tissue Int 1996;58:320–325.

Dornemann TM, McMurray RG, Renner JB, Anderson JJ. Effects of high-intensity resistance exercise on bone mineral density and muscle strength of 40–50 year-old women. J Sports Med Phys Fitness 1997;37(4):246–251.

Freudenheim JL, Johnson NE, Smith EL. Relationships between usual nutrient intake and bone mineral content of women 35–65 years of age: longitudinal and cross-sectional analysis. Am J Clin Nutr 1986;44:863–876.

Huang BK, Golden LA, Tarjan G, et al. Insulin-like growth factor I production is essential for anabolic effects of thyroid hormone in osteoblasts. J Bone Miner Res 2000;15(2):188–197.

Kraemer WJ, Volek JS, Bush JA, et al. Hormonal responses to consecutive days of heavy-resistance exercise with or without nutritional supplementation. J Appl Physiol 1998;85(4):1544–1555.

Orwell ES. The effects of dietary protein insufficiency and excess on skeletal health. Bone 1992;13:343–350.

Parkhouse WS, Coupland DC, Li C, Vanderhoek KJ. IGF-1 bioavailability is increased by resistance training in older women with low bone mineral density. Mech Ageing Dev 2000;113(2):75–83.

Poortmans JR, Dellalieux O. Do regular high-protein diets have potential health risks on kidney function in athletes? Int J Sports Nutr 2000;10(1):28–38.

Porter KH, Johnson MA. Dietary protein supplementation and recovery from femoral fracture. Nutr Rev 1999;56(11):337–340.

Schurch M, Rizzoli R, Slosman D, et al. Protein supplements increase serum insulin-like growth factor-1 levels and attenuate proximal femur bone loss in patients with recent hip fracture. Ann Intern Med 1998;128:801–809.

Zaragoza R, Renau-Piqueras J, Portioles M, et al. Rats fed a prolonged high-protein diet show an increase in nitrogen metabolism and liver megamitochondria. Arch Biochem Biophys 1987;258(2): 426–435.

 Current Controversy: Protein Intake

Although recent scientific research has provided some support for the idea that regular strength training increases dietary protein needs, these data indicate any benefit appears to plateau at protein intakes around 1.5 g/kg/day. In contrast, there are some data suggesting that much greater protein intakes enhance muscle size and strength gains even further; however, it is possible that these latter studies were confounded by interacting effects from exogenous anabolic agent use and/or by variable training/peaking preparations due to the timing of competitions held during the data collection. Despite these experimental limitations, many strength athletes are convinced that these high-protein intakes are advantageous. If so, it should be possible not only to document this in a controlled setting, but also to clearly describe the underlying mechanism(s) responsible. This needs to be done before such high-protein intakes can be recommended.

Dragan I, Vasiliu A, Georgescu E. Effects of increased supply of protein on elite weight-lifters. In: Galesloot TE, Tinbergen BJ, eds. Milk Proteins '84. Wageningen, The Netherlands: Pudoc, 1985: 99–103.

Laritcheva KA, Yalavaya NI, Shubin VI, Smornov PV. Study of energy expenditure and protein needs of top weight lifters. In: Parizkova J, Rogozkin VA, eds. Nutrition, Physical Fitness & Health. Baltimore: University Park Press, 1978:155–163.

SUMMARY

Many factors appear to affect the dietary protein needs of strength athletes. Current experimental data indicate that a dietary protein intake of about 1.5–2.0 g/kg/day should be sufficient for strength athletes. However, this may not be so if energy and/or carbohydrate intake is insufficient. This latter concern is possible for many female athletes and for both genders if dieting or extreme training energy expenditures occur. Other high-risk groups include those with elevated baseline requirements such as the elderly and anyone who is experiencing rapid growth (children, adolescents, and women who are pregnant). Areas that need to be clarified involve not only which nutrients/compounds affect the anabolic response induced by strength exercise, but also the best timing of intake relative to strength exercise and, of course, the underlying mechanisms responsible. Finally, it appears that the timing of nutrient/compound ingestion relative to a weight-training session could be an extremely fruitful research area to pursue. As the details regarding how nutrition can alter the response of muscle to strength training become unraveled, it is likely that it will not only be possible to enhance athletic performance but it will also be possible to improve the quality of life for significant numbers of the population and at the same time lower substantial health care costs in the elderly.

AUTHOR'S RECOMMENDATION

Based on scientific research the typical protein intake of strength athletes should be approximately 1.5–2.0 g/kg/day. Although some data indicate protein type may be important, this topic is controversial and until more data become available the best advice is to consume a mixture of protein types. Finally, evidence is beginning to accumulate suggesting that the availability of amino acids (especially the indispensable amino acids) and carbohydrate during the immediate post-exercise period may play a significant role in subsequent muscle growth. Therefore, it is recommended that strength athletes attempt to ensure an optimal anabolic environment by consuming a protein/carbohydrate source both before and after their training sessions. Precise recommendations are not possible yet, but it appears that a few indispensable amino acids may limit the post-exercise anabolic response. If so, assuming that one's energy and insulin supply are adequate, only small quantities of certain indispensable amino acids may be needed to maximize muscle growth.

FUTURE RESEARCH

Clearly, the RDA should be different for athletes versus sedentary individuals. This is evident particularly as it applies to bodybuilding and other strength-power athletes. Also, the notion that high-protein diets confer harm to various organs warrants further investigation. Nonetheless, at this point there is no evidence to support such a claim. The notion that certain protein sources are superior for promoting muscle protein accretion is an idea worth investigating. For instance, many athletes anecdotally (i.e., trial and error approach) believe that animal sources such as beef and chicken as well as protein found in many of the popular meal replacement powders (usually consisting of whey protein concentrate) are superior to other sources (i.e., plant sources) with regards to the promotion of lean mass gains. In the clinical arena, future research efforts might examine the establishment of protein requirements for those being treated clinically with various wasting diseases. Acquired immune deficiency syndrome (AIDS), burn patients, sepsis, trauma victims, those recovering from surgery, and patients in injury rehabilitation could greatly benefit from an increased intake of protein and calories.

REFERENCES

1. von Liebig J. Animal Chemistry or Organic Chemistry in Its Application to Physiology. Gregory G (Translator). London: Taylor & Walton, 1842.
2. Lemon PWR. Effects of exercise on dietary protein requirements. Int J Sports Nutr 1998;8:426–447.
3. Rennie MJ. Physical exertion, amino acid and protein metabolism, and protein requirements. In: The Role of Protein and Amino Acids in Sustaining and Enhancing Performance. Washington, DC: Institute of Medicine, National Academy Press, 1999:243–253.
4. US Food and Nutrition Board. Recommended Dietary Allowances. Washington, DC: National Academy Press, 1989.
5. Åstrand P-O, Rodahl K. Textbook of Work Physiology. New York: McGraw-Hill, 1977.
6. Food and Agricultural Organization, World Health Organization, and United Nations University: Energy and Protein Requirements. Geneva: World Health Organization, 1985, Tech Rep Ser 724.
7. Lemon PWR. Effects of exercise on protein metabolism. In: Maughan RJ, ed. Nutrition in Sport. Oxford: Blackwell Science, 2000:133–152.
8. Young VR. Adult amino acid requirements: the case for a major revision in current recommendations. J Nutr 1994;124:1517S–1523S.
9. Young VR. Amino acid flux and requirements: Counterpoint tentative estimates are feasible and necessary. In: The Role of Protein and Amino Acids in Sustaining and Enhancing Performance. Washington, DC: Institute of Medicine, National Academy Press, 1999:217–242.
10. Milward DJ. Inherent difficulties in defining amino acid requirements. In: The Role of Protein and Amino Acids in Sustaining and Enhancing Performance. Washington, DC: Institute of Medicine, National Academy Press, 1999:169–216.
11. Munro HN. Carbohydrate and fat as factors in protein utilization and metabolism. Physiol Rev 1951;31:449–488.
12. Montoye HJ. Energy costs of exercise and sport. In: Maughan RJ, ed. Nutrition in Sport. Oxford: Blackwell Science, 2000:53–72.
13. American College of Sports Medicine. Encyclopedia of Sports Sciences and Medicine. New York: MacMillan, 1971:1128–1129.
14. Hultman E, Greenhaff PL. Carbohydrate metabolism in exercise. In: Maughan RJ, ed. Nutrition in Sport. Oxford: Blackwell Science, 2000:85–96.
15. Lemon PWR, Mullin JP. Effect of initial muscle glycogen levels on protein catabolism during exercise. J Appl Physiol 1980;48:624–629.
16. Wagenmakers AJM. Amino acid metabolism in exercise. In: Maughan RJ, ed. Nutrition in Sport. Oxford: Blackwell Science, 2000:119–132.
17. Henley EC, Kuster JM. Protein quality evaluation by protein digestibility-corrected amino acid scoring. Food Tech 1994;48:74–77.
18. Campbell WW, Barton Jr ML, Cyr-Campbell D, et al. Effects of an omnivorous diet compared with a lacto-ovovegetarian diet on resistance-training-induced changes in body composition and skeletal muscle in older men. Am J Clin Nutr 1999;70:1032–1039.
19. Lands LC, Grey VL, Smountas AA. Effect of supplementation with a cysteine donor on muscular performance. J Appl Physiol 1999;87:1381–1385.

20. Demling RH, DeSanti L. Effect of a hypercaloric diet, increased protein intake, and resistance training on lean mass gains and fat mass loss in overweight police officers. Ann Nutr Metab 2000;44:21–29.

21. Appicelli P, Ziegenfuss T, Lowery L, et al. Does type of dietary protein supplementation affect muscle strength/size gains in adult bodybuilders? Can J Appl Physiol 1995;20(suppl):1P.

22. Boirie Y, Dandin M, Gachon P, et al. Slow and fast dietary protein differently modulate postprandial protein accretion. Proc Nat Acad Sci 1997;94:14930–14935.

23. Stein TP, Schluter MD, Leskiw MJ, Boden G. Attenuation of the protein wasting associated with bed rest by branched-chain amino acids. Nutrition 1999;15:656–660.

24. Rasmussen BB, Tipton KD, Miller SL, et al. An oral essential amino acid-carbohydrate supplement enhances muscle protein anabolism after resistance exercise. J Appl Physiol 2000;88:386–392.

25. Antalikova J, Jankela J, Baranovska M. The effect of branched chain amino acids on protein synthesis in two skeletal muscles of Japanese quail. Physiol Res 1999;48:59–63.

26. Anthony JC, Anthony TG, Layman DK. Leucine supplementation enhances skeletal muscle recovery in rats following exercise. J Nutr 1999;129:1102–1106.

27. van Loon LJC, Saris WHM, Verhagen H, Wagenmakers AJM. Plasma insulin responses after ingestion of different amino acid or protein mixtures with carbohydrate. Am J Clin Nutr 2000;72:96–105.

28. van Loon LJC, Saris WHM, Kruijshoop M, Wagenmakers AJM. Maximizing postexercise muscle glycogen synthesis: carbohydrate supplementation and the application of amino acid or protein hydrolysate mixtures. Am J Clin Nutr 2000;72:106–111.

29. Di Luigi L, Guidetti L, Pigozzi F, et al. Acute amino acids supplementation enhances pituitary responsiveness in athletes. Med Sci Sports Exerc 1999;31:1748–1754.

30. Colker-Carlon M, Swain MA, Fabrucini B, et al. Effects of supplemental protein on body composition and muscular strength in healthy athletic male adults. Curr Therapeutic Res 2000;61:19–28.

31. Antonio J, Street C. Glutamine: a potentially useful supplement for athletes. Can J Appl Physiol 1999;24:1–14.

32. White TP, Brooks GA. [U-^{14}C] glucose, -alanine, and leucine oxidation in rats at rest and two intensities of running. J Appl Physiol 1981;241:E155–E165.

33. Lemon PWR, Nagle FJ, Mullin JP, Benevenga NJ. In vivo leucine oxidation at rest and during two intensities of exercise. J Appl Physiol 1982;53:947–954.

34. Babij P, Matthews SM, Rennie MJ. Changes in blood ammonia, lactate, and amino acids in relation to workload during bicycle ergometer exercise in man. Eur J Appl Physiol 1983;50:405–411.

35. Kasperek GJ, Snider RD. Effect of exercise intensity and starvation on the activation of branched-chain keto acid dehydrogenase by exercise. Am J Physiol 1987;252:E33–E37.

36. Wagenmakers AJM, Beckers EJ, Brouns F, et al. Carbohydrate supplementation, glycogen depletion, and amino acid metabolism during exercise. Am J Physiol 1991;260:E883–E890.

37. Tarnopolsky MA, Atkinson SA, MacDougall JD, et al. Whole body leucine metabolism during and after resistance exercise in fed humans. Med Sci Sports Exerc 1991;23:326–333.

38. Fern EB, Bielinski RN, Schutz Y. Effects of exaggerated amino acid and protein supply in man. Experientia 1991;47:168–172.

39. Lemon PWR, Tarnopolsky MA, MacDougall JD, Atkinson SA. Protein requirements and muscle mass/strength changes during intensive training in novice bodybuilders. J Appl Physiol 1992;73:767–775.

40. Tarnopolsky MA, Atkinson SA, MacDougall JD, et al. Evaluation of protein requirements for trained strength athletes. J Appl Physiol 1992;73:1986–1995.

41. Greenhaff PL. Creatine. In: Maughan RJ, ed. Nutrition in Sport. Oxford: Blackwell Science, 2000:367–378.

42. Schulte JN, Noreen EE, Bachman LD, et al. Does creatine monohydrate supplementation enhance muscle development due to a super-training effect? Med Sci Sports Exerc 2000;32(suppl):S135.

43. Ingwall JS, Weiner CD, Morales MF, et al. Specificity of creatine in the control of muscle protein synthesis. J Cell Biol 1974;63:145–151.

44. Haussinger D, Roth ER, Lang F, Gerok W. Cellular hydration state: an important determinant of protein catabolism in health and disease. Lancet 1993;341:1330–1332.

45. Dangott B, Schultz E, Mozdziak PE. Dietary creatine monohydrate supplementation increases satellite cell mitotic activity during compensatory hypertrophy. Int J Sports Med 2000;21:13–16.

46. Bhasin S, Storer TW, Berman N, et al. The effects of supraphysiologic doses of testosterone on muscle size and strength in normal men. N Engl J Med 1996;335:1–7.

47. Cahill GF Jr. Starvation in man. N Engl J Med 1970;282:668–675.

48. Dohm GL, Hecker AL, Brown WE, et al. Adaptation of protein metabolism to endurance training. Biochem J 1977;164:705–708.

49. Henderson SA, Black AL, Brooks GA. Leucine turnover in trained rats during exercise. Am J Physiol 1985;249:E137–E144.

50. Layman DK, Paul GL, Olken MH. Amino acid metabolism during exercise. In: Wolinsky I, Hickson JF, eds. Nutrition in Exercise and Sport. 2nd ed. Boca Raton, FL: CRC Press, 1994:123–137.

51. Hood DA, Terjung RL. Effect of endurance training on leucine oxidation in perfused rat skeletal muscle. Am J Physiol 1987;253:E648–656.

52. Tarnopolsky MA, MacDougall JD, Atkinson SA. Influence of protein intake and training status on nitrogen balance and lean body mass. J Appl Physiol 1988;64:187–193.

53. Phillips SM, Tipton KD, Ferrando AA, Wolfe RR. Resistance training reduces the acute exercise-induced increase in muscle protein turnover. Am J Physiol 1999;276:E118–E124.

54. Newham DJ, Jones DA, Clarkson PM. Repeated high-force eccentric exercise: effects on muscle pain and damage. J Appl Physiol 1987;63:1381–1386.

55. Tarnopolsky LJ, MacDougall JD, Atkinson SA, et al. Gender differences in substrate for endurance exercise. J Appl Physiol 1990;68:302–308.

56. Phillips SM, Atkinson SA, Tarnopolsky MA, MacDougall JD. Gender differences in leucine kinetics and nitrogen balance in endurance athletes. J Appl Physiol 1993;75:2134–2141.

57. Tarnopolsky MA, Atkinson SA, Phillips SM, MacDougall JD. Carbohydrate loading and metabolism during exercise in men and women. J Appl Physiol 1995;78:1360–1368.

58. Cortright RN, Koves TR. Sex differences in substrate metabolism and energy homeostasis. Can J Appl Physiol 2000;25:288–311.

59. Tarnopolsky MA. Gender differences in substrate metabolism during endurance exercise. Can J Appl Physiol 2000;25:312–327.

60. Tapscott EB, Kasperek GJ, Dohm GL. Effect of training on muscle protein turnover in male and female rats. Biochem Med 1982;27:254–259.

61. Amelink GJ, Kamp HH, Barr PR. Creatine kinase isoenzyme profiles after exercise in the rat: sex-linked differences in leakage of CK-MM. Pflugers Arch 1988;412:417–421.

62. Barr PR, Amelink GJ, Oldenburg B, Blankenstein MA. Prevention of exercise-induced muscle membrane damage by oestradiol. Life Sci 1988;42:2677–2681.

63. Tiidus PM. Estrogen and gender effects on muscle damage, inflammation, and oxidative stress. Can J Appl Physiol 2000;25:274–287.

64. Lamont LS, Lemon PWR, Bruot BC. Menstrual cycle and exercise effects on protein catabolism. Med Sci Sports Exerc 1987;19:106–110.

65. Welle S, Thornton C, Jozefowicz R, Statt M. Myofibrillar protein synthesis in young and old men. Am J Physiol 1993;264:E693–E698.

66. Fiatarone MA, Marks EC, Ryan ND, et al. High intensity strength training in nonagenarians: effects on skeletal muscle. J Am Med Assoc 1990;263:3029–3034.

67. Yarasheski KE, Pak-Loduca J, Hasten DL, et al. Resistance exercise training increases mixed muscle protein synthesis rate in frail men and women > 76 yr old. Am J Physiol 1999;277:E118–E125.

68. Bos C, Benamouzig R, Bruhat A, et al. Short-term protein and energy supplementation activates nitrogen kinetics and accretion in poorly nourished elderly subjects. Am J Clin Nutr 2000;71:1129–1137.

69. Fiatarone Singh MA, Ding W, Manfredi TJ, et al. Insulin-like growth factor I in skeletal muscle after weight lifting exercise in frail elders. Am J Physiol 1999;277:E135–E143.

70. Welle S, Thornton CA. High-protein meals do not enhance myofibrillar synthesis after resistance exercise in 62–75-yr-old men and women. Am J Physiol 1998;274:E677–E683.

71. Arnal MA, Mosoni L, Boirie Y, et al. Protein pulse feeding improves protein retention in elderly women. Am J Clin Nutr 1999;69:1202–1208.

72. Arnal MA, Mosoni L, Boirie Y, et al. Protein pulse feeding does not affect protein retention in young women. J Nutr 2000;130:1700–1704.
73. Lemon PWR. Nutrition for the muscular development of young athletes. In: Gisolfi CV, Lamb DR, eds. Youth, Exercise, and Sport. Carmel, CA: Benchmark Press, 1989:369–400.
74. Roemmich RN, Sinning WE. Sport-seasonal changes in body composition, growth, power, and strength of adolescent wrestlers. Int J Sports Med 1996;17:92–99.
75. Roemmich RN, Sinning WE. Weight loss and wrestling training: effects on nutrition, growth, maturation, body composition, and strength. J Appl Physiol 1997;82:1751–1759.
76. Roemmich RN, Sinning WE. Weight loss and wrestling training: effects on growth-related hormones. J Appl Physiol 1997;82:1760–1764.
77. Ivy JL, Katz AL, Culter CL, et al. Muscle glycogen synthesis after exercise: effect of time of carbohydrate ingestion. J Appl Physiol 1988;64:1480–1485.
78. Ivy J. Optimization of glycogen stores. In: Maughan RJ, ed. Nutrition in Sport. Oxford: Blackwell Science, 2000:97–111.
79. Biolo G, Maggi SP, Williams BD, et al. Increased rates of muscle protein turnover and amino acid transport after resistance exercise in humans. Am J Physiol 1995;268:E514–E520.
80. MacDougall JD, Gibala MJ, Tarnopolsky MA, et al. The time course of elevated muscle protein synthesis following heavy resistance exercise. Can J Appl Physiol 1995;20:480–486.
81. Phillips SM, Tipton KD, Aarsland A, et al. Mixed muscle protein synthesis and breakdown after resistance exercise in humans. Am J Physiol 1997;273:E99–E107.
82. Roy BD, Tarnopolsky MA, MacDougall JD, et al. Effect of glucose supplement timing on protein metabolism after resistance training. J Appl Physiol 1997;82:1882–1888.
83. Roy BD, Fowles JR, Hill R, Tarnopolsky MA. Macronutrient intake and whole body protein metabolism following resistance exercise. Med Sci Sports Exerc 2000;32:1412–1418.
84. Farrell PA, Fedele MJ, Vary TC, et al. Effects of intensity of acute-resistance exercise on rates of protein synthesis in moderately diabetic rats. J Appl Physiol 1998;85:2291–2297.

Subject Index

Page numbers in *italics* indicate figures. Page numbers followed by "t" indicate tables.

Achlorhydria, folate deficiency with, 146
Acquired immunodeficiency syndrome, whey protein and, 124, 188
ACTH. *See* Adrenocorticotropin hormone
Additives, food, nutritional supplements, distinguishing, 4–5
Adenine nucleotide, recovery and, *248*
Adenosine triphosphate, 44, 46, 101
  energy contribution from, *45*
Adipocyte
  lipolysis, *87*
  size of, 86
Adipose tissue
  fat-soluble vitamins, 139
  lipoprotein lipase, insulin sensitivity, 35
Adrenocorticotropin hormone, 242
Adrostenediol, 163–167
Adulterated, nutritional supplement categorized as, 5
Aerobics, energy cost, 21
Alanyl-glutamine, 127
Albumin clearances, with creatine, 56
Alcohol consumption, 2
  effect on biotin, 145
  folic acid deficiency from, 146
  pantothenic acid deficiency from, 144
  pyridoxine and, 143
  thiamin, 139
  vitamin C deficiency from, 147
Alertness, protein and, 33–34
Alkaline, effect of creatine on, 56
Almonds, as source of boron, 61
Alopecia, from biotin deficiency, 145
Alpha-ketoglutarate, 115–116
  animal studies, 116
  human studies, 116
  safety, toxicity, 116
Alpha-ketoisocaproate, 120–121
  animal studies, 120–121
  beta-hydroxy-betamethylbutyrate, 58
  human studies, 121
  safety, toxicity, 121
Alpha-lactalbumin, whey, 121, 187
Alpha-tocopherol, sources of, 267
Amenorrhea, as sign of overtraining, 201
Amino acid-sucrose ingestion, effect of, *310*
Amino acids, 3, 126–127, 205–206
  branched-chain, 117–118, 282
    animal studies, 117
    human studies, 117–118, 282
    safety, toxicity, 118, 282
  as growth hormone enhancers, 168–169
  metabolism, folic acid, 146
  protein requirements and, *304*

in synthesis of creatine, 47
tyrosine, protein, relationship between, 34
Amphetamine, 86
Amplitude of movement, decreased, as sign of overtraining, 201
Anabolic, defined, 15
Anabolic Steroid Control Act of 1990, 162
Anabolic steroids. *See* Androgens
Androgens, *8*, 160–179
  biosynthesis of, *95*
  pathways, *163*
  prohormones, 162–167
    androstenediol, 163–167
    androstenedione, 163–167
  risks associated with, 161
Androstenediol, 163–167
  antiviral response, 193
Androstenedione, *7*, 162–167
  older men and, 162
Anemia
  with deficiency of vitamin B12, 144
  with folic acid deficiency, 146
  megaloblastic, with folic acid deficiency, 146
  with vitamin E deficiency, 149
Angular stomatitis, from riboflavin deficiency, 141
Anorectic agents, 86
Anorexia
  from biotin deficiency, 145
  as sign of overtraining, 201
  from vitamin A deficiency, 155
Anti-convulsants, pyridoxine and, 143
Antibiotics, long-term, vitamin K deficiency from, 154
Anticatabolics, 111–136
  alanyl-glutamine, 127
  alpha-ketoglutarate, 115–116
    safety, toxicity, 116
  alpha-ketoisocaproate, 120–121
    safety, toxicity, 121
  alpha-lactalbumin, whey, 121
  amino acid mixtures, 126–127
  branched-chain amino acids, 117–118
    animal studies, 117
    human studies, 117–118
    safety, toxicity, 118
  casein, 121, 124–125
    animal studies, 124–125
    human studies, 125
    potential carcinogenic effects, 125
    safety, toxicity, 125
  cystine, in whey, 122
  glutamine, 113–115

animal studies, 113–114
glucose regulation, 115
glycogen storage, 112
human studies, 114
safety, toxicity, 115
insulin-like growth factor-1/somatomedin C, 124
leucine, 118–120
  animal studies, 119
  human studies, 119–120
  safety, toxicity, 120
lysine, in whey, 122
methionine, in whey, 122
milk protein isolates, 125–126
  animal studies, 125
  human studies, 125–126
  insulin-like growth factor, 126
  safety, toxicity, 126
ornithine-alpha-ketoglutarate, 116
  animal studies, 116
  human studies, 116
peptides, 127
peritonitis, 127
phosphoprotein, from milk. *See* Casein
recommendations, 128
soy isoflavones, cardioprotective benefits of, 127–130
soy protein, 127–130
structured lipids, 126
valine, 117
vitamin E, 138
whey, 120, 121–122, 124
  animal studies, 122–123
  for cystic fibrosis, 122
  for HIV/AIDS, 124
  human studies, 123–124
  safety, toxicity, 124
Anticoagulants, NSAIDs and, 250
Anticonvulsants
  effect on biotin, 145
  impaired vitamin D absorption with, 153
Antioxidants, 183–187, 264, 266–267
  beta carotene, 268
  co-enzyme Q10, 271
  conjugated linoleic acid, 271
  copper, 270
  endogenous, functions, 262
  exercise performance, 265
  iron, 270
  lipoic acid, 271
  manganese, 270
  mechanism of, 273–275
  minerals, 269–270
  mitochondrial oxygen processing, 262

317